Update on Prenatal Diagnosis and Maternal Fetal Medicine

Update on Prenatal Diagnosis and Maternal Fetal Medicine

Editor

Roland Axt-Fliedner

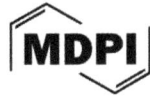

Basel • Beijing • Wuhan • Barcelona • Belgrade • Novi Sad • Cluj • Manchester

Editor
Roland Axt-Fliedner
Justus-Liebig University
Giessen
Germany

Editorial Office
MDPI
St. Alban-Anlage 66
4052 Basel, Switzerland

This is a reprint of articles from the Special Issue published online in the open access journal *Journal of Clinical Medicine* (ISSN 2077-0383) (available at: https://www.mdpi.com/journal/jcm/special_issues/Prenatal_Maternal_Fetal).

For citation purposes, cite each article independently as indicated on the article page online and as indicated below:

Lastname, A.A.; Lastname, B.B. Article Title. *Journal Name* **Year**, *Volume Number*, Page Range.

ISBN 978-3-0365-9598-6 (Hbk)
ISBN 978-3-0365-9599-3 (PDF)
doi.org/10.3390/books978-3-0365-9599-3

© 2023 by the authors. Articles in this book are Open Access and distributed under the Creative Commons Attribution (CC BY) license. The book as a whole is distributed by MDPI under the terms and conditions of the Creative Commons Attribution-NonCommercial-NoDerivs (CC BY-NC-ND) license.

Contents

About the Editor ix

Preface xi

Jens Kjeldsen-Kragh, Gregor Bein and Heidi Tiller
Pregnant Women at Low Risk of Having a Child with Fetal and Neonatal Alloimmune Thrombocytopenia Do Not Require Treatment with Intravenous Immunoglobulin
Reprinted from: *J. Clin. Med.* **2023**, *12*, 5492, doi:10.3390/jcm12175492 1

Corinna Keil, Siegmund Köhler, Benjamin Sass, Maximilian Schulze, Gerald Kalmus, Michael Belfort, et al.
Implementation and Assessment of a Laparotomy-Assisted Three-Port Fetoscopic Spina Bifida Repair Program
Reprinted from: *J. Clin. Med.* **2023**, *12*, 5151, doi:10.3390/jcm12155151 11

Annisa Dewi Nugrahani, Sidik Maulana, Kevin Dominique Tjandraprawira, Dhanny Primantara Johari Santoso, Dani Setiawan, Adhi Pribadi, et al.
Analysis of Clinical Profiles and Echocardiographic Cardiac Outcomes in Peripartum Cardiomyopathy (PPCM) vs. PPCM with Co-Existing Hypertensive Pregnancy Disorder (HPD-PPCM) Patients: A Systematic Review and Meta-Analysis
Reprinted from: *J. Clin. Med.* **2023**, *12*, 5303, doi:10.3390/jcm12165303 23

Ladina Vonzun, Romana Brun, Nora Gadient-Limani, Marcel André Schneider, Theresia Reding, Rolf Graf, et al.
Serum Pancreatic Stone Protein Reference Values in Healthy Pregnant Women: A Prospective Cohort Study
Reprinted from: *J. Clin. Med.* **2023**, *12*, 3200, doi:10.3390/jcm12093200 39

Marios Mamalis, Tamara Koehler, Ivonne Bedei, Aline Wolter, Johanna Schenk, Ellyda Widriani, et al.
Comparison of the Results of Prenatal and Postnatal Echocardiography and Postnatal Cardiac MRI in Children with a Congenital Heart Defect
Reprinted from: *J. Clin. Med.* **2023**, *12*, 3508, doi:10.3390/jcm12103508 49

Razvan Ciortea, Andrei Mihai Malutan, Carmen Elena Bucuri, Costin Berceanu, Maria Patricia Rada, Cristina Mihaela Ormindean, et al.
Amniocentesis—When It Is Clear That It Is Not Clear
Reprinted from: *J. Clin. Med.* **2023**, *12*, 454, doi:10.3390/jcm12020454 59

Ivonne Alexandra Bedei, Thierry A. G. M. Huisman, William Whitehead, Roland Axt-Fliedner, Michael Belfort and Magdalena Sanz Cortes
Fetal Brain Tumors, a Challenge in Prenatal Diagnosis, Counselling, and Therapy
Reprinted from: *J. Clin. Med.* **2023**, *12*, 58, doi:10.3390/jcm12010058 73

Anthea de Sainte Fare, Ivonne Bedei, Aline Wolter, Johanna Schenk, Ellydda Widriani, Corinna Keil, et al.
The Value of Delta Middle Cerebral Artery Peak Systolic Velocity for the Prediction of Twin Anemia-Polycythemia Sequence—Analysis of a Heterogenous Cohort of Monochorionic Twins
Reprinted from: *J. Clin. Med.* **2022**, *11*, 7541, doi:10.3390/jcm11247541 85

Ladina Vonzun, Ladina Rüegg, Julia Zepf, Ueli Moehrlen, Martin Meuli and
Nicole Ochsenbein-Kölble
Are Cervical Length and Fibronectin Predictors of Preterm Birth after Fetal Spina Bifida Repair?
A Single Center Cohort Study
Reprinted from: *J. Clin. Med.* **2023**, *12*, 123, doi:10.3390/jcm12010123 97

Fanny Tevaearai, Maike Katja Sachs, Samia El-Hadad, Ladina Vonzun, Ueli Moehrlen,
Luca Mazzone, et al.
Stage 2: The Vaginal Flora in Women Undergoing Fetal Spina Bifida Repair and Its Potential
Association with Preterm Rupture of Membranes and Preterm Birth
Reprinted from: *J. Clin. Med.* **2022**, *11*, 7038, doi:10.3390/jcm11237038 107

Marios Mamalis, Ivonne Bedei, Bjoern Schoennagel, Fabian Kording, Justus G. Reitz,
Aline Wolter, et al.
The Evolution and Developing Importance of Fetal Magnetic Resonance Imaging in the
Diagnosis of Congenital Cardiac Anomalies: A Systematic Review
Reprinted from: *J. Clin. Med.* **2022**, *11*, 7027, doi:10.3390/jcm11237027 115

Iris Soveral, Laura Guirado, Maria C. Escobar-Diaz, María José Alcaide,
Josep Maria Martínez, Víctor Rodríguez-Sureda, et al.
Cord Blood Cardiovascular Biomarkers in Left-Sided Congenital Heart Disease
Reprinted from: *J. Clin. Med.* **2022**, *11*, 7119, doi:10.3390/jcm11237119 125

Julia Murlewska, Oskar Sylwestrzak, Maria Respondek-Liberska, Mark Sklansky and
Greggory Devore
Longitudinal Surveillance of Fetal Heart Failure Using Speckle Tracking Analysis
Reprinted from: *J. Clin. Med.* **2022**, *11*, 7102, doi:10.3390/jcm11237102 139

Laila Miserre, Sandra Wienzek-Lischka, Andreas Mann, Nina Cooper, Sentot Santoso,
Harald Ehrhardt, et al.
ABO Incompatibility between the Mother and Fetus Does Not Protect against Anti-Human
Platelet Antigen-1a Immunization by Pregnancy
Reprinted from: *J. Clin. Med.* **2022**, *11*, 6811, doi:10.3390/jcm11226811 145

Daria Salloum, Paweł Jan Stanirowski, Aleksandra Symonides, Paweł Krajewski,
Dorota Bomba-Opoń and Mirosław Wielgoś
Enlarged Abdominal Lymph Node as a Cause of Polyhydramnios in the Course of Congenital
Neonatal Leukaemia: A Case Report and Review of the Literature on Foetal Abdominal
Tumours with Coexisting Polyhydramnios
Reprinted from: *J. Clin. Med.* **2022**, *11*, 6598, doi:10.3390/jcm11216598 159

Adrianna Kondracka, Ilona Jaszczuk, Dorota Koczkodaj, Bartosz Kondracki,
Karolina Frąszczak, Anna Oniszczuk, et al.
Analysis of Circulating C19MC MicroRNA as an Early Marker of Hypertension and
Preeclampsia in Pregnant Patients: A Systematic Review
Reprinted from: *J. Clin. Med.* **2022**, *11*, 7051, doi:10.3390/jcm11237051 167

Xiaona Xu, Baoying Ye, Min Li, Yuanqing Xia, Yi Wu and Weiwei Cheng
The UA Doppler Index, Plasma HCY, and Cys C in Pregnancies Complicated by Congenital
Heart Disease of the Fetus
Reprinted from: *J. Clin. Med.* **2022**, *11*, 5962, doi:10.3390/jcm11195962 183

Hee-Sun Kim, Soo-Young Oh, Geum Joon Cho, Suk-Joo Choi, Soon Cheol Hong,
Ja-Young Kwon, et al.
A Predictive Model for Large-for-Gestational-Age Infants among Korean Women with
Gestational Diabetes Mellitus Using Maternal Characteristics and Fetal Biometric Parameters
Reprinted from: *J. Clin. Med.* **2022**, *11*, 4951, doi:10.3390/jcm11174951 193

Ivonne Alexandra Bedei, Alexander Graf, Karl-Philipp Gloning, Matthias Meyer-Wittkopf,
Daria Willner, Martin Krapp, et al.
Is Fetal Hydrops in Turner Syndrome a Risk Factor for the Development of Maternal Mirror Syndrome?
Reprinted from: *J. Clin. Med.* 2022, 11, 4588, doi:10.3390/jcm11154588 203

Miriam Potrony, Antoni Borrell, Narcís Masoller, Alfons Nadal,
Leonardo Rodriguez-Carunchio, Karmele Saez de Gordoa Elizalde, et al.
Lethal Congenital Contracture Syndrome 11: A Case Report and Literature Review
Reprinted from: *J. Clin. Med.* 2022, 11, 3570, doi:10.3390/jcm11133570 211

Luca Zaninović, Marko Bašković, Davor Ježek and Ana Katušić Bojanac
Validity and Utility of Non-Invasive Prenatal Testing for Copy Number Variations and Microdeletions: A Systematic Review
Reprinted from: *J. Clin. Med.* 2022, 11, 3350, doi:10.3390/jcm11123350 223

Zagorka Milovanović, Dejan Filimonović, Ivan Soldatović and Nataša Karadžov Orlić
Can Thyroid Screening in the First Trimester Improve the Prediction of Gestational Diabetes Mellitus?
Reprinted from: *J. Clin. Med.* 2022, 11, 3916, doi:10.3390/jcm11133916 239

Jens Kjeldsen-Kragh and Åsa Hellberg
Noninvasive Prenatal Testing in Immunohematology—Clinical, Technical and Ethical Considerations
Reprinted from: *J. Clin. Med.* 2022, 11, 2877, doi:10.3390/jcm11102877 251

Bartosz Czuba, Piotr Tousty, Wojciech Cnota, Dariusz Borowski, Agnieszka Jagielska,
Mariusz Dubiel, et al.
First-Trimester Fetal Hepatic Artery Examination for Adverse Outcome Prediction
Reprinted from: *J. Clin. Med.* 2022, 11, 2095, doi:10.3390/jcm11082095 263

Maria Isabel Alvarez-Mora, Ines Agusti, Robin Wijngaard, Estefania Martinez-Barrios,
Tamara Barcos, Aina Borras, et al.
Evaluation of FMR4, FMR5 and FMR6 Expression Levels as Non-Invasive Biomarkers for the Diagnosis of Fragile X-Associated Primary Ovarian Insufficiency (FXPOI)
Reprinted from: *J. Clin. Med.* 2022, 11, 2186, doi:10.3390/jcm11082186 275

Carlo Bieńkowski, Małgorzata Aniszewska, Monika Kowalczyk, Jolanta Popielska,
Konrad Zawadka, Agnieszka Ołdakowska, et al.
Analysis of Preventable Risk Factors for *Toxoplasma gondii* Infection in Pregnant Women: Case-Control Study
Reprinted from: *J. Clin. Med.* 2022, 11, 1105, doi:10.3390/jcm11041105 285

Rui Gilberto Ferreira, Carolina Rodrigues Mendonça, Carolina Leão de Moraes,
Fernanda Sardinha de Abreu Tacon, Lelia Luanne Gonçalves Ramos,
Natalia Cruz e Melo, et al.
Ultrasound Markers for Complex Gastroschisis: A Systematic Review and Meta-Analysis
Reprinted from: *J. Clin. Med.* 2021, 10, 5215, doi:10.3390/jcm10225215 293

About the Editor

Roland Axt-Fliedner

Professor Roland Axt-Fliedner, MD, is a full academic professor leading the division of fetal medicine and therapy at Justus-Liebig University, University Hospital Gießen&Marburg, Germany, born in Frankfurt/Main, Germany. His clinical and scientific interests are high-risk pregnancies and the management of fetal abnormalities. He is affiliated with one of Germany's biggest pediatric heart centres; thus, cardiovascular fetal abnormalities have become one of his topics of interest. Advanced cardiovascular imaging research using new ultrasound techniques as well as fetal MRI within international collaborations are some of his major scientific directions. Fetal therapy as an evolving field makes up part of the clinical setting in his unit, and therapy of fetal open spina bifida is another topic of major clinical and scientific interest.

Preface

This Special Issue is dedicated to fetal and maternal surveillance during pegancy and manuscripts comprise a wide range of topics from fetal to maternal medicine.

Fetal medicine is a complex undertaking that involves a multidisciplinary team for prenatal diagnosis and fetal therapy. Several issues, including ethical and legal considerations, are particular to fetal medicine; fetal treatment centers may provide solutions to some of these.

Advanced ultrasound sonography has allowed not only for more detailed examinations of the anatomy but also for cardiovascular and other organ function in the fetus. Sonography and genetic analysis also enable prenatal diagnosis to be carried out through accessing the fetus for selected therapies in utero. In the beginning, these treatments were limited to lethal diseases. However, certain diseases leading to severe disability have also become indications for in utero treatment in recent years. Extensive studies are dedicated to looking for proper therapies to ameliorate these diseases. Today, different strategies have been scientifically evaluated to treat fetal tissue directly or administrate substances through maternal blood indirectly. Based on the invasiveness for the mother and fetus, fetal therapies could be divided into four categories, including non-invasive (medicine administration), minimally invasive (blood transfusion, shunt placement, balloon valvuloplasty, radiofrequency ablation, laser coagulation and fetoscopy surgery), invasive (open surgery) and experimental therapies (stem cell and gene therapy).

Further, continuing improvements in diagnosis and genetic testing bring new insights to professionals and involved families.

Roland Axt-Fliedner
Editor

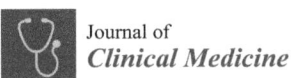

Journal of
Clinical Medicine

Review

Pregnant Women at Low Risk of Having a Child with Fetal and Neonatal Alloimmune Thrombocytopenia Do Not Require Treatment with Intravenous Immunoglobulin

Jens Kjeldsen-Kragh [1,2,*], Gregor Bein [3,4] and Heidi Tiller [5,6]

1. Department of Clinical Immunology and Transfusion Medicine, University and Regional Laboratories, Akutgatan 8, 221 85 Lund, Sweden
2. Department of Laboratory Medicine, University Hospital of North Norway, 9019 Tromsø, Norway
3. Institute for Clinical Immunology, Transfusion Medicine and Hemostasis, Justus-Liebig-University, 35392 Giessen, Germany; gregor.bein@immunologie.med.uni-giessen.de
4. German Center for Feto-Maternal Incompatibility, University Hospital Giessen and Marburg, Campus Giessen, 35392 Giessen, Germany
5. Department of Obstetrics and Gynecology, University Hospital of North Norway, 9019 Tromsø, Norway; heidi.tiller@uit.no
6. Women's Health and Perinatology Research Group, Department of Clinical Medicine, UiT The Arctic University of Norway, 9019 Tromsø, Norway
* Correspondence: jkk@jkkmedical.com

Abstract: Fetal and neonatal alloimmune thrombocytopenia (FNAIT) is a rare condition in which maternal alloantibodies to fetal platelets cause fetal thrombocytopenia that may lead to intracranial hemorrhage (ICH). Off-label intravenous immunoglobulin (IVIg) has for 30 years been the standard of care for pregnant women who previously have had a child with FNAIT. The efficacy of this treatment has never been tested in a placebo-controlled clinical trial. Although IVIg treatment may improve the neonatal outcome in women who previously have had a child with FNAIT-associated ICH, the question is whether IVIg is necessary for all immunized pregnant women at risk of having a child with FNAIT. The results from some recent publications suggest that antenatal IVIg treatment is not necessary for women who are (1) HPA-1a-immunized and HLA-DRB3*01:01-negative, (2) HPA-1a-immunized with a previous child with FNAIT but without ICH or (3) HPA-5b-immunized. If IVIg is not used for these categories of pregnant women, the amount of IVIg used in pregnant women with platelet antibodies would be reduced to less than $1/4$ of today's use. This is important because IVIg is a scarce resource, and the collection of plasma for the treatment of one pregnant woman is not only extremely expensive but also requires tremendous donor efforts.

Keywords: pregnancy; alloimmunization; intracranial hemorrhage; intravenous immunoglobulin; platelet antibodies

Citation: Kjeldsen-Kragh, J.; Bein, G.; Tiller, H. Pregnant Women at Low Risk of Having a Child with Fetal and Neonatal Alloimmune Thrombocytopenia Do Not Require Treatment with Intravenous Immunoglobulin. *J. Clin. Med.* **2023**, *12*, 5492. https://doi.org/10.3390/jcm12175492

Academic Editor: Rubén Barakat

Received: 19 July 2023
Revised: 17 August 2023
Accepted: 21 August 2023
Published: 24 August 2023

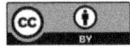

Copyright: © 2023 by the authors. Licensee MDPI, Basel, Switzerland. This article is an open access article distributed under the terms and conditions of the Creative Commons Attribution (CC BY) license (https://creativecommons.org/licenses/by/4.0/).

1. Introduction

Fetal and neonatal alloimmune thrombocytopenia (FNAIT) is a rare but potentially severe fetal–maternal condition in which maternal alloantibodies to paternally inherited platelet antigens cause thrombocytopenia in the fetus/newborn. Thus, there is resemblance to the pathogenesis of hemolytic disease of the fetus and newborn (HDFN) where an RhD-negative mother can be RhD-immunized if she gives birth to an RhD-positive child. FNAIT, however, differs from HDFN, as immunization against paternally inherited platelet antigens more often occurs in the first incompatible pregnancy and severe clinical outcomes are seen even in firstborns [1].

The true Incidence of FNAIT is not known but has been estimated at around 1 in 1500 pregnancies [1]. The clinical spectrum varies from mild thrombocytopenia to severe intracranial hemorrhage (ICH), which has been estimated to occur in around 1 in

10,000 unselected pregnancies [2]. In Caucasians, antibodies to human platelet antigen (HPA)-1a account for approximately 80% of FNAIT cases [1] and HPA-5b antibodies have been considered to be implicated in around 15% of the cases [3]. In some Asian populations, however, the majority of antibodies detected in suspected FNAIT cases are HPA-5b antibodies followed by HPA-4b antibodies [4].

For more than 30 years, it has been known that the propensity to develop antibodies against HPA-1a is closely associated with HLA-DRB3*01:01 [5]. Recently it was shown that the risk of having a neonate with severe FNAIT is extremely low for an HPA-1a-immunized, HLA-DRB3*01:01-negative mother [6].

The HPA-1a/b polymorphism is located on the $\beta 3$ integrin chain of the $\alpha IIb\beta 3$ complex that constitutes the platelets' fibrinogen receptor. As the $\beta 3$ chain forms heterodimers with the αV chain of the endothelial cells' vitronectin receptor, HPA-1a antibodies also bind to endothelial cells. This may have pathophysiological importance as HPA-1a antibodies that are specific for the $\alpha V\beta 3$ complex are suggested to play a key role in women who have given birth to a child with ICH [7]. However, it is not fully understood if or how such subgroups of HPA-1a antibodies relate to ICH risk, and the clinical use of such antibody analyses has not been tested in prospective studies. Whether the quantification of maternal HPA-1a antibody levels could be useful to predict the risk of ICH is also not known. Therefore, based on current knowledge, the only known ICH risk predictor is an obstetric history with FNAIT.

According to early reports, ICH occurs in 10–30% of FNAIT cases [8–11]. Moreover, as the recurrence rate was reported to be very high in subsequent pregnancies and the severity was believed to increase compared to that of the previous affected fetus/infant, similar to in HDFN [8,12], the need for fetal bleeding prophylaxis became obvious. However, due to the rarity of ICH in FNAIT cases, there are many uncertainties regarding the natural history of FNAIT. For this reason, the scientific community has relied heavily on data from retrospective case series collected by fetal–maternal medicine specialists, neonatologists and reference laboratories spanning two or more decades. This implies fragmentary clinical data, a lack of appropriate control groups and reduced antibody avidity due to repeated thaw and freeze cycles of historic sera.

In this review, we will critically examine the scientific foundation for today's management of FNAIT, and we will suggest that the majority of pregnant women at risk of having a child with FNAIT may not necessarily need the currently applied treatment with intravenous immunoglobulin (IVIg).

2. Intravenous Immunoglobulin Is the Predominant Treatment for Platelet-Immunized Women

In a landmark paper by Bussel and co-workers from 1988 [13], they reported the results of IVIg treatment (IVIg 1 g/kg/week) in seven pregnant women who previously had had a child with FNAIT. In all children, the platelet count was higher than in their older FNAIT-affected sibling. This paper was subsequently followed by a large number of reports where IVIg, with or without corticosteroids, was used for pregnant women at risk of FNAIT in their newborn. Many of these studies were case reports and case series, while some were randomized clinical trials (RCT) where IVIg was tested against IVIg plus corticosteroids or where different doses of IVIg were compared; for an overview, see Rayment et al., 2011 [14] or Winkelhorst et al., 2017 [15].

Surprisingly, despite decades of usage of IVIg in platelet-immunized women, it is still unknown how IVIg works. Several potential mechanisms of IVIg in platelet-immunized pregnant women were recently summarized by Wabnitz and co-workers [16].

Due to the rarity of FNAIT, it is a considerable challenge to conduct an RCT. Unfortunately, a placebo-controlled RCT demonstrating the efficacy of IVIg treatment for risk pregnancies has never been conducted. Consequently, the off-label usage of IVIg has become the standard treatment for pregnant women who previously have had a child with FNAIT. This treatment modality has become so rooted that it is integrated into several clinical guidelines for the management of risk pregnancies [17–19]. Today, it has even been considered unethical to conduct a placebo-controlled RCT to demonstrate IVIg's efficacy [14].

Although IVIg treatment is usually considered safe, significant side effects have been reported, such as aseptic meningitis, renal failure, hemolytic anemia and thrombotic complications [20,21]. More than 80% of women experience headache during treatment, which has a non-negligible adverse impact on life quality [20].

3. The Traditional View on the Severity of FNAIT in Subsequent Pregnancies

Due to the high recurrence rate of severe FNAIT, the efficacy of IVIg has been evaluated by comparing the neonatal outcome in an index pregnancy with the outcome of a subsequent IVIg-treated pregnancy. These studies have indicated that IVIg treatment of women with platelet antibodies is efficient in preventing fetal/neonatal ICH; for details, see Winkelhorst et al., 2017 [15]. Thus, the reported efficacy of IVIg relies on the assumption that the neonatal outcome becomes worse in subsequent incompatible pregnancies, similar to in HDFN. This assumption is based on a frequently referenced study by Radder et al. [22]. In this study, the risk of ICH was calculated to be greater than 70% if the mother previously had had a child with ICH, and 7% if the previous FNAIT-affected sibling did not suffer with ICH. However, these calculations were based on retrospective data from case reports and smaller observational series where samples from the mother and child had been sent to a platelet immunology laboratory on the suspicion of FNAIT. For such retrospective studies, there is a potential risk of publication bias—cases where a woman has given birth to two or more children with FNAIT-associated ICH are more likely to be published than cases where the neonatal outcome of a subsequent pregnancy had a more benign course than the previous. Thus, there is considerable uncertainty regarding this estimate of the ICH recurrence rate and severity of FNAIT in subsequent pregnancies. Ideally, this should be evaluated in a population of pregnant women not treated with IVIg, where the risk of selection bias is minimal.

4. Identification of Less Severe Courses of FNAIT

The view that FNAIT becomes more severe in subsequent pregnancies has been challenged by observations from Norway. Prospective data have shown that the levels of HPA-1a antibodies in most multigravida women declined during pregnancy [23], and that the neonatal platelet count in $2/3$ of subsequent HPA-1a-immunized pregnancies increase or remain unchanged [24]. Furthermore, as IVIg only has a very small role in the Norwegian FNAIT management strategy, the neonatal outcome of Norwegian women with platelet antibodies represents the best available data on the natural history of FNAIT. Assuming that IVIg is efficient in preventing anti-HPA-1a-associated ICH, one would expect the neonatal outcome of platelet-immunized pregnancies in Norway to be worse than in other countries where IVIg is used for this category of patients. This question was addressed in a recent study [25] where the neonatal outcome of platelet-immunized women not treated with IVIg was compared with the outcome of women who received IVIg during pregnancy [15]. The pregnant women were stratified according to their previous obstetric history. Women with a prior child with anti-HPA-1a-associated ICH were categorized as "high-risk" pregnancies, whereas women with a prior child with FNAIT without ICH were categorized as "low-risk" pregnancies. In the group of high-risk pregnancies, there were five cases of fetal/neonatal ICH among ninety IVIg-treated pregnancies, equivalent to 5.6% (95% confidence interval (CI): 2.4–12.4%), and two cases among seven children (29%, 95% CI: 8.2–64.1%) from non-IVIg-treated pregnancies ($p = 0.08$). Among the low-risk pregnancies, 2 of 313 IVIg-treated women gave birth to children with ICH (0.6%, 95% CI: 0.2–2.3%), as opposed to 0 cases (0.0%, 95% CI: 0.0–5.7%) among 64 children from non-IVIg-treated pregnancies ($p = 1.00$) [25]. This study is considered to provide the hitherto most reliable data for the evaluation of IVIg treatment in low-risk pregnancies. As the neonatal outcome of low-risk pregnancies in Norway did not seem to be less favorable than in the IVIg-treated control group [15], it seems reasonable to question if IVIg treatment is really necessary for all HPA-1a-immunized pregnant women who previously have had a child with FNAIT but without ICH. However, it is important to emphasize that non-IVIg treatment in Norway is not the same as no intervention. When the risk of FNAIT is recognized before birth, several measures are taken according to Norwegian clinical guidelines, including delivery by caesarean section 1–2 weeks prior to term if the maternal HPA-1a antibody concentration is >3 IU/mL as well as prompt transfusion with compatible platelets to the newborn; for details, see Tiller et al., 2020 [26].

Antibodies against HPA-5b have for years been considered the second most common platelet antibody responsible for FNAIT. This notion was challenged by Alm and coworkers in a recent study from Gießen, Germany [3]. Neither data retrieved from the literature, nor retrospective data from 761 pairs of maternal/fetal samples from the platelet immunology laboratory in Gießen, supported the hypothesis that HPA-5b antibodies cause severe thrombocytopenia or bleeding complications in the fetus/newborn [3].

The HPA-5b antigen is far more immunogenic than, for instance, the HPA-1a antigen, and consequently, around 2% of pregnant women are HPA-5b-immunized as compared to only 0.2% who are HPA-1a-immunized [3]. Thus, it is questionable if HPA-5b antibodies can cause fetal/neonatal thrombocytopenia, or whether the presence of maternal HPA-5b antibodies in a thrombocytopenic newborn is merely coincidental [3].

In a recent Dutch cohort study [27], there were four cases with severe fetal/neonatal bleeding among 40 HPA-5b-immunized women with an incompatible fetus. Interestingly, they also reported [27] the neonatal outcomes of eight HPA-5b-negative women with high levels of HPA-5b antibodies where there was no HPA-5b incompatibility between the mother and fetus. Of these eight children, there was one child with ICH and one child with thrombocytopenia and skin bleeding; none of these children suffered from any other clinical condition known to be associated with thrombocytopenia or ICH [27]. Hence, the incidence of severe bleeding, including ICH, among HPA-5b-incompatible immunized pregnancies (4 of 40) was not higher than among HPA-5b compatible pregnancies (1 of 8). Furthermore, the prevalence of maternal HPA-5b antibodies in pregnancies from 105 neonates with ICH (1.9% [28]) was not different from the prevalence of maternal HPA-5b antibodies in the healthy controls (1.96% [3]), calling into question the causal role of HPA-5b antibodies in ICH.

Despite the fact that up to 2% of all women who have been pregnant are HPA-5b-immunized, we have only been able to find one single case report of thrombocytopenia after the transfusion of a plasma unit containing HPA-5b antibodies [29]. This finding supports the notion that HPA-5b antibodies do not cause severe neonatal thrombocytopenia and thus that IVIg treatment is probably not necessary for pregnant women who are HPA-5b-immunized.

Although the association between HPA-1a immunization and HLA-DRB3*01:01 has been known for decades, the neonatal outcome has only recently been studied in HPA-1a-immunized women who are HLA-DRB3*01:01-positive and -negative, respectively. A systematic review and metanalysis was conducted by the International Collaboration for Transfusion Medicine Guidelines (ICTMG), which included four prospective and five retrospective studies [6]. In none of the four prospective studies (representing > 150,000 pregnant women) were there any HPA-1a-immunized, HLA-DRB3*01:01-negative women who gave birth to a severely thrombocytopenic child (platelet count < 50×10^9/L). In the five retrospective studies, there were 13 severely thrombocytopenic newborns, of whom 2 suffered with ICH. These two cases were from a retrospective study that reported data from a large French reference laboratory over a 25-year period [30]. Clinical information about these two children with ICH was unfortunately not available. It is therefore not known if these two cases had concurrent neonatal or obstetric risk factors for ICH. Moreover, the grading of the bleeding was not reported; thus, it is not known if the ICH was of clinical importance or if it was an incidental finding, as ICH has been found in 26% of unselected asymptomatic newborns delivered by the vaginal route [31]. The metanalysis showed that the odds ratio for giving birth to a severely thrombocytopenic child, given the mother is HPA-1a-immunized, is only 0.08 if she is also HLA-DRB3*01:01-negative.

HLA-DRB3*01:01 typing is relevant for a pregnant woman who has been identified as HPA-1a-negative by virtue of being a blood donor or if she has a sister who previously had a child with FNAIT. The results from the systematic review and metanalysis conducted by ICTMG indicate that no special follow-up during pregnancy would be necessary. Even if she should develop HPA-1a antibodies during pregnancy, it is unlikely that the levels of HPA-1a antibodies will be high enough to produce significant thrombocytopenia in the fetus/newborn and treatment with IVIg should therefore not be necessary.

5. What Are the Risks of Not Treating Low-Risk Pregnancies with IVIg?

Based on the more recent data presented above [3,6,25], we suggest that pregnant women who are:

- HPA-1a-immunized and HLA-DRB3*01:01-negative;
- HPA-1a-immunized with a previous child with FNAIT but without ICH;
- HPA-5b-immunized;

should be categorized as "low-risk" pregnancies for having a fetus/child with ICH, and we would suggest that these women generally should not be treated with IVIg during pregnancy.

Critics may say that there still is a risk that low-risk women give birth to a child with ICH if IVIg is not administered during pregnancy, although this risk is low. There are not many cases in the literature that have described a low-risk woman not treated with IVIg who has had a child with ICH [32–35]. It is of course not possible to guarantee that a woman at low risk will not have a fetus/child with ICH, but the real question is whether this case could have been avoided if IVIg had been administered to the pregnant woman. IVIg treatment is also no guarantee for preventing ICH. There are several reports describing treatment failures [15,36,37]. IVIg treatment was initially introduced for high-risk pregnancies, i.e., cases where a woman previously had had a child with FNAIT-associated ICH. As these initial studies showed that the majority of these IVIg-treated women did not give birth to a child with ICH, it was assumed that IVIg treatment of low-risk pregnancies would also prevent ICH from happening. We question this assumption because there are no significant clinical or epidemiological data to support the usage of IVIg in low-risk pregnancies.

Although ICH is a known complication of FNAIT, Refsum et al. demonstrated that FNAIT only accounts for a minority of the neonatal clinical conditions which can cause ICH [28]. They analyzed 105 maternal samples obtained after searching a national register for neonates with ICH born after 32 weeks and found three platelet-immunized women. In addition to one woman with HPA-1a antibodies (1%), there were two women with HPA-5b antibodies (1.9%), which is similar to the percentage of HPA-5b-immunized women that would be expected by chance in a random population of pregnant women. Furthermore, in 194 consecutive ICH fetuses (FNAIT excluded), Coste et al. [38] screened for variants of the *COL4A1/COL4A2* genes, which have been associated with ICH, and identified pathogenic variants in 19%. Thus, fetal ICH is a highly heterogeneous condition and the probability of coincidence between fetal/neonatal ICH and maternal HPA antibodies is therefore high.

In the recent Norwegian study, none of the sixty-four women with low-risk pregnancies gave birth to a child with ICH, and fetal/neonatal ICH was only detected in two of seven high-risk pregnancies [25]. These data indicate that subsequent pregnancies of women who have had a fetus or newborn with FNAIT but without ICH usually have benign courses, and that the recurrence rate of FNAIT-associated ICH is lower than previously reported. Although some concerns have been raised regarding the Norwegian study [39], it provides the hitherto most reliable data regarding the efficacy of IVIg in low-risk pregnancies.

The natural history of pregnant HPA-5b-immunized women carrying an HPA-5b-incompatible fetus is not known. However, the clinical course of FNAIT in HPA-5b-immunized women has generally been considered as less severe than that of anti-HPA-1a-associated FNAIT. In addition, indirect evidence [29], as well as the recent study by Alm et al. [3], has questioned if HPA-5b antibodies can cause severe thrombocytopenia and argues that the association between neonatal ICH and HPA-5b-alloimmunisation is coincidental. Although ICH can occur in the fetus/child of an HPA-5b-immunized woman who is not treated with IVIg, a causal relationship with the presence of HPA-5b-antibodies is unlikely. The association could just be coincidental, similar to the case reported by de Vos and co-workers [27], where an HPA-5b-immunized mother without fetal–maternal incompatibility gave birth to a child with ICH.

As explained above, it is highly unlikely that a pregnant woman who is HPA-1a-immunized and HLA-DRB3*01:01-negative will have a fetus/child with ICH [6]. Thus, if an HLA-DRB3*01:01-negative mother gives birth to a child with ICH, this would more likely be coincidental than causal.

Since the study by Ernstsen et al. [25] is based on results from Norway, it could be questioned if these results can be extrapolated to other populations and ethnicities. However, despite this methodological weakness, the level of evidence for using IVIg treatment in low-risk pregnancies is much lower than the level of evidence for the opposite—that IVIg is not necessary in these pregnancies.

In the very rare scenario where an HPA-5b-immunized or an HPA-1a-immunized, HLA-DRB3*01:01-negative pregnant woman previously has had a child with FNAIT-suspected ICH, the counselling of the woman can be challenging. As such cases would be extremely rare, there are no data from the literature that could be used as guidance for the clinical management during pregnancy. The question in such rare cases is whether or not the ICH in the previous sibling was causally related to the mother's alloantibodies; this is a question that rarely can be answered on an individual level. In this setting, the decision about prenatal IVIg treatment should be determined by the woman together with her physician.

6. Abstaining from IVIg Treatment for Low-Risk Pregnancies Would Significantly Reduce the Amount of IVIg Used for Women with Platelet Antibodies

The percentage of the three categories of low-risk pregnancies among pregnancies at risk of FNAIT in general can be calculated as follows:

1. HPA-1a-immunized women with a previous child without ICH. Based on the data from Ernstsen and co-workers [25], 80% of all subsequent pregnancies of HPA-1a-immunized women belonged to the low-risk category (of a total of 474 women, 375 belonged to the low-risk group). Given that 80% of all FNAIT cases are associated with HPA-1a antibodies, approximately 64% (80% × 80%) will belong to the low-risk group.
2. HPA-5b-immunized women. If 15% of FNAIT cases are associated with HPA-5b antibodies, and if we assume that all HPA-5b-immunized women belong to the low-risk category, there will be an additional 15% of all FNAIT cases that can be considered as low-risk pregnancies.
3. HPA-1a-negative and HLA-DRB3*01:01-negative women. As these women only rarely become immunized, the majority of women belonging to this category will be identified by virtue of being HPA-1a-typed as a potential platelet donor or because they have a sister who has had a child with FNAIT. Hence, this group will be negligible compared to the other two groups of low-risk pregnancies.

If we changed the current clinical practice and stopped treating low-risk pregnancies with IVIg, we could reduce the use of IVIg in FNAIT by 79% (64% + 15%). This is important, first, because there is a worldwide shortage of IVIg [40]; secondly, because IVIg treatment is extremely costly (the IVIg used for treating one low-risk woman costs more than USD 150,000 or USD 300,000 depending on whether the dosage is 1 or 2 g/kg/week—see Table 1 for details); and thirdly, because the collection of plasma for the manufacture of IVIg requires tremendous donor efforts (>4 or 8 man-months for the collection of plasma for treating one low-risk woman, depending on the dosage of IVIg; Table 1).

Table 1. Cost of treating one woman with a low-risk pregnancy.

Monetary costs		
Body weight [41]	a	76 kg
No. of treatment weeks [42]	b	20
Dose of IVIg per week [14,42]	c	1–2 g/kg/week *
Total dose of IgG	d = a × b × c	1520–3040 g *
Price for IgG [43]	e	USD 100/g
Price for total dose of IgG	d × e	USD 152,000–304,000 *
Donor engagement		
Amount of plasma per plasmapheresis [44]	f	0.7 L
Amount of extractable IgG per L plasma [44,45]	g	5 g/L
Amount of plasma for treatment of one woman	h = d/g	304–608 L *
No. of apheresis procedures for treatment of one woman	i = h/f	869
Time for one apheresis procedure [46]	j	1.5 h
No. of apheresis hours for treatment of one woman	k = i × j	652–1303 h *
One man-month	l	80
No. of man-months for treatment of one woman	k/l	4–8 *

* The recommended dose used for treating low-risk pregnancies varies from 2 g of IVIg/kg/week in the US to 1 g/kg/week in most European countries. IVIg: intravenous immunoglobulin. IgG: immunoglobulin G.

As explained above, none of the 64 low-risk HPA-1a-immunized women gave birth to a child with ICH [25]. In addition, we have questioned the relevance of IVIg for HPA-5b-immunized women as well as HLA-DRB3*01:01-negative HPA 1a-immunized women. Consistent with the current programs of IVIg prophylaxis, all three categories of low-risk pregnancies would be treated with IVIg. Hence, according to a conservative assumption, it would be necessary to treat > 50 low-risk pregnancies to prevent one case of ICH. Thus, depending on the dose of IVIg, it would be necessary to use 76 or 152 kg IVIg for the prevention of one case of ICH, equivalent to USD 7,600,000 or USD 15,200,000 and 16.9 or 33.8 man-years in donor engagement (Table 1). We do not know of any other medical condition where such high costs are used for the prevention or cure of one case.

7. Conclusions

Here, we argue that the IVIg treatment of all pregnant women with a low risk of FNAIT results in significant overtreatment and with limited clinical benefit. Better tools for risk predictions, other than an individual's FNAIT history, are urgently needed. The question of whether the risk of ICH in anti-HPA-1a-immunized women can be better predicted by in vitro methods, such as the identification of HPA-1a antibodies that bind to $\alpha V\beta 3$ integrin [8] or afucosylated HPA-1a antibodies [47], must be addressed in a large prospective international collaborative trial. Finally, we suggest that the relevant scientific communities critically scrutinize available evidence for the efficacy of IVIg treatment of low-risk pregnancies and be open to revise current treatment guidelines for the prenatal management of FNAIT.

Author Contributions: J.K.-K. conceptualized and wrote the first draft of the manuscript. H.T. and G.B. revised the various versions of the manuscript and approved the final version. All authors have read and agreed to the published version of the manuscript.

Funding: This research received no external funding.

Conflicts of Interest: J.K.-K. belongs to a group of founders and owners of Prophylix AS—a Norwegian biotech company that has produced a hyperimmune antihuman platelet antigen (HPA)-1a immunoglobulin G (IgG) (NAITgam) for the prevention of HPA-1a-alloimmunisation and fetal and neonatal alloimmune thrombocytopenia (FNAIT). J.K.-K. is also a consultant for Rallybio and Janssen Pharmaceuticals. H.T. reports previous payment from Prophylix AS related to a patent on a monoclonal HPA-1a antibody and has been funded as a research consultant by Janssen Pharmaceuticals since August 2021. H.T. is the local study site principal investigator in an ongoing multicenter natural history study on FNAIT sponsored by Rallybio. G.B. is investigator in a study to evaluate the safety, efficacy, pharmacokinetics and pharmacodynamics of nipocalimab administered to pregnant women at high risk for early-onset severe hemolytic disease of the fetus and newborn, sponsored by Janssen Pharmaceuticals. G.B. reports consultancy fees from Janssen Pharmaceuticals for participating on the advisory board on FNAIT.

References

1. De Vos, T.W.; Winkelhorst, D.; de Haas, M.; Lopriore, E.; Oepkes, D. Epidemiology and management of fetal and neonatal alloimmune thrombocytopenia. *Transfus. Apher. Sci.* **2020**, *59*, 102704. [CrossRef]
2. Kamphuis, M.M.; Paridaans, N.P.; Porcelijn, L.; Lopriore, E.; Oepkes, D. Incidence and consequences of neonatal alloimmune thrombocytopenia: A systematic review. *Pediatrics* **2014**, *133*, 715–721. [CrossRef]
3. Alm, J.; Duong, Y.; Wienzek-Lischka, S.; Cooper, N.; Santoso, S.; Sachs, U.J.; Kiefel, V.; Bein, G. Anti-human platelet antigen-5b antibodies and fetal and neonatal alloimmune thrombocytopenia; incidental association or cause and effect? *Br. J. Haematol.* **2022**, *198*, 14–23. [CrossRef]
4. Ohto, H.; Miura, S.; Ariga, H.; Ishii, T.; Fujimori, K.; Morita, S. The natural history of maternal immunization against foetal platelet alloantigens. *Transfus. Med.* **2004**, *14*, 399–408. [CrossRef]
5. Valentin, N.; Vergracht, A.; Bignon, J.D.; Cheneau, M.L.; Blanchard, D.; Kaplan, C.; Reznikoff-Etievant, M.F.; Muller, J.Y. HLA-DRw52a is involved in alloimmunization against PL-A1 antigen. *Hum. Immunol.* **1990**, *27*, 73–79. [CrossRef]
6. Kjeldsen-Kragh, J.; Fergusson, D.A.; Kjaer, M.; Lieberman, L.; Greinacher, A.; Murphy, M.F.; Bussel, J.; Bakchoul, T.; Corke, S.; Bertrand, G.; et al. Fetal/neonatal alloimmune thrombocytopenia: A systematic review of impact of HLA-DRB3*01:01 on fetal/neonatal outcome. *Blood Adv.* **2020**, *4*, 3368–3377. [CrossRef]
7. Santoso, S.; Wihadmadyatami, H.; Bakchoul, T.; Werth, S.; Al-Fakhri, N.; Bein, G.; Kiefel, V.; Zhu, J.; Newman, P.J.; Bayat, B.; et al. Antiendothelial alphavbeta3 Antibodies Are a Major Cause of Intracranial Bleeding in Fetal/Neonatal Alloimmune Thrombocytopenia. *Arter. Thromb. Vasc. Biol.* **2016**, *36*, 1517–1524. [CrossRef]
8. Bussel, J.B. Neonatal alloimmune thrombocytopenia (NAIT): A prospective case accumulation study. *Pediatr. Res.* **1988**, *23*, 337a.
9. Pearson, H.A.; Shulman, N.R.; Marder, V.J.; Cone, T.E., Jr. Isoimmune Neonatal Thrombocytopenic Purpura. *Clin. Ther. Consid. Blood* **1964**, *23*, 154–177. [CrossRef]
10. Blanchette, V.S. Neonatal alloimmune thrombocytopenia: A clinical perspective. *Curr. Stud. Hematol. Blood Transfus.* **1988**, *54*, 112–126.
11. Mueller-Eckhardt, C.; Kiefel, V.; Grubert, A.; Kroll, H.; Weisheit, M.; Schmidt, S.; Mueller-Eckhardt, G.; Santoso, S. 348 cases of suspected neonatal alloimmune thrombocytopenia. *Lancet* **1989**, *1*, 363–366. [CrossRef] [PubMed]
12. Shulman, N.R.; Jordan, J.V.J. Platelet immunology. In *Hemostasis and Thrombosis: Basic Principles and Clinical Practice*; Colman, R.W., Hirsh, J., Manier, V.J., Salzman, E.W., Eds.; J.B. Lippincott: Philadelphia, PE, USA, 1982; pp. 274–342.
13. Bussel, J.B.; Berkowitz, R.L.; McFarland, J.G.; Lynch, L.; Chitkara, U. Antenatal treatment of neonatal alloimmune thrombocytopenia. *N. Engl. J. Med.* **1988**, *319*, 1374–1378. [CrossRef]
14. Rayment, R.; Brunskill, S.J.; Soothill, P.W.; Roberts, D.J.; Bussel, J.B.; Murphy, M.F. Antenatal interventions for fetomaternal alloimmune thrombocytopenia. *Cochrane Database Syst. Rev.* **2011**, *5*, CD004226. [CrossRef] [PubMed]
15. Winkelhorst, D.; Murphy, M.F.; Greinacher, A.; Shehata, N.; Bakchoul, T.; Massey, E.; Baker, J.; Lieberman, L.; Tanael, S.; Hume, H.; et al. Antenatal management in fetal and neonatal alloimmune thrombocytopenia: A systematic review. *Blood* **2017**, *129*, 1538–1547. [CrossRef] [PubMed]
16. Wabnitz, H.; Khan, R.; Lazarus, A.H. The use of IVIg in fetal and neonatal alloimmune thrombocytopenia—Principles and mechanisms. *Transfus. Apher. Sci.* **2020**, *59*, 102710. [CrossRef] [PubMed]
17. National Blood Authority. Australia. Available online: https://www.blood.gov.au/system/files/documents/Fetal-and-neonatal-alloimmune-thrombocytopenia-FNAIT-CV3.pdf (accessed on 15 August 2023).
18. Regan, F.; Lees, C.C.; Jones, B.; Nicolaides, K.H.; Wimalasundera, R.C.; Mijovic, A. Prenatal Management of Pregnancies at Risk of Fetal Neonatal Alloimmune Thrombocytopenia (FNAIT): Scientific Impact Paper No. 61. *BJOG Int. J. Obstet. Gynaecol.* **2019**, *126*, e173–e185. [CrossRef] [PubMed]
19. Winkelhorst, D.; Oepkes, D.; Lopriore, E. Fetal and neonatal alloimmune thrombocytopenia: Evidence based antenatal and postnatal management strategies. *Expert. Rev. Hematol.* **2017**, *10*, 729–737. [CrossRef]
20. Rossi, K.Q.; Lehman, K.J.; O'Shaughnessy, R.W. Effects of antepartum therapy for fetal alloimmune thrombocytopenia on maternal lifestyle. *J. Matern. Fetal Neonatal Med.* **2015**, *29*, 1783–1788. [CrossRef]

21. Cherin, P.; Cabane, J. Relevant criteria for selecting an intravenous immunoglobulin preparation for clinical use. *BioDrugs* **2010**, *24*, 211–223. [CrossRef]
22. Radder, C.M.; Brand, A.; Kanhai, H.H. Will it ever be possible to balance the risk of intracranial haemorrhage in fetal or neonatal alloimmune thrombocytopenia against the risk of treatment strategies to prevent it? *Vox Sang* **2003**, *84*, 318–325. [CrossRef]
23. Killie, M.K.; Husebekk, A.; Kjeldsen-Kragh, J.; Skogen, B. A prospective study of maternal anti-HPA 1a antibody level as a potential predictor of alloimmune thrombocytopenia in the newborn. *Haematologica* **2008**, *93*, 870–877. [CrossRef] [PubMed]
24. Tiller, H.; Husebekk, A.; Skogen, B.; Kjeldsen-Kragh, J.; Kjaer, M. True risk of fetal/neonatal alloimmune thrombocytopenia in subsequent pregnancies: A prospective observational follow-up study. *BJOG Int. J. Obstet. Gynaecol.* **2016**, *123*, 738–744. [CrossRef] [PubMed]
25. Ernstsen, S.L.; Ahlen, M.T.; Johansen, T.; Bertelsen, E.L.; Kjeldsen-Kragh, J.; Tiller, H. Antenatal intravenous immunoglobulins in pregnancies at risk of fetal and neonatal alloimmune thrombocytopenia: Comparison of neonatal outcome in treated and nontreated pregnancies. *Am. J. Obs. Gynecol.* **2022**, *227*, 506.e1–506.e12. [CrossRef] [PubMed]
26. Tiller, H.; Ahlen, M.T.; Akkok, C.A.; Husebekk, A. Fetal and neonatal alloimmune thrombocytopenia—The Norwegian management model. *Transfus. Apher. Sci.* **2020**, *59*, 102711. [CrossRef]
27. de Vos, T.W.; Porcelijn, L.; Hofstede-van Egmond, S.; Pajkrt, E.; Oepkes, D.; Lopriore, E.; van der Schoot, C.E.; Winkelhorst, D.; de Haas, M. Clinical characteristics of human platelet antigen (HPA)-1a and HPA-5b alloimmunised pregnancies and the association between platelet HPA-5b antibodies and symptomatic fetal neonatal alloimmune thrombocytopenia. *Br. J. Haematol.* **2021**, *195*, 595–603. [CrossRef]
28. Refsum, E.; Hakansson, S.; Mortberg, A.; Wikman, A.; Westgren, M. Intracranial hemorrhages in neonates born from 32 weeks of gestation-low frequency of associated fetal and neonatal alloimmune thrombocytopenia: A register-based study. *Transfusion* **2018**, *58*, 223–231. [CrossRef]
29. Warkentin, T.E.; Smith, J.W.; Hayward, C.P.; Ali, A.M.; Kelton, J.G. Thrombocytopenia caused by passive transfusion of anti-glycoprotein Ia/IIa alloantibody (anti-HPA-5b). *Blood* **1992**, *79*, 2480–2484. [CrossRef]
30. Delbos, F.; Bertrand, G.; Croisille, L.; Ansart-Pirenne, H.; Bierling, P.; Kaplan, C. Fetal and neonatal alloimmune thrombocytopenia: Predictive factors of intracranial hemorrhage. *Transfusion* **2016**, *56*, 59–66. [CrossRef]
31. Looney, C.B.; Smith, J.K.; Merck, L.H.; Wolfe, H.M.; Chescheir, N.C.; Hamer, R.M.; Gilmore, J.H. Intracranial hemorrhage in asymptomatic neonates: Prevalence on MR images and relationship to obstetric and neonatal risk factors. *Radiology* **2007**, *242*, 535–541. [CrossRef]
32. Giovangrandi, Y.; Daffos, F.; Kaplan, C.; Forestier, F.; Mac Aleese, J.; Moirot, M. Very early intracranial haemorrhage in alloimmune fetal thrombocytopenia. *Lancet* **1990**, *336*, 310. [CrossRef]
33. Kuhn, M.J.; Couch, S.M.; Binstadt, D.H.; Rightmire, D.A.; Morales, A.; Khanna, N.N.; Long, S.D. Prenatal recognition of central nervous system complications of alloimmune thrombocytopenia. *Comput. Med. Imaging Graph.* **1992**, *16*, 137–142. [CrossRef] [PubMed]
34. Lipitz, S.; Ryan, G.; Murphy, M.F.; Robson, S.C.; Haeusler, M.C.; Metcalfe, P.; Kelsey, H.; Rodeck, C.H. Neonatal alloimmune thrombocytopenia due to anti-P1A1 (anti-HPA-1a): Importance of paternal and fetal platelet typing for assessment of fetal risk. *Prenat. Diagn.* **1992**, *12*, 955–958. [CrossRef] [PubMed]
35. Khouzami, A.N.; Kickler, T.S.; Callan, N.A.; Shumway, J.B.; Perlman, E.J.; Blakemore, K.J. Devastating sequelae of alloimmune thrombocytopenia: An entity that deserves more attention. *J. Matern. Fetal Med.* **1996**, *5*, 137–141. [CrossRef]
36. Bussel, J.B.; Berkowitz, R.L.; Hung, C.; Kolb, E.A.; Wissert, M.; Primiani, A.; Tsaur, F.W.; Macfarland, J.G. Intracranial hemorrhage in alloimmune thrombocytopenia: Stratified management to prevent recurrence in the subsequent affected fetus. *Am. J. Obs. Gynecol.* **2010**, *203*, 135.e1–135.e14. [CrossRef] [PubMed]
37. Matusiak, K.; Patriquin, C.J.; Deniz, S.; Dzaja, N.; Smith, J.W.; Wang, G.; Nazy, I.; Kelton, J.G.; Arnold, D.M. Clinical and laboratory predictors of fetal and neonatal alloimmune thrombocytopenia. *Transfusion* **2022**, *62*, 2213–2222. [CrossRef]
38. Coste, T.; Vincent-Delorme, C.; Stichelbout, M.; Devisme, L.; Gelot, A.; Deryabin, I.; Pelluard, F.; Aloui, C.; Leutenegger, A.L.; Jouannic, J.M.; et al. COL4A1/COL4A2 and inherited platelet disorder gene variants in fetuses showing intracranial hemorrhage. *Prenat. Diagn.* **2022**, *42*, 601–610. [CrossRef] [PubMed]
39. Bussel, J.B.; Vander Haar, E.L.; Berkowitz, R.L. Fetal and Neonatal Alloimmune Thrombocytopenia in 2022. *Am. J. Obstet. Gynecol.* **2023**, *228*, 759. [CrossRef]
40. Pharmaceutical Technology. Available online: https://www.pharmaceutical-technology.com/features/immune-globulin-shortages/ (accessed on 15 August 2023).
41. Verywellfit. Available online: https://www.verywellfit.com/average-weight-for-a-woman-statistics-2632138 (accessed on 15 August 2023).
42. Pacheco, L.D.; Berkowitz, R.L.; Moise, K.J., Jr.; Bussel, J.B.; McFarland, J.G.; Saade, G.R. Fetal and neonatal alloimmune thrombocytopenia: A management algorithm based on risk stratification. *Obs. Gynecol.* **2011**, *118*, 1157–1163. [CrossRef]
43. Available online: https://www.howmuchisit.org/how-much-does-ivig-cost/ (accessed on 15 August 2023).
44. Buchacher, A.; Curling, J.M. Current Manufacturing of Human Plasma lmmunoglobulin G. In *Biopharmaceutical Processing Development, Design, and Implementation of Manufacturing Process*; Jagschies, G., Lindskog, E., Lacki, K., Galliher, P., Eds.; Elsevier: Amsterdam, The Netherlands; Oxford, UK; Cambridge, UK, 2018; pp. 857–876.

45. Radosevich, M.; Burnouf, T. Intravenous immunoglobulin G: Trends in production methods, quality control and quality assurance. *Vox Sang.* **2010**, *98*, 12–28. [CrossRef]
46. Miller-Keystone Blood Center. Available online: https://www.giveapint.org/ufaqs/how-long-does-it-take-to-donate-plasma/ (accessed on 15 August 2023).
47. Kapur, R.; Kustiawan, I.; Vestrheim, A.; Koeleman, C.A.; Visser, R.; Einarsdottir, H.K.; Porcelijn, L.; Jackson, D.; Kumpel, B.; Deelder, A.M.; et al. A prominent lack of IgG1-Fc fucosylation of platelet alloantibodies in pregnancy. *Blood* **2014**, *123*, 471–480. [CrossRef]

Disclaimer/Publisher's Note: The statements, opinions and data contained in all publications are solely those of the individual author(s) and contributor(s) and not of MDPI and/or the editor(s). MDPI and/or the editor(s) disclaim responsibility for any injury to people or property resulting from any ideas, methods, instructions or products referred to in the content.

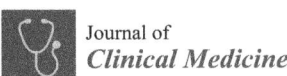

Article

Implementation and Assessment of a Laparotomy-Assisted Three-Port Fetoscopic Spina Bifida Repair Program

Corinna Keil [1,*], Siegmund Köhler [1], Benjamin Sass [2], Maximilian Schulze [3], Gerald Kalmus [4], Michael Belfort [5,6], Nicolas Schmitt [4], Daniele Diehl [7], Alice King [6,8], Stefanie Groß [7], Caitlin D. Sutton [9], Luc Joyeux [6,8], Mirjam Wege [10], Christopher Nimsky [2], Wiliam E. Whitehead [6,11], Eberhard Uhl [12], Thierry A. G. M. Huisman [13], Bernd A. Neubauer [7], Stefanie Weber [14], Helmut Hummler [10], Roland Axt-Fliedner [15] and Ivonne Bedei [15]

1 Department of Prenatal Medicine and Fetal Therapy, Philipps University, 35043 Marburg, Germany
2 Department of Neurosurgery, Philipps University, 35043 Marburg, Germany
3 Department of Neuroradiology, Philipps University, 35043 Marburg, Germany
4 Department of Anesthesiology and Intensive Care Medicine, Philipps University, 35043 Marburg, Germany
5 Department of Obstetrics and Gynecology, Texas Children's Hospital, Baylor College of Medicine, Houston, TX 77030, USA
6 Texas Children's Fetal Center, Texas Children's Hospital, Baylor College of Medicine, Houston, TX 77030, USA
7 Department of Pediatric Neurology, Justus-Liebig University Giessen, 35392 Giessen, Germany
8 Division of Pediatric Surgery, Department of Surgery, Texas Children's Hospital, Baylor College of Medicine, Houston, TX 77030, USA
9 Department of Pediatric Anesthesiology, Perioperative, and Pain Medicine, Texas Children's Hospital, Baylor College of Medicine, Houston, TX 77030, USA
10 Division of Neonatology, University Children's Hospital Marburg, 35043 Marburg, Germany
11 Department of Neurosurgery, Texas Children's Hospital, Baylor College of Medicine, Houston, TX 77030, USA
12 Department of Neurosurgery, Justus-Liebig University, 35390 Giessen, Germany
13 Edward B. Singleton Department of Radiology, Texas Children's Hospital, Baylor College of Medicine, Houston, TX 77030, USA
14 Division of Pediatric Nephrology and Transplantation, University Children's Hospital Marburg, 35043 Marburg, Germany
15 Department of Prenatal Medicine and Fetal Therapy, Justus-Liebig University Giessen, 35390 Giessen, Germany
* Correspondence: corinna.keil@med.uni-marburg.de

Abstract: Open spina bifida (OSB) is a congenital, non-lethal malformation with multifactorial etiology. Fetal therapy can be offered under certain conditions to parents after accurate prenatal diagnostic and interdisciplinary counseling. Since the advent of prenatal OSB surgery, various modifications of the original surgical techniques have evolved, including laparotomy-assisted fetoscopic repair. After a two-year preparation time, the team at the University of Giessen and Marburg (UKGM) became the first center to provide a three-port, three-layer fetoscopic repair of OSB via a laparotomy-assisted approach in the German-speaking area. We point out that under the guidance of experienced centers and by intensive multidisciplinary preparation and training, a previously described and applied technique could be transferred to a different setting.

Keywords: open spina bifida; fetal therapy; fetoscopic repair; standardized training

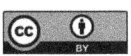

1. Objective

The incidence of open spina bifida (OSB) is approximately 4.9 per 10,000 live births in Europe and 3.17 in the USA [1,2].

Affected persons typically present with a Chiari 2 malformation and subsequent supratentorial ventriculomegaly, leading to postnatal ventriculo-peritoneal shunt interventions with associated morbidity (e.g., infections, obstructions). Furthermore, they suffer from impaired sensory-motor function of the lower extremities, orthopedic deformities, limitations in bladder and bowel function, and sexual dysfunction depending on the type and level of the lesion [3]. Intrauterine damage to the neuronal OSB structures occurs in two steps [4]. This natural history has been called the "two-hit hypothesis". The "first hit" is the actual congenital anomaly that results from the lack of closure of the neural tube in the embryonic period. The "second hit" results from direct trauma to the neuronal tissue from fetal movement and from exposure to toxic substances in the amniotic fluid during intrauterine life [5].

The rationale for prenatal therapy is based on the idea of preventing the "second hit" by closing the defect in the second trimester by limiting or reducing the severity of the associated Chiari 2 malformation. The preclinical scientific evidence for this rationale was provided by the experimental work in fetal sheep undertaken by Harrison and colleagues in San Francisco in the 1990s that ultimately culminated in the human randomized controlled trial named the Management of Myelomeningocele Study (MOMS trial) [4]. This trial demonstrated an improvement in motor function and a decrease in hydrocephalus and its shunt rate in children who underwent prenatal closure of OSB. The open surgical approach was a combination of a lower abdominal transverse laparotomy and large hysterotomy at which time the defect was closed using an adaptation of the postnatal neurosurgical technique [6–8]. The average gestational age at the time of delivery was 34.1 weeks with 13% delivering before 30 weeks. Delivery via C-section was and remains mandatory with this approach and all further pregnancies [9–11].

In an attempt to reduce prematurity and maternal complications, different techniques have been developed. One such technique is a laparotomy-assisted, exteriorized uterus, fetoscopic closure. This has also been called the "hybrid method". Another minimally invasive technique is the totally percutaneous laparoscopic approach [12–15]. Similar fetal and infant outcomes have been demonstrated for both techniques as compared to the MOMS trial (preservation of motor function, reduced degree of hydrocephalus). However, there are differences in the preterm birth rate, neonatal outcomes (respiratory distress syndrome and need for NICU management), and the effectiveness of the closure (leakage of cerebrospinal fluid). Later gestational age at delivery was reported for the hybrid technique in comparison to the open and transcutaneous approach that may be attributed to the fixation of the membranes before trocar insertion. Other reasons are less manipulation of the membranes and uterine environment due to the precise placement of the ports directly on the uterus and the gentle hand-held positioning of the fetus. However, these laparoscopic techniques have undergone several modifications making comparison of outcomes difficult [16–19].

The "International Fetoscopic Myelomeningocele Repair Consortium" was founded in 2017 to compare the results of these laparoscopic approaches. The consortium was an association of international centers with demonstrated expertise in fetoscopic OSB surgery. The aim of the consortium was to evaluate the feto-maternal outcome of the various fetoscopic methods, and in so doing advance the potential for training of new fetal centers by more experienced centers [20,21].

2. What Is the Aim of This Current Study?

To report on our experience and then based on the IDEAL recommendations confirm the replication of the safety of this hybrid fetoscopic method, as already reported by other centers [22,23]. Other studies report the outcome of small groups of patients (seven cases, one case) but do not describe the implementation of the surgical approach or the establishment of a multidisciplinary team [24,25]. As part of our training, we were supervised directly by experts from the fetal team of TCH; in addition, essential requirements had to be met prior to the start of the surgery to join the consortium [20].

3. Material and Methods

The University Hospital Giessen and Marburg (UKGM) had some experience in prenatal therapy of OSB using the totally percutaneous laparoscopic procedure [26]. Structures and multidisciplinary teams were already in place for the interdisciplinary care of patients.

After an in-depth comparison of different techniques, the team decided on the safe and effective "hybrid fetoscopic approach" due to the improved rates of prematurity, fewer maternal risks, and the potential for vaginal delivery [14,20].

In 2019, interdisciplinary preparations for the implementation of the "hybrid procedure" began by gathering different subspecialties involved in the pre- and postnatal care of patients with OSB at the UKGM. Regular meetings took place, followed by the development of treatment concepts in the individual subgroups: diagnostics (neuroradiology, prenatal ultrasound (US), genetics), surgical therapy (gynecology, neurosurgery, prenatal diagnostics, anesthesia), and follow-up care (neonatology, neuropediatric). The surgical team began extensive simulator training as well as surgical staff training [27]. In addition, other disciplines were included in the care structure (pediatric orthopedics, urology and nephrology, obstetrics, and human genetics).

Due to the SARS-CoV-2 pandemic, visits to international training centers for external training following in-house training were not feasible. Therefore, expert exchange and counseling took place through virtual/online platforms.

With online observation of live operations (USA, Spain) and one-to-one exchange between the cooperating disciplines, the preparations were intensified. During the training process, virtual step-by-step exchange and assistance in OSB repair were accompanied by extensive debriefing. Before the first in-vivo OSB repair according to the criteria of the consortium, we fulfilled the full catalog of requirements that was set up to qualify for participation in the "International Fetoscopic Myelomeningocele Repair Consortium" [20].

A clinical trial (prospective cohort study) was approved by institutional review boards in Giessen (161/20) and Marburg (195/20), as well as registration in the German Registry for Clinical Trials (DRKS00026102). After completing the preparations (total time 20 months), the team joined the "International Fetoscopic Myelomeningocele Repair Consortium" in March 2021. The team was supported by centers from the USA (Texas Children Hospital, Houston, TX, USA), Belgium (University Hospital of Leuven, Leuven), and Spain (Clinica Val d'Hebron, Barcelona).

4. Results

In July 2021, the first case was performed at UKGM in accordance with the criteria of the international consortium and under the guidance of Prof. Michael Belfort, TCH, Baylor College of Medicine (Houston, TX, USA). Since then, a total of 20 patients have been treated at UKGM (as of 07/23). Seven operations were performed with the physical presence of at least one member of the TCH team, with anesthesia, neurosurgery, and neuroradiology guidance from designated experts from the multidisciplinary fetal team of TCH. The "International Fetoscopic Myelomeningocele Repair Consortium" was closed in the summer of 2022 and by then ten cases had been performed at UKGM. Currently, a total of 13 departments at UKGM are involved in the care of OSB (Figure 1). The center offers the complete spectrum of pre-, peri-, and postnatal care for OSB, starting with prenatal diagnosis and therapy with infant follow-up extending to 72 months of life.

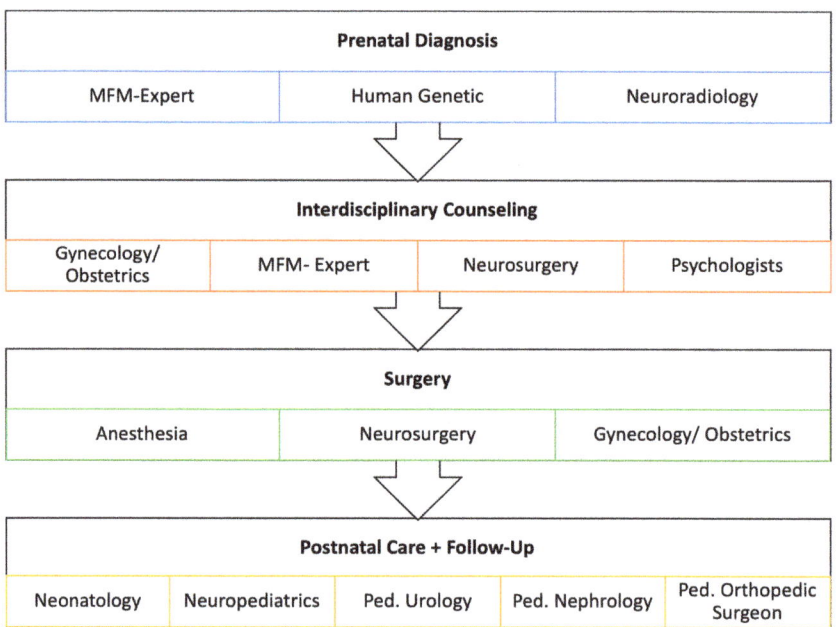

Figure 1. Interdisciplinary team at UKGM: 13 departments are involved in the care of OSB. The center offers the complete spectrum of pre-, peri-, and postnatal care for OSB.

We have a standardized protocol for tracking maternal-fetal data. The prospective study records all data collected at each stage of treatment, which are described in detail in the following sections. Figure 2 gives an overview of neuropediatric follow-up as an example.

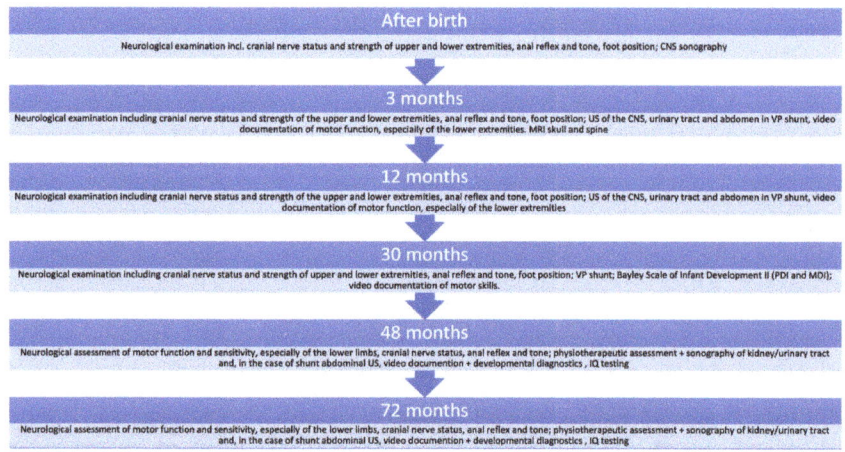

Figure 2. UKGM's own long-term follow-up: parents are asked to attend regular neuropediatric checkups, MRI imaging is dependent on the child's clinical condition, but at least once a year. Children are followed up until 72 months of age in a standardized protocol.

4.1. Diagnostics

Prenatal diagnosis of the fetus includes a detailed fetal anomaly scan, a fetal echocardiogram and central nervous system (CNS)-focused 2D/3D ultrasound, assessment of the anatomic level of the lesion, fetal motor function as described by Carreras [28], evaluation of the posterior fossa and supratentorial structures (e.g., Corpus callosum, ventricular size), and detailed evaluation of any additional CNS anomalies.

OSB nowadays can be detected already in the first trimester. Findings that are suggestive are the "crash sign", absence of intracranial translucency (IT), and the ratio between brain stem diameter (BS) and its distance to the occipital bone (BSOB) (BS/BSOB ratio). This allows timely presentation in a referral center to further specialized US and MRI to classify the lesion and allow for early fetal therapy already in the second trimester [29–31].

Invasive genetic diagnosis including karyotype, chromosomal microarray (CMA), and whole exome sequencing (WES) is offered to all patients. A normal karyotype is mandatory for all patients who pursue fetal therapy at our center.

In terms of prenatal imaging, we regard ultrasound and fetal magnetic resonance imaging (MRI) as complementary modalities. MRI adds important prognostic information for detecting brain anomalies, e.g., abnormalities of the ventricular wall such as heterotopias, and abnormalities of the corpus callosum and the cavum septi pellucidi. Secondly, MRI is useful in confirming our inclusion criteria (e.g., hindbrain herniation), delineates the anatomy, rules out other associated anomalies, and, unlike sonography, is independent of confounding factors such as maternal habitus, fetal position, and bone artifacts [32,33]. Per protocol, hindbrain herniation below the level of the foramen magnum is mandatory for prenatal surgery and must be confirmed on MRI. In addition, MRI adds specific information on any associated findings of Chiari malformation, not accessible on prenatal US (e.g., tectal beaking, cerebellar towering, medullary kinking) as well as further information on anomalies of the corpus callosum [34,35]. Follow-up MRI after in utero repair assesses the integrity of the repair and the potential need for postnatal hydrocephalus treatment [36]. Neuroradiologists should be familiar with either pediatric or fetal MRI. Furthermore, the fetal imaging protocols need subspeciality expertise for the set up. Most standard MRI scanners have very standard and consequently limited fetal imaging protocols. Therefore, optimization on fetal MRI protocol is a continuous process and needs close cooperation by experienced centers and collaboration with the vendors.

4.2. Parental Counseling

After completion of all diagnostic steps, parents are counseled by neuropediatric experts regarding the OSB spectrum and resulting limitations and changes in child development. Furthermore, contact with the German support group spina bifida and hydrocephalus (ASBH) is offered [37].

All parents receive the offer of psychological counseling by dedicated psychologists. They provide continuous assistance to the parents from preoperative counseling to neonatal treatment. The low-threshold psychological counseling focuses on reducing anxiety and perceived helplessness through reframing, providing information, and instructing relaxation techniques or using process- and embodiment-focused techniques. Helpful handling of the situation by the entire family, especially the siblings, is discussed or, if necessary, contacts for further help in the home environment are arranged [38].

The surgical team (prenatal diagnostics, neurosurgery, gynecology) consults with the parents regarding the options for OSB management (pre-/postnatal) depending on the feto-maternal conditions. Inclusion criteria for prenatal surgery are based on modified MOMS criteria (see Table 1) [39].

Table 1. Inclusion and exclusion criteria according to the modified MOMS criteria.

Inclusion Criteria	Exclusion Criteria
<ul><li>Maternal age > 18 years</li><li>Singleton pregnancy</li><li>Myelomeningocele/Myeloschisis at level T1 through S1</li><li>Evidence of hindbrain herniation in fetal MRI</li><li>Gestational age of 19–26 + 0 weeks at surgery</li><li>Normal karyotype</li></ul>	<ul><li>A fetal anomaly unrelated to OSB</li><li>Severe kyphosis >/= 30°</li><li>Obesity, Body mass index (kg/m^2) > 40</li><li>Placenta previa or placental abruption</li><li>Risk of preterm birth (including short cervix (<20 mm, previous preterm birth)</li><li>Current or planned cervical cerclage or history of cervical weakness</li><li>Previous spontaneous singleton delivery prior to 37 weeks</li><li>Maternal hypertension that would increase the risk of pre-eclampsia or preterm delivery</li><li>Chronic hypertension with end organ damage and new onset hypertension in current pregnancy</li><li>Maternal-fetal Rh isoimmunization, Kell sensitization</li><li>History of neonatal alloimmune thrombocytopenia</li><li>Maternal HIV or hepatitis-B status positive, known hepatitis-C positivity (screening is not required)</li><li>Uterine anomaly (large or multiple fibroids, mullerian duct abnormality)</li><li>Patient does not have social support person</li><li>Inability to comply with the travel and follow-up requirements of the trial</li><li>Patient does not meet other psychosocial criteria</li></ul>

4.3. OSB Surgery

Inpatient admission starts 2–3 days prior to the procedure. During this time, further assessments are made by the neonatology, anesthesia, and psychological teams. Preparation for surgery is carried out as described in our standardized protocol including steroid administration (betamethason 2 × 12 mg im.), preoperative prophylactic tocolysis (atosiban and indomethacin), and antibiotics (cefazolin or if allergic clindamycin).

Surgery is performed by a multidisciplinary team consisting of two gynecologists, one neurosurgeon, one fetal medicine specialist (for fetal surveillance), an anesthetic team monitoring the mother and fetus, and a dedicated nursing team and operating room scrub staff.

First, a low transverse laparotomy is performed, followed by externalization of the uterus. Amniotic membranes are sutured to the uterine wall, and a total of three ports are inserted using the Seldinger technique. Amniotic fluid is removed and replaced with humidified, warmed carbon dioxide. The spinal cord is released sharply, and a bovine Durapatch is applied. After preparing a muscle and skin flap, they are separately closed. After completing suturing, carbon dioxide is removed, and the uterus is refilled with sterile Ringer's acetate solution. Trocars are removed and defects are closed with transmural sutures. After repositioning the uterus, the maternal abdomen is closed in a standardized way (Figure 3).

The surgery is performed by a gynecologist with special expertise in oncologic and gynecological laparoscopy, a gynecologist/obstetric expert, and a neurosurgeon. Laparotomy and placement and removement of the ports are performed by the GYN/OBS team. Together with the maternal-fetal medicine specialist, they manage the fetal positioning. The maternal-fetal medicine specialist provides fetal surveillance by monitoring umbilical blood flow and heart rate, and, in addition, measures ductus venosus (DV) and arteria cerebri media (a.c.m.) flow at determined timepoints during surgery. The fetoscopic OSB repair is performed under the guidance of the neurosurgeon in collaboration with the gynecological laparoscopic specialist.

The surgical approach is based on the technique published by the TCH team. The main difference is the three-port instead of the two-port technique [14,40]. Single steps of the repair are presented in Table 2, which also gives an overview of associated problems and possible solutions.

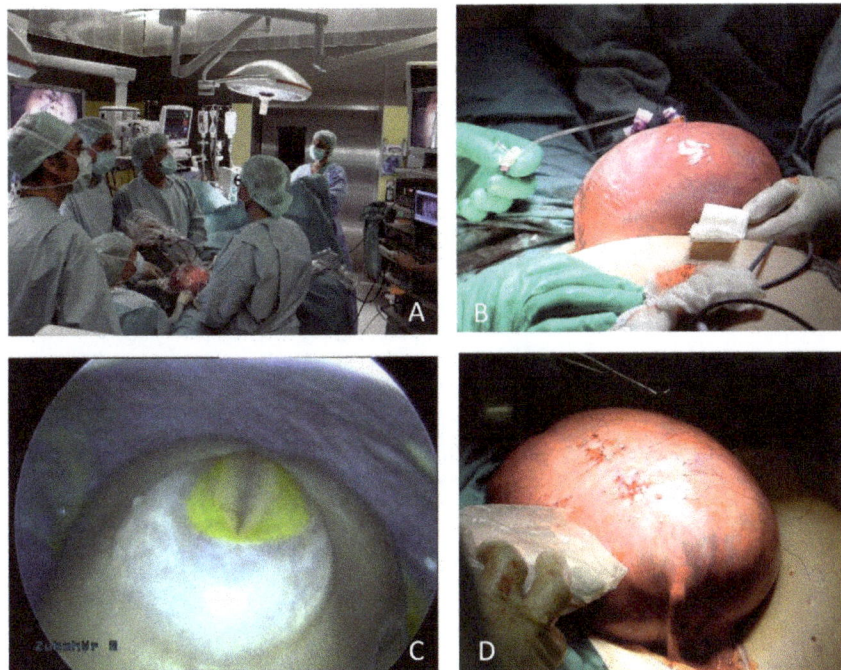

Figure 3. (**A**): Multidisciplinary team during laparotomy-assisted fetoscopic approach (**B**): Exteriorized uterus with 3 ports (**C**): Fetoscopic view on Myelomeningocele (**D**): Uterus after port removal.

Table 2. Systematic illustration of the laparotomy-assisted fetoscopic approach for prenatal OSB repair. For each step, the associated problems and possible solutions are described in detail.

Surgical Step	Problem	Solution
Low transverse laparotomy, externalisation of the uterus	Laparotomy is too small, which can lead to compression of the uterine artery, affecting feto-placental perfusion	Extend laparotomy
Placing 3 Ports (12 French, 10 French)	Incorrect port placement will result in difficulty in visualising and accessing the fetal OSB and may compromise surgical closure.	Careful port placement considering placenta, fetal position and operative environment.
	Alteration of placenta/fetus/myometral vessels	Careful sonographic visualisation of (intra-)uterine structures (placenta, fetus, vessels)
Removing amniotic fluid	Can lead to fetal heart alteration	Careful monitoring of fetal heart rate, slow remove
Uterine carbon dioxide insufflation (10 ± 2 mm Hg)	Gas needs to be humidified and warmed, otherwise there is an increased risk of premature rupture of the membranes. Moderate uterine pressure and moisturisation prevents fetal acidaemia	Additional Intermittent irrigation of membranes with sterile solution during OSB repair

Table 2. Cont.

Surgical Step	Problem	Solution
Fetal positioning	Can lead to fetal heart alteration, lack of positioning can complicate surgery or make it impossible.	Immediate cessation of fetal manipulation, ongoing fetal monitoring
		Intrauterine resuscitation of the fetus by administration of epinephrine (0.01 mg/kg)
Fetal anesthesia	Can lead to fetal heart alteration, fetal death caused by inccorect dose/application	Assesment of estimated preoperative fetal weight by experienced investigator
(fentanyl 10 ug/kg, cis-atracurium 0.6 mg/kg, atropine 0.03 mg/kg)- every 60 min during OSB repair		Monitoring and administration of fetal anaesthesia using four-eyes principle (MFM and anesthesia)
		Subcutaneous administration under direct vision only
Releasing spinal cord	Too close to skin	May develop inclusion cysts causing severe functional deterioration
	Excessive distance to skin	Injury to the neuronal structures
Preparation muscle flap	Not enough muscle mobilised/present	Close as much muscle as possible
Preparation skin flap	Not enough skin mobilised/present	Relaxing skin incisions lateral of the defect
Placing bovine dura patch	Patch too small/wide/big	Patch preparation according to defect size from MRI/US
Single sutures muscle	Low proportion of muscle	Close as much muscle as possible
Continous closure of the skin	Thin/fragile skin	Relaxing skin incisions lateral of the defect
End of CO_2-insufflation and instillation of sterile solution	Too much gas/too less sterile solution	Sonographic monitoring of refill
Removal of 3 ports and closure of the myometrial defect	Suture of fetal structures during closure	Controlled suture under sonographic guidance
	Insufficient closure	Uterine loss of amniotic fluid

The laparotomy-assisted fetoscopic approach required a realignment of the surgical skills of all team members as well as scrub staff. Through continuous interdisciplinary training, multidisciplinary interaction, enhancement of skills by expert exchange, and external supervision, a multidisciplinary team was created that met the requirements to cover the complex needs of patients with OSB.

The anesthetic management for this surgical procedure consists of a combination of general endotracheal anesthesia administered to the pregnant patient and direct intramuscular anesthesia administered to the fetus. The approach to anesthesia must account for both maternal and fetal considerations, as both are undergoing distinct surgical interventions, and hemodynamics must be tightly maintained to optimize both maternal and fetal conditions. Any physiologic changes due to anesthetic management (i.e., ventilation, hemodynamic control, and medication administration) impact both unique patients directly or indirectly. To optimize surgical conditions, significant uterine relaxation is required, particularly during phases of direct manipulation of the uterus. Tocolysis is typically achieved using volatile anesthetics combined with other agents (e.g., magnesium sulfate, atosiban, indomethacin). Magnesium sulfate can contribute to postoperative weakness and/or residual neuromuscular blockade when long-acting neuromuscular blocking agents are used, and quantitative neuromuscular blockade monitoring can be useful. Due to the known risk of postoperative pulmonary edema in the context of fetal surgery, a restrictive fluid regimen is used. Both the significant fluid restriction as well as many tocolytic agents can impact maternal and fetal hemodynamic stability, so advanced hemodynamic monitoring is used during surgery and for up to 48 h postoperatively [41–43]. A multimodal postoperative analgesic strategy, often including the use of neuraxial analgesia and/or fascial plane blocks, is critical to facilitate early recovery.

The patient receives close postoperative maternal-fetal monitoring, and regular multidisciplinary rounds take place. In an uneventful course, the mother is discharged at day 5–6 after surgery. Ambulatory monitoring is provided weekly by the local OB/Gyn provider and the maternal-fetal medicine specialist at UKGM every 4 weeks. Postoperative follow-up at the center includes sonographic evaluation, including detailed neurosonography, fetal growth evaluation, presence/degree of chorionic amnion separation (CAS), amniotic fluid volume assessment, and measurement of the cervical length. An MRI is performed 6 weeks after the fetal surgery to document regression of hindbrain herniation and quality of the OSB closure. If prenatal inpatient admission is necessary, the patient is ideally transferred to UKGM.

4.4. Delivery and Postnatal Care

Delivery should take place in our center, and this is part of the prenatal counseling. In case patients have to travel a long distance, relocation is offered at around 36 weeks if there is no threat of preterm delivery or CAS > 50%. In case of admission to a local hospital, a transfer is organized whenever feasible. In case of emergency (premature rupture of the membranes, threat of preterm delivery), which impedes traveling, patients should present immediately at the closest tertiary care center. UKGM provides guidance and additional information.

At UKGM, we ensure that the choice of delivery mode is based on obstetric indications.

Postnatal care of the newborn is interdisciplinary in terms of neonatology, neurosurgery, and neuropediatrics. Diagnostics include clinical examination, ultrasound, advanced imaging, and the involvement of pediatric orthopedics, urology, and nephrology.

After discharge, the family is referred to a neuropediatric center close to home, as well as to an integrated aftercare model for outpatient treatment for chronically ill patients, which includes various aspects (nursing, social pedagogy, psychology, etc.) and enables central organization and coordination, aiming for close-to-home connections to specialized institutions and seamless transitions between inpatient and outpatient care.

As part of the center's own follow-up, parents are asked to attend regular neuropediatric checkups, MRI imaging is dependent on the child's clinical condition but is performed at least once a year. Children are followed up until 72 months of age in a standardized protocol (Figure 2). We plan to expand follow-up through adolescence and into adulthood. The cost of the surgery is EUR 12,050 and is covered by the German National Health Service. Diagnostic and follow-up costs are also covered; therefore, the procedure is accessible to all families.

5. Discussion

The implementation of a fetal surgery program for myelomeningocele repair required multidisciplinary collaboration in the setting of a comprehensive program for the care of patients with OSB at UKGM. One challenge we faced internally was in connecting several subspecialties that otherwise have few points of interaction with each other. This required a rethinking of previous treatment concepts.

Structured training by experienced centers played a crucial role in supporting this fetoscopic program and breaking new ground. Joyeux et al. were able to show that the "learning curve" takes longer with the hybrid technique than with standard hysterotomy, which underscores the need for structured training by experienced centers. This study shows that standardized and structured training with the help and supervision of experienced centers is an appropriate and feasible method for supporting a new center in establishing this surgical procedure [17].

A new surgical innovation must be feasible, effective, and safe and needs continuous evaluation. Referring to the IDEAL framework recommendations, the implementation of the laparotomy-assisted three-port, three-layer fetoscopic repair of OSB fulfills IDEAL Stage 2a. Hereby, a new procedure is performed in a single center under close monitoring and data recruitment [22].

It is essential that full transparency with appropriate oversight exist in any such program, regardless of whether it is a new program or an experienced one. Fetal surgery is not yet a well-regulated field worldwide and in order to ensure the highest level of quality, safety, and patient care the highest ethical standards must be maintained. In this, we have made a commitment to our patients and to our colleagues (national and international) to collect and publish the short-, medium- and long-term outcomes of all children and mothers who receive antenatal surgery at UKGM under our standardized protocol. The manuscript of the results of the first 20 cases performed at UKGM is currently in preparation.

The successful establishment of prenatal OSB surgery at the UKGM is the result of a careful strategic and tactical plan, set up and implemented over years, which was driven by the desire to improve the maternal and fetal outcomes of patients with OSB. Using an intense interdisciplinary exchange, a willingness to learn from each other, and the help of external expert coaching, is reflected in the current program at UKGM. In the future, we are looking forward to continuing the interdisciplinary expert exchange and we are committed to the further development and enhancement of the long-term follow-up of our patients in order to improve patient care.

Author Contributions: Conceptualization, C.K., S.K., B.S., E.U., B.A.N., R.A.-F. and I.B.; Methodology, C.K., S.K., M.S., G.K., M.B., N.S., D.D., S.G., C.N., E.U., B.A.N., S.W., H.H., R.A.-F. and I.B.; Validation, M.S.; Investigation, C.K., B.S., G.K., M.B., N.S., D.D., S.G., M.W., C.N., H.H., R.A.-F. and I.B.; Writing—original draft, C.K. and I.B.; Writing—review & editing, S.K., B.S., M.S., M.B., N.S., D.D., A.K., C.D.S., L.J., M.W., W.E.W., E.U., T.A.G.M.H., S.W., H.H. and R.A.-F.; Supervision, M.B., A.K., C.D.S., L.J., W.E.W. and T.A.G.M.H. All authors have read and agreed to the published version of the manuscript.

Funding: This research received no external funding.

Institutional Review Board Statement: The study was conducted in accordance with the Declaration of Helsinki, and approved by the Institutional Review Board in Giessen (161/20, date of approval: 9 March 2020) and Marburg (195/20, date of approval: 12 November 2020).

Informed Consent Statement: Informed consent was obtained from all subjects involved in the study.

Data Availability Statement: Data available on request because of privacy/ethical restrictions.

Conflicts of Interest: The authors declare no conflict of interest.

References

1. Khoshnood, B.; Loane, M.; Walle, H.; Arriola, L.; Addor, M.-C.; Barisic, I.; Beres, J.; Bianchi, F.; Dias, C.; Draper, E.; et al. Long term trends in prevalence of neural tube defects in Europe: Population based study. *BMJ* **2015**, *351*, h5949. [CrossRef]
2. Canfield, M.A.; Mai, C.T.; Wang, Y.; O'Halloran, A.; Marengo, L.K.; Olney, R.S.; Borger, C.L.; Rutkowski, R.; Fornoff, J.; Irwin, N.; et al. The Association Between Race/Ethnicity and Major Birth Defects in the United States, 1999–2007. *Am. J. Public Health* **2014**, *104*, e14–e23. [CrossRef]
3. Bowman, R.M.; McLone, D.G.; Grant, J.A.; Tomita, T.; Ito, J.A. Spina Bifida Outcome: A 25-Year Prospective. *Pediatr. Neurosurg.* **2001**, *34*, 114–120. [CrossRef]
4. Meuli, M.; Meuli-Simmen, C.; Yingling, C.D.; Hutchins, G.M.; Hoffman, K.M.; Harrison, M.R.; Adzick, N.S. Creation of myelomeningocele in utero: A model of functional damage from spinal cord exposure in fetal sheep. *J. Pediatr. Surg.* **1995**, *30*, 1028–1033. [CrossRef]
5. Meuli, M.; Meuli-Simmen, C.; Hutchins, G.M.; Seller, M.J.; Harrison, M.R.; Adzick, N.S. The spinal cord lesion in human fetuses with myelomeningocele: Implications for fetal surgery. *J. Pediatr. Surg.* **1997**, *32*, 448–452. [CrossRef]
6. Adzick, N.S.; Thom, E.A.; Spong, C.Y.; Brock, J.W.; Burrows, P.K.; Johnson, M.P.; Howell, L.J.; Farrell, J.A.; Dabrowiak, M.E.; Sutton, L.N.; et al. A Randomized Trial of Prenatal versus Postnatal Repair of Myelomeningocele. *N. Engl. J. Med.* **2011**, *364*, 993–1004. [CrossRef]
7. Tulipan, N.; Wellons, J.C.; Thom, E.A.; Gupta, N.; Sutton, L.N.; Burrows, P.K.; Farmer, D.; Walsh, W.; Johnson, M.P.; Rand, L.; et al. Prenatal surgery for myelomeningocele and the need for cerebrospinal fluid shunt placement. *PED* **2015**, *16*, 613–620. [CrossRef]
8. Farmer, D.L.; Thom, E.A.; Brock, J.W.; Burrows, P.K.; Johnson, M.P.; Howell, L.J.; Farrell, J.A.; Gupta, N.; Adzick, N.S. The Management of Myelomeningocele Study: Full cohort 30-month pediatric outcomes. *Am. J. Obstet. Gynecol.* **2018**, *218*, 256.e1–256.e13. [CrossRef]
9. Johnson, M.P.; Bennett, K.A.; Rand, L.; Burrows, P.K.; Thom, E.A.; Howell, L.J.; Farrell, J.A.; Dabrowiak, M.E.; Brock, J.W.; Farmer, D.L.; et al. The Management of Myelomeningocele Study: Obstetrical outcomes and risk factors for obstetrical complications following prenatal surgery. *Am. J. Obstet. Gynecol.* **2016**, *215*, 778.e1–778.e9. [CrossRef]

10. Wilson, R.D.; Johnson, M.P.; Flake, A.W.; Crombleholme, T.M.; Hedrick, H.L.; Wilson, J.; Adzick, N.S. Reproductive outcomes after pregnancy complicated by maternal-fetal surgery. *Am. J. Obstet. Gynecol.* **2004**, *191*, 1430–1436. [CrossRef]
11. Soni, S.; Moldenhauer, J.S.; Spinner, S.S.; Rendon, N.; Khalek, N.; Martinez-Poyer, J.; Johnson, M.P.; Adzick, N.S. Chorioamniotic membrane separation and preterm premature rupture of membranes complicating in utero myelomeningocele repair. *Am. J. Obstet. Gynecol.* **2016**, *214*, 647.e1–647.e7. [CrossRef]
12. Lapa, D.A.; Chmait, R.H.; Gielchinsky, Y.; Yamamoto, M.; Persico, N.; Santorum, M.; Gil, M.M.; Trigo, L.; Quintero, R.A.; Nicolaides, K.H. Percutaneous fetoscopic spina bifida repair: Effect on ambulation and need for postnatal cerebrospinal fluid diversion and bladder catheterization. *Ultrasound Obstet. Gyne* **2021**, *58*, 582–589. [CrossRef]
13. Kohl, T. Percutaneous minimally invasive fetoscopic surgery for spina bifida aperta. Part I: Surgical technique and perioperative outcome. *Ultrasound Obs. Gynecol.* **2014**, *44*, 515–524. [CrossRef]
14. Belfort, M.A.; Whitehead, W.E.; Shamshirsaz, A.A.; Bateni, Z.H.; Olutoye, O.O.; Olutoye, O.A.; Mann, D.G.; Espinoza, J.; Williams, E.; Lee, T.C.; et al. Fetoscopic Open Neural Tube Defect Repair: Development and Refinement of a Two-Port, Carbon Dioxide Insufflation Technique. *Obstet. Gynecol.* **2017**, *129*, 734–743. [CrossRef]
15. Graf, K.; Kohl, T.; Neubauer, B.A.; Dey, F.; Faas, D.; Wanis, F.A.; Reinges, M.H.T.; Uhl, E.; Kolodziej, M.A. Percutaneous minimally invasive fetoscopic surgery for spina bifida aperta. Part III: Neurosurgical intervention in the first postnatal year: Fetoscopic surgery for SBA: Part III. *Ultrasound Obstet. Gynecol.* **2016**, *47*, 158–161. [CrossRef]
16. Verweij, E.J.; Vries, M.C.; Oldekamp, E.J.; Eggink, A.J.; Oepkes, D.; Slaghekke, F.; Spoor, J.K.H.; Deprest, J.A.; Miller, J.L.; Baschat, A.A.; et al. Fetoscopic myelomeningocele closure: Is the scientific evidence enough to challenge the gold standard for prenatal surgery? *Prenat. Diagn.* **2021**, *41*, 949–956. [CrossRef]
17. Joyeux, L.; De Bie, F.; Danzer, E.; Russo, F.M.; Javaux, A.; Peralta, C.F.A.; De Salles, A.A.F.; Pastuszka, A.; Olejek, A.; Van Mieghem, T.; et al. Learning curves of open and endoscopic fetal spina bifida closure: Systematic review and meta-analysis. *Ultrasound Obstet. Gynecol.* **2020**, *55*, 730–739. [CrossRef]
18. Joyeux, L.; De Bie, F.; Danzer, E.; Van Mieghem, T.; Flake, A.W.; Deprest, J. Safety and efficacy of fetal surgery techniques to close a spina bifida defect in the fetal lamb model: A systematic review. *Prenat. Diagn.* **2018**, *38*, 231–242. [CrossRef]
19. Chmait, R.H.; Monson, M.A.; Chon, A.H. Advances in Fetal Surgical Repair of Open Spina Bifida. *Obstet. Gynecol.* **2023**, *141*, 505–521. [CrossRef]
20. Sanz Cortes, M.; Lapa, D.A.; Acacio, G.L.; Belfort, M.; Carreras, E.; Maiz, N.; Peiro, J.L.; Lim, F.Y.; Miller, J.; Baschat, A.; et al. Proceedings of the First Annual Meeting of the International Fetoscopic Myelomeningocele Repair Consortium: International Fetoscopic Myelomeningocele Repair Consortium. *Ultrasound Obstet. Gynecol.* **2019**, *53*, 855–863. [CrossRef]
21. Sanz Cortes, M.; Chmait, R.H.; Lapa, D.A.; Belfort, M.A.; Carreras, E.; Miller, J.L.; Brawura Biskupski Samaha, R.; Sepulveda Gonzalez, G.; Gielchinsky, Y.; Yamamoto, M.; et al. Experience of 300 cases of prenatal fetoscopic open spina bifida repair: Report of the International Fetoscopic Neural Tube Defect Repair Consortium. *Am. J. Obstet. Gynecol.* **2021**, *225*, 678.e1–678.e11. [CrossRef]
22. Hirst, A.; Philippou, Y.; Blazeby, J.; Campbell, B.; Campbell, M.; Feinberg, J.; Rovers, M.; Blencowe, N.; Pennell, C.; Quinn, T.; et al. No Surgical Innovation Without Evaluation: Evolution and Further Development of the IDEAL Framework and Recommendations. *Ann. Surg.* **2019**, *269*, 211–220. [CrossRef]
23. Miller, J.L.; Groves, M.L.; Ahn, E.S.; Berman, D.J.; Murphy, J.D.; Rosner, M.K.; Wolfson, D.; Jelin, E.B.; Korth, S.A.; Keiser, A.M.; et al. Implementation Process and Evolution of a Laparotomy-Assisted 2-Port Fetoscopic Spina Bifida Closure Program. *Fetal Diagn. Ther.* **2021**, *48*, 603–610. [CrossRef]
24. Arthuis, C.; James, S.; Bussieres, L.; Hovhannisyan, S.; Corroenne, R.; Ville, Y.; Stirnemann, J.J. Laparotomy-Assisted 2-Port Fetoscopic Repair of Spina Bifida Aperta: Report of a Single-Center Experience in Paris, France. *Fetal Diagn. Ther.* **2022**, *49*, 377–384. [CrossRef]
25. Pastuszka, A.; Zamłyński, M.; Horzelski, T.; Zamłyński, J.; Horzelska, E.; Maruniak-Chudek, I.; Marzec, A.; Paprocka, J.; Gazy, P.; Koszutski, T.; et al. Fetoscopic Myelomeningocoele Repair with Complete Release of the Tethered Spinal Cord Using a Three-Port Technique: Twelve-Month Follow-Up—A Case Report. *Diagnostics* **2022**, *12*, 2978. [CrossRef]
26. Degenhardt, J.; Schürg, R.; Winarno, A.; Oehmke, F.; Khaleeva, A.; Kawecki, A.; Enzensberger, C.; Tinneberg, H.-R.; Faas, D.; Ehrhardt, H.; et al. Percutaneous minimal-access fetoscopic surgery for spina bifida aperta. Part II: Maternal management and outcome. *Ultrasound Obstet. Gynecol.* **2014**, *44*, 525–531. [CrossRef]
27. Joyeux, L.; Basurto, D.; Eastwood, M.; Javaux, A.; De Bie, F.; Vergote, S.; Devlieger, R.; De Catte, L.; Van Calenbergh, F.; Belfort, M.A.; et al. OC10.01: A novel training program for fetoscopic spina bifida repair. *Ultrasound Obstet. Gynecol.* **2020**, *56*, 27. [CrossRef]
28. Carreras, E.; Maroto, A.; Illescas, T.; Meléndez, M.; Arévalo, S.; Peiró, J.L.; García-Fontecha, C.G.; Belfort, M.; Cuxart, A. Prenatal ultrasound evaluation of segmental level of neurological lesion in fetuses with myelomeningocele: Development of a new technique: Functional ultrasound in MMC. *Ultrasound Obstet. Gynecol.* **2016**, *47*, 162–167. [CrossRef]
29. Ushakov, F.; Sacco, A.; Andreeva, E.; Tudorache, S.; Everett, T.; David, A.L.; Pandya, P.P. Crash sign: New first-trimester sonographic marker of spina bifida. *Ultrasound Obstet. Gynecol.* **2019**, *54*, 740–745. [CrossRef]
30. Chaoui, R.; Benoit, B.; Mitkowska-Wozniak, H.; Heling, K.S.; Nicolaides, K.H. Assessment of intracranial translucency (IT) in the detection of spina bifida at the 11–13-week scan. *Ultrasound Obstet. Gynecol.* **2009**, *34*, 249–252. [CrossRef]

31. Sirico, A.; Raffone, A.; Lanzone, A.; Saccone, G.; Travaglino, A.; Sarno, L.; Rizzo, G.; Zullo, F.; Maruotti, G.M. First trimester detection of fetal open spina bifida using BS/BSOB ratio. *Arch. Gynecol. Obstet.* **2020**, *301*, 333–340. [CrossRef]
32. Trigo, L.; Eixarch, E.; Bottura, I.; Dalaqua, M.; Barbosa, A.A.; De Catte, L.; Demaerel, P.; Dymarkowski, S.; Deprest, J.; Lapa, D.A.; et al. Prevalence of supratentorial anomalies assessed by magnetic resonance imaging in fetuses with open spina bifida. *Ultrasound Obstet. Gynecol.* **2022**, *59*, 804–812. [CrossRef]
33. Mufti, N.; Sacco, A.; Aertsen, M.; Ushakov, F.; Ourselin, S.; Thomson, D.; Deprest, J.; Melbourne, A.; David, A.L. What brain abnormalities can magnetic resonance imaging detect in foetal and early neonatal spina bifida: A systematic review. *Neuroradiology* **2022**, *64*, 233–245. [CrossRef]
34. Egloff, A.; Bulas, D. Magnetic Resonance Imaging Evaluation of Fetal Neural Tube Defects. *Semin. Ultrasound CT MRI* **2015**, *36*, 487–500. [CrossRef]
35. Davidson, J.R.; Uus, A.; Matthew, J.; Egloff, A.M.; Deprez, M.; Yardley, I.; De Coppi, P.; David, A.; Carmichael, J.; Rutherford, M.A. Fetal body MRI and its application to fetal and neonatal treatment: An illustrative review. *Lancet Child. Adolesc. Health* **2021**, *5*, 447–458. [CrossRef]
36. Zarutskie, A.; Guimaraes, C.; Yepez, M.; Torres, P.; Shetty, A.; Sangi-Haghpeykar, H.; Lee, W.; Espinoza, J.; Shamshirsaz, A.A.; Nassr, A.; et al. Prenatal brain imaging for predicting need for postnatal hydrocephalus treatment in fetuses that had neural tube defect repair in utero. *Ultrasound Obstet. Gynecol.* **2019**, *53*, 324–334. [CrossRef]
37. Flint, G.A.; Lammers, W.; Mitnick, D.G. Emotional Freedom Techniques. *J. Aggress. Maltreatment Trauma* **2006**, *12*, 125–150. [CrossRef]
38. Craig, G. The EFT manual. EFT: Emotional Freedom Technique: A Universal Healing Aid. Retrieved 15 January 2001. Available online: http://www.emofree.com/freestuff.htm (accessed on 6 August 2023).
39. Sacco, A.; Ushakov, F.; Thompson, D.; Peebles, D.; Pandya, P.; De Coppi, P.; Wimalasundera, R.; Attilakos, G.; David, A.L.; Deprest, J. Fetal surgery for open spina bifida. *Obstet. Gynecol.* **2019**, *21*, 271–282. [CrossRef]
40. Espinoza, J.; Shamshirsaz, A.A.; Sanz Cortes, M.; Pammi, M.; Nassr, A.A.; Donepudi, R.; Whitehead, W.E.; Castillo, J.; Johnson, R.; Meshinchi, N.; et al. Two-port, exteriorized uterus, fetoscopic meningomyelocele closure has fewer adverse neonatal outcomes than open hysterotomy closure. *Am. J. Obstet. Gynecol.* **2021**, *225*, 327.e1–327.e9. [CrossRef]
41. Ferschl, M.; Ball, R.; Lee, H.; Rollins, M.D. Anesthesia for In Utero Repair of Myelomeningocele. *Anesthesiology* **2013**, *118*, 1211–1223. [CrossRef]
42. Ring, L.E.; Ginosar, Y. Anesthesia for Fetal Surgery and Fetal Procedures. *Clin. Perinatol.* **2019**, *46*, 801–816. [CrossRef]
43. Hoagland, M.A.; Chatterjee, D. Anesthesia for fetal surgery. *Paediatr. Anaesth.* **2017**, *27*, 346–357. [CrossRef]

Disclaimer/Publisher's Note: The statements, opinions and data contained in all publications are solely those of the individual author(s) and contributor(s) and not of MDPI and/or the editor(s). MDPI and/or the editor(s) disclaim responsibility for any injury to people or property resulting from any ideas, methods, instructions or products referred to in the content.

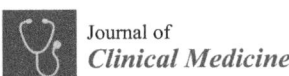

Systematic Review

Analysis of Clinical Profiles and Echocardiographic Cardiac Outcomes in Peripartum Cardiomyopathy (PPCM) vs. PPCM with Co-Existing Hypertensive Pregnancy Disorder (HPD-PPCM) Patients: A Systematic Review and Meta-Analysis

Annisa Dewi Nugrahani [1,2,*], Sidik Maulana [3], Kevin Dominique Tjandraprawira [2], Dhanny Primantara Johari Santoso [1,2], Dani Setiawan [2], Adhi Pribadi [2], Amillia Siddiq [2], Akhmad Yogi Pramatirta [2], Muhammad Alamsyah Aziz [2] and Setyorini Irianti [2]

1. Department of Obstetrics and Gynecology, Faculty of Medicine, University of Padjadjaran, Dr. Slamet General Hospital Garut, Bandung 45363, West Java, Indonesia; dhannydsog18@gmail.com
2. Department of Obstetrics and Gynecology, Faculty of Medicine, University of Padjadjaran, Dr. Hasan Sadikin General Hospital, Bandung 45363, West Java, Indonesia; kevin14007@mail.unpad.ac.id (K.D.T.); danisetiawan0323@gmail.com (D.S.); priana1001@gmail.com (A.P.); amel2000id@yahoo.com (A.S.); dryogipramatirta@gmail.com (A.Y.P.); alamsyahaziz9119@gmail.com (M.A.A.); dririanti0901@gmail.com (S.I.)
3. Nursing Internship Program, University of Padjadjaran, Sumedang 45363, West Java, Indonesia; sidik17001@mail.unpad.ac.id
* Correspondence: annisanugrahani99@gmail.com or annisa16005@mail.unpad.ac.id; Tel.: +62-821-1664-5912 or +62-821-1898-6852

Abstract: Peripartum cardiomyopathy (PPCM) is a form of new-onset heart failure that has a high rate of maternal morbidity and mortality. This was the first study to systematically investigate and compare clinical factors and echocardiographic findings between women with PPCM and co-incident hypertensive pregnancy disorders (HPD-PPCM) and PPCM-only women. We followed the Preferred Reporting Items for Systematic Review and Meta-Analysis (PRISMA) framework. We used four databases and a single search engine, namely PubMed/Medline, Scopus, Web of Science, and Cochrane. We used Cochrane Risk of Bias (RoB) 2.0 for quality assessment. Databases were searched for relevant articles published from 2013 to the end of April 2023. The meta-analysis used the DerSimonian–Laird random-effects model to analyze the pooled mean difference (MD) and its p-value. We included four studies with a total of 64,649 participants and found that systolic blood pressure was significantly more likely to be associated with the PPCM group than the HPD-PPCM group (SMD = -1.63) (95% CI; $-4.92, 0.28$, $p = 0.01$), while the other clinical profiles were not significant. HPD-PPCM was less likely to be associated with LVEF reduction (SMD = -1.55, [CI: -2.89, -0.21], $p = 0.02$). HPD-PPCM was significantly associated with less LV dilation (SMD = 1.81; 95% (CI 0.07–3.01), $p = 0.04$). Moreover, HPD-PPCM was less likely to be associated with relative wall thickness reduction (SMD = 0.70; 95% CI (-1.08–-0.33), $p = 0.0003$). In conclusion, PPCM and HPD-PPCM shared different clinical profiles and remodeling types, which may affect each disease's response to pharmacological treatment. Patients with HPD-PPCM exhibited less eccentric remodeling and seemed to have a higher chance of recovering their LV ejection fraction, which means they might not benefit as much from ACEi/ARB and beta-blockers. The findings of this study will guide the development of guidelines for women with PPCM and HPD-PPCM from early detection to further management.

Keywords: echocardiography; hypertensive pregnancy disorder; peripartum cardiomyopathy; PPCM

Citation: Nugrahani, A.D.; Maulana, S.; Tjandraprawira, K.D.; Santoso, D.P.J.; Setiawan, D.; Pribadi, A.; Siddiq, A.; Pramatirta, A.Y.; Aziz, M.A.; Irianti, S. Analysis of Clinical Profiles and Echocardiographic Cardiac Outcomes in Peripartum Cardiomyopathy (PPCM) vs. PPCM with Co-Existing Hypertensive Pregnancy Disorder (HPD-PPCM) Patients: A Systematic Review and Meta-Analysis. *J. Clin. Med.* 2023, 12, 5303. https://doi.org/10.3390/jcm12165303

Academic Editors: Dinesh K. Kalra and Attila Nemes

Received: 6 June 2023
Revised: 15 July 2023
Accepted: 9 August 2023
Published: 15 August 2023

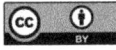

Copyright: © 2023 by the authors. Licensee MDPI, Basel, Switzerland. This article is an open access article distributed under the terms and conditions of the Creative Commons Attribution (CC BY) license (https://creativecommons.org/licenses/by/4.0/).

1. Introduction

Peripartum cardiomyopathy (PPCM) is defined as a form of new-onset heart failure with reduced left ventricular ejection fraction (LVEF) during the peripartum period in the absence of other identified etiologies [1]. In the United States (US), this cardiomyopathy affects 1/1000 to 1/4000 pregnancies. The consequences are devastating for both mothers and infants. PPCM accounts for 5% of heart transplants in women in the United States, as an alternative treatment is not offered in the majority of the world [2]. In underdeveloped countries, up to 25% of mothers with PPCM die within 5 years [3], with neonatal mortality rates ranging from 50% to 75% [4,5].

The etiology of PPCM is enigmatic. There have been numerous hypotheses proposed, including viral myocarditis, autoimmunity, and fetal microchimerism. In 1938, Hull and Hidden [6] discovered a link between postpartum heart failure and hypertensive heart disease when they discovered that >85% of instances of "toxic" postpartum heart disease were related to hypertension, which was double the frequency reported in their control group. PE has frequently been recognized as an independent risk factor for the development of PPCM since the publication of these important studies [7–9]. Hypertensive pregnancy disorder (HPD), including preeclampsia, is a significant risk factor for PPCM since women with preeclampsia have a 10–20 times higher risk of PPCM than non-hypertensive controls [6]. While an anti-angiogenic state could theoretically provide a relationship between the two disorders, not all women with HPD have superimposed PPCM [10,11]. Identifying preeclamptic women at high risk of PPCM may lead to focused quality improvement care initiatives, allowing for the early identification of this cardiomyopathy and reducing the burden of unfavorable outcomes associated with late presentation [12]. However, the risk factors for PPCM in HPD women are still not widely known.

Given that less than 20% of women with PPCM have co-incident HPD including preeclampsia, understanding the impact of HPD on PPCM outcomes should assist clinicians in anticipating complications and counseling patients more accurately [13]. Preeclampsia and other HPD-related structural cardiac alterations, including left ventricular concentric remodeling and diastolic dysfunction, may influence the clinical course of women with PPCM. A previous study showed that when PPCM was aggravated with preeclampsia or another HPD (HPD-PPCM group), the pattern of LV remodeling was noticeably different than in PPCM alone. Greater LV dilatation and a decrease in relative LV wall thickness were observed in patients with PPCM only, which was consistent with the traditional "eccentric" LV remodeling. In contrast, neither LV dilation nor a decrease in relative wall thickness were linked with the decline in LV ejection fraction (LVEF) in patients with HPD-PPCM, which was more compatible with a concentric pattern of LV remodeling [3–5]. While various small studies with contradictory results have addressed the impact of HPD on PPCM outcomes [7–9,12,14–16], only two studies reported with sample sizes of less than 40 patients specifically focused on co-incident preeclampsia [14,15].

To the best of our knowledge, there have been no systematic reviews or meta-analyses comparing echocardiographic findings and their associated sociodemographic and clinical factors between women with PPCM and co-incident HPD (HPD-PPCM) and those with PPCM and no HPD (PPCM). It is postulated that PPCM and HPD-PPCM share different types of remodeling, which may affect each disease's response to pharmacological treatment. A previous study revealed that different types of remodeling have clinical biomarkers and phenotypes that are distinctly different. Moreover, compared to patients with eccentric LV remodeling, people with concentric LV remodeling might not benefit as much from angiotensin-converting enzyme inhibitors, angiotensin receptor blockers, and beta-blockers [7–9,14–16].

Thus, this study aims to systematically investigate and compare clinical factors and echocardiographic findings between women with PPCM and co-incident HPD (HPD-PPCM) and those with PPCM, which has never been reported before. Since there have been no published guidelines for managing women with PPCM comprehensively, this study intends to guide the development of further provisions and guidelines for women with PPCM worldwide, from early detection to further management, in order to reduce the burden of unfavorable outcomes associated with late presentation of PPCM and PPCM with co-existing HPD including preeclampsia (HPD-PPCM).

2. Materials and Methods

2.1. Study Design

This study was presented as a systematic review and meta-analysis. The systematic review followed PRISMA and the Cochrane Collaboration's reporting item for systematic reviews and meta-analyses [17]. PROSPERO registered this study with CRD number (CRD42023428302).

2.2. Eligibility Criteria

This systematic review's inclusion criteria adhered to the PECO (Population, Exposure, Comparison, Outcome) approach. Women with PPCM with or without the co-existence of hypertensive pregnancy disorder (HPD) comprised the study population. The exposure or prognostic factors were risk factors. We extracted information on the following clinical risk factors potentially associated with PPCM and superimposed PPCM among women with HPD (HPD-PPCM), which are: maternal age, gravidity, tobacco use, chronic hypertension history, baseline systolic blood pressure, baseline diastolic blood pressure, and medical therapy initiated after diagnosis (furosemide and beta-blocker). This study compares the risk factors and echocardiographic findings as outcomes in PPCM vs. HPD-PPCM patients. The primary outcome of echocardiographic findings was a composite of cardiovascular indicators that may describe the severity of PPCM and type of remodeling such as left ventricular ejection fraction (LVEF) reduction, left ventricular (LV) dilation, and relative wall thickness reduction.

Studies were included if they were published in peer-reviewed journals, contained original quantitative data, and were written in English. Review and abstract-only articles were also excluded. No restrictions were placed on the publication date of studies. Studies were identified through searching electronic databases, scanning reference lists, and consulting with experts in the field.

2.3. Search Strategy and Study Selection

To identify relevant studies for this systematic review and meta-analysis, a comprehensive search of multiple databases was conducted. This search strategy was applied to the PubMed/Medline, Scopus, Web of Science, and Cochrane databases, which were reviewed from their inception up to April 2023. For the purpose of the current review, cases described as preeclampsia, eclampsia, chronic hypertension, gestational hypertension, and chronic hypertension with superimposed preeclampsia were grouped as HPD-PPCM.

The search strategy was developed using a combination of keywords and MeSH terms related to PPCM, preeclampsia (PE), and echocardiographic findings. The search terms used are described in Supplementary File S1. The 'related articles' feature and reference lists of included articles were also searched to identify additional relevant studies. Two independent reviewers (ADN and SM) screened all articles for eligibility, and any discrepancies were resolved through discussion with a third reviewer (DPJS). Studies were included if they contained original quantitative data regarding factors and echocardiographic outcomes of PPCM and HPD-PPCM. After the screening had been completed, the reference manager automatically removed duplicates of the article using Mendeley (Mendeley Ltd., New York, NY, USA).

2.4. Data Analysis and Quality Assessment

Three authors (ADN, DPJS, and SM) independently extracted data using a standardized data extraction form that included details for risk factors which are maternal age, gravidity, tobacco use, chronic hypertension history, baseline systolic blood pressure, baseline diastolic blood pressure, and medical therapy initiated after diagnosis (furosemide and beta-blocker) as well as echocardiographic findings which are left ventricular ejection fraction (LVEF) reduction, left ventricular (LV) dilation, and relative wall thickness reduction. First, we thoroughly read the studies to identify relevant text related to our research question. Next, we identified recurring themes and categories from the data. We used an iterative process to refine these themes and ensure they accurately represent the data. In cases of disagreement between two authors, a third author (DPJS) served as a mediator.

We evaluated the quality of the non-randomized clinical trials using Cochrane Reviews for Nonrandomized Studies of Intervention (ROBINS-I). Two authors independently evaluated the mentioned studies (ADN and SM). During the evaluation, the following factors were considered: bias resulting from the randomization process, bias resulting from deviation from the intended intervention, bias resulting from missing outcome data, bias in the measurement of the outcome, and bias in the selection of the reported results. Discourse addressed divergent perceptions regarding the quality of the study.

2.5. Statistical Analysis

This meta-analysis was performed using RevMan (RevMan International, Inc., New York, NY, USA), Comprehensive Meta-Analysis (CMA) for statistical analysis (Biostat Inc., Englewood, CO, USA), and Jamovie. We calculated pooled effect size estimates as mean differences with 95% confidence intervals using the DerSimonan–Laird method formula (CI). The inconsistency index (I^2) and subgroup analysis using the Chi-square test were used to assess potential reasons for heterogeneity. An I^2 of more than 50% and a p-value lower than 0.05 were considered significant for heterogeneity [18]. A random-effects model accounted for interstudy variability regardless of study heterogeneity [18–20]. We decided to assess statistical significance using a two-tailed p-value of 0.05.

3. Results

3.1. Study Selection

An initial search was conducted in electronic databases, including Scopus, PubMed/Medline, Web of Science, and Cochrane, which yielded a total of 5903 articles. After removing 151 articles due to duplication, the remaining 5080 articles were screened for eligibility. Of those, five studies were evaluated to determine eligibility and a full-text article was excluded from subsequent analysis since it did not present the outcome of interest (this paper separated PPCM with chronic hypertension and PPCM with preeclampsia) [14,15,21,22]. Ultimately, four studies were included in the analysis. Figure 1 illustrates the selection process for identifying the studies included in this review.

3.2. Characteristics of Included Studies

The included studies in this systematic review and meta-analysis were similar in terms of study design and country of origin. Among the four studies included, three were retrospective studies, and one a was prospective study. The majority of the studies were conducted in the United States of America (USA) (two studies), in addition to South Africa (one study) and Sweden (one study), indicating that currently, this type of study is rare and is still focusing on developed countries' populations. This study included a total of 64,649 participants. The age distribution of the study participants ranged from 15 to 55 years old. The patterns of study designs and data included in this review provide a comprehensive understanding of the comparison of sociodemographic factors, clinical factors, and echocardiographic outcomes among PPCM vs. HPD-PPCM patients. There were no significant differences in the characteristics of maternal age at diagnosis and gravidity between the PPCM and HPD-PPCM groups in all the included studies (Table 1).

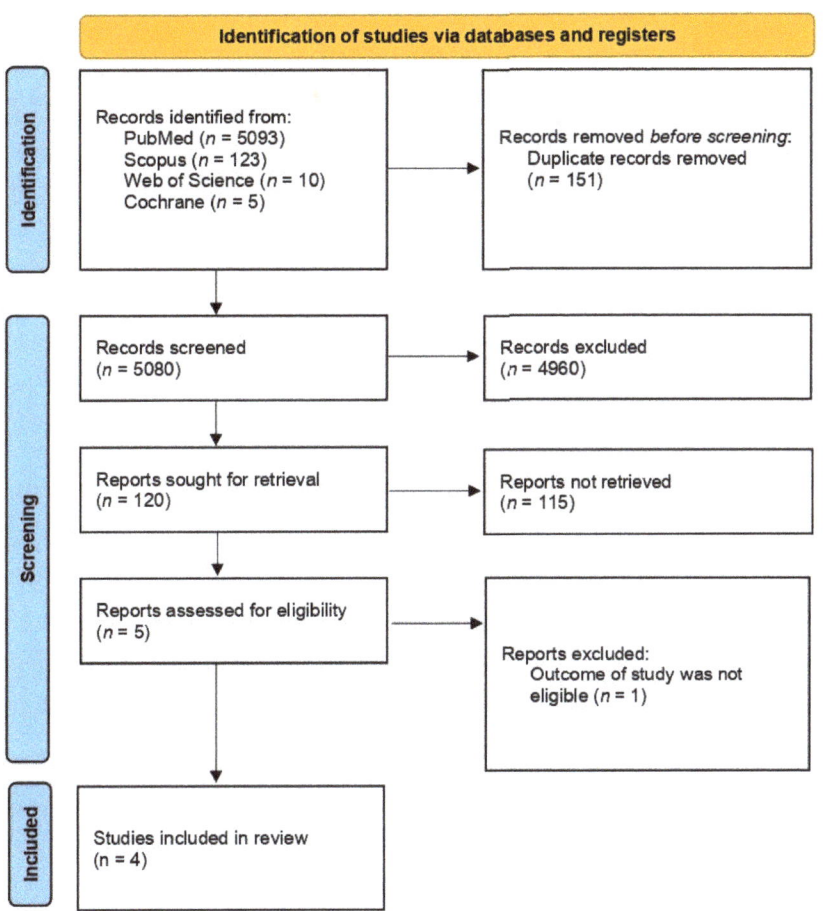

Figure 1. PRISMA flow diagram.

Table 1. Characteristics of included studies ($n = 4$ studies).

Study	PPCM		HPD-PPCM		p-Value
	Mean (SD)	N	Mean (SD)	N	
Design					
Barasa et al. (2017) [14]	Retrospective cohort				
Lindley et al. (2017) [15]	Retrospective cohort				
Ntusi et al. (2015) [22]	Retrospective cohort				
Malhamé et al. (2019) [21]	Prospective cohort				
Sociodemographic Profiles					
Location					
Barasa et al. (2017) [14]	Sweden				
Lindley et al. (2017) [15]	USA				
Ntusi et al. (2015) [22]	USA				
Malhamé et al. (2019) [21]	South Africa				

Table 1. Cont.

Study	PPCM		HPD-PPCM		p-Value
	Mean (SD)	N	Mean (SD)	N	
Maternal Age at Diagnosis					
Lindley et al. (2017) [15]	29.30 (5.090)	22	27.40 (7.40)	17	
Ntusi et al. (2015) [22]	31.50 (7.50)	30	29.60 (6.60)	53	0.90
Malhamé et al. (2019) [21]	30.20 (5.80)	64,220	31.80 (6.80)	283	
Gravidity					
Lindley et al. (2017) [15]	3.10 (1.90)	22	2.60 (2.20)	17	0.13
Ntusi et al. (2015) [22]	2.40 (0.70)	30	2.20 (0.60)	53	
Tobacco Use	(Even, Total)		(Event, Total)		
Lindley et al. (2017) [15]	4	22	4	17	
Malhamé et al. (2019) [21]	8	283	1143	64,220	0.10
Ntusi et al. (2015) [22]	7	30	5	53	

Note: PPCM (peripartum cardiomyopathy); HPD-PPCM (peripartum cardiomyopathy with co-existing hypertensive pregnancy disorder comorbidities); USA (United States of America); SD (standard deviation). p-value was created through meta-analysis.

3.3. Risk of Bias

Based on the risk of bias assessment using ROBINS-I, there are two studies with moderate risk, one study with serious risk, and one study with a critical risk of bias. The risk of bias domain with moderate level was dominated by D1 (bias due to confounding), D2 (bias due to selection of participants), D6 (bias in measurements of outcomes), and D7 (bias in reported results). The serious risk bias was due to D2 (bias due to the selection of participants) and D4 (bias due to deviations from intended interventions). The critical risk of bias study was due to critical D2 (bias due to selection of participants) Moreover, the risk of bias was dominated by D1 (bias due to confounding) and D6 (bias in measurement of outcomes) (see Figure 2).

3.4. Study Outcomes

3.4.1. Clinical Profiles

Chronic Hypertension

Similar to tobacco use analysis, three studies (Lindley et al., Ntusi et al., and Malhame et al.) [15,21,22] included an analysis of baseline history of chronic hypertension in their studies. Figure 3 reveals that chronic hypertension was more likely to influence the PPCM group rather than the HPD-PPCM group (RR = 0.73) [95% CI; 0.17,3.05, $p = 0.67$], which may favor diseases' outcomes, although not significant. A high heterogeneity was also identified ($I^2 = 81\%$, $p = 0.005$).

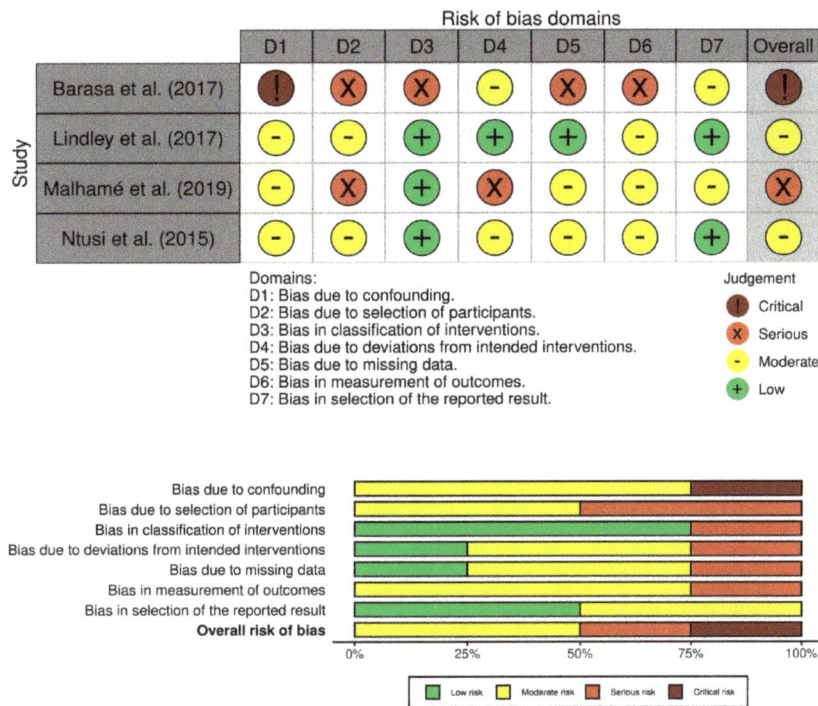

Figure 2. Risk of bias assessment with ROBINS-I [14,15,21,22].

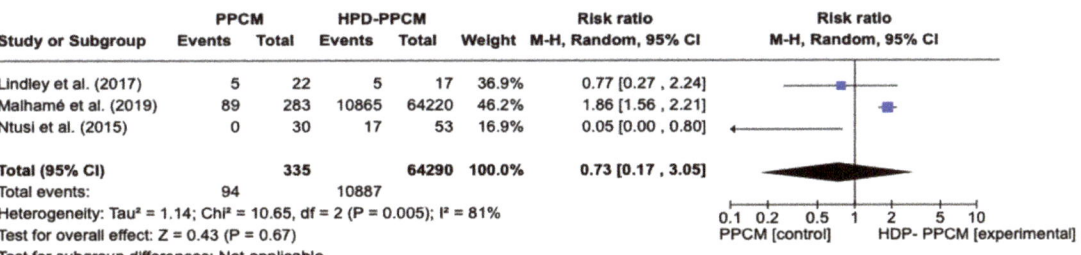

Figure 3. Forest plot of the impact of chronic hypertension on PPCM vs. HPD-PPCM [15,21,22].

Systolic Blood Pressure (SBP)

Only two studies (Lindley et al. and Ntusi et al.) [15,22] included an analysis of baseline systolic blood pressure in their studies. Figure 4 revealed that systolic blood pressure was significantly more likely to less influence the PPCM group rather than the HPD-PPCM group (SMD = -1.63 [95% CI; $-4.92, 0.28$, $p = 0.01$], which may favor diseases' outcome significantly. A high heterogeneity was also identified ($I^2 = 88\%$, $p = 0.004$).

Study or Subgroup	PPCM Mean	SD	Total	HPD-PPCM Mean	SD	Total	Weight	Std. mean difference IV, Random, 95% CI	Std. mean difference IV, Random, 95% CI
Lindley et al. (2017)	130	14.7	22	151	27.1	17	49.0%	-0.98 [-1.65 , -0.31]	
Ntusi et al. (2015)	105.9	16.2	30	162.3	28.4	53	51.0%	-2.26 [-2.83 , -1.69]	
Total (95% CI)			52			70	100.0%	-1.63 [-2.89 , -0.38]	

Heterogeneity: Tau² = 0.72; Chi² = 8.08, df = 1 (P = 0.004); I² = 88%
Test for overall effect: Z = 2.55 (P = 0.01)
Test for subgroup differences: Not applicable

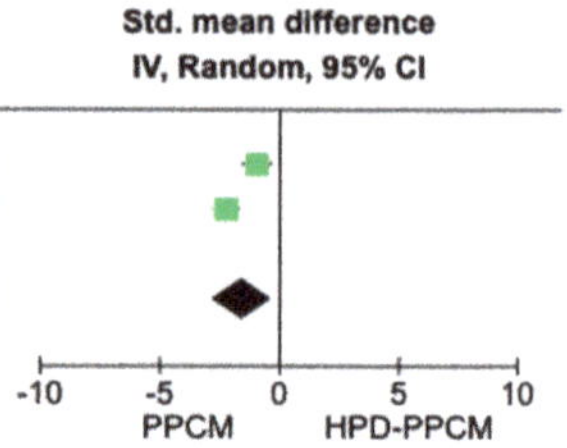

Figure 4. Forest plot thehe impact of systolic blood pressure on PPCM vs. HPD-PPCM [15,22].

Diastolic Blood Pressure

Only two studies (Lindley et al. and Ntusi et al.) [15,22] included an analysis of baseline diastolic blood pressure in their studies. Figure 5 revealed that diastolic blood pressure was less likely to influence the PPCM group rather than the HPD-PPCM group with (SMD = -2.32) [95% CI; $-4.92, 0.28$, $p = 0.08$], which may favor diseases' outcome, although not significant. A high heterogeneity was identified ($I^2 = 96\%$, $p = <0.00001$).

Study or Subgroup	PPCM Mean	SD	Total	HPD-PPCM Mean	SD	Total	Weight	Std. mean difference IV, Random, 95% CI	Std. mean difference IV, Random, 95% CI
Lindley et al. (2017)	82	8.7	22	97	20.1	17	50.1%	-1.00 [-1.67 , -0.32]	
Ntusi et al. (2015)	63.5	9.6	30	105	12.1	53	49.9%	-3.65 [-4.37 , -2.92]	
Total (95% CI)			52			70	100.0%	-2.32 [-4.92 , 0.28]	

Heterogeneity: Tau² = 3.39; Chi² = 27.61, df = 1 (P < 0.00001); I² = 96%
Test for overall effect: Z = 1.75 (P = 0.08)
Test for subgroup differences: Not applicable

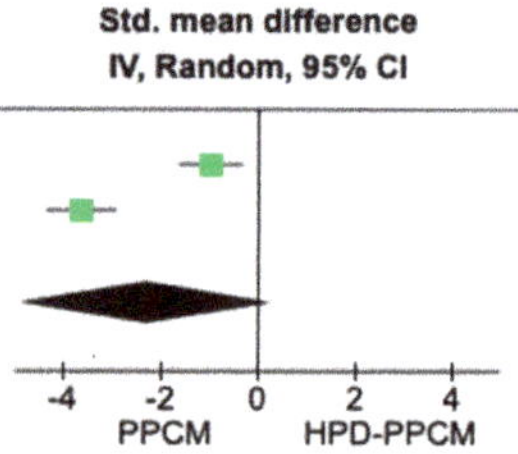

Figure 5. Forest plot of the impact of diastolic blood pressure on PPCM vs. HPD-PPCM [15,22].

Medical Therapy Initiated after Diagnosis (Furosemide)

Only Lindley et al. and Ntusi et al. [15,22] included an analysis of the initiation of furosemide in their studies. Although not significant, Figure 6 revealed that furosemide was more likely used in HPD-PPCM patients after diagnosis (RR = 2.08) [95% CI; 0.71, 8.34, $p = 0.10$], which may favor the disease's outcome. A high heterogeneity was identified ($I^2 = 78\%$, $p = 0.03$).

Study or Subgroup	PPCM Events	Total	HPD-PPCM Events	Total	Weight	Risk ratio M-H, Random, 95% CI	Risk ratio M-H, Random, 95% CI
Lindley et al. (2017)	12	55	12	71	44.0%	1.29 [0.63 , 2.65]	
Ntusi et al. (2015)	30	30	17	53	56.0%	3.04 [2.06 , 4.47]	
Total (95% CI)		85		124	100.0%	2.08 [0.87 , 4.97]	
Total events:	42		29				

Heterogeneity: Tau² = 0.31; Chi² = 4.59, df = 1 (P = 0.03); I² = 78%
Test for overall effect: Z = 1.66 (P = 0.10)
Test for subgroup differences: Not applicable

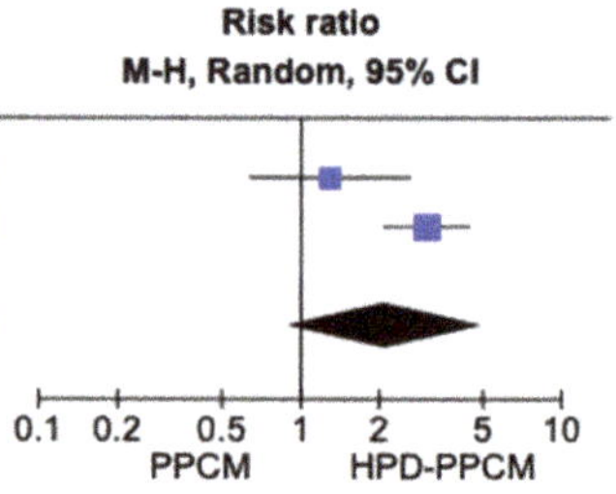

Figure 6. Forest plot of the impact of furosemide on PPCM vs. HPD-PPCM initiated after diagnosis [15,22].

Medical Therapy Initiated after Diagnosis (Beta-Blocker)

Similar to previous analyses of furosemide initiation after diagnosis, only two studies (Lindley et al. and Ntusi et al.) [15,22] included an analysis of the initiation of beta-blockers in their studies. Figure 7 revealed that beta-blocker was more likely used in HPD-PPCM patients after diagnosis, although not significant (RR = 2.44) [95% CI; 0.71, 8.34, $p = 0.16$], which may favor diseases' outcomes. A high heterogeneity was identified (I^2 = 89%, p = 0.003).

PPCM
HPD-PPCM
Risk ratio
Risk ratio
Study or Subgroup
Events
Total
Events
Total
Weight
M-H, Random, 95% CI
M-H, Random, 95% CI
Lindley et al. (2017) 17 77 15 88 49.2% 1.30 [0.69 , 2.42]
Ntusi et al. (2015) 28 30 11 53 50.8% 4.50 [2.63 , 7.68]
Total (95% CI) 107 141 100.0% 2.44 [0.71 , 8.34]
Total events: 45 26
Heterogeneity: Tau² = 0.70; Chi² = 8.97, df = 1 (P = 0.003); I² = 89%
Test for overall effect: Z = 1.42 (P = 0.16)
Test for subgroup differences: Not applicable
0.1 0.2 0.5 1 2 5 10
PPCM
HPD-PPCM

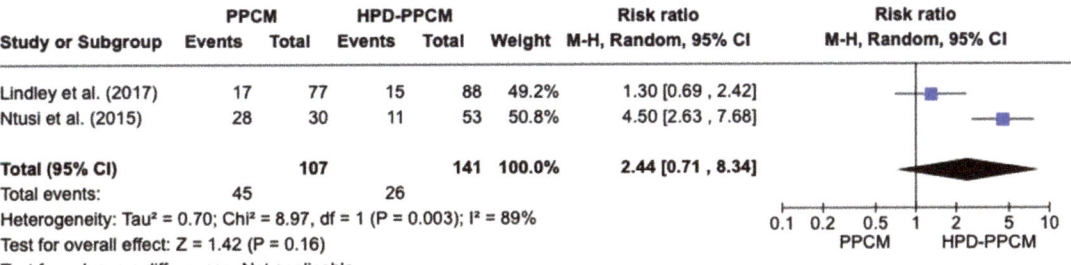

Figure 7. Forest plot of the impact of beta blocker on PPCM vs. HPD-PPCM Initiated after Diagnosis [15,22].

3.4.2. Echocardiographic Findings

The Impact of PPCM vs. HPD-PPCM on LVEF Reduction

In the LVEF outcome analysis consisting of all studies included, HPD-PPCM was less likely to have LVEF reduction compared to the PPCM group with SMD = −1.55 [95% CI: −2.89, −0.21] (Figure 8), and it was considered significant (p = 0.02). Moreover, a high heterogeneity was identified (I^2 = 90%, p < 0.00001).

PPCM
HPD-PPCM
Std. mean difference
Std. mean difference
Study or Subgroup
Mean
SD
Total
Mean
SD
Total
Weight
IV, Random, 95% CI
IV, Random, 95% CI
Barasa et al 38.3 7.9 14 59.4 4.3 10 28.7% -3.06 [-4.30 , -1.81]
Lindley et al 27.3 10.5 22 29.6 8.7 17 35.2% -0.23 [-0.87 , 0.40]
Ntusi et al 23.8 8.3 30 49.9 18.7 53 36.1% -1.64 [-2.15 , -1.12]
Total (95% CI) 66 80 100.0% -1.55 [-2.89 , -0.21]
Heterogeneity: Tau² = 1.22; Chi² = 20.13, df = 2 (P < 0.0001); I² = 90%
Test for overall effect: Z = 2.27 (P = 0.02)
Test for subgroup differences: Not applicable
-4 -2 0 2 4
PPCM
HPD-PPCM

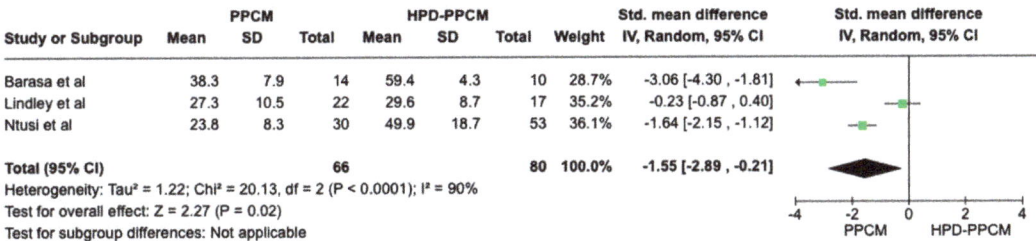

Figure 8. Forest plot of the impact of PPCM vs. HPD-PPCM on LVEF reduction [14,15,22].

The Impact of PPCM vs. HPD-PPCM on LV Dilation

Two studies were included in the analysis of LV dilation. Lindley et al. [15] showed that HPD-PPCM only was not associated with LV dilation; meanwhile, Ntusi et al. [22] showed that HPD-PPCM was related to greater LV dilation. Figure 9 is a forest plot depicting that HPD-PPCM was significantly associated with less LV dilation, with SMD = 1.81; 95% CI (0.07–3.01)] and p = 0.04. However, a high heterogeneity was identified (I^2 = 82%, p = 0.02).

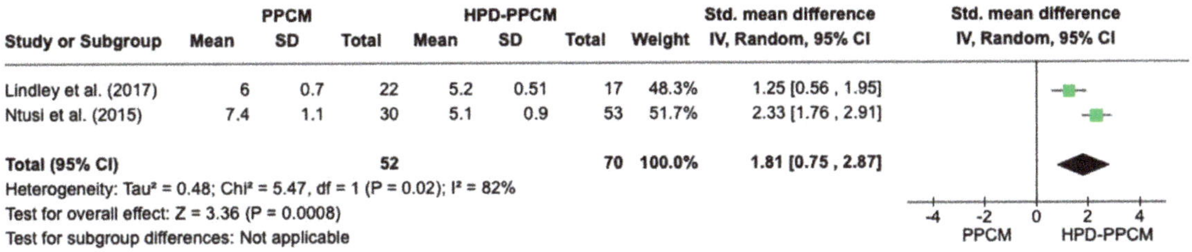

PPCM
HPD-PPCM
Std. mean difference
Std. mean difference
Study or Subgroup
Mean
SD
Total
Mean
SD
Total
Weight
IV, Random, 95% CI
IV, Random, 95% CI
Lindley et al. (2017) 6 0.7 22 5.2 0.51 17 48.3% 1.25 [0.56 , 1.95]
Ntusi et al. (2015) 7.4 1.1 30 5.1 0.9 53 51.7% 2.33 [1.76 , 2.91]
Total (95% CI) 52 70 100.0% 1.81 [0.75 , 2.87]
Heterogeneity: Tau² = 0.48; Chi² = 5.47, df = 1 (P = 0.02); I² = 82%
Test for overall effect: Z = 3.36 (P = 0.0008)
Test for subgroup differences: Not applicable
-4 -2 0 2 4
PPCM
HPD-PPCM

Figure 9. Forest plot of the impact of PPCM vs. HPD-PPCM on LV dilation [15,22].

The Impact of PPCM vs. HPD-PPCM on Relative Wall Thickness Reduction

Both Lindley et al. and Ntusi et al. [15,22] showed that HPD-PPCM patients were less likely to develop a reduction in relative wall thickness. Figure 10 is a forest plot depicting that HPD-PPCM was less likely and the PPCM group was more likely to have a relative wall thickness reduction [SMD = 0.70; 95% CI (−1.08–−0.33)], with p = 0.0003. No heterogeneity was identified (I^2 = 0%, p = 0.0003).

Study or Subgroup	PPCM Mean	PPCM SD	PPCM Total	HPD-PPCM Mean	HPD-PPCM SD	HPD-PPCM Total	Weight	Std. mean difference IV, Fixed, 95% CI
Lindley et al. (2017)	0.35	0.06	22	0.41	0.09	17	32.7%	−0.79 [−1.45, −0.13]
Ntusi et al. (2015)	1.2	0.3	30	1.4	0.3	53	67.3%	−0.66 [−1.12, −0.20]
Total (95% CI)			52			70	100.0%	−0.70 [−1.08, −0.33]

Heterogeneity: Chi² = 0.10, df = 1 (P = 0.75); I² = 0%
Test for overall effect: Z = 3.65 (P = 0.0003)
Test for subgroup differences: Not applicable

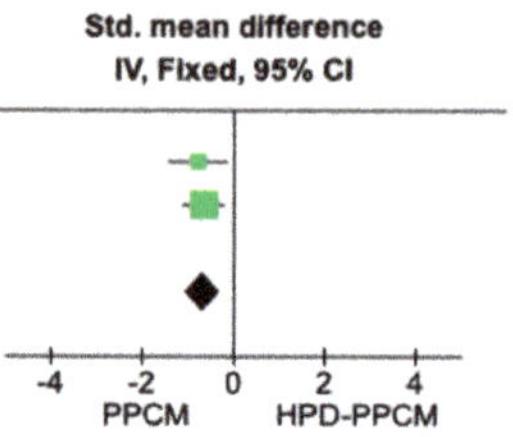

Figure 10. Forest plot of the impact of PPCM vs. HPD-PPCM on relative wall thickness reduction [15,22].

4. Discussion

4.1. Principal Findings

PPCM is a new onset of heart failure that has a high rate of maternal morbidity and mortality [1–5]. Preeclampsia and other HPD-related structural cardiac alterations, including left ventricular concentric remodeling and diastolic dysfunction, may influence the clinical course of women with PPCM. We focused on investigating the comparison of echocardiographic findings and their associated sociodemographic and clinical factors between women with PPCM and co-incident HPD (HPD-PPCM) and those with PPCM and no HPD (PPCM). This study revealed that systolic blood pressure was significantly more likely to influence the PPCM group rather than the HPD-PPCM group (SMD = −1.63) [95% CI; −4.92, 0.28, p = 0.01], which may favor diseases' outcome significantly, while the other sociodemographic or clinical profiles were not considered significant. To illustrate risk factors for HPD-PPCM vs. PPCM's course of the disease, our study reported that HPD-PPCM was associated with older or more advanced maternal age, a greater number of gravidity, tobacco use, and chronic hypertension rather than the PPCM-only group, although they were not significant. Medical therapy such as furosemide and beta-blockers were more likely used in HPD-PPCM patients after diagnosis and might favor the disease's course, although not significant.

Hypertensive pregnancy disorder was found in 37% of women with PPCM, while PPCM was found in 22% of these women, compared to an average worldwide background rate of 5% [2,23]. Preeclampsia is a common hypertensive pregnancy disease that has been linked to short-term and long-term cardiovascular dysfunction-related postpartum morbidity and mortality in both [12,23–28]. Preeclampsia amplifies the systemic angiogenic imbalance that develops in PPCM [29]. Soluble FLT1 (sFLT1) is one of the VEGF inhibitors secreted by the placenta in human beings, resulting in angiogenic imbalance and high blood pressure as one of its manifestations [29]. Although sFLT1 levels are higher in patients with preeclampsia than in controls, they are higher in women with PPCM [29]. After delivery, sFLT1 levels rapidly decrease. Even in the absence of pregnancy, exogenous sFlt1 was sufficient to induce severe systolic dysfunction in an in vivo study. Furthermore, preeclampsia patients have significantly higher sFlt1 levels, which is probably considered a high-risk factor for PPCM [15]. These findings are in line with our study, which revealed that systolic and diastolic blood pressure is less likely to influence the PPCM group rather than HPD-PPCM due to the basic nature of each disease, and HPD-PPCM patients tend to have a higher mean baseline blood pressure.

Based on echocardiology findings, HPD-PPCM was significantly less likely to have LVEF reduction compared to the PPCM group, with SMD −0.67 [95% CI: −3.04, 1.71] (p = 0.02). HPD-PPCM was significantly associated with less LV dilation, with SMD = 1.81;

95% CI (0.07–3.01)] and $p = 0.04$. Moreover, HPD-PPCM was less likely, and the PPCM group was more likely to have a relative wall thickness reduction [SMD = 0.70; 95% CI (-1.08–-0.33)], with $p = 0.0003$. PPCM and HPD-PPCM share different types of remodeling, which may affect each disease's response to pharmacological treatment. These findings suggest that in PPCM patients with HPD, the patterns of LV remodeling and LV function recovery were noticeably different and considered to share different pathophysiology mechanisms. Patients with HPD-PPCM exhibited less eccentric remodeling (more concentric) and seemed to have a higher chance of recovering their LV ejection fraction.

Although it has been demonstrated that decreases in radial, circumferential, and longitudinal strain occur before an ejection fraction loss, preeclampsia and HPD are associated with afterload-driven left ventricular concentric remodeling and impaired diastolic function [12,15,22]. The left ventricle is more likely to be affected by the rise in afterload that comes with hypertension than the right ventricle. However, HPD-PPCM patients seem to have a higher chance of recovering their LV ejection fraction, as mentioned, which might be due to more aggressive optimization of heart failure therapies in concomitant HPD-PPCM circumstances rather than PPCM-only patients.

When hypertension is resolved (with the removal of an increased afterload), recovery of LV function and reverse remodeling in HPD-PPCM may occur more in individuals with dilated cardiomyopathy than from other causes. Reverse remodeling has been seen in various series of PPCM-affected women up to 2–5 years after diagnosis [24,30]. Based on an earlier study, HPD-PPCM patients were more likely to exhibit symptoms of 'conventional' dilated cardiomyopathies, including more severe biventricular dysfunction, frequent electrocardiographic changes like left bundle branch block, and a higher frequency of family history of cardiomyopathy [31,32].

Moreover, a previous study revealed that different types of remodeling have clinical biomarkers and phenotypes that are distinctly different. In PPCM, a previous study found that compared to two control groups of women with prior severe preeclampsia and prior uncomplicated pregnancies, respectively, who were matched on age and year of index delivery, women with PPCM had significantly higher levels of sFlt-1, PlGF, copeptin, and NT-proBNP and more frequently detectable cathepsin D (CD) activity. However, prior systematic reviews on PPCM diagnosis using biomarkers and echocardiography have demonstrated that no parameter has consistently performed well across all investigations. In numerous trials, echocardiographic parameters—including strain profiles and biomarkers—proved important in predicting the prognosis of patients with PPCM [33,34]. We propose that further investigation would be needed to evaluate the association between the predictive value of biomarkers, genetics, polymorphism, and PPCM vs. HPD-PPCM. Moreover, the genetic foundations of PPCM are still poorly understood. In addition, a study conducted by Goli et al. in 2021 [35] showed some genetic overlap between PPCM and dilated cardiomyopathy, indicating that PPCM may benefit from gene-specific therapy strategies being explored for dilated cardiomyopathy. A total of 10% of women with PPCM had TTN variations that are truncating (TTNtvs). There were no appreciable differences in the timing of presentation after delivery, the prevalence of preeclampsia, or the rates of clinical recovery. A case of PPCM with predominately diastolic dysfunction was reported by Ballo et al. [36] and was treated with bromocriptine to inhibit prolactin. Through removing the cleaved form of prolactin despite activating the cleaving enzyme, bromocriptine, a dopamine agonist that decreases prolactin production, may improve outcomes in patients with peripartum cardiomyopathy. The study also discovered that bromocriptine therapy reduced the development of PPCM in animals lacking STAT3 and improved the cardiac output function in women with PPCM. Bromocriptine prevents prolactin production from the pituitary, which suppresses lactation. However, its utilization in acute PPCM is not linked to any substantial adverse effects, including no thromboembolism occurrences. Additional research is required to report the clinical outcomes of newborns whose mothers use this treatment [37]. However, none of our included studies compared any biomarkers, genetics, and polymorphisms, as well as bromocriptine utilization in PPCM vs. HPD-PPCM.

When patients are successfully up-titrated, the point estimates of the hazard ratio are lower in eccentric hypertrophy than in concentric hypertrophy. The Valsartan Heart Failure Trial (Val-HeFT) study revealed that valsartan significantly reduced relative and absolute risk in patients with the largest LV internal diastolic dimensions [32]. A previous study also postulated that in addition to ejection percentage, the shape of the left ventricle may also have an impact on how well beta-blockers and angiotensin-converting enzyme inhibitor (ACEi)/angiotensin receptor blockers (ARBs) respond to up-titration. Moreover, compared to patients with eccentric LV remodeling, people with concentric LV remodeling (HPD-PPCM) might not benefit as much from angiotensin-converting enzyme inhibitors, angiotensin receptor blockers, and beta-blockers [7–9,14–16].

4.2. The Implication for Clinical Practice

Identifying preeclamptic women at high risk of PPCM may lead to focused quality improvement care initiatives. This condition leads to the early identification of this cardiomyopathy and reduces the burden of unfavorable outcomes associated with late presentation. Moreover, this meta-analysis study also gives insight. PPCM and HPD-PPCM share different types of remodeling, which may affect each disease's response to pharmacological treatment. Compared to patients with eccentric LV remodeling, people with concentric LV remodeling might not benefit as much from angiotensin-converting enzyme inhibitors, angiotensin receptor blockers, and beta-blockers. The findings in this study will guide the development of guidelines for women with PPCM worldwide, from early detection to further management, in order to lessen the burden of unfavorable outcomes associated with the late presentation of PPCM and HPD-PPCM.

4.3. Strength and Limitations

To the best of our knowledge, this is the first systematic review or meta-analysis comparing clinical factors and echocardiographic findings between women with PPCM and co-incident HPD (HPD-PPCM) and those with PPCM and no HPD (PPCM); that is the primary strength of this study. This study also uses a careful assessment of the reviewed studies' risk of bias. However, several limitations should be acknowledged. First, after bias was assessed, the results showed that most studies have a moderate risk of bias, with one study having a serious risk of bias and the other study having a critical risk of bias. The risk of bias domain with moderate level was dominated by D1 (bias due to confounding), D2 (bias due to selection of participants), D6 (bias in measurements of outcomes), and D7 (bias in reported results). Moreover, the risk of bias was dominated by D1 (bias due to confounding) and D6 (bias in measurement of outcomes). Thus, it has quite an effect on the overall biased results. Second, the study was limited to be performed in USA and Africa. Therefore, this study could not be generalized to other countries. Third, this study was limited to the number of included studies due to a lack of studies that reported the comparison of PPCM vs. HPD-PPCM clinical profiles and echocardiographic outcomes. Not all studies reported clinical profiles, such as medical therapy initiated after diagnosis. Only a few studies reported the use of ACEi/ARBs. Thus, only furosemide and beta-blocker use were reported by related studies. Therefore, only a few outcomes can be performed with meta-analysis.

5. Conclusions

PPCM and HPD-PPCM share different clinical profiles as well as types of remodeling, which may affect each disease's response to pharmacological treatment. Systolic blood pressure was significantly more likely associated with the PPCM group than the HPD-PPCM group, while the other clinical profiles were not significant. HPD-PPCM was less likely to have LVEF reduction, less LV dilation, and was less likely to have a relative wall thickness reduction. In PPCM patients with HPD, the patterns of LV remodeling and LV function recovery were noticeably different and considered to share different pathophysiology mechanisms. Patients with HPD-PPCM exhibited less eccentric remodeling (more concentric) and seemed to have a higher chance of recovering their LV ejection fraction, which might not benefit as much with angiotensin-converting enzyme inhibitors, angiotensin receptor blockers, and beta-blockers. The findings in this study will guide the development of guidelines for women with PPCM worldwide, from early detection to further management, in order to lessen the burden of unfavorable outcomes associated with the late presentation of PPCM and HPD-PPCM. However, further studies are needed to emphasize the intricate connection between PPCM and HPD, as well as meta-analysis regarding the clinical outcomes of PPCM after follow-up.

Supplementary Materials: The following supporting information can be downloaded at: https://www.mdpi.com/article/10.3390/jcm12165303/s1, File S1: Searching strategy.

Author Contributions: Conceptualization, A.D.N., S.M. and D.P.J.S.; methodology, A.D.N. and S.M.; software, A.D.N. and S.M.; validation, A.D.N., S.M., D.P.J.S. and D.S.; formal analysis, A.D.N.; investigation, A.D.N. and S.M.; resources, A.D.N., S.M. and D.P.J.S.; data curation, A.D.N. and S.M.; writing—original draft preparation, A.D.N., S.M. and D.P.J.S.; writing—review and editing, A.D.N., S.M., K.D.T., D.P.J.S. and D.S.; visualization, A.D.N.; supervision, A.P., A.S., A.Y.P., M.A.A. and S.I.; project administration, A.D.N. and S.M.; funding acquisition, A.D.N. and D.S. All authors have read and agreed to the published version of the manuscript.

Funding: The Article Processing Charge (APC) was funded by the Directorate of Research and Community Engagement, University of Padjadjaran, Bandung, Indonesia.

Informed Consent Statement: Not applicable.

Data Availability Statement: More data are available from the author. Please contact the corresponding author for more data.

Acknowledgments: The great gratitude to Department Obstetrics and Gynecology, Faculty of Medicine, University of Padjadjaran/Dr. Hasan Sadikin General Hospital.

Conflicts of Interest: The authors declare no conflict of interest.

References

1. Sliwa, K.; Hilfiker-Kleiner, D.; Petrie, M.C.; Mebazaa, A.; Pieske, B.; Buchmann, E.; Regitz-Zagrosek, V.; Schaufelberger, M.; Tavazzi, L.; van Veldhuisen, D.J.; et al. Current state of knowledge on aetiology, diagnosis, management, and therapy of peripartum cardiomyopathy: A position statement from the Heart Failure Association of the European Society of Cardiology Working Group on peripartum cardiomyopathy. *Eur. J. Heart Fail.* **2010**, *12*, 767–778. [CrossRef] [PubMed]
2. Bello, N.; Rendon, I.S.H.; Arany, Z. The relationship between pre-eclampsia and peripartum cardiomyopathy: A systematic review and meta-analysis. *J. Am. Coll. Cardiol.* **2013**, *62*, 1715–1723. [CrossRef] [PubMed]
3. Sliwa, K.; Skudicky, D.; Bergemann, A.; Candy, G.; Puren, A.; Sareli, P. Peripartum cardiomyopathy: Analysis of clinical outcome, left ventricular function, plasma levels of cytokines and Fas/APO-1. *J. Am. Coll. Cardiol.* **2000**, *35*, 701–705. [CrossRef] [PubMed]
4. Clark, S.J.; Kahn, K.; Houle, B.; Arteche, A.; Collinson, M.A.; Tollman, S.M.; Stein, A. Young children's probability of dying before and after their mother's death: A rural South African population-based surveillance study. *PLoS Med.* **2013**, *10*, e1001409. [CrossRef] [PubMed]
5. Fett, J.; Murphy, J. Infant survival in Haiti after maternal death from peripartum cardiomyopathy. *Int. J. Gynecol. Obstet.* **2006**, *94*, 135–136. [CrossRef] [PubMed]
6. Hull, E.; Hidden, E. Postpartal heart failure. *South Med. J.* **1938**, *31*, 265–270. [CrossRef]
7. Amos, A.M.; Jaber, W.A.; Russell, S.D. Improved outcomes in peripartum cardiomyopathy with contemporary. *Am. Heart J.* **2006**, *152*, 509–513. [CrossRef]
8. Witlin, A.G.; Mabie, W.C.; Sibai, B.M. Peripartum cardiomyopathy: An ominous diagnosis. *Am. J. Obstet. Gynecol.* **1997**, *176*, 182–188. [CrossRef]
9. Gunderson, E.P.; Croen, L.A.; Chiang, V.; Yoshida, C.K.; Walton, D.; Go, A.S. Epidemiology of peripartum cardiomyopathy: Incidence, predictors, and outcomes. *Obstet. Gynecol.* **2011**, *118*, 583–591. [CrossRef]
10. Levine, R.J.; Maynard, S.E.; Qian, C.; Lim, K.-H.; England, L.J.; Yu, K.F.; Schisterman, E.F.; Thadhani, R.; Sachs, B.P.; Epstein, F.H.; et al. Circulating angiogenic factors and the risk of preeclampsia. *N. Engl. J. Med.* **2004**, *350*, 672–683. [CrossRef]
11. Damp, J.; Givertz, M.M.; Semigran, M.; Alharethi, R.; Ewald, G.; Felker, G.M.; Bozkurt, B.; Boehmer, J.; Haythe, J.; Skopicki, H.; et al. Relaxin-2 and soluble Flt1 levels in peripartum cardiomyopathy: Results of the multicenter IPAC study. *JACC Heart Fail.* **2016**, *4*, 380–388. [CrossRef] [PubMed]

12. McNamara, D.M.; Elkayam, U.; Alharethi, R.; Damp, J.; Hsich, E.; Ewald, G.; Modi, K.; Alexis, J.D.; Ramani, G.V.; Semigran, M.J.; et al. Clinical outcomes for peripartum cardiomyopathy in North America: Results of the IPAC study (Investigations of Pregnancy-Associated Cardiomyopathy). *J. Am. Coll. Cardiol.* **2015**, *66*, 905–914. [CrossRef] [PubMed]
13. Isezuo, S.A.; Abubakar, S.A. Epidemiologic profile of peripartum cardiomyopathy in a tertiary care hospital. *Ethn. Dis.* **2007**, *17*, 228–233. [PubMed]
14. Barasa, A.; Goloskokova, V.; Ladfors, L.; Patel, H.; Schaufelberger, M. Symptomatic recovery and pharmacological management in a clinical cohort with peripartum cardiomyopathy. *J. Matern.-Fetal Neonatal Med.* **2017**, *31*, 1342–1349. [CrossRef] [PubMed]
15. Lindley, K.J.; Conner, S.N.; Cahill, A.G.; Novak, E.; Mann, D.L. Impact of preeclampsia on clinical and functional outcomes in women with peripartum cardiomyopathy. *Circ. Heart Fail.* **2017**, *10*, e003797. [CrossRef]
16. Demakis, J.G.; Rahimtoola, S.H. Peripartum cardiomyopathy. *Circulation* **1971**, *44*, 964–968. [CrossRef]
17. Page, M.J.; McKenzie, J.E.; Bossuyt, P.M.; Boutron, I.; Hoffmann, T.C.; Mulrow, C.D.; Shamseer, L.; Tetzlaff, J.M.; Akl, E.A.; Brennan, S.E.; et al. The PRISMA 2020 statement: An updated guideline for reporting systematic reviews. *BMJ* **2021**, *372*, 71. [CrossRef]
18. Higgins, J.P.T.; Thompson, S.G.; Deeks, J.J.; Altman, D.G. Measuring inconsistency in meta-analyses. *BMJ* **2003**, *327*, 557–560. [CrossRef]
19. Riley, R.D.; Moons, K.G.M.; Snell, K.I.E.; Ensor, J.; Hooft, L.; Altman, D.G.; Hayden, J.; Collins, G.S.; Debray, T.P.A. A guide to systematic review and meta-analysis of prognostic factor studies. *BMJ* **2019**, *364*, k4597. [CrossRef]
20. Peters, J.L.; Sutton, A.J.; Jones, D.R.; Abrams, K.R.; Rushton, L. Contour-enhanced meta-analysis funnel plots help distinguish publication bias from other causes of asymmetry. *J. Clin. Epidemiol.* **2008**, *61*, 991–996. [CrossRef]
21. Malhamé, I.; Dayan, N.; Moura, C.S.; Samuel, M.; Vinet, E.; Pilote, L. Peripartum cardiomyopathy with co-incident preeclampsia: A cohort study of clinical risk factors and outcomes among commercially insured women. *Pregnancy Hypertens.* **2019**, *17*, 82–88. [CrossRef] [PubMed]
22. Ntusi, N.B.A.; Badri, M.; Gumedze, F.; Sliwa, K.; Mayosi, B.M. Pregnancy-associated heart failure: A comparison of clinical presentation and outcome between hypertensive heart failure of pregnancy and idiopathic peripartum cardiomyopathy. *PLoS ONE* **2015**, *10*, e0133466. [CrossRef] [PubMed]
23. Kamiya, C.A.; Kitakaze, M.; Ishibashi-Ueda, H.; Nakatani, S.; Murohara, T.; Tomoike, H.; Ikeda, T. Different characteristics of peripartum cardiomyopathy between patients complicated with and without hypertensive disorders—Results from the japanese nationwide survey of peripartum cardiomyopathy. *Circ. J.* **2011**, *75*, 1975–1981. [CrossRef] [PubMed]
24. Ersbøll, A.S.; Johansen, M.; Damm, P.; Rasmussen, S.; Vejlstrup, N.G.; Gustafsson, F. Peripartum cardiomyopathy in Denmark: A retrospective, population-based study of incidence, management and outcome. *Eur. J. Heart Fail.* **2017**, *19*, 1712–1720. [CrossRef]
25. Lewey, J.; Levine, L.D.; Elovitz, M.A.; Irizarry, O.C.; Arany, Z. Importance of early diagnosis in peripartum cardiomyopathy. *Hypertension* **2020**, *75*, 91–97. [CrossRef] [PubMed]
26. Behrens, I.; Basit, S.; Lykke, J.A.; Ranthe, M.F.; Wohlfahrt, J.; Bundgaard, H.; Melbye, M.; Boyd, H.A. Hypertensive disorders of pregnancy and peripartum cardiomyopathy: A nationwide cohort study. *PLoS ONE* **2019**, *14*, e0211857. [CrossRef]
27. Hilfiker-Kleiner, D.; Kaminski, K.; Podewski, E.; Bonda, T.; Schaefer, A.; Sliwa, K.; Forster, O.; Quint, A.; Landmesser, U.; Doerries, C.; et al. A cathepsin D-cleaved 16 kDa form of prolactin mediates postpartum cardiomyopathy. *Cell* **2007**, *128*, 589–600. [CrossRef]
28. Khurana, S.; Liby, K.; Buckley, A.R.; Ben-Jonathan, N. Proteolysis of human prolactin: Resistance to cathepsin D and formation of a nonangiostatic, C-terminal 16K fragment by thrombin1. *Endocrinology* **1999**, *140*, 4127–4132. [CrossRef]
29. Patten, I.S.; Rana, S.; Shahul, S.; Rowe, G.C.; Jang, C.; Liu, L.; Hacker, M.R.; Rhee, J.S.; Mitchell, J.; Mahmood, F.; et al. Cardiac angiogenic imbalance leads to peripartum cardiomyopathy. *Nature* **2012**, *485*, 333–338. [CrossRef]
30. Shahul, S.; Rhee, J.; Hacker, M.R.; Gulati, G.; Mitchell, J.D.; Hess, P.; Mahmood, F.; Arany, Z.; Rana, S.; Talmor, D. Subclinical left ventricular dysfunction in preeclamptic women with preserved left ventricular ejection fraction: A 2D speckle-tracking imaging study. *Circ. Cardiovasc. Imaging* **2012**, *5*, 734–773. [CrossRef]
31. Melchiorre, K.; Sutherland, G.R.; Watt-Coote, I.; Liberati, M.; Thilaganathan, B. Severe myocardial impairment and chamber dysfunction in preterm preeclampsia. *Hypertens. Pregnancy* **2010**, *31*, 454–471. [CrossRef]
32. Jackson, A.M.; Petrie, M.C.; Frogoudaki, A.; Laroche, C.; Gustafsson, F.; Ibrahim, B.; Mebazaa, A.; Johnson, M.R.; Seferovic, P.M.; Regitz-Zagrosek, V.; et al. Hypertensive disorders in women with peripartum cardiomyopathy: Insights from the ESC EORP PPCM Registry. *Eur. J. Heart Fail.* **2021**, *23*, 2058–2069. [CrossRef]
33. Ersbøll, A.S.; Goetze, J.P.; Johansen, M.; Hauge, M.G.; Sliwa, K.; Vejlstrup, N.; Gustafsson, F.; Damm, P. Biomarkers and their relation to cardiac function late after peripartum cardiomyopathy. *J. Card. Fail.* **2021**, *27*, 168–175. [CrossRef] [PubMed]
34. Sanusi, M.; Momin, E.S.; Mannan, V.; Kashyap, T.; Pervaiz, M.A.; Akram, A.; Khan, A.A.; Elshaikh, A.O. Using echocardiography and biomarkers to determine prognosis in peripartum cardiomyopathy: A systematic review. *Cureus* **2022**, *14*, e26130. [CrossRef] [PubMed]
35. Goli, R.; Li, J.; Brandimarto, J.; Levine, L.D.; Riis, V.; McAfee, Q.; DePalma, S.; Haghighi, A.; Seidman, J.G.; Seidman, C.E.; et al. Genetic and phenotypic landscape of peripartum cardiomyopathy. *Circulation* **2021**, *143*, 1852–1862. [CrossRef] [PubMed]

36. Ballo, P.; Betti, I.; Mangialavori, G.; Chiodi, L.; Rapisardi, G.; Zuppiroli, A. Peripartum Cardiomyopathy Presenting with Predominant Left Ventricular Diastolic Dysfunction: Efficacy of Bromocriptine. *Case Rep. Med.* **2012**, *2012*, 476903. [CrossRef]
37. Badianyama, M.; Das, P.K.; Gaddameedi, S.R.; Saukhla, S.; Nagammagari, T.; Bandari, V.; Mohammed, L. A Systematic Review of the Utility of Bromocriptine in Acute Peripartum Cardiomyopathy. *Cureus* **2021**, *13*, e18248. [CrossRef]

Disclaimer/Publisher's Note: The statements, opinions and data contained in all publications are solely those of the individual author(s) and contributor(s) and not of MDPI and/or the editor(s). MDPI and/or the editor(s) disclaim responsibility for any injury to people or property resulting from any ideas, methods, instructions or products referred to in the content.

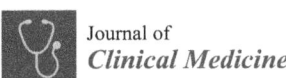

Journal of
Clinical Medicine

Article

Serum Pancreatic Stone Protein Reference Values in Healthy Pregnant Women: A Prospective Cohort Study

Ladina Vonzun [1,2,*,†], Romana Brun [1,2,*,†], Nora Gadient-Limani [3], Marcel André Schneider [2,4], Theresia Reding [2,4], Rolf Graf [2,4], Perparim Limani [2,4,‡] and Nicole Ochsenbein-Kölble [1,2,‡]

1. Department of Obstetrics, University Hospital of Zurich, Frauenklinikstrasse 10, 8091 Zurich, Switzerland
2. Faculty of Medicine, University of Zurich, Rämistrasse 71, 8091 Zurich, Switzerland
3. Department of Obstetrics and Gynaecology, Cantonal Hospital Baden, 5404 Baden, Switzerland
4. Department of Surgery & Transplantation, Swiss Hepatopancreatobiliary Laboratory, University Hospital Zurich, Raemistrasse 100, CH-8091 Zurich, Switzerland
* Correspondence: ladina.vonzun@usz.ch (L.V.); romana.brun@usz.ch (R.B.); Tel.: +41-44-255-11-11
† These authors contributed equally to this work.
‡ These authors contributed equally to this work.

Abstract: Background: In non-pregnant populations, pancreatic stone protein (PSP) has been reported to have a higher diagnostic performance for identifying severe inflammatory and infectious disease than other established biomarkers. Objective: To generate reference values for serum PSP in pregnancy and compare them to the values of the general healthy population. Design: A prospective cohort study. Setting: A single center. Population: Healthy women with singleton and multiple pregnancies. Methods: This is a prospective single-center cohort study. Between 2013 and 2021, samples of 5 mL peripheral blood were drawn from 440 healthy pregnant women. Therein, 393 cases were singletons and 47 were multiple pregnancies. Serum PSP levels were measured by specific enzyme-linked immunosorbent assay. The main outcome measures were serum PSP level (ng/mL) reference values in healthy pregnant women. Results: The mean PSP reference values in women with singleton pregnancies were 7.9 ± 2.6 ng/mL (95% CI; 2.69–13.03 ng/mL). The PSP values in women with multiple pregnancies (9.17 ± 3.06 ng/mL (95% CI; 3.05–15.28 ng/mL)) were significantly higher (p = 0.001). The PSP values in the first trimester (6.94 ± 2.53 ng/mL) were lower compared to the second (7.42 ± 2.21 ng/mL) and third trimesters (8.33 ± 2.68 ng/mL, p = 0.0001). Subgroup analyses in singletons revealed no correlations between PSP values, maternal characteristics, and pre-existing medical conditions. Conclusion: The PSP values in healthy pregnant women (4–12 ng/mL) were in the range of the reference values of the general healthy population (8–16 ng/mL). This insight blazes a trail for further clinical studies on the use of PSP as a potential novel biomarker for the early detection of pregnancy-related diseases such as chorioamnionitis.

Keywords: PSP; pancreatic stone protein; pregnancy; reference values

1. Introduction

Pancreatic stone protein (PSP) is a C-type lectin protein that triggers polymorphonuclear cell activation and has shown proinflammatory activity in vitro [1]. Under physiological conditions, pancreatic stone protein (PSP) is predominantly produced in the pancreas and gut. Both preclinical and clinical trials demonstrated increased PSP levels in inflammatory diseases with or without infection [1–3]. Current evidence shows that PSP is an accurate diagnostic and prognostic marker in critically ill patients and helps in discerning the risk of developing sepsis, the severity of peritonitis, and in predicting mortality in intensive care unit patients [1,2,4–6]. The diagnostic performance of PSP, alone and in combination with other markers or clinical scores, was evaluated further in several studies conducted in adults, children, and neonates, in both intensive care units (ICUs)

Citation: Vonzun, L.; Brun, R.; Gadient-Limani, N.; Schneider, M.A.; Reding, T.; Graf, R.; Limani, P.; Ochsenbein-Kölble, N. Serum Pancreatic Stone Protein Reference Values in Healthy Pregnant Women: A Prospective Cohort Study. *J. Clin. Med.* **2023**, *12*, 3200. https://doi.org/10.3390/jcm12093200

Academic Editor: Valerio Gaetano Vellone

Received: 31 March 2023
Revised: 18 April 2023
Accepted: 27 April 2023
Published: 29 April 2023

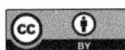

Copyright: © 2023 by the authors. Licensee MDPI, Basel, Switzerland. This article is an open access article distributed under the terms and conditions of the Creative Commons Attribution (CC BY) license (https://creativecommons.org/licenses/by/4.0/).

and emergency departments [7]. PSP has been reported to have a higher diagnostic performance in identifying sepsis than other established biomarkers such as procalcitonin (PCT), interleukin 6 (IL-6), and C-reactive protein (CRP) [7,8]. Despite extensive research, no novel biomarkers have been identified in order to detect sepsis in an early clinical stage and with a high degree of diagnostic accuracy. In contrast, CRP is a clinically well-characterized inflammatory marker widely measured in the diagnosis of infectious diseases. Additionally, PCT has been evaluated in the last decade as a marker of bacteremia. Even if CRP and PCT are commonly used in the context of the diagnosis of sepsis, both have shown suboptimal performance [8,9]. Combining PSP with PCT in a bio-score significantly improves the ability to diagnose neonatal early-onset sepsis [10]. So far, only one study exists regarding PSP in pregnant women, postulating PSP to be a suitable marker for the assessment of renal function in pregnancy [11].

PSP reference values of 8–16 ng/mL have been described in general non-obstetric healthy populations [9]. Increased PSP values up to 20–50 ng/mL have been observed in patients with benign disorders such as diabetes mellitus [12]. In patients with septic conditions PSP exceeds 100 ng/mL [1].

Since its first description as a potential infection biomarker in patients after trauma, PSP has repeatedly been shown to perform superiorly to CRP, and at least as well as PCT, in identifying patients with infectious diseases [1,6]. In contrast to PCT, no cut-off threshold value has yet been defined for its clinical use [13]. A systematic review obtained raw data from five observational studies and performed a meta-analysis at the individual patient level in order to explore the performance of PSP in detecting infectious diseases. The eligible studies were performed in different countries and included acutely diseased patients from emergency departments or intensive care units. The resulting cohort of 631 hospitalized adult patients encompassed an important proportion (42%) of patients without infection, which makes it the largest analysis of PSP [13]. This systematic review with meta-analysis concludes that a cut-off value of 44.18 ng/mL PSP performs better than CRP or PCT across the considered studies. The combination of PSP with CRP further enhances its accuracy [13].

Additionally, PSP was assessed to differentiate between burn- and infection-related inflammation [2]. Burn victims' state of hyperinflammation triggers infectious complications. However, microbiological cultures provide results with a delay of 48–72 h following the sampling of patient material. Both of these factors postpone the initiation of targeted antimicrobial and intensive care therapy. Blood biomarkers are supposed to support the clinician's diagnostic and therapeutic decision-making processes but often fail in that respect due to lack of sensitivity, specificity, availability or affordability. With regard to this, altered levels of pro-inflammatory markers secondary to trauma or surgery still present a major problem in that they are prone to interfere with the clinical identification of infectious events [2]. In another study, the first 14 days of serum PSP in a cohort of 90 severely burned patients ($\geq 15\%$ total body surface area) were analyzed to assess PSP-discriminatory accuracy in order to differentiate sterile systemic inflammation from infectious/septic clinical courses as compared to current clinically established inflammatory biomarkers (WBCs, CRP, PCT) [2]. This study evaluated the temporal course of PSP serum levels before the clinically diagnosed septic event. It concludes that PSP demonstrates high discriminatory ability in the timely identification of evolving sepsis and septic shock in patients with acute severe burns. Its steep increase allows sepsis detection up to 72 h before clinically overt deterioration, thus outperforming CRP- and PCT-based protocols for sepsis diagnosis [2].

To date, no reference values for pregnant women have been reported. Since pregnancy features complex immunological conditions, pregnant women are more susceptible to infections and inflammatory diseases [14,15]. Therefore, their PSP values might differ from those measured in general healthy populations.

The aim of this study was to evaluate physiological serum levels of the novel biomarker PSP throughout different time points in singleton and multiple pregnancies and to compare these values to the reference values of the general healthy population.

2. Methods

This is a prospective, single-centered cohort study assessing reference values of PSP in pregnancy.

2.1. Study Population

From 2013 to 2021, 440 healthy pregnant women were recruited. According to the study protocol, a minimum of seven women per week of gestation were included for determination of the reference values.

Healthy women with a singleton (N = 393) or multiple (N = 47) pregnancy, and who were older than 18 years, were included in this study. Each woman was included once only. Women with pathological conditions such as premature ruptures of the membranes (PPROM), amniotic infection syndrome (AIS), preeclampsia (PE), and viral (hepatitis B virus, hepatitis C virus, human immunodeficiency virus or coronavirus) or confirmed bacterial infections were excluded. Information on demographics, maternal age, body mass index (BMI), week of gestation, parity, pregnancy history, and comorbidities was collected.

2.2. Generation of Reference Values for Pregnant Women

The generation of PSP reference values in healthy pregnant women was based on the values retrieved from the healthy singleton pregnancies of this study population. Outliers were previously excluded as per outlier testing (N = 3).

In a second stage analysis, PSP values from multiple pregnancies were compared to reference values of the general healthy population (median: 10.8 ng/mL, interquartile range (IQR): 9.0–12.5) previously published by Schlapbach et al. [9].

2.3. Sample Collection and Processing

Peripheral blood (5 mL) was drawn from each participant. Following the arrival of the blood sample in the laboratory, serum PSP levels were measured by enzyme-linked immunosorbent assay (ELISA), as previously described [1,16]. All laboratory measurements were performed in triplicates. Excessive material was stored and catalogued in a central, anonymous biobank (at $-80\ °C$ temperature).

2.4. Data Analysis

Statistical significance was defined as $p < 0.05$ and all tests were 2-sided. Numerical variables were summarized as mean ± standard deviation (SD) or median with interquartile range (IQR) as appropriate and were compared by Student's t-test/ANOVA or Wilcoxon's rank-sum test/Kruskal–Wallis test as appropriate. The normal distribution of data was evaluated with the Shapiro–Wilk test. A multivariate regression analysis was performed where necessary. The correlation between numerical variables was assessed with Pearson's correlation coefficient. Outliers were identified using the boxplot method (above Q3 + 1.5xIQR or below Q1—1.5xIQR) with extreme outliers defined as above Q3 + 3xIQR or below Q1—3xIQR. Categorical variables are presented as number (N) and percentage (%), and were compared with Fisher's exact test. R V4.0.2 and R-Studio V1.3.1093 (R Foundation for Statistical Computing, Vienna, Austria) were used for statistical analyses, calculations, and graphical representations.

2.5. Ethics Approval and Registration

The study was conducted in accordance with the approval of the local Ethic Commission (KEK-ZH-No. 2014-0046.). Written consent was received from all women before participating in this study. Primary international registry Clinicaltrials.gov ID NCT02247297, Swiss National Clinical Trials Portal SNCTP000000290.

3. Results

Baseline demographics and characteristics of the study population are shown in Table 1.

Table 1. Baseline characteristics of singleton and multiple pregnancies.

	Singleton Pregnancy (N = 390)	Multiple Pregnancy (N = 47)	p-Value	Total (N = 440)
PSP Mean ± SD [ng/m]	7.86 ± 2.59	9.17 ± 3.06	0.001	8.26 ± 4.13
Maternal Age Mean ± SD [years]	32.9 ± 5.29	35.1 ± 4.17	0.001	33.1 ± 5.22
Parity Mean ± SD	2.12 ± 1.34	2.32 ± 1.32	0.33	2.14 ± 1.34
BMI Mean ± SD [kg/m^2]	23.8 ± 5.19	24.2 ± 4.87	0.59	23.8 ± 5.15
Ethnicity [N (%)]			0.42	
Afro-Caribbean	17 (4.4%)	2 (4.3%)		19 (4.3%)
Asian	23 (5.9%)	1 (2.1%)		24 (5.5%)
Caucasian	283 (72.1%)	40 (85.1%)		323 (73.4%)
Mediterranean	38 (9.7%)	4 (8.5%)		42 (9.5%)
Mixed	7 (1.8%)	0 (0.0%)		7 (1.6%)
Oriental	24 (6.2%)	0 (0.0%)		24 (5.5%)

Abbreviations: pancreatic stone protein (PSP), standard deviation (SD), body mass index (BMI).

3.1. Singleton Pregnancies

Mean PSP values in all healthy singleton pregnancies were 8.15 ± 4.23 ng/mL with a median of 7.66 (IQR: 6.10, 9.50) and were right-skewed ($p \leq 0.001$) due to three outliers >40 ng/mL without apparent clinical reason or explanation by the analysis procedure for these high values. Of the remaining 390 patients, mean PSP values were 7.86 ± 2.59 ng/mL (95% CI; 2.69–13.03 ng/mL) (Figure 1).

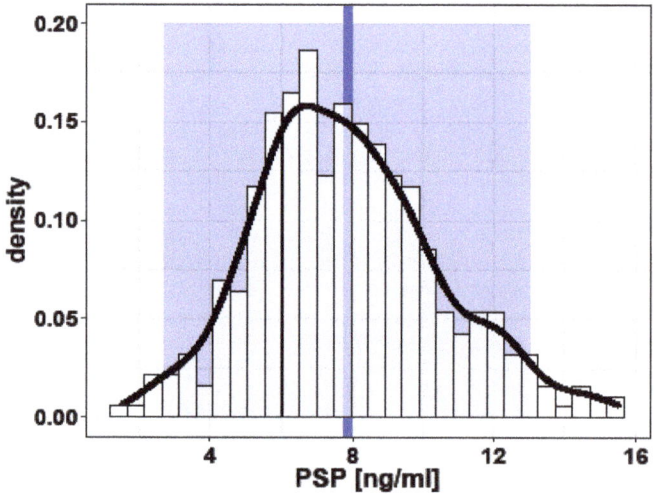

Figure 1. Density plot of pancreas stone protein (PSP) serum values in singleton pregnancies independent of the trimester of pregnancy. Blue line: mean overall PSP value 7.86 ng/mL. Blue square: 95% confidential interval (CI) (2.69 to 13.03 ng/mL). Black curve: density curve.

Figure 2 shows the course of PSP levels in singleton pregnancies throughout pregnancy.

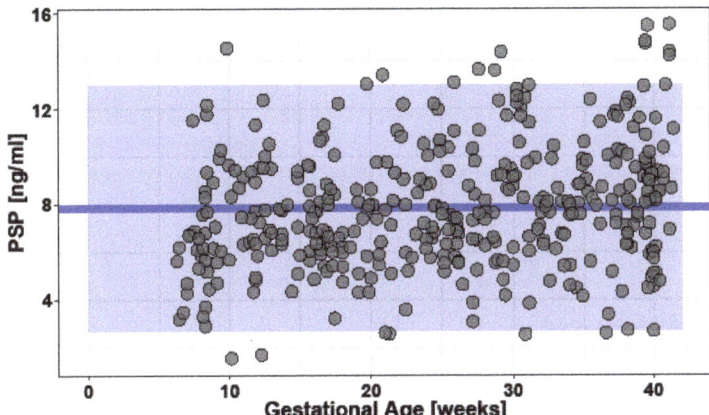

Figure 2. Scatter plot of pancreatic stone protein (PSP) values in singleton pregnancies according to gestational age (3 outliers not displayed). Blue line: mean overall PSP value 7.86 ng/mL. Blue square: 95% confidential interval (CI) (2.69 to 13.03 ng/mL).

PSP values in the first trimester (6.94 ± 2.53 ng/mL) were lower compared to the second (7.42 ± 2.21 ng/mL) and third trimesters (8.33 ± 2.68 ng/mL, $p = 0.0001$) (Figure 3).

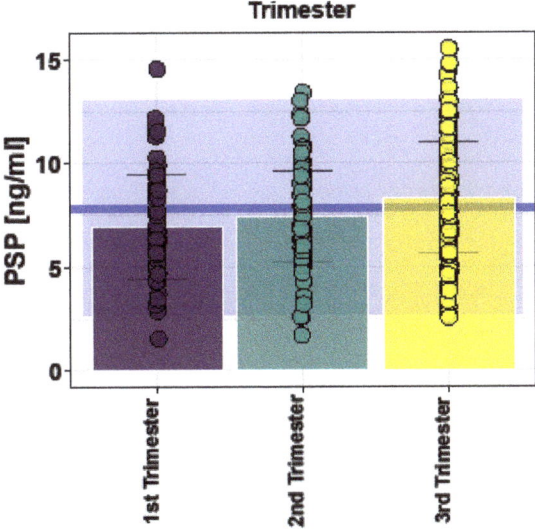

Figure 3. Bar plot of pancreatic stone protein (PSP) values in singleton pregnancies grouped according to trimester (Mean ± standard deviation (SD)). 1. Trimester 6.96 ± 2.5 ng/mL, 2. Trimester 7.43 ± 2.21 ng/mL, 3. Trimester 8.34 ± 2.69 ng/mL. Blue line: mean overall PSP value 7.86 ng/mL. Blue square: 95% confidential interval (CI) (2.69 to 13.03 ng/mL).

A comparison of gestational age to PSP level showed a correlation ($R = 0.22$, $p \leq 0.0010$).

No correlation between PSP values and BMI ($R = -0.06$, $p = 0.22$) or maternal age ($R = 0.08$, $p = 0.11$) was observed. Furthermore, no statistical difference in PSP values and women's parity ($p = 0.59$) and ethnicity ($p = 0.50$), nor in women with and without comorbidities, was noted (Table 2).

Table 2. Comparison between pancreatic stone protein (PSP) in 390 healthy singleton pregnancies with and without comorbidities.

Comorbidities	Singleton Pregancy [N (%)]	PSP Values Mean ± SD [ng/m]	p-Value
Thyroid disorders			
Hypothyroidism	18 (4.6%)	7.10 ± 2.51	0.43
Hyperthyroidism	3 (0.8%)	10.45 ± 3.41	0.20
no	369 (94.6%)	7.87 ± 2.57	
Gestational diabetes			
Diet	64 (16.3%)	6.76 ± 1.91	0.99
Insulin therapy	8 (2.1%)	7.84 ± 2.78	0.44
no	318 (81.5%)	7.89 ± 2.56	
Cardiac disease			
yes	13 (3.3%)	8.38 ± 1.81	0.45
no	377 (96.7%)	7.84 ± 2.61	
Rheumatologic disease			
yes	8 (2.1%)	7.31 ± 2.06	0.55
no	382	7.87 ± 2.60	
Hematologic disease			
yes	13 (3.3%)	8.10 ± 2.40	0.73
no	377 (96.7%)	7.85 ± 2.59	
Nicotine Abuse			
yes	13 (3.3%)	8.10 ± 2.40	0.73
no	377 (96.7%)	7.85 ± 2.59	

3.2. Multiple Pregnancies

Mean PSP values in the 47 healthy women with multiple pregnancies were 9.17 ± 3.06 ng/mL (95% CI; 3.05–15.28 ng/mL). No difference in PSP values in the different trimesters ($p = 0.69$) was observed and PSP levels showed no correlation to gestational age ($R = 0.075$, $p = 0.62$). Subgroup analysis revealed that maternal age is correlated with PSP values in women with multiple pregnancies ($R = 0.31$, $p = 0.04$). No relevant influence of further baseline characteristics and comorbidities on PSP levels were found in multiple pregnancies. Furthermore, no difference in the chorionicity of the multiple pregnancies and PSP values was observed ($p = 0.52$). However, PSP serum values were significantly increased in women with multiple pregnancies compared to singleton pregnancies ($p = 0.001$) (Figure 4).

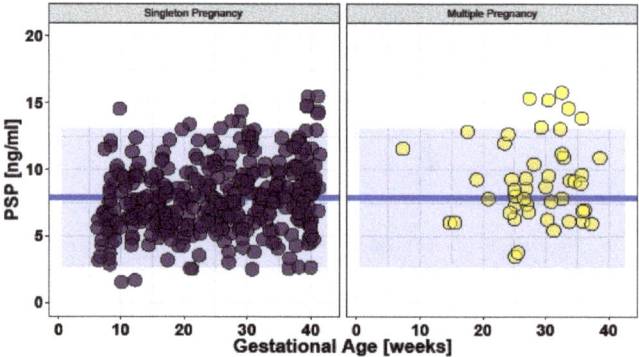

Figure 4. Bar plot of PSP values grouped in singleton vs. multiple pregnancies (3 outliers not displayed). Blue line: mean overall PSP value in healthy pregnant women 7.86 ng/mL. Blue square: 95% CI (2.69 to 13.03 ng/mL).

A comparison of PSP serum values in healthy pregnant women with singleton (median: 7.66 ng/mL, IQR: 6.10, 9.50) and multiple (median: 8.73 ng/mL, IQR: 6.88, 11.1) pregnancies with reference values of the general healthy population (median: 10.8 ng/mL, IQR: 9.0–12.5) revealed no relevant differences (p = 0.21 and p = 0.52, respectively).

4. Discussion

4.1. Main Findings

This study reports the physiological course of PSP serum values in healthy pregnant women. The reference values obtained in women with singleton 8 ± 3 ng/mL and multiple 9 ± 3 ng/mL pregnancies are comparable to the values in the healthy general population of 8–16 ng/mL [9]. Therefore, this study blazes a trail for the potential use of PSP as a novel biomarker in pregnant women in corresponding clinical situations, such as inflammatory or infectious diseases.

4.2. Interpretation

PSP was introduced as a potential infection biomarker in patients after trauma (Ref: Keel, 2009). Since then, several studies have repeatedly shown that PSP performs superiorly to CRP and at least as well as PCT in identifying patients with infectious diseases [1,6]. A systematic review obtained raw data from five observational studies and carried out a meta-analysis at the individual patient level to explore the performance of PSP in detecting infectious diseases. The conclusion drawn across the considered studies is that, at a cut-off value of 44.18 ng/mL, PSP performs better than CRP or the combination of PSP with CRP further enhances its accuracy [13]. The diagnostic accuracy for the diagnosis of sepsis of PSP, CRP, and PCT were reported to be similar [8]. They report that serial measurements of biomarker revealed that blood PSP levels increased incrementally 3 days before the clinical diagnosis of nosocomial sepsis in critically ill patients, potentially allowing the early detection of sepsis before the appearance of signs and symptoms [8]. Some aspects of the clinical use of PSP deserve detailed considerations. Knowledge about norm values of PSP is of importance since the performance of various biomarkers (e.g., leucocytes) differs in the case of pregnancy compared to in the general population due to modified immune response in pregnant women [17]. The immune system of pregnant women is modulated by complex mechanisms to allow the genetically and immunologically foreign fetus to thrive and prosper [17]. Consequently, the immunologic response in pregnancy is altered leading to decreased stress response [17] which might cause altered PSP values throughout pregnancy. On the other hand, immunological modifications render pregnant women more susceptible to infections [14,15,17].

A further aspect is the increased glomerular filtration rate in pregnancy [18]. PSP, being a low molecular weight protein of 14–19 kilodaltons (kDa), crosses the glomerular basement membrane and undergoes reabsorption in the proximal renal tubules [19]. Whereas glomerular filtration rate is known to increase throughout pregnancy, reabsorption in the proximal renal tubes remains constant [17]. This renal loss of PSP could result in the rather low values in comparison with the known values of the general population.

Another consideration is that our study shows a significant rise in PSP values along with increasing gestational age. This observation might be important in terms of the interpretation of PSP values as a novel biomarker in pregnancy. Schlapbach et al. reported relevant age-dependent variations of PSP values and emphasized the practical need for different thresholds for PSP [9]. In this context, it might be possible that PSP thresholds for detecting pregnancy-related diseases may even need to be adapted during the course of pregnancy, even if the differences in references between the trimesters found in this study were clinically irrelevant

Moreover, PSP values observed in healthy pregnant women did not show any correlation with pre-existing non-infectious medical conditions such as cardiac, autoimmune, renal, and diabetic conditions. Earlier studies revealed that urinary PSP values increase markedly in patients with various renal diseases, particularly also in diabetic nephropathies [19]. At the same time, PSP serum levels were described to rise in patients with diabetes mellitus [12,16]. However, these observations were independent from the glomerular filtration rate and, rather, led back to an augmented PSP secretion by the kidney itself as well as an inflammatory response of the infiltrated beta cells of the pancreas [12,16]. We could not undermine these observations. Eventually, in our cohort, the close follow-up and the rigorous control of pre-existing medical conditions as well as gestational diabetes during pregnancy, may explain our findings. The sole correlation observed was the correlation with PSP levels and maternal age in multiple pregnancies. To date, we do not have a plausible explanation for this observation. However, there is no clinical relevance of the absolute value differences.

4.3. Strengths and Limitations

This study presents PSP norm references in the first prospective cohort of healthy pregnant women. PSP values were measured under clearly defined clinical and laboratory criteria, conditions under which data are reproducible. Based on this large dataset, we report that the novel biomarker PSP measured in pregnant women is comparable to values measured in the general healthy population. This study, however, does not answer the question of whether PSP really holds its promise as a novel clinical biomarker in obstetric pathological conditions and is clearly not designed to provide thresholds or cut-offs for pathologies. Therefore, we are currently designing further clinical trials to evaluate PSP values in pregnant women diagnosed with pathological diseases.

5. Conclusions

PSP serum values in healthy pregnant women (4–12 ng/mL) correspond to the reference values of the general population (8–16 ng/mL). This insight blazes a trail for further clinical studies on the use of PSP as a potentially novel biomarker for early detection of pregnancy-related conditions such as chorioamnionitis.

Author Contributions: Conceptualization: N.G.-L., N.O.-K., R.G. and P.L. Methodology: N.G.-L., N.O.-K., P.L., R.B., L.V. and M.A.S.; Investigation: N.G.-L., L.V., R.B. and T.R.; Visualization: T.R. and M.A.S.; Funding acquisition: R.G. and P.L.; Project administration: N.O.-K., P.L., R.B. and L.V.; Supervision: N.O.-K., P.L. and R.G.; Writing—original draft: L.V. and R.B.; Writing—review and editing: P.L., N.O.-K., R.G., T.R., M.A.S. and N.G.-L.; All authors have read and agreed to the published version of the manuscript.

Funding: The study was supported by the Gebert Rüf Foundation granted to RG. This is strictly a non-profit foundation. The foundation decided to fund our project in 2012. Our funding application at the Geberet Rüf Foundation underwent an external review process with scientists who are experts in this field.

Institutional Review Board Statement: The study was conducted in accordance with the Declaration of Helsinki, and approved by the Medical Ethics Commission of the Canton Zurich, Switzerland via a peer-reviewed process (Kantonale Ethikkommission Zurich). Swiss National Clinical Trials Portal SNCTP000000290; Institution Ethical Board Approval ID: KEK-ZH-Nr. 2014-0046. Clinicaltrials.gov ID: NCT02247297.

Informed Consent Statement: Informed consent was obtained from all subjects involved in the study.

Data Availability Statement: Data are available in the main text.

Acknowledgments: We would like to thank Anja Zabel, Rong Chen, and Leandro Manciana for their excellent technical support.

Conflicts of Interest: The authors declare no conflict of interest.

Abbreviations

AIS	amniotic inflammatory syndrome
BMI	Body mass index
CRP	C-reactive protein
ELISA	Enzyme Linked Immunosorbent Assay

PE	preeclampsia
IL-6	interleukin 6
IQR	Interquartile range
PCT	procalcitonin
PSP	Pancreatic stone protein
SD	Standard deviation
SNCTP	Swiss National Clinical Trials Portal

References

1. Keel, M.; Härter, L.; Reding, T.; Sun, L.K.; Hersberger, M.; Seifert, B.; Bimmler, D.; Graf, R. Pancreatic stone protein is highly increased during posttraumatic sepsis and activates neutrophil granulocytes. *Crit. Care Med.* **2009**, *37*, 1642–1648. [CrossRef] [PubMed]
2. Klein, H.J.; Niggemann, P.; Buehler, P.K.; Lehner, F.; Schweizer, R.; Rittirsch, D.; Fuchs, N.; Waldner, M.; Steiger, P.; Giovanoli, P.; et al. Pancreatic Stone Protein Predicts Sepsis in Severely Burned Patients Irrespective of Trauma Severity: A Monocentric Observational Study. *Ann. Surg.* **2020**, *276*, e1179–e1186. [CrossRef] [PubMed]
3. Scherr, A.; Graf, R.; Bain, M.; Christ-Crain, M.; Müller, B.; Tamm, M.; Stolz, D. Pancreatic stone protein predicts positive sputum bacteriology in exacerbations of COPD. *Chest* **2013**, *143*, 379–387. [CrossRef] [PubMed]
4. Llewelyn, M.J.; Berger, M.; Gregory, M.; Ramaiah, R.; Taylor, A.L.; Curdt, I.; Lajaunias, F.; Graf, R.; Blincko, S.J.; Drage, S.; et al. Sepsis biomarkers in unselected patients on admission to intensive or high-dependency care. *Crit. Care* **2013**, *17*, R60. [CrossRef] [PubMed]
5. García de Guadiana-Romualdo, L.; Albaladejo-Otón, M.D.; Berger, M.; Jiménez-Santos, E.; Jiménez-Sánchez, R.; Esteban-Torrella, P.; Rebollo-Acebes, S.; Hernando-Holgado, A.; Ortín-Freire, A.; Trujillo-Santos, J. Prognostic performance of pancreatic stone protein in critically ill patients with sepsis. *Biomark. Med.* **2019**, *13*, 1469–1480. [CrossRef] [PubMed]
6. Gukasjan, R.; Raptis, D.A.; Schulz, H.U.; Halangk, W.; Graf, R. Pancreatic stone protein predicts outcome in patients with peritonitis in the ICU. *Crit. Care Med.* **2013**, *41*, 1027–1036. [CrossRef] [PubMed]
7. Eggimann, P.; Que, Y.A.; Rebeaud, F. Measurement of pancreatic stone protein in the identification and management of sepsis. *Biomark. Med.* **2019**, *13*, 135–145. [CrossRef] [PubMed]
8. Pugin, J.; Daix, T.; Pagani, J.L.; Morri, D.; Giacomucci, A.; Dequin, P.F.; Guitton, C.; Que, Y.A.; Zani, G.; Brealey, D.; et al. Serial measurement of pancreatic stone protein for the early detection of sepsis in intensive care unit patients: A prospective multicentric study. *Crit. Care* **2021**, *25*, 151. [CrossRef] [PubMed]
9. Schlapbach, L.J.; Giannoni, E.; Wellmann, S.; Stocker, M.; Ammann, R.A.; Graf, R. Normal values for pancreatic stone protein in different age groups. *BMC Anesthesiol.* **2015**, *15*, 168. [CrossRef] [PubMed]
10. Schlapbach, L.J.; Graf, R.; Woerner, A.; Fontana, M.; Zimmermann-Baer, U.; Glauser, D.; Giannoni, E.; Roger, T.; Müller, C.; Nelle, M.; et al. Pancreatic stone protein as a novel marker for neonatal sepsis. *Intensive Care Med.* **2013**, *39*, 754–763. [CrossRef] [PubMed]
11. Zhu, X.; Dong, B.; Reding, T.; Peng, Y.; Lin, H.; Zhi, M.; Han, M.; Graf, R.; Li, L. Association of Serum PSP/REG Ialpha with Renal Function in Pregnant Women. *Biomed. Res. Int.* **2019**, *2019*, 6970890. [CrossRef] [PubMed]
12. Yang, J.; Li, L.; Raptis, D.; Li, X.; Li, F.; Chen, B.; He, J.; Graf, R.; Sun, Z. Pancreatic stone protein/regenerating protein (PSP/reg): A novel secreted protein up-regulated in type 2 diabetes mellitus. *Endocrine* **2015**, *48*, 856–862. [CrossRef] [PubMed]
13. Prazak, J.; Irincheeva, I.; Llewelyn, M.J.; Stolz, D.; García de Guadiana Romualdo, L.; Graf, R.; Reding, T.; Klein, H.J.; Eggimann, P.; Que, Y.A. Accuracy of pancreatic stone protein for the diagnosis of infection in hospitalized adults: A systematic review and individual patient level meta-analysis. *Crit. Care* **2021**, *25*, 182. [CrossRef] [PubMed]
14. Mor, G.; Cardenas, I. The immune system in pregnancy: A unique complexity. *Am. J. Reprod. Immunol.* **2010**, *63*, 425–433. [CrossRef] [PubMed]
15. Kourtis, A.P.; Read, J.S.; Jamieson, D.J. Pregnancy and infection. *N. Engl. J. Med.* **2014**, *370*, 2211–2218. [CrossRef] [PubMed]
16. Li, L.; Jia, D.; Graf, R.; Yang, J. Elevated serum level of pancreatic stone protein/regenerating protein (PSP/reg) is observed in diabetic kidney disease. *Oncotarget* **2017**, *8*, 38145–38151. [CrossRef] [PubMed]
17. Hill, C.C.; Pickinpaugh, J. Physiologic changes in pregnancy. *Surg. Clin. N. Am.* **2008**, *88*, 391–401, vii. [CrossRef] [PubMed]
18. Cheung, K.L.; Lafayette, R.A. Renal physiology of pregnancy. *Adv. Chronic. Kidney Dis.* **2013**, *20*, 209–214. [CrossRef] [PubMed]
19. Sobajima, H.; Niwa, T.; Shikano, M.; Naruse, S.; Kitagawa, M.; Nakae, Y.; Ishiguro, H.; Kondo, T.; Hayakawa, T. Urinary excretion of pancreatic stone protein in diabetic nephropathy. *Intern. Med.* **1998**, *37*, 500–503. [CrossRef] [PubMed]

Disclaimer/Publisher's Note: The statements, opinions and data contained in all publications are solely those of the individual author(s) and contributor(s) and not of MDPI and/or the editor(s). MDPI and/or the editor(s) disclaim responsibility for any injury to people or property resulting from any ideas, methods, instructions or products referred to in the content.

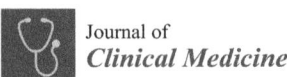

Article

Comparison of the Results of Prenatal and Postnatal Echocardiography and Postnatal Cardiac MRI in Children with a Congenital Heart Defect

Marios Mamalis *, Tamara Koehler, Ivonne Bedei, Aline Wolter, Johanna Schenk, Ellyda Widriani and Roland Axt-Fliedner *

Division of Prenatal Medicine & Fetal Therapy, Department of Obstetrics & Gynecology, Justus-Liebig-University Giessen, 35390 Giessen, Germany
* Correspondence: marios.mamalis@yahoo.com (M.M.); roland.axt-fliedner@gyn.med.uni-giessen.de (R.A.-F.)

Abstract: Objective: In fetuses with suspicion of congenital heart disease (CHD), assessment by segmental fetal echocardiography is of great importance. This study sought to examine the concordance of expert fetal echocardiography and postnatal MRI of the heart at a high-volume paediatric heart centre. Methods: The data of two hundred forty-two fetuses have been gathered under the condition of full pre- and postnatal and the presence of a pre- and postnatal diagnosis of CHD. The haemodynamically leading diagnosis was determined for each test person and was then sorted into diagnostic groups. The diagnoses and diagnostic groups were used for the comparison of diagnostic accuracy in fetal echocardiography. Results: All comparisons between the diagnostic methods for detection of congenital heart disease showed an "almost perfect" (Cohen's Kappa > 0.9) strength of agreement for the diagnostic groups. The diagnosis made by prenatal echocardiography showed a sensitivity of 90–100%, a specificity and a negative predictive value of 97–100%, and a positive predictive value of 85–100%. The diagnostic congruence resulted in an "almost perfect" strength of agreement for all evaluated diagnoses (transposition of great arteries, double outlet right ventricle, hypoplastic left heart, tetralogy of Fallot, atrioventricular septal defect). An agreement of Cohen's Kappa > 0.9 was achieved for all groups, with exception of the diagnosis of double outlet right ventricle (0.8) in prenatal echocardiography compared to postnatal echocardiography. This study came to the result of a sensitivity of 88–100%, a specificity and negative predictive value of 97–100%, and a positive predictive value of 84–100%. The performance of cardiac magnetic resonance imaging (MRI) as an additional measure to echocardiography had an added value in the description of the malposition of the great arteries when diagnosed with double outlet right ventricle and in the detailed description of the anatomy of the lung circulation. Conclusions: Prenatal echocardiography could be shown to be a reliable method for detection of congenital heart disease when regarding the slightly lower accuracy of diagnosis for double outlet right ventricle and right heart anomalies. Furthermore, the impact of examiner experience and the consideration of follow-up examinations for further improvement of diagnosis accuracy may not be underestimated. The main advantage of an additional MRI is the possibility to obtain a detailed anatomic description of the blood vessels of the lung and the outflow tract. The conduction of further studies that include false-negative and false-positive cases, and studies that are not set within the high-risk-group, as well as studies in a less specialized setting, would allow the completion and investigation of possible differences and discrepancies when comparing the results that have been obtained in this study.

Keywords: congenital heart disease; echocardiography; postnatal cardiac MRI

1. Introduction

Congenital heart defects (CHD) represent a group of congenital anomalies difficult to characterize prenatally. For this reason, an antenatally suspected congenital heart defect

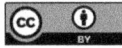

(CHD) via a fetal echocardiography is postnatally confirmed by a postnatal echocardiography and, on some occasions, postnatal cardiac magnetic resonance imaging (MRI) is adjunctively required.

In this retrospective explorative analysis, we describe our experience in the clinical management of two hundred forty-two fetuses with suspected congenital heart defects (CHD) referred to our unit for diagnosis and management over a five-year period.

The objective of this study is to assess whether and to what extent the prenatal echocardiography is a reliable method for diagnosis of several CHD and if postnatal cardiac MRI provides additional diagnostic value.

2. Methods

During a five-year study period from 2012 to 2017, there have been two hundred forty-two cases with suspected CHD referred to our fetal medicine unit (FMU) at the University Hospital of Giessen and Marburg (UKGM) for diagnosis and further management. All individuals, in addition to prenatal echocardiography, have underwent postnatal echocardiography and postnatal cardiac MRI examination, when indicated. Prenatal and postnatal echocardiography have been performed in accordance to published guidelines [1–3].

Statistical analysis was performed by the Institute of Biostatistics at Justus-Liebig University Giessen. The interpretation of results has been based on Cohen's Kappa coefficient and the concordance rate of Landis and Koch. The congenital heart defects' spectrum that has been met in our patient's collective is demonstrated in Table 1. The level of significance when testing concordance for all Cohen's Kappa scores has been a: 5%. Additionally, the Bonferroni correction method and p-value have been utilized. Overall results are presented as descriptive data. Sensitivity (SEN) and specificity (SPE), and positive (PPV) and negative predictive values (NPV) were calculated.

Table 1. Classification of congenital heart defects in current study.

Congenital Heart Disease	Diagnosis
Conotruncal and outflow tract anomalies	• Transposition of great arteries (TGA) • Double outlet left ventricle (DOLV) • Double outlet right ventricle (DORV) • Truncus arteriosus communis (TAC)
Anomalies of left heart	• Aortic valve stenosis • Hypoplastic left heart (HLH) • Interruption of the aortic arch—aortic arch hypoplasia
Anomalies of right heart	• Insufficiency of the tricuspid valve • Atresia of the tricuspid valve • Pulmonary valve stenosis • Atresia of pulmonary valve (PAT) • Absent pulmonary valve • Ebstein anomaly • Tetralogy of Fallot (TOF)
Septal defects	• Ventricular septal defect (VSD) • Atrial septal defect (ASD) • Atrioventricular septal defect (AVSD)
Complex CHD	• Univentricular heart (UVH) • Isomerism: L-isomerism, R-isomerism
Other anomalies	• Ectopia cordis • cardiac tumours

3. Results

Two hundred forty-two cases were included in the study. Twenty-four cases were excluded due to termination of pregnancy; seven intrauterine demises occurred. Two hundred eleven cases remained for final analysis.

Table 2 shows the overall prevalence of CHD in our cohort. The strength of agreement for CHD in the different groups has been evaluated (Table 3). Comparing the several CHD in the prenatal-postnatal echocardiography group, the anomalies of right heart and complex CHD have shown the lowest strength of agreement (Cohen's Kappa: 0.92). For conotruncal and outflow tract anomalies, and septal defects, the strength of agreement has been 0.93 and for left heart anomalies, 0.96.

Table 2. Frequency of congenital heart defects in present collective.

	Prenatal Echocardiography (%)	Postnatal Echocardiography (%)
Conotruncal/anomalies of outflow tract	21.4	21.5
Transposition of great arteries	9	9.6
Double outlet left ventricle	0.6	0.6
Double outlet right ventricle	10.7	10.2
Anomalies of left heart	26.6	28.3
Stenosis of the aortic valve	3.4	4
Hypoplastic left heart	19.8	20.3
Interrupted aortic arch	0.6	0.6
Hypolastic aortic arch	2.8	3.4
Anomalies of right heart	21	22.7
Insufficiency of tricuspid valve	0.6	1.1
Atresia of tricuspid valve	1.7	2.3
Stenosis of pulmonary valve	2.3	2.3
Pulmonary atresia	1.7	2.3
Absent pulmonary valve	1.1	1.1
Ebstein anomaly	0.6	0.6
Tetralogy of Fallot	13	13
Septal defects	19.2	17
Atrial septal defect	0	0.6
Ventricular septal defect	3.4	2.8
Atrioventricular septal defect	15.8	13.6
Complex CHD	7.9	6.8
Univentricular heart	6.2	5.1
L-isomerismus	1.1	1.1
R-isomerismus	0.6	0.6
Other anomalies	5.1	5.1
Ectopia cordis	1.1	1.1
Tumours	1.1	1.1
Number of patients	177	177

The lowest strength of agreement has been indicated for septal defects in the prenatal echocardiography-MRI group (Cohen's Kappa: 0.91). The anomalies of right heart and complex CHD have shown a concordance of Cohen's Kappa as high as 0.94 and the conotruncal and outflow tract anomalies' Cohen's Kappa has been 0.95. The left heart anomalies have demonstrated the second highest strength of agreement (Cohen's Kappa: 0.98) below the "Other anomalies" group.

Table 3. Strength of agreement; comparison among prenatal echocardiography, postnatal echocardiography and cardiac MRI.

Diagnosis	Concordance (Cohen's Kappa)		
	Prenatal-Postnatal Echocardiography	Prenatal Echocardiography-MRI	Postnatal Echocardiography-MRI
Conotruncal and outflow tract anomalies	0.933	0.946	0.974
Anomalies of left heart	0.957	0.98	0.98
Anomalies of right heart	0.917	0.941	0.971
Septal defects	0.924	0.913	1
Complex defects	0.917	0.942	0.936
Other anomalies	1	1	1

In the postnatal echocardiography-postnatal MRI group, the diagnosis of septal defects has been "perfectly" concordant. The left heart anomalies have shown a concordance rate of 0.98 and the conotruncal and outflow tract anomalies, and right heart anomalies have similarly achieved high concordance (Cohen's Kappa: 0.97).

The comparison of the precision of the diagnosis via different diagnostic methods by utilized Cohen's Kappa has proved to have a significance of $p < 0.001$ in all cases. After implying the Bonferroni correction, all tests for CHD have proved significance.

In Table 4, the predictive parameters for CHD via prenatal echocardiography, compared to postnatal echocardiography, are demonstrated; "Other anomalies" have achieved a positive predictive value (PPV) of 100%. Conotruncal and outflow tract anomalies, and right and left heart anomalies have shown a positive predictive value (PPV) higher than 94%. A low PPV score of 88% and 86% could be reported for septal defects and complex CHD, respectively. In all groups, a PPV higher than 97% has been achieved. The lowest sensitivity (SEN) has been shown for right heart anomalies (90%), while the rest of CHD have demonstrated high sensitivity (SEN) and specificity (SPE) scores (Table 5).

Table 4. Sensitivity (SEN), specificity (SPE), positive (PPV) and negative predictive value (NPV) for diagnosis in the prenatal echocardiography. Reference: The postnatal echocardiography. N = 177.

	Prenatal Echocardiography				
	Prevalence of Prenatal Echocardiography (%)	SEN (%)	SPE (%)	PPV (%)	NPV (%)
Conotruncal and outflow tract anomalies	21.5	94.7	98.6	94.7	98.6
Anomalies of left heart	26.6	94	100	100	97.7
Anomalies of right heart	20.9	90	99.3	97.3	97.1
Septal defects	19.2	100	97.3	88.2	100
Complex congenital heart defects	8.5	100	98.8	85.7	100
Other anomalies	5.1	100	100	100	100

In the prenatal echocardiography-MRI group, the right heart anomalies group has shown the lowest sensitivity (SEN) (90%). Prenatal echocardiography has been proved to provide a high accuracy for diagnosis of left heart anomalies, conotruncal and outflow tract anomalies, and "Other anomalies", as SEN lies as high as 97.5%, 95.8%, and 100%, respectively. Similarly, specificity (SPE) has shown a very high score (>97%) for all CHD. The conotruncal and outflow tract anomalies, septal defects, and complex CHD have reached a specificity (SPE) of 97.9–99%. For left heart anomalies, right heart anomalies, and "Other anomalies", the SPE has been 100%. Right heart anomalies, despite low SEN, have demonstrated a PPV score of 100%. PPV scores for conotruncal and outflow tract anomalies have been 95.8%, and 100% for left heart anomalies, right heart anomalies, and "Other anomalies". Septal defects have possessed the lowest PPV score of 85.7%. Negative predictive value (NPV) has reached a high score (>97%). Septal defects, complex CHD, and "Other anomalies" have reached a negative predictive value (NPV) of 100%.

Table 5. Sensitivity (SEN), specificity (SPE), positive (PPV) and negative predictive value (NPV) for diagnosis in the prenatal echocardiography. Reference: Postnatal cardiac. MRI: 108.

	Prenatal Echocardiography				
	Prevalence Prenatal (%)	SEN (%)	SPE (%)	PPV (%)	NPV (%)
Conotruncal and outflow tract anomalies	22.2	95.8	98.8	95.8	98.8
Left heart anomalies	36.1	97.5	100	100	98.6
Right heart anomalies	18.1	90.9	100	100	97.7
Septal defects	13	100	97.9	85.7	100
Complex congenital heart defects	9.3	100	99	90	100
Other anomalies	2.8	100	100	100	100

The postnatal echocardiography-MRI group has achieved an "almost perfect" strength of agreement in all CHD. A Cohen's Kappa score of 1 has been shown for septal defects and "Other anomalies", 0.98 for conotruncal and outflow tract anomalies, and 0.97 for right heart abnormalities. The lowest rate has been related to complex CHD with Cohen's Kappa (0.94). For all groups, there is a statistical significance for Cohen's Kappa before and after the Bonferroni correction. For conotruncal and outflow tract anomalies, and left heart anomalies, an SEN score of 100% and an SPE higher than 98% could be achieved. For right heart anomalies, an SEN of 95.5% for postnatal echocardiography has been shown. The lowest SEN of 89% has been related to complex CHD, and it has represented the only one with a score lower than 95%. A high SPE (98%) has been achieved in all groups. For right heart anomalies, septal defects, complex CHD, and "Other anomalies", an SPE of 100% has been achieved. For conotruncal and outflow tract anomalies, and left heart anomalies, an SPE higher than 98% has been shown (Table 6). The right heart anomalies, septal defects and "Other anomalies" have achieved a PPV of 100%. Moreover, the conotruncal and outflow tract anomalies, left heart anomalies, septal defects, and "Other anomalies" have shown an NPV as high as 100%. The right heart anomalies with an NPV of 99% indicate that there is 1% chance of a false-negative result.

Table 6. Sensitivity, specificity, positive and negative predictive value for the diagnosis in postnatal echocardiography. Reference: Diagnosis in cardiac MRI. N = 108.

	Postnatal Echocardiography and MRI				
	Prevalence Postnatal (%)	SEN (%)	SPE (%)	PPV (%)	NPV (%)
Conotruncal and outflow tract anomalies	23.1	100	98.8	96	100
Anomalies of left heart	38	100	98.5	97.6	100
Anomalies of right heart	19.4	95.5	100	100	98.9
Septal defects	11.1	100	100	100	100
Complex CHD	7.4	88.9	100	100	99
Other anomalies	2.8	100	100	100	100

The concordance of transposition of great arteries (TGA), double outlet right ventricle (DORV), hypoplastic left heart (HLH), tetralogy of Fallot (ToF), and atrioventricular septum defect (AVSD) in the prenatal-postnatal echocardiography group has been "almost perfect" achieving Cohen's Kappa higher than 0.8 (Table 7). Double outlet right ventricle (DORV) has been the only entity with a Cohen's Kappa score lower than 0.9. In the prenatal echocardiography-MRI group, double outlet right ventricle (DORV) and atrioventricular septal defect (AVSD) have achieved an "almost perfect" classification with a Cohen's Kappa score lower than 0.9. In case of transposition of great arteries (TGA), hypoplastic left heart (HLH), and tetralogy of Fallot (ToF), the concordance rate has been 1. A same pattern is used to evaluate the concordance of transposition of great arteries (TGA), double outlet right ventricle (DORV), hypoplastic left heart (HLH), tetralogy of Fallot (ToF), and atrioventricular septal defect (AVSD) in the postnatal echocardiography-MRI group. For a concordance with a score higher than 0.9 for all and specifically for AVSD, a rate of 1 has been shown. For all groups, a statistical significance could be shown, which was consistent after Bonferroni correction.

Table 7. Strength of agreement; comparison among prenatal echocardiography, postnatal echocardiography and cardiac MRI.

	Concordance (Cohen's Kappa)		
	Prenatal and Postnatal Echocardiography	Prenatal Echocardiography and MRI	Postnatal Echocardiography and MRI
Transposition of great arteries	0.967	1	0.918
Double outlet right ventricle	0.849	0.927	0.927
Hypoplastic left heart	0.982	1	0.976
Tetralogy of Fallot	0.950	1	0.960
Atrioventricular septal defect	0.910	0.913	1

Table 8 shows the quality criteria SEN and SPE for TGA, DORV, HLH, ToF, and AVSD in the prenatal-postnatal echocardiography group. Diagnosis of DORV has achieved the lowest sensitivity of 88.9%. The rest have achieved an SEN higher than 94%. Particularly, TGA and ToF have been as high as 95%. HLH has shown an SEN of 97%, while AVSD, 100%. All groups have presented an SPE higher than 97%, while TGA and HLH have had an SPE as high as 100%. Similarly, ToF has shown an SPE of 99.4%. The lowest SPE has corresponded to DORV (98.1%) and AVSD (97.4%). The PPV has been 85% for DORV and AVSD, while the PPV was 95% for ToF and 100% for TGA and HLH. The NPV for all CHD has achieved a score higher than 98%. The lowest NPV has corresponded to DORV (98.7%). For the rest, the NPV has been as high as almost 100%.

Table 8. Sensitivity, specificity, positive (PPV) and negative predictive value (NPV) for the diagnosis in the prenatal echocardiography. Reference: Diagnosis in the postnatal echocardiography. N = 177.

	Prenatal Echocardiography				
	Prevalence (%)	SEN (%)	SPE (%)	PPV (%)	NPV (%)
Transposition of great arteries	9	94.1	100	100	99.4
Double outlet right ventricle	10.7	88.9	98.1	84.2	98.7
Hypoplastic left heart	19.8	97.2	100	100	99.3
Tetralogy of Fallot	13	95.7	99.4	95.7	99.4
Atrioventricular septal defect	15.8	100	97.4	85.7	100

Table 9 shows that the quality criteria used for the prenatal echocardiography-postnatal MRI group have represented a high overall SPE (>97%); in particular for AVSD, as high as 98% and for DORV, almost 99%. The rest have had an SPE of 100%. For TGA, HLH, and ToF, no false-positive diagnoses have been made. DORV has had the lowest SEN score (93.8%), whereas for TGA, HLH, ToF, and AVSD, an SEN score of 100% could be achieved. The NPV has been as high as 99% for DORV, representing the lowest score; the scores for the rest of CHD have achieved as high as 100%, reflecting the high reliability of prenatal echocardiography for these CHD. The PPV for AVSD has been 86% and was the lowest. On the contrary, DORV achieved a PPV score of 94%, and an even higher score has been achieved for TGA, HLH, and ToF, reaching 100%.

Table 9. Sensitivity, specificity, positive and negative predictive value for diagnosis in the prenatal echocardiography. Reference: Diagnosis in cardiac MRI. N = 108.

	Prenatal Echocardiography				
	Prevalence Prenatal (%)	SEN (%)	SPE (%)	PPV (%)	NPV (%)
Transposition of great arteries	5.6	100	100	100	100
Double outlet right ventricle	14.8	93.8	98.9	93.8	98.9
Hypoplastic left heart	26.9	100	100	100	100
Tetralogy of Fallot	13.9	100	100	100	100
Atrioventricular septal defect	13	100	97.9	85.7	100

In Table 10, only the CHD with a prenatal number of individuals more than fifteen (N > 15) are demonstrated, in order to minimize a possible misleading effect on the results of smaller groups. The exceptions to these are TGA and AVSD in cardiac MRI, whose numbers in prenatal and postnatal echocardiography have been adequate. The postnatal echocardiography has achieved for different entities an SPE of 98%. It has performed for TGA, DORV, and HLH, an SPE of 99% and for TOF and AVSD, 100%. An SEN for DORV and ToF has been as high as 93%, which is lower compared to TGA, HLH, and AVSD (SEN 100%). On the whole, postnatal echocardiography has performed detection higher than 93% of the Individuals with congenital heart diseases. The postnatal echocardiography has shown an NPV higher than 98%. For DORV and ToF, an NPV has been as high as 100%. A PPV of 86% has been shown for TGA; being the lowest. A total of 14% of individuals with suspicion of TGA have had none. It is important to notice that this low PPV could be in association with the small number of individuals. The rest have shown a PPV higher than 93%. The PPV for DORV has been 94% and for HHL, 97%. In the case of ToF and AVSD, PPV has been 100%.

Table 10. Sensitivity, specificity, positive and negative predictive value in the postnatal echocardiography. Reference: Diagnosis in cardiac MRI. N = 108.

	Postnatal Echocardiography and MRI				
	Prevalence Postnatal (%)	SEN (%)	SPE (%)	PPV (%)	NPV (%)
Transposition of Great arteries	6.5	100	99	85.7	100
Double outlet right ventricle	14.8	93.8	98.9	93.8	98.9
Hypoplastic left heart	26.9	100	98.8	96.6	100
Tetralogy of Fallot	13	93.3	100	100	98.9
Atrioventricular septal defect	11.1	100	100	100	100

4. Discussion

Firstly, we wanted to examine agreement between fetal prenatal and postnatal echocardiography. The results show that prenatal echocardiography is a reliable diagnostic tool for conotruncal and outflow tract anomalies, left heart anomalies, and "Other anomalies"; though, with a higher rate of false-positive diagnosis for septal defects and CHD. Similarly, an additional postnatal echocardiography may be reasonable in the case of right heart anomalies, as this is indicated by the low strength of agreement and high false-negative rate in this group. Regarding the group of diagnoses TGA, DORV, HLH, ToF, and AVSD, it shows an almost perfect agreement, with 6% remaining; though, prenatally undetected and an increased risk of false-negative diagnosis for DORV, which reaches 12%. In addition, DORV shows a higher rate of false-positive diagnosis when compared to rest.

Secondly, we studied the agreement between prenatal echocardiography and postnatal MRI. The rate of prenatally undetected fetuses with CHD was, in general, low, especially for left heart anomalies, excepting right heart anomalies with a higher false-negative rate. However, right heart anomalies have demonstrated the highest PPV score in this group, indicating in this manner, a low risk of false-positive diagnosis. The highest risk of false-negative diagnosis has been shown in the case of right heart anomalies. The number of cases for MRI for TGA and AVSD has been lower than 15, and we have followed a careful interpretation of these results taking into consideration the reduced reliability of these results (Table 7). An increased rate of false-positive diagnosis has been shown for AVSD.

Thirdly, we found that the agreement in the postnatal echocardiography-postnatal MRI group has been almost perfect (Tables 3 and 7). This proves that the echocardiography in postnatal life is a reliable tool. The complex CHD have shown the lowest strength of agreement and the highest rate of false-negative diagnosis reaching 11%.

This retrospective study leads to the conclusion that the prenatal echocardiography is a reliable diagnostic tool for both making and excluding a diagnosis of CHD. A reliable prenatal echocardiography permits an interdisciplinary approach for parental counselling. In that manner, it is possible for paediatricians and paediatric surgeons to involve, and make a plan for the delivery in, a tertiary hospital [4]. This leads to better outcomes [5–7]. This cohort has proven an "almost perfect" strength of agreement for all CHD in three groups. The left heart anomalies have the highest rate of strength of agreement in prenatal echocardiography and in the postnatal diagnostic methods. The second highest rate of concordance has been achieved by the group of conotruncal and outflow tract anomalies and it is in the same line with Gottliebson et al. [8]. Moreover, Gottliebson et al. have demonstrated a high detection rate for the conotruncal anomalies and for complex CHD such as univentricular heart and heterotaxy syndrome.

Regarding the group of diagnoses TGA, DORV, HLH, ToF, and AVSD, HLHS has demonstrated the highest strength of agreement in all groups (Table 7), and it is in agreement with the results of the left heart anomalies. DORV has demonstrated a high risk of increased false-negative diagnosis in prenatal echocardiography, when compared to postnatal echocardiography, and this is in line with Bensemlali et al. [9], who reported that DORV, and specifically the definition of malposition-type of great arteries, is challenging, and in 80% of cases, it can be correctly detected [9,10]; results which agree with the current study, in which in two cases with correct-detected DORV, the position of great arteries have had to be adjusted (TGA-type or Fallot-type). Regarding right heart anomalies and DORV, the high rate of false-negative diagnosis should be taken into consideration and in case of negative diagnosis, eventually a re-evaluation should be considered. The risk of false-negative diagnosis is related to the lack of re-evaluation or treatment [11]. Right heart anomalies similarly have demonstrated a higher false-negative rate in the prenatal echocardiography when this compared to postnatal MRI and in these cases, individuals are at risk of unnecessary treatments or even termination [11].

Mainly due to a high NPV, only a small number of individuals face a false-negative diagnosis. On the contrary, the risk of a false-positive diagnosis mainly for septal defects, complex CHD, and TGA, DORV, HLH, ToF, and AVSD is higher. The prenatal echocardiography has shown a low SEN score for DORV compared with rest. The false-positive rate in this group varied up to 15% for complex CHD. This may lead to unnecessary tests with consequent parents' disquiet or even misleading decision to termination of pregnancy [12]. The CHD with a lower PPV and positive diagnosis requires, therefore, re-evaluation and adequate counselling of parents [13]. In the present study, due to the small number of individuals (N < 15) with CHD and "Other anomalies", bias is possible. These results show common features with those of the study about precision of echocardiographic diagnosis in early pregnancy from Pike et al. [14] with an SPE of 97.3%, a PPV of 81.2%, and an NPV as high as 100%. A SEN has reached 100% in the study of Pike et al. [14], and it has been higher than in the present study (90–100%). The difference in the current study lies with the evaluation of findings of the whole pregnancy. Pike et al. [14] recommend a follow-up after 20 weeks to increase the reliability of the diagnosis. Bakiler et al. [15] could demonstrate a high SPE of 98% and predictive values higher than 90%; though, with a SEN of 42%, there is a lower reliability for detection than in the present study. In the current study, there have been generally shown higher scores than in the study of Gottliebson et al. [8]; SPE and NPV of 82–100% and SEN and PPV of 83–100%. However, it is important to take into consideration the time period of the study of Gottliebson et al., which took place from 1998 to 2003, and that it is easier to achieve better results in more recent Cohort than in older ones. Therefore, the results of the present study, that took place from 2012 to 2017 are based on better technical equipment.

The study had some limitations. Firstly, in this retrospective approach the results correspond to a collective with a CHD and they cannot be applied to general population. Our collective has been a "high risk population" that had been referred to our referral centre for final diagnosis and delivery to our maternity unit with direct connection to the paediatric cardiology centre. Ascertainment rate, therefore, was high in our study, however there are CHD cases identified prenatally born outside our centre, which have not undergone MRI examination postnatally. Individuals with milder forms of CHD that have been delivered at local hospitals have been excluded from this study because of unavailable data. Secondly, due to retrospective design of present study and focus on prenatally diagnosed CHD, this study is not able to make a reliable statement about false-negative and false-positive diagnosis. Thirdly, intrauterine demise and termination of pregnancy have been excluded from the present study. Fourthly, it is important to mention that the restricted number of Individuals in some cases could potentially lead to bias. The results in these cases should either compared with other studies with a greater number of Individuals or re-evaluated in future larger studies. Fifthly, the expertise of fetal medicine and fetal cardiology specialists in our unit has contributed to the achieved accurate results [14,16,17].

5. Conclusions

The careful observation and evaluation of the results of the current study leads to the conclusion that the prenatal echocardiography represents a reliable method of detection and exclusion of CHD. It is important to mention that the experience of the examiner and eventually a follow-up to adjust the diagnosis in some cases are essential. The greatest reliability could be shown for the anomalies of the left heart and specifically for hypoplastic left heart in the present study. The anomalies of the right heart, on the contrary, have shown the highest rate of false-negative diagnosis. Septal defects have possessed the highest rate of false-positive diagnosis. The greatest challenge for an accurate diagnosis has been related to DORV due to its extreme anatomical variability and frequent association with complex abnormalities. This study shows that cardiac MRI is an additional diagnostic tool for the detailed study of the vascular anatomy and pulmonary supply. In general, it is recommended to re-evaluate the results of the present study in future studies with "low risk collective" and examiners with varying experience. Further studies with a greater number of individuals are essential for comparing and verifying our results. Additionally, it would be interesting to assess in future studies the concordance in relation to gestational week and evaluate the best time to detect progressive CHD. Lastly in case of a prospective study it would be meaningful to include false-positive and false-negative results.

Author Contributions: M.M. was responsible for writing original draft preparation. M.M. and R.A.-F. was responsible for writing—review and editing, while the rest of Authors (T.K., I.B., A.W., J.S. and E.W.) for validation and investigation. All authors have read and agreed to the published version of the manuscript.

Funding: This research received no external funding.

Institutional Review Board Statement: The study was conducted in accordance with the Declaration of Helsinki, and approved by the Institutional Review Board (Ethics approval Committee Justus Giessen University) (protocol number 169/17).

Informed Consent Statement: Informed consent was obtained from all subjects involved in the study.

Data Availability Statement: Data is unavailable due to privacy or ethical restrictions.

Conflicts of Interest: The authors declare no conflict of interest.

References

1. Chaoui, R.; Heling, K.; Mielke, G.; Hofbeck, M.; Gembruch, U. Quality standards of the DEGUM for performance of fetal echocardiography. *Ultrashall Med.* **2008**, *29*, 197–200. [CrossRef] [PubMed]
2. Herberg, U. Functional Echocardiography for Neonatologists-Consensus based Recommendations of the German Association for Pediatric Cardiology and the German Association for Neonatology and Pediatric Intensive Care. *Z. Fur Geburtshilfe Und Neonatol.* **2020**, *224*, 160–161.
3. Schuster, A.; Thiele, H.; Katus, H.; Werdan, K.; Eitel, I.; Zeiher, A.M.; Baldus, S.; Rolf, A.; Kelle, S. Kompetenz und Innovation in der kardiovaskulären MRT: Stellungnahme der Deutschen Gesellschaft für Kardiologie–Herzund Kreislaufforschung Deutsche Gesellschaft für Kardiologie-Herzund Kreislaufforschung. *Kardiologe* **2021**, *15*, 471–479. [CrossRef]
4. Eronen, M. Outcome of fetuses with heart disease diagnosed in utero. *Arch. Dis. Child. Fetal Neonatal Ed.* **1997**, *77*, F41–F46. [CrossRef] [PubMed]
5. Seale, A.N.; Carvalho, J.S.; Gardiner, H.M.; Mellander, M.; Roughton, M.; Simpson, J.; Tometzki, A.; Uzun, O.; Webber, S.A.; Daubeney, P.E.F.; et al. Total anomalous pulmonary venous connection: Impact of prenatal diagnosis. *Ultrasound Obstet. Gynecol.* **2012**, *40*, 310–318. [CrossRef] [PubMed]
6. Donofrio, M.T.; Levy, R.J.; Schuette, J.J.; Skurow-Todd, K.; Sten, M.-B.; Stallings, C.; Pike, J.I.; Krishnan, A.; Ratnayaka, K.; Sinha, P.; et al. Specialized delivery room planning for fetuses with critical congenital heart disease. *Am. J. Cardiol.* **2013**, *111*, 737–747. [CrossRef] [PubMed]
7. Penny, D.J.; Shekerdemian, L.S. Management of the neonate with symptomatic congenital heart disease. *Arch. Dis. Child. Fetal Neonatal Ed.* **2001**, *84*, F141–F145. [CrossRef] [PubMed]
8. Gottliebson, W.M.; Border, W.L.; Franklin, C.M.; Meyer, R.A.; Michelfelder, E.C. Accuracy of fetal echocardiography: A cardiac segment-specific analysis. *Ultrasound Obstet. Gynecol. Off. J. Int. Soc. Ultrasound Obstet. Gynecol.* **2006**, *28*, 15–21. [CrossRef] [PubMed]
9. Bensemlali, M.; Stirnemann, J.; Le Bidois, J.; Lévy, M.; Raimondi, F.; Hery, E.; Stos, B.; Bessières, B.; Boudjemline, Y.; Bonnet, D. Discordances between pre-natal and post-natal diagnoses of congenital heart diseases and impact on care strategies. *J. Am. Coll. Cardiol.* **2016**, *68*, 921–930. [CrossRef] [PubMed]
10. Gedikbasi, A.; Oztarhan, K.; Gul, A.; Sargin, A.; Ceylan, Y. Diagnosis and prognosis in double-outlet right ventricle. *Am. J. Perinatol.* **2008**, *25*, 427–434. [CrossRef] [PubMed]
11. Herrmann, F.; Neuerburg-Heusler, D.; Nissen, P. Statistische Grundbegriffe für die Validierung diagnostischer Verfahren. Ein Beitrag zur Qualitätssicherung am Beispiel der Doppler-Sonographie. *Ultraschall Med.* **1986**, *7*, 59–69. [CrossRef]
12. Molinaro, A.M. Diagnostic tests: How to estimate the positive predictive value. *Neuro-Oncol. Pract.* **2015**, *2*, 162–166. [CrossRef]
13. Bender, R.; Lange, S. Die Vierfeldertafel. *DMW-Dtsch. Med. Wochenschr.* **2007**, *132*, e12–e14. [CrossRef] [PubMed]
14. Pike, J.I.; Krishnan, A.; Donofrio, M.T. Early fetal echocardiography: Congenital heart disease detection and diagnostic accuracy in the hands of an experienced fetal cardiology program. *Prenat. Diagn.* **2014**, *34*, 790–796. [CrossRef] [PubMed]
15. Bakiler, A.R.; Ozer, E.A.; Kanik, A.; Kanit, H.; Aktas, F.N. Accuracy of prenatal diagnosis of congenital heart disease with fetal echocardiography. *Fetal Diagn. Ther.* **2007**, *22*, 241–244. [CrossRef] [PubMed]
16. Novaes, J.Y.; Zamith, M.M.; Araujo Junior, E.; de Sá Barreto, E.Q.; Barros, F.S.; Moron, A.F. Screening of congenital heart diseases by three-dimensional ultrasound using spatiotemporal image correlation: Influence of professional experience. *Echocardiography* **2016**, *33*, 99–104. [CrossRef] [PubMed]
17. Meyer-Wittkopf, M.; Schönfeld, B.; Cooper, S.G.; Sholler, G.F. Correlation between fetal cardiac diagnosis by obstetric and pediatric cardiologist sonographers and comparison with postnatal findings. *Ultrasound Obstet. Gynecol.* **2001**, *17*, 392–397. [CrossRef] [PubMed]

Disclaimer/Publisher's Note: The statements, opinions and data contained in all publications are solely those of the individual author(s) and contributor(s) and not of MDPI and/or the editor(s). MDPI and/or the editor(s) disclaim responsibility for any injury to people or property resulting from any ideas, methods, instructions or products referred to in the content.

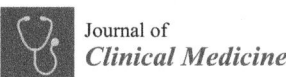

Article

Amniocentesis—When It Is Clear That It Is Not Clear

Razvan Ciortea [1], Andrei Mihai Malutan [1], Carmen Elena Bucuri [1], Costin Berceanu [2], Maria Patricia Rada [1], Cristina Mihaela Ormindean [1,*] and Dan Mihu [1]

[1] 2nd Department of Obstetrics and Gynaecology, "Iuliu Hațieganu" University of Medicine and Pharmacy, 400012 Cluj-Napoca, Romania
[2] Department of Obstetrics and Gynecology, Emergency University Hospital Craiova, The University of Medicine and Pharmacy of Craiova, 200642 Craiova, Romania
* Correspondence: cristina.mihaela.prodan@gmail.com; Tel.: +40-72-360-1422

Abstract: A fetus identified to be at risk for chromosomal abnormalities may benefit from identification of genetic defects through amniocentesis. Although the risks associated with amniocentesis are considered to be minimal, being an invasive procedure it is not completely without complications. Background and Objectives: The current study aims to identify correlations between blood contamination of samples collected during amniocentesis and certain factors dependent on the instruments used (thickness of the needle used to aspirate the fluid), the location of the placenta, and uterine vascularity (more pronounced in multiparous patients). Materials and Methods: The study included 190 patients in the second trimester of pregnancy who met one of the criteria for invasive prenatal diagnosis (age over 35 years, high risk in first trimester screening, history of pregnancies with genetic abnormalities, etc.). The amniotic fluid samples collected from these patients were analyzed in terms of blood contamination of the amniotic fluid aspirated with maternal cells Results: Of the patients in whom the procedure was performed using 21 G size needles, 16 samples (13.33% of the total) were contaminated. None of the samples collected from patients where a 20 G needle was used were contaminated. There was a statistically significant association between the lack of contamination and the use of Doppler ultrasound in multiparous patients with anterior placenta in whom a 21-gauge needle was used for amniocentesis. Conclusions: There is an increased rate of sample contamination (statistically significant) when using 21 G needle sizes and a significant difference in contamination between primiparous and multiparous patients, with contamination being more frequent in multiparous patients. The use of Doppler ultrasonography may benefit the procedure, as the contamination rate was significantly reduced when used during amniocentesis.

Keywords: amniocentesis; contamination; technique; needle gauge; doppler; pregnancy; risk

Citation: Ciortea, R.; Malutan, A.M.; Bucuri, C.E.; Berceanu, C.; Rada, M.P.; Ormindean, C.M.; Mihu, D. Amniocentesis—When It Is Clear That It Is Not Clear. *J. Clin. Med.* 2023, 12, 454. https://doi.org/10.3390/jcm12020454

Academic Editor: Roland Axt-Fliedner

Received: 27 November 2022
Revised: 26 December 2022
Accepted: 1 January 2023
Published: 6 January 2023

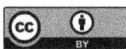

Copyright: © 2023 by the authors. Licensee MDPI, Basel, Switzerland. This article is an open access article distributed under the terms and conditions of the Creative Commons Attribution (CC BY) license (https://creativecommons.org/licenses/by/4.0/).

1. Introduction

Amniocentesis is an invasive procedure performed primarily in the second trimester of pregnancy to establish a prenatal diagnosis [1,2]. It was first performed in 1967, and by the mid-1970s it was accepted as a tool used for prenatal diagnosis [3]. It involves obtaining fetal cells from the amniotic fluid by ultrasonographically guided puncture of the amniotic sac. A fetal ultrasound is performed prior to amniocentesis to confirm fetal viability, gestational age, number of fetuses, placental location, amniotic fluid volume, fetal anatomical survey, uterine cavity abnormalities, or presence of fibroids. The procedure is performed to identify any fetal chromosomal anomalies [2,4]. A fetus identified to be at risk for chromosomal abnormalities may benefit from identification of genetic defects through amniocentesis. On the one hand this helps the family in making an informed decision on whether or not to continue the course of pregnancy, preparation for delivery, and neonatal prognosis, and on the other hand it helps the physician in making a diagnosis [1,5].

The indications for amniocentesis may vary depending on the geographical region, medical centre, personal, or family history of the patient or risk factors identified for each individual patient. Patients over 35 years of age, those with a family history of genetic abnormalities, patients with a history of children with different genetic syndromes, pregnancies in which abnormalities are ultrasonographically identified, and pregnancies with positive screening for abnormalities may benefit from this diagnostic procedure [1,2,6].

Since 2015, the number of pregnant patients undergoing this type of invasive investigation has started to progressively and steadily decrease due to the development of non-invasive methods of prenatal testing (NIPT) that involve the identification of fetal DNA from maternal blood. Based on sequencing of cell-free fetal DNA (cff DNA) from maternal plasma (NIPT), professional societies have issued their present positions on non-invasive testing regarding Down syndrome (trisomy 21), in addition to other autosomal aneuploidies (trisomy 18 and 13 [7–10]). All existing statements emphasize that NIPT should not be offered as a diagnostic test for fetal aneuploidy. Many declarations also insist that there is lacking evidence for NIPT to be used as a screening test in a wide population, even though of late there have been some studies that validate good performance in women at average risk. DNA sequenced represents a combination of maternal and fetal cell-free DNA, with the latter actually originating from the placenta, thus rendering NIPT for common autosomal aneuploidies less than fully accurate [11]. A positive result (beckoning a supposed aneuploidy) may be created by factors other than an aneuploid fetal karyotype, therefore including placental mosaicism, a vanishing twin or a maternal tumor; false alarms are foreseeable [12].

NIPT is a much more accurate examination for common autosomal aneuploidies than cFTS. Nevertheless, a positive NIPT result should not be looked upon as a concluding diagnosis, as the placenta contributes to the cff DNA. Women should consequently be advised to have a positive result confirmed through invasive testing, if possible, by amniocentesis [13].

Therefore, amniocentesis and chorionic villus sampling remain the preferred methods of diagnosis [5,14]. Although the risks associated with amniocentesis are considered to be minimal, being an invasive procedure, it is not completely without complications. These include loss of amniotic fluid, which can occur both during and after the test. Most often this disappears within a week, but in rare cases it may continue throughout pregnancy increasing the maternal and fetal risk for infection, fetal compromise (cardiac compression) and preterm birth [2,4,5]. Another complication associated with amniocentesis, described in the literature, is fetal injury during maneuvering, which is why amniotic sac puncture is performed under ultrasonographic guidance. One of the most feared complications is pregnancy loss, but the rate of pregnancy loss after amniocentesis is less than 1% [2,3,5].

A recent study shows that the complication rate associated with amniocentesis may be related to the thickness of the needle used to perform the procedure, the number of punctures performed, the puncture performed transplacentally and, last but not least, the experience of the operator. Literature data show a need for at least 30 procedures performed annually to maintain manuality in performing the diagnostic maneuver, as well as to minimise risks related to the experience of the performer [2,5].

Contamination of amniotic fluid collected during amniocentesis with maternal cells has been identified to be responsible for diagnostic errors as early as 1976 [15]. The maternal cells are thought to be artificially introduced into the amniotic fluid sample, as a result of placental bleeding during amniocentesis [16], but they also can be maternal cells from all tissues that are punctured during the procedure. In 1983 Benn et al. [17] reported a decrease in the contamination rate of samples by removing the first millilitres of amniotic fluid collected, with a 2.5-fold lower contamination rate [15,18].

The current study aims to identify correlations between blood contamination of samples collected during amniocentesis and certain factors dependent on the instruments used (thickness of the needle used to aspirate the fluid), the location of the placenta, and uterine vascularity (more pronounced in multiparous patients).

2. Materials and Methods

The present study is a prospective cohort study, carried out in the period 2016–2021 in the Obstetrics-Gynecology Clinic "Dominic Stanca" Cluj Napoca, Romania. The study included 190 patients in the second trimester of pregnancy (between 16 and 19 weeks of gestation) who met one of the criteria for invasive prenatal diagnosis (age over 35 years, high risk in prenatal screening, history of pregnancies with genetic abnormalities, family history, pregnancies with ultrasonographic anomalies). Patients where the procedure was performed using needles with other sizes (18 or 22 G), patients with increased risk of amniotic fluid contamination (uterine fibroid located in the anterior uterine wall, patients with haematological pathologies, and those with changes in coagulation parameters), and also patients who required multiple punctures for amniotic fluid collection, or the ones in which the procedure needed to be repeated, were not included in the study Figure 1.

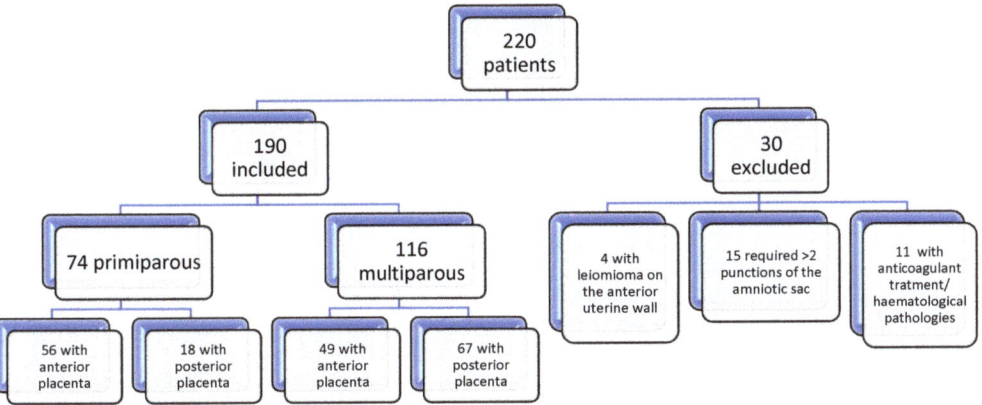

Figure 1. Inclusion and exclusion criteria for patients.

This prospective cohort research was conducted after obtaining the approval of the Ethics Commission of the University of Medicine and Pharmacy "Iuliu Hațieganu" Cluj Napoca (73/22.03.2016) and the informed consent of the patients included in the study group.

The amniotic fluid samples collected from these patients were analyzed in terms of blood contamination of the amniotic fluid aspirated with maternal cells and an attempt was made to make associations according to the following parameters: thickness of the needle used to perform amniocentesis (20–21 G), location of the placenta (at the level of the anterior/posterior uterine wall), uterine vascularization (parity-primipara/multipara).

The analysis was performed on patients who met one of the three criteria, two of the three criteria, or all three criteria. For the latter, additionally data were also analysed according to whether or not Doppler ultrasound was performed.

The technique of performing amniocentesis involves preparation of the patient's tegument and its disinfection with antiseptic solution, followed by puncture of the tegument, under ultrasonographic guidance, Doppler mode was employed only during the insertion of the needle in order to choose a less vascularized area of the uterus or placenta, using needles with sizes between 20–21 G until the amniotic sac is punctured. Once penetrated into the cavity, 15–30 mL of amniotic fluid is aspirated, none of the aspirated fluid is disposed. The collected sample is then sent to the laboratory for fetal karyotype analysis. For establishing the contamination of the collected samples the test method used involves the numerical analysis of short repetitive sequences specific to each individual, called STRs, through QF-PCR (Quantitative Fluorescence—PCR) technique, which is based on multiplex-PCR amplification using fluorescent labelling. DNA extraction was performed from the processed sample, followed by PCR reaction using the Devyser Compact v3 kit. PCR products were migrated through capillary electrophoresis using the ABI3500 Genetic Analyzer. Interpretation was performed using GeneMapper analysis software. Fetal and maternal STR markers were analysed in parallel and contamination of the amniotic fluid sample with maternal cells was analyzed. Prenatal sampling procedures carry a risk of including maternal cells alongside the envisioned fetal sample. This risk has been empirically calculated as approximately 0.5% in amniotic fluid sampling, 1–2% in chorionic villi sampling, and can possibly be higher, reliant on the method used for invasive sampling. The markers present in the putative fetal DNA sample (derived from cultured or uncultured cells from amniotic fluid, cord blood, chorionic villi, or products of conception) are compared to those from a maternal DNA sample (from a maternal blood specimen). By inspecting these samples in parallel and associating the relative ratios of alleles at each individual marker, it is possible to estimate the presence and level of contaminating maternal cells in the fetal sample. The finding of MCC does not automatically dictate that a repeat invasive sampling procedure be recommended or performed. The mere presence of MCC does not impede diagnostic testing, while the test employed is robust to the level of contamination observed. Common cutoffs include 10% for SNP oligonucleotide analysis (SOMA) and 15% for direct sequencing-based tests [19]. These common cutoffs are the ones we used in our assessments.

We have excluded visual analyzing of samples because data from the literature show that even in macroscopically clear samples maternal cells can be identified. Amniotic fluid samples contamination with maternal cells, depending on the proportion of maternal cells identified, can reduce the accuracy of the result, and may also lead to the impossibility of interpreting the sample.

For amniocentesis, 20 G needles were used in 70 patients who met the inclusion criteria between 2016 and 2018 and 21 G needles in 120 patients who met the inclusion criteria for our study between 2019 and 2021. Amniocentesis procedures were performed either with a 120 mm 20-gauge (G) needle specific for amniocentesis and chorionic villous sampling (Egemen International Amniocentesis Needle, İzmir, Turkey), or with a 120 mm 21 G amniocentesis needle (Wallace Amniocentesis Needles, Cooper Surgical, Trumbull, CT, USA). Both needles are provided with an adjustable stopper to determine insertion depth, and with a female luer lock connector to collect the amniotic fluid through a syringe.

Statistical processing of the data was performed using the χ^2 (chi-square) statistical test. The significance threshold for the statistical test used was $\alpha = 0.05$ (5%) and risks were also calculated (RE—risk in the exposed, RN—risk in the unexposed and RR—relative risk or risk ratio).

3. Results

From May 2016 to July 2021, more than 200 diagnostic amniocenteses were performed in our institution, and of these a significant sample, 190 patients, consented for enrollment in the study.

The location of the placenta was in the anterior uterine wall in 55% of the study participants, the rest (45% of the patients) had the placenta located in the posterior uterine wall. In terms of uterine vascularity during pregnancy, a variable directly influenced by the parity of the patients, 38% of those included in the study group were primiparous, and the remaining 62% of patients were multiparous.

Samples were analyzed according to the fulfillment of one to all three criteria (thickness of the needle used to perform amniocentesis, location of the placenta, uterine vascularization).

3.1. One of Three Criteria Used

Of the total 190 patients included in the study, in 120 (63.16%) amniocentesis was performed using a 21 G needle and in 70 (36.84%) the procedure was performed using a 20 G needle. Of the patients in whom the procedure was performed using 21 G size needles, 16 samples (13.33% of the total) were contaminated. None of the samples collected from patients where a 20 G needle was used were contaminated. There was a statistically significant association between the use of a 21 G needle for amniotic sac puncture and contamination of collected samples ($p = 0.0035$) Figure 2.

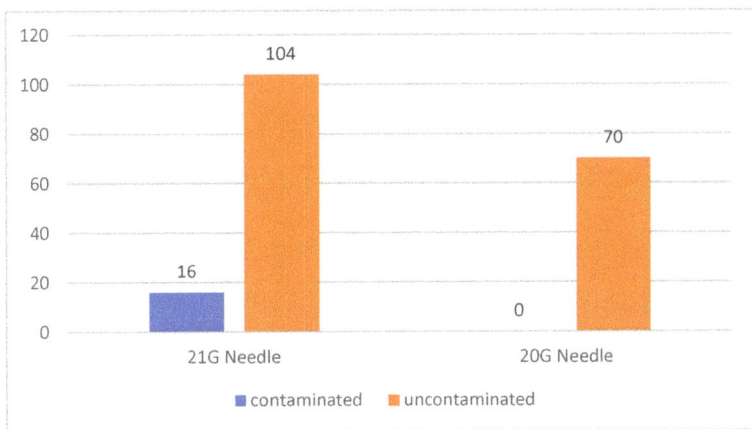

Figure 2. Number of contaminated versus uncontaminated samples according to the size of needle used for amniocentesis.

In the patients included in the study, the contamination of the samples was analyzed taking into account the location of the placenta in the anterior or posterior uterine wall; thus from the group of 190 patients, in 105 of them (55.26%) the placenta was located anteriorly, out of which when performing amniocentesis in a group of 34 patients the sample was collected by punctioning across the placental tissue, and in 85 (44.74%) the placenta was located posteriorly. Of the patients with anterior placenta, in 13 patients (6.84% of the total) the sample collected was contaminated. Amongst patients with posterior placenta, only three patients (1.58% of the total) had contaminated samples. No statistically significant association could be observed between placental position and contamination of samples collected for prenatal diagnosis ($p = 0.0546$, RE = 12.38, RN = 3.53, RR = 3.51).

The last criterion for data analysis considered was the number of previous pregnancies of the patients, thus out of the group of 190 patients, 116 of them (61.05%) were multiparous and 74 (38.95%) were primiparous. Of the multiparous patients, in 14 patients (7.37% of the total) the samples collected showed contamination, and of the primiparous patients, in 2 of them (1.05% of the total) the samples were classified as contaminated. A statistically significant association was observed for sample contamination in multiparous versus primiparous patients ($p = 0.0456$) Figure 3.

3.2. Two of the Three Criteria Used

A total of 105 patients had placenta located in the anterior uterine wall; in 80 of them (76.19%) amniocentesis was performed using 21 G needles, and in 27 patients the sample was collected by punctioning across the placenta. In the other study participants, a number of 25 patients (23.81%), out of which in 7 cases the sample was collected through placental punctioning, the operation was performed with 20 G needles. Of the patients in whom 21 G needles were used for amniocentesis, in 13 patients (12.38% of all patients with anteriour placenta) the samples were contaminated. In none of the patients in whom amniotic sac puncture was performed using 20 G needles was there contamination of the samples. There was a statistically significant association between the use of a 21 G needle to perform amniocentesis and contamination of samples obtained from patients with previous placenta ($p = 0.0226$) Figure 4.

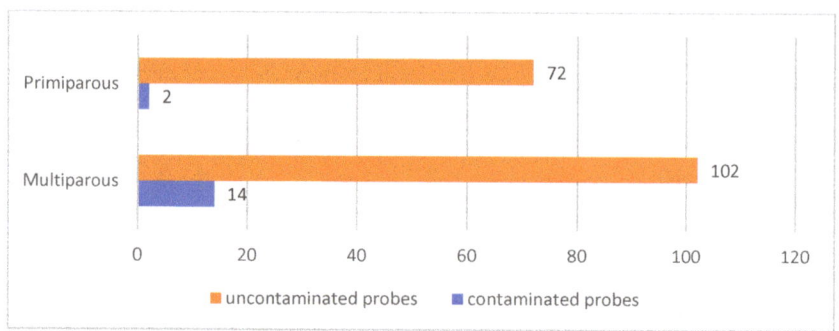

Figure 3. Number of contaminated versus uncontaminated samples according to vascularity during pregnancy (multiparous versus primiparous) regardless of needle gauge used.

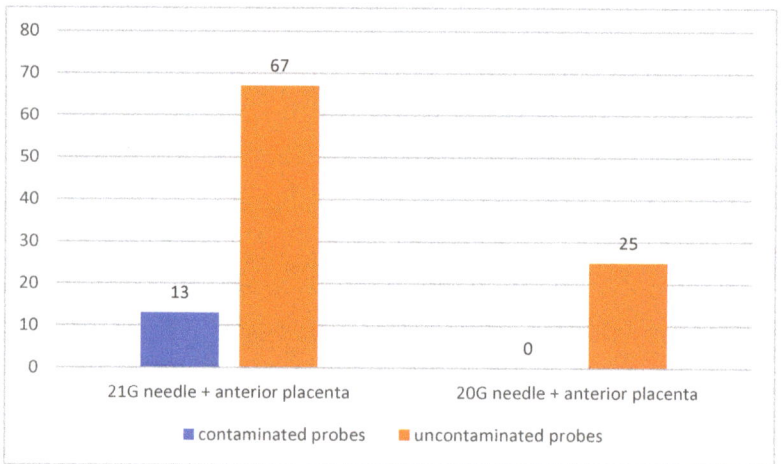

Figure 4. Sample contamination in patients with anteriorly located placenta correlated with the size of the needle used for sampling.

The correlation between patient parity and the size of the needle used to perform the maneuver was also analyzed. Out of the total 116 multiparous patients, in 74 of them (63.79%) amniocentesis was performed using a 21 G needle and in 42 of them (36.21%) a 20 G needle was used for the maneuver. Among the patients in whom 21 G needle was used for amniotic fluid collection, samples collected from 14 patients (12.07% of all multiparous patients) were contaminated, but there were no contaminated samples in patients in whom 20 G needle was used. There was a statistically significant association between the use of a 21 G needle for amniocentesis in multiparous patients and contamination of amniotic fluid samples ($p = 0.007$) Figure 5.

A correlation was also sought between the use of a 21 G needle and multiparity for amniocentesis. Thus, out of the total of 120 patients in whom a 21 G needle was used for amniocentesis, 74 (61.67%) were multiparous and 46 (38.33%) were primiparous. Of the multiparous patients, 14 patients (11.67% of the total number of patients who used a 21-gauge needle for amniocentesis) had contaminated samples, and of the primiparous patients, only two samples had maternal cell contamination (1.67% of the total number of patients who used a 21-gauge needle for amniocentesis). A statistically significant association was observed between the use of a 21 G needle for amniocentesis and contamination of samples collected from multiparous patients ($p = 0.0448$) Figure 6.

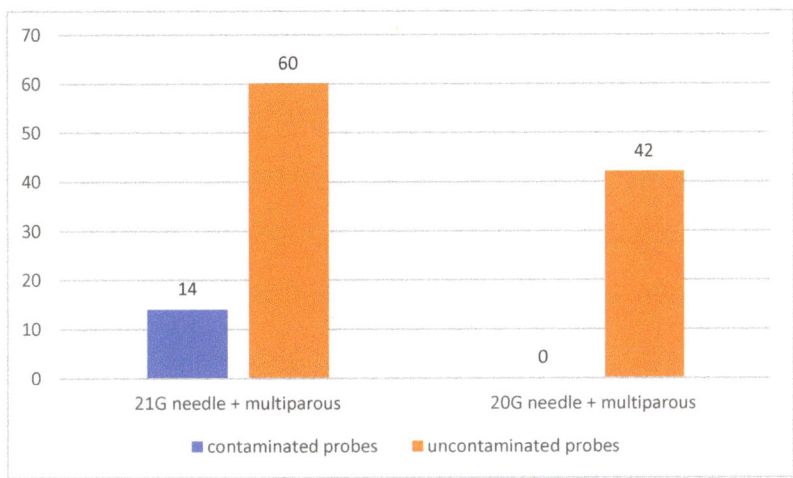

Figure 5. Contamination of samples based on multiparity and different gauge of needle used for collection.

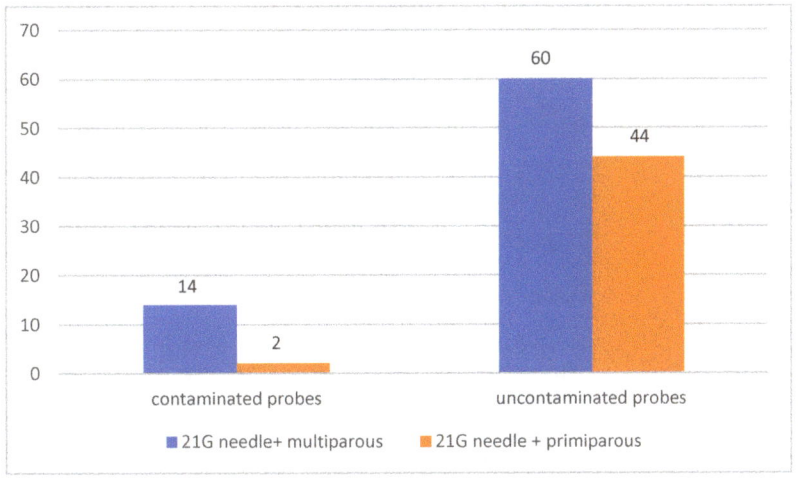

Figure 6. Sample contamination based on parity with 21 G needle.

In patients who met two of the three criteria established, correlations were also sought between anterior placental location and patient parity, placental location at the posterior uterine wall and multiparity or primiparity, multiparity and anterior or posterior placental location, and primiparity and anterior or posterior placental location, posterior location of the placenta and size of needle used for amniocentesis (20 G or 21 G), use of 21 G needle and location of the placenta in the anterior or posterior uterine wall, and primiparity of the patient and thickness of needle used (20 G or 21 G), with no statistically significant associations between these criteria.

3.3. All of the Three Criteria Used

The presence of a statistically significant association between the use of a 21 G needle in multiparous patients and the location of the placenta in the anterior uterine wall compared to the use of 20 G needles in primiparous patients and a location of the placenta in the posterior uterine wall was analyzed.

Out of the total of 49 multiparous patients with anterior placenta in whom amniotic sac puncture was performed using 21 G needles, in 23 patients the punction was realised across the placenta, and in 11 of them (22.45% of them) maternal cells were identified present in the collected samples. None of the samples collected from primiparous patients in whom the placenta was identified in the posterior uterine wall and a 20 G needle was used to puncture the amniotic sac showed contamination.

There was a statistically significant association between the use of a 21 G needle for amniocentesis in multiparous patients with anteriorly located placenta and contamination of amniotic puncture samples ($p = 0.0454$) Figure 7.

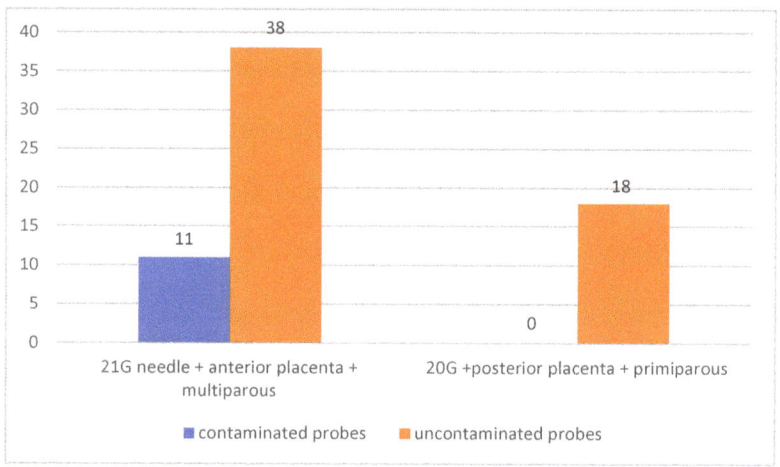

Figure 7. Contamination of samples according to the use of a 21 G needle in multiparous patients with placenta located at the anterior uterine wall compared to the use of 20 G needles in primiparous patients with placenta located at the posterior uterine wall.

For patients who met all three criteria, we also looked for correlations between the size of the needle used (20 G or 21 G), the anterior location of the placenta in multiparous patients, the size of the needle used (20 G or 21 G), the anterior location of the placenta in primiparous patients, the use of 21 G needles, the anterior location of the placenta and the parity of the patients, and the use of 21 G needles. Posterior location of the placenta and parity of the patients and correlations were also sought between needle size used for amniocentesis (21 G), parity (primiparous and multiparous) and anterior or posterior location of the placenta, but no statistically significant associations could be found to correlate these criteria with contamination of amniocentesis samples ($p > 0.05$). Using these conditions it was however observed that 21 G needles were used for all samples collected that showed contamination.

Further research was carried out to find ways in which the amniocentesis procedure could be improved to avoid contamination. Thus, the use of Doppler ultrasound during the maneuver was attempted and the data were then analyzed using the same statistical tests and reference intervals.

We looked for a difference between performing or not performing Doppler ultrasound and contamination of samples obtained from multiparous patients with placenta located in the anterior uterine wall and in whom 21 G needles were used for amniocentesis.

Of the total 49 multiparous patients with anterior placenta in whom 21 G needles were used for amniotic fluid collection, in 39 of them (79.59%) the collection was performed under Doppler ultrasonographic guidance and in 10 of them (20.41%) using only grayscale

(2 D) ultrasonography. Of the patients in whom Doppler ultrasonography was used, in two patients (4.08% of the total multiparous patients with anterior placenta in whom 21 needle was used for amniocentesis) maternal cells were identified in the samples collected. Of the patients in whom Doppler ultrasound was not used, nine patients (18.37% of all multiparous patients with previous placenta in whom a 21-gauge needle was used for amniocentesis) showed contamination in the samples collected.

There was a statistically significant association between the lack of contamination and the use of Doppler ultrasound in multiparous patients with anterior placenta in whom a 21-gauge needle was used for amniocentesis ($p < 0.0001$) Figure 8.

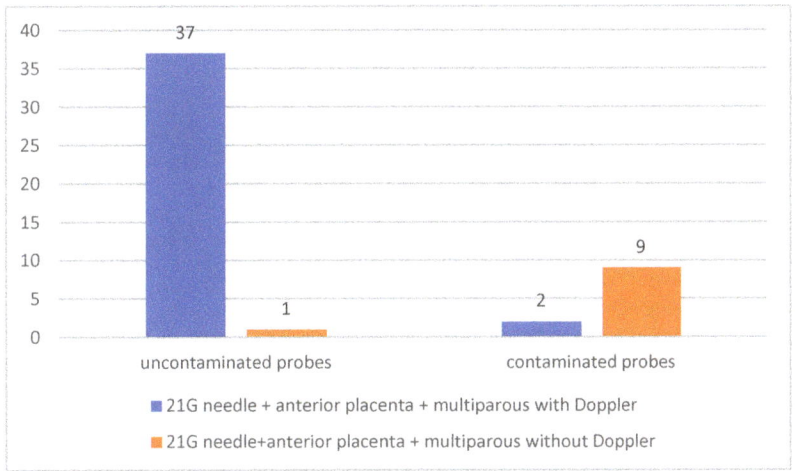

Figure 8. Use of Doppler ultrasound and reduction in contamination of samples collected using 21 G needles in multiparous patients with anteriorly located placenta.

This method has also been tested to improve amniocentesis performance using 21 G needles in primiparous patients with placenta located at the anterior uterine wall was also tested. Thus, out of a total of 31 primiparous patients with anterior placenta in whom 21 G needles were used for amniocentesis, Doppler ultrasound was performed in 27 of them (87.10%) and not in 4 of them (12.90%). None of the patients in whom Doppler ultrasound was used had contaminated samples, and of the patients in whom Doppler ultrasound was not used, two patients (6.45% of all primiparous patients with previous placenta in whom 21 G needle was used for amniocentesis) had contaminated samples.

There was a statistically significant association between lack of contamination and the use of Doppler ultrasound in primiparous patients with previous placenta in whom a 21-gauge needle was used for amniocentesis ($p = 0.0146$) Figure 9.

Comparative analysis of the group of patients with placenta located in the anterior uterine wall who underwent amniocentesis using 21 G size needles and Doppler ultrasound to perform amniocentesis showed that out of the total 66 patients, 39 of them (59.09%) were multiparous and 27 (40.91%) were primiparous. Among the multiparous patients, two patients (3.03% of those in whom previous placental location was detected in which 21 G needle was used for amniocentesis and Doppler ultrasound was used) had samples contaminated with maternal cells. None of the samples collected from primiparous patients were contaminated. No statistical significance was found ($p = 0.6$).

The reduction in contamination of samples collected during amniocentesis using 21 G needles and Doppler ultrasound was also analyzed for posterior placental location in both primiparous and multiparous patients.

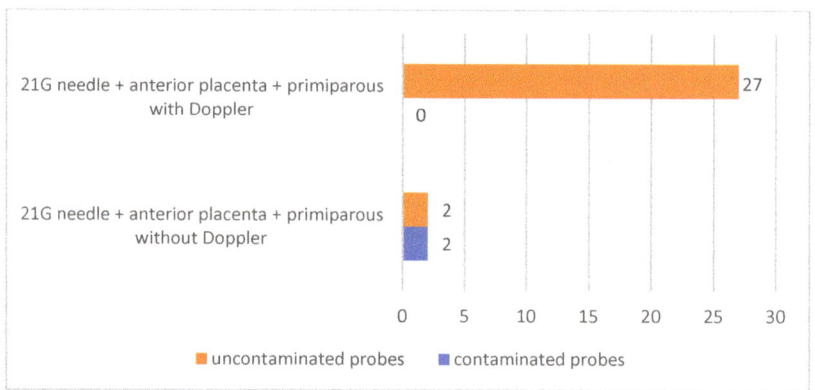

Figure 9. Association between lack of contamination of samples by performing amniocentesis using Doppler ultrasound.

Of the total 25 multiparous patients with posterior placenta in whom 21 G needles were used for amniocentesis, 18 of them (72.00%) benefited from the use of Doppler ultrasonography and in seven (28.00%) it was not used. None of the patients in whom Doppler ultrasound was performed had contaminated samples. Of the patients in whom Doppler ultrasound was not performed, in three patients (12.00% of the total of multiparous patients with posterior placenta in whom 21 needles were used for amniocentesis) the samples showed maternal cell contamination.

There was a statistically significant association between the lack of contamination of amniotic fluid samples collected and the use of Doppler ultrasound in multiparous patients with posterior placenta in whom a 21 G needle was used for amniocentesis ($p = 0.0152$) Figure 10.

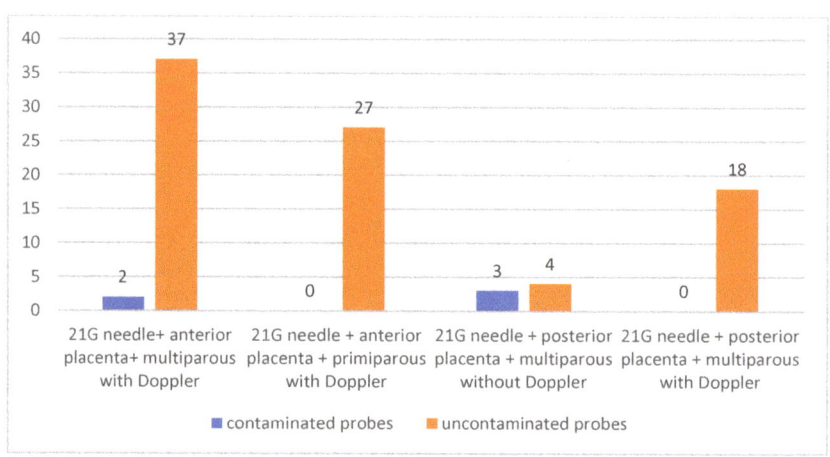

Figure 10. Reduction in contamination of amniocentesis samples using Doppler ultrasound.

The existence of statistically significant associations between the use of 21 G needles, placenta with posterior uterine wall insertion, primiparous patients, the existence of a difference between primiparous and multiparous patients, and the non-use of Doppler ultrasound during the maneuver was also investigated, without identifying the existence of statistically significant correlations.

Data and results from the present study are listed in Table 1.

Table 1. Study results. R_E—Exposed risk, R_N—unexposed risk, RR—relative risk.

Studied Criteria	Contaminated Probes	Uncontaminated Probes	p Value	R_E	R_N	RR
21 G Needle	16	104	0.0035	13.33	0	-
20 G Needle	0	70				
Multiparous	14	102	0.0456	12.07	2.703	4.466
Primiparous	2	72				
21 G needle + anterior placenta	13	67	0.0226	16.25	0	-
20 G needle + anterior placenta	0	25				
21 G needle + multiparous	14	60	0.007	18.92	0	-
20 G needle + multiparous	0	42				
21 G needle + multiparous	14	60	0.0448	18.92	4.348	4.351
21 G needle + primiparous	2	44				
21 G needle + anterior placenta + multiparous	11	38	0.0454	22.45	0	-
20 G needle + posterior placenta + primiparous	0	18				
21 G needle + anterior placenta + multiparous with Doppler	37	2	<0.0001	94.87	10	9.487
21 G needle + anterior placenta + multiparous without Doppler	1	9				
21 G needle + anterior placenta + primiparous with Doppler	27	0	0.0146	100	50	2
21 G needle + anterior placenta + primiparous without Doppler	2	2				
21 G needle + anterior placenta + multiparous with Doppler	2	37	0.6909	5.128	0	-
21 G needle + anterior placenta + primiparous with Doppler	0	27				
21 G needle + posterior placenta + multiparous without Doppler	3	4	0.0152	42.86	0	-
21 G needle + postrerior placenta + multiparous with Doppler	0	18				

4. Discussion

Amniocentesis is currently the most widely used antenatal diagnostic method. Over time, the way of performing the maneuver has been improved in order to reduce the risks associated with amniotic sac puncture, but these risks, although considered minimal, must be known by the couple undergoing such a procedure [3,6]. Amniocentesis is a minor surgical procedure, usually performed in the second trimester of pregnancy to ensure that an optimal number of fetal cells are extracted from the amniotic fluid [1,15]. Amniocentesis is associated with higher rates of successful, clear taps, and lower rates of bloody taps (reduced from 2.4% to 0.8%) when performed under direct ultrasound control with continuous needle tip visualization. Best practice is that ultrasound scanning during the procedure be performed by the person inserting the needle [18]. When we also utilize the Doppler function, we enhance the safety of the maneuver, taking into account the added possibility of visualization of increased flow through some parts of the placenta, which can then be avoided. This is one of the major advantages of the Doppler feature. Additional advantage consists of avoiding a major complication, specifically puncturing the umbilical cord, which is certainly better visualized through Doppler examination, precisely useful in oligohydramnios situations where the cord has less freedom of motion. One of the ways to evaluate the success of this procedure is by assessing the postprocedural abortion rate which reaches 0.6% for ultrasound-guided maneuvers. Another criterion used to assess the success of the procedure is the quality of the specimen extracted, as contamination with maternal cells can lead to diagnostic errors [15,16].

Most studies in the literature have focused on how to perform amniocentesis in order to reduce the risks associated with the maneuver and very few studies have focused on the association between the size of needles used to perform amniotic sac puncture and the occurrence of complications. In this direction, the aim of our study was to identify the increased risk of specimen contamination taking into account both maternal factors (placental location, parity) and extrinsic factors (instruments used to perform the procedure, more specifically the size of needles used to perform amniocentesis). At the same time, a method to reduce the risk of contamination of the samples by using Doppler examination during the procedure was analyzed. Current research results show a significant association between maternal cell contamination of amniotic fluid samples collected during amniocentesis and the use of fine needles of smaller diameter (21 G). This finding is supported by two studies: the first one was published by Peter A. Benn and Lillian Y.F. Hsu [17] and identified a higher rate of contamination of samples obtained after puncture of the amniotic sac using needles larger than 20 G, and the second one was conducted by Apostolos P., Athanasiadis et al. [20] who demonstrate that the use of smaller needle diameters (22 G) causes greater trauma to tissues during amniocentesis, primarily through the longer duration of the amniotic fluid aspiration process. At the same time, the present study identified a higher risk of contamination associated with the use of small puncture needles (21 G), regardless of the patient's parity (primiparous or multiparous). The use of larger gauge needles (20 G) shortens the time to perform the procedure, but is associated with a higher rate of amniotic fluid leakage postprocedurally [21]. This hypothesis is demonstrated through an experimental study design by Devlieger R et al. who tested amniotic fluid leakage in patients undergoing Caesarean section at term [22].

There are conflicting data in the literature regarding the increased risk of contamination associated with placental location at the uterine cavity walls. The findings of the study led by Hockstein et al. [23] show a lack of association between the risk of contamination of collected amniotic fluid samples and placental location in the uterine cavity. In contrast, research by Nub et al. [16] found a significantly higher rate of maternal cells in samples collected from patients with placenta located in the anterior uterine wall. This hypothesis is also supported by the studies performed by Pergamentet al. [23] and Giorlandino C et al. [24]. They concluded that the frequency of contaminated samples was higher in three different situations: when the collection was performed transplacentally, when more punctures of the amniotic sac were required for collection, and when the maneuver was performed by a less experienced physician [25]. The present study shows a significant association between the amniotic fluid contamination and the anterior location of the placenta, thus an increased rate of contamination in association with transplacental amniotic fluid collection. The risk of contamination is further increased by two factors: when the placenta is located on the anterior wall and when the amniotic fluid extraction is performed using small (21 G) needles. Apostolos P. Athanasiadis et al. [20] and Uludag S [26] supported the hypothesis in which the use of 20 G needles for amniocentesis reduces intrauterine bleeding and therefore amniotic fluid contamination.

Another risk factor for samples contamination is the parity of patients, showing a significant association between multiparity and frequency of contamination.

In this research the usefulness of Doppler ultrasound during amniocentesis was investigated, demonstrating a reduction in contamination through its use. This hypothesis is in addition to Jennifer Weida et al. [15] and Benn et al. [17] studies that showed a significant 2.5-fold reduction in the frequency of contamination after removal of the first 1–2 mL of aspirated amniotic fluid.

One of the strengths of the present study is the large number of patients included in the study, with 190 patients undergoing invasive genetic testing. Also, the analysis of the contaminated samples with maternal cells taking into account all the criteria, considering the fact that the literature data analyses the factors separately, is another strength of the current research. Data from the present study show a significant reduction in the risk of contamination while using Doppler ultrasound for identifying uteroplacental circulation during amniocentesis, regardless of the size of the needle used to perform the puncture.

The present study has some limitations, among which we mention the impossibility to quantify the degree of contamination of the samples in order to assess the risk of false positive or negative results. Also, the existence of a correlation between the size of the needle used to perform the maneuver and the number of maternal cells identified in the sample analyzed was not possible.

5. Conclusions

There is an increased rate of sample contamination (statistically significant) when using 21 G needle sizes and a significant difference in contamination between primiparous and multiparous patients, with contamination being more frequent in multiparous patients. There was a significantly higher rate of contamination of samples associated with amniotic sac puncture using 21 G needles, as opposed to the contamination rate observed when larger gauge needles (20 G) were used. The contamination rate was significantly higher in multiparous patients when 21 G needles were used. In multiparous patients, contamination of collected samples is more frequent when 21 G needles are used for maneuvering.

A higher rate of contamination is observed in multiparous patients with a previously located placenta in whom 21 G needles were used to collect amniotic fluid for prenatal diagnosis.

The use of Doppler ultrasonography clearly benefits the procedure, as the contamination rate was significantly reduced when used during amniocentesis regardless of the factors favoring contamination present. Thus, it is our strong belief that only Doppler ultrasound should accompany amniocentesis procedures. This hypothesis should open opportunities for future research into the usefulness of Doppler studies during invasive diagnostic maneuvers.

Author Contributions: Conceptualization, R.C. and D.M.; methodology, A.M.M. and C.B.; software, C.M.O.; validation, R.C., C.E.B. and C.M.O.; formal analysis, M.P.R.; investigation, R.C.; resources, R.C.; data curation, C.E.B.; writing—original draft preparation, C.M.O.; writing—review and editing, C.M.O.; visualization, D.M. and C.B.; supervision, R.C.; project administration, R.C.; funding acquisition, R.C. All authors have read and agreed to the published version of the manuscript.

Funding: This research received no external funding.

Institutional Review Board Statement: The study was conducted in accordance with the Declaration of Helsinki, and approved by Ethics Commission of the University of Medicine and Pharmacy "Iuliu Hațieganu" Cluj Napoca (73/22.03.2016).

Informed Consent Statement: Informed consent was obtained from all subjects involved in the study.

Data Availability Statement: Not applicable.

Conflicts of Interest: The authors declare no conflict of interest.

References

1. Jummaat, F.; Ahmad, S.; Ismail, N.A.M. 5-Year review on amniocentesis and its maternal fetal complications. *Horm. Mol. Biol. Clin. Investig.* **2019**, *40*, 20190006. [CrossRef] [PubMed]
2. Ghi, T.; Sotiriadis, A.; Calda, P.; Costa, F.D.S.; Raine-Fenning, N.; Alfirevic, Z.; McGillivray, G. International Society of Ultrasound in Obstetrics and Gynecology (ISUOG) ISUOG Practice Guidelines: Invasive procedures for prenatal diagnosis. *Ultrasound Obstet. Gynecol.* **2016**, *48*, 256–268. [CrossRef] [PubMed]
3. Anandakumar, C.; Wong, Y.C.; Annapoorna, V.; Arulkumaran, S.; Chia, D.; Bongso, A.; Ratnam, S.S. Amniocentesis and Its Complications. *Aust. New Zealand J. Obstet. Gynaecol.* **1992**, *32*, 97–99. [CrossRef] [PubMed]
4. Carlson, L.M.; Vora, N.L. Prenatal Diagnosis: Screening and Diagnostic Tools. *Obstet. Gynecol. Clin. N. Am.* **2017**, *44*, 245–256. [CrossRef] [PubMed]
5. Goto, M.; Nakamura, M.; Takita, H.; Sekizawa, A. Study for risks of amniocentesis in anterior placenta compared to placenta of other locations. *Taiwan J. Obstet. Gynecol.* **2021**, *60*, 690–694. [CrossRef]
6. Seeds, J.W. Diagnostic mid trimester amniocentesis: How safe? *Am. J. Obstet. Gynecol.* **2004**, *191*, 607–615. [CrossRef]
7. Benn, P.; Borrell, A.; Cuckle, H.; Dugoff, L.; Gross, S.; Johnson, J.-A.; Maymon, R.; Odibo, A.; Schielen, P.; Spencer, K.; et al. Prenatal Detection of Down Syndrome using Massively Parallel Sequencing (MPS): A rapid response statement from a committee on behalf of the Board of the International Society for Prenatal Diagnosis, 24 October 2011. *Prenat. Diagn.* **2012**, *32*, 1–2. [CrossRef]

8. Gregg, A.R.; Gross, S.; Best, R.; Monaghan, K.; Bajaj, K.; Skotko, B.; Thompson, B.; Watson, M. ACMG statement on noninvasive prenatal screening for fetal aneuploidy. *Anesth. Analg.* **2013**, *15*, 395–398. [CrossRef]
9. Langlois, S.; Brock, J.-A.; Wilson, R.D.; Audibert, F.; Carroll, J.; Cartier, L.; Gagnon, A.; Johnson, J.-A.; MacDonald, W.; Murphy-Kaulbeck, L.; et al. RETIRED: Current Status in Non-Invasive Prenatal Detection of Down Syndrome, Trisomy 18, and Trisomy 13 Using Cell-Free DNA in Maternal Plasma. *J. Obstet. Gynaecol. Can.* **2013**, *35*, 177–181. [CrossRef] [PubMed]
10. Royal College of Obstetricians & Gynaecologists. Non-invasive Prenatal Testing for Chromosomal Abnormality using Maternal Plasma DNA. *RCOG Sci. Impact Pap.* **2014**, *15*, 1–14.
11. Taglauer, E.; Wilkins-Haug, L.; Bianchi, D. Review: Cell-free fetal DNA in the maternal circulation as an indication of placental health and disease. *Placenta* **2014**, *35*, S64–S68. [CrossRef] [PubMed]
12. Bianchi, D.W.; Platt, L.D.; Goldberg, J.D.; Abuhamad, A.Z.; Sehnert, A.J.; Rava, R.P. Genome-Wide Fetal Aneuploidy Detection by Maternal Plasma DNA Sequencing. *Obstet. Gynecol.* **2012**, *119*, 890–901. [CrossRef] [PubMed]
13. Dondorp, W.; De Wert, G.; Bombard, Y.; Bianchi, D.W.; Bergmann, C.; Borry, P.; Chitty, L.S.; Fellmann, F.; Forzano, F.; Hall, A.; et al. Non-invasive prenatal testing for aneuploidy and beyond: Challenges of responsible innovation in prenatal screening. Summary and recommendations. *Eur. J. Hum. Genet.* **2015**, *23*, 1438–1450. [CrossRef] [PubMed]
14. Srouji, S.S.; Carr, D.B.; Gardella, C.M.; Benedetti, T.; Tait, J.F. The Effect of Common Clinical Contaminants on Amniotic Fluid Fluorescence Polarization Results. *Obstet. Gynecol.* **2004**, *104*, 1237–1243. [CrossRef]
15. Weida, J.; Patil, A.S.; Schubert, F.P.; Vance, G.; Drendel, H.; Reese, A.; Dlouhy, S.; Bai, S.; Lee, M.J. Prevalence of maternal cell contamination in amniotic fluid samples. *J. Matern. Neonatal Med.* **2017**, *30*, 2133–2137. [CrossRef] [PubMed]
16. Nufl, S.; Brebaum, D.; Grond-Ginsbach, C. Maternal cell contamination in amniotic fluid samples as a consequence of the sampling technique. *Hum. Genet.* **1994**, *93*, 121–124.
17. Benn, P.A.; Hsu, L.Y.F.; Karp, L.E. Maternal cell contamination of amniotic fluid cell cultures: Results of a U.S. nationwide survey. *Am. J. Med. Genet.* **1983**, *15*, 297–305. [CrossRef]
18. Alfirevic, Z.; Navaratnam, K.; Mujezinovic, F. Amniocentesis and chorionic villus sampling for prenatal diagnosis. *Cochrane Database Syst. Rev.* **2017**, *2017*, CD003252. [CrossRef]
19. Buchovecky, C.M.; Nahum, O.; Levy, B. Assessment of Maternal Cell Contamination in Prenatal Samples by Quantitative Fluorescent PCR (QF-PCR). *Methods Mol. Biol.* **2019**, *1885*, 117–127. [CrossRef]
20. Athanasiadis, A.P.; Pantazis, K.; Goulis, D.G.; Chatzigeorgiou, K.; Vaitsi, V.; Assimakopoulos, E.; Tzevelekis, F.; Tsalikis, T.; Bontis, J.N. Comparison between 20G and 22G needle for second trimester amniocentesis in terms of technical aspects and short-term complications. *Prenat. Diagn.* **2009**, *29*, 761–765. [CrossRef]
21. Daum, H.; Ben David, A.; Nadjari, M.; Zenvirt, S.; Helman, S.; Yanai, N.; Meiner, V.; Yagel, S.; Frumkin, A.; Rafid, S.S.; et al. Role of late amniocentesis in the era of modern genomic technologies. *Ultrasound Obstet. Gynecol.* **2019**, *53*, 676–685. [CrossRef]
22. Devlieger, R.; Gratacos, E.; Ardon, H.; Vanstraelen, S.; Deprest, J. Factors influencing the flow rate through a surgical defect in human fetal membranes. *Prenat. Diagn.* **2002**, *22*, 201–205. [CrossRef] [PubMed]
23. Hockstein, S.; Chen, P.X.; Thangavelu, M.; Pergament, E. Factors Associated With Maternal Cell Contamination in Amniocentesis Samples as Evaluated by Fluorescent In Situ Hybridization. *Obstet. Gynecol.* **1998**, *92*, 551–556. [CrossRef] [PubMed]
24. Giorlandino, C.; Gambuzza, G.; D'Alessio, P.; Santoro, M.L.; Gentili, P.; Vizzone, A. Blood contamination of amniotic fluid after amniocentesis in relation to placental location. *Prenat. Diagn.* **1996**, *16*, 180–182. [CrossRef]
25. Welch, R.A.; Salem-Elgharib, S.; Wiktor, A.E.; Van Dyke, D.L.; Blessed, W.B. Operator experience and sample quality in genetic amniocentesis. *Am. J. Obstet. Gynecol.* **2006**, *194*, 189–191. [CrossRef]
26. Uludag, S.; Aydin, Y.; Ibrahimova, F.; Madazli, R.; Sen, C. Comparison of complications in second trimester amniocentesis performed with 20G, 21G and 22G needles. *J. Périnat. Med.* **2010**, *38*, 597–600. [CrossRef]

Disclaimer/Publisher's Note: The statements, opinions and data contained in all publications are solely those of the individual author(s) and contributor(s) and not of MDPI and/or the editor(s). MDPI and/or the editor(s) disclaim responsibility for any injury to people or property resulting from any ideas, methods, instructions or products referred to in the content.

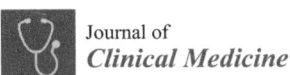

Case Report

Fetal Brain Tumors, a Challenge in Prenatal Diagnosis, Counselling, and Therapy

Ivonne Alexandra Bedei [1,2], Thierry A. G. M. Huisman [3], William Whitehead [4], Roland Axt-Fliedner [1], Michael Belfort [5] and Magdalena Sanz Cortes [2,*]

1 Department of Prenatal Diagnosis and Fetal Therapy, Justus-Liebig University Giessen, 35392 Giessen, Germany
2 Division of Fetal Therapy and Surgery, Department of Obstetrics and Gynecology, Texas Children's Hospital Fetal Center, Baylor College of Medicine, Houston, TX 77030, USA
3 Edward B. Singleton Department of Radiology, Texas Children's Hospital, Baylor College of Medicine, Houston, TX 77030, USA
4 Department of Neurosurgery, Baylor College of Medicine, Houston, TX 77030, USA
5 Department of Obstetrics and Gynecology, Texas Children's Hospital Pavilion for Women, Baylor College of Medicine, Houston, TX 77030, USA
* Correspondence: magdalena.sanzcortes@bcm.edu

Abstract: Fetal brain tumors are a rare entity with an overall guarded prognosis. About 10% of congenital brain tumors are diagnosed during fetal life. They differ from the postnatally encountered pediatric brain tumors with respect to location and tumor type. Fetal brain tumors can be benign or malignant and infiltrate or displace adjacent brain structures. Due to their high mitotic rate, they can show rapid growth. Outcome depends on age of diagnosis, size, and histological tumor type. Findings like polyhydramnios and macrocephaly encountered on routine ultrasound are frequently associated. Detailed prenatal anomaly scan and subsequent fetal magnetic resonance imaging (MRI) may identify the brain tumor and its severity. Both maternal and fetal prognosis should be included in prenatal counselling and decision making.

Keywords: fetal brain tumor; macrocephaly; teratoma; hydrocephalus; prenatal imaging

1. Introduction

Fetal brain tumors (FBT) are very rare. They occur in 0.34/1,000,000 live births and account for 10% of all antenatal tumors [1–5]. About 10% of congenital brain tumors are diagnosed during fetal life [4,6]. In comparison to tumors appearing in the pediatric population, they differ in location, histological type, clinical behavior and prognosis [1,4,5,7,8]. Whereas pediatric tumors are mostly infratentorial, FBTs originate typically in the supratentorial region [1,3,9]. Teratomas are the most frequently encountered intracranial tumors in the prenatal period, occurring in about half of the reported cases, in contrast to pilocytic astrocytomas, malignant gliomas and medulloblastoma which are typically found in the pediatric age group [1,3,9–12].

Depending on the tumor type, diagnosis is usually made in the late second or third trimester [2,3,10]. Intraparenchymal tumors like teratomas, gliomas and embryonal tumors are often characterized by their rapid growth and infiltration of the surrounding brain tissue [7]. Fetal brain tumors most often occur in isolation but can be part of a genetic/tumor predisposition syndrome like Gorlin syndrome (medulloblastoma), Li-Fraumeni syndrome (glioblastoma), Pallister Hall syndrome (hypothalamic hamartoma), neurofibromatosis (astrocytoma) or Rhabdoid predisposition syndrome (ATRT, medulloblastoma, choroid plexus tumors and former PNET) [7,13]. Prognosis is generally poor with a postnatal survival rate varying between 16% and 28% [1,2,9]. Outcome depends on the tumor histological type, growth behavior and the timing of occurrence/diagnosis relative to the gestational age [9]. Limited by the fact that definitive histopathological confirmation is only made after birth, prenatal counselling is difficult and relies on prenatal imaging, combining detailed ultrasound (US) and complementary Magnetic Resonance Imaging (MRI) as well as multiple biometric and clinical parameters. MRI helps to confirm and refine diagnosis and adds valuable predictive information about outcome. Counselling should be multidisciplinary and include both, fetal prognosis, and possible maternal complications.

2. Case Series

We present four fetuses with matching prenatal US and MRI diagnosis of FBTs presenting at our high complexity tertiary referral center between 2011–2019. Goal of this case series is to familiarize physicians with the various primary brain tumors that can be encountered on prenatal imaging and the respective value of US and MRI to narrow down differential diagnosis.

Case 1: A 35-year-old G1P1 was diagnosed at 18 weeks and 6 days gestational age with a fetal brain mass of unclear etiology at her referring institution. Outside fetal MRI showed a 2.5 × 4.2 × 3.9 cm suprasellar, predominantly solid, partially cystic midline mass lesion elevating the floor of the third ventricle, high grade compression and displacement of the mesencephalon and brainstem with resultant supratentorial ventriculomegaly and macrocephaly (Figure 1A,B).

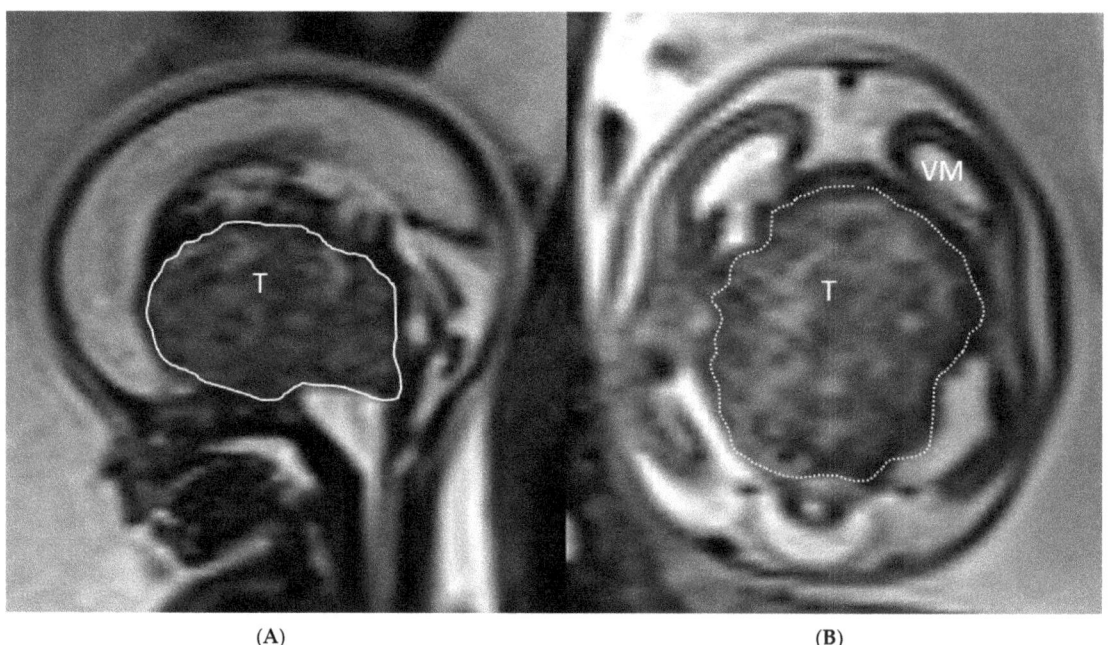

(A) (B)

Figure 1. (A,B): Ultrafast T2-weighted fetal MR image showing a 3.9 cm suprasellar mixed solid-cystic, suprasellar mass lesion compressing the brainstem (BS), mesencephalon (M) and elevating and compressing the third ventricle with resultant supratentorial ventriculomegaly (VM). Imaging characteristics most compatible with a teratoma (T).

Follow-up ultrasound at 20 weeks and one day showed a rapid enlargement in the predominantly solid component of the intracranial mass, measuring 5 cm × 6.3 cm × 7 cm, macrocephaly with a head circumference (HC) of 285 mm (>5SD above the mean) and polyhydramnios (amniotic fluid index, AFI: 26 cm) (Figure 2A,B).

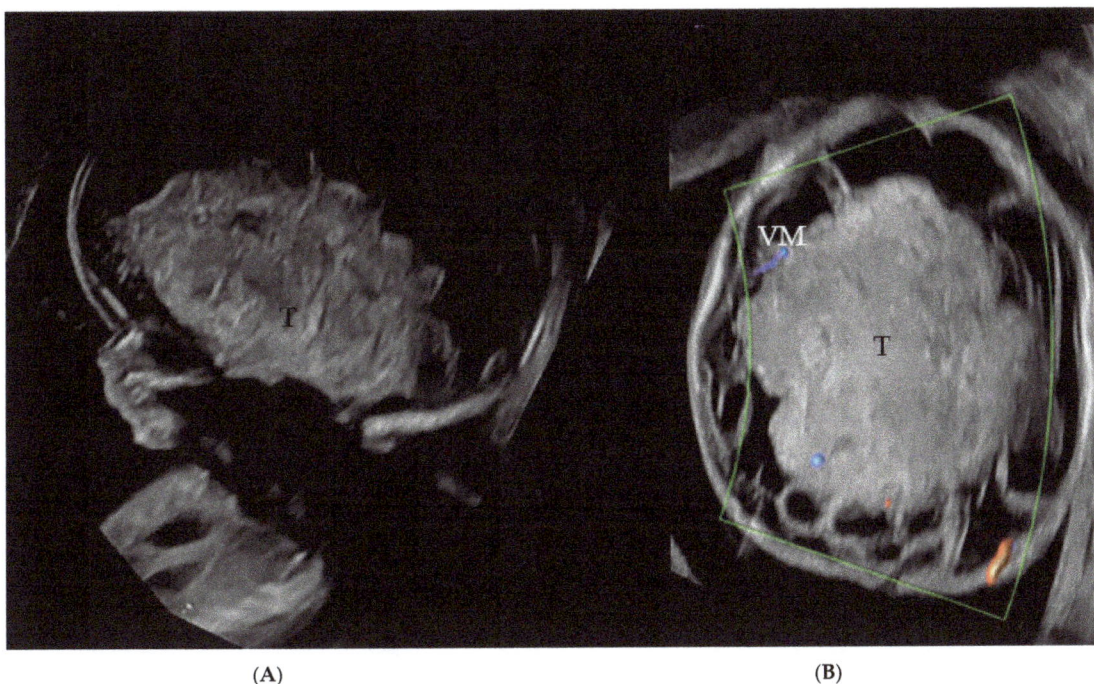

(A)　　　　　　　　　　　　　　　　　　(B)

Figure 2. (**A**,**B**): US showing a 5 × 6.3 × 7 cm predominantly hyperechogenic solid midline mass lesion, centered in the suprasellar region (T). High grade supratentorial ventriculomegaly (VM) is noted.

Prominent arterial feeders originating from the middle cerebral artery (MCA) were noted. The MCA peak systolic velocity was >2 MoM (multiple of the median) suggesting a high cardiac output status or fetal anemia. Cardiothoracic ratio was normal. There were no signs of fetal hydrops. Based on the imaging characteristics a germ cell tumor, e.g., teratoma was considered the most likely diagnosis. The parents received extensive multidisciplinary counselling on fetal prognosis and potential maternal complications, mostly due to the large head size. They opted for palliative/comfort care at delivery. Pregnancy was complicated by a preterm premature rupture of membranes (PPROM) with subsequent delivery at 25 weeks outside of our institution. The newborn died at 1 h of life. Histopathological results and mode of delivery are unfortunately unavailable.

Case 2: A 17-year-old G1P0 was referred at 35 weeks and 5 days of gestation to our institution. Ultrasound showed a highly perfused mass lesion located in the posterior fossa associated with hydrocephalus, macrocephaly (HC 366.3 mm, >5 SD above the mean) and mildly increased amniotic fluid volume (AFI 23 cm). On fetal MRI, a well perfused posterior fossa infratentorial mixed solid and cystic mass lesion was seen associated with moderate to marked supratentorial hydrocephalus. Cystic elements of the lesion were seen herniating through the tentorial incisura into the supratentorial compartment. Diffusion weighted imaging (DWI) showed restricted diffusion within the solid tumor component, which could be indicative of a medulloblastoma versus an atypical terato-rhabdoid tumor (ATRT) (Figure 3A–D).

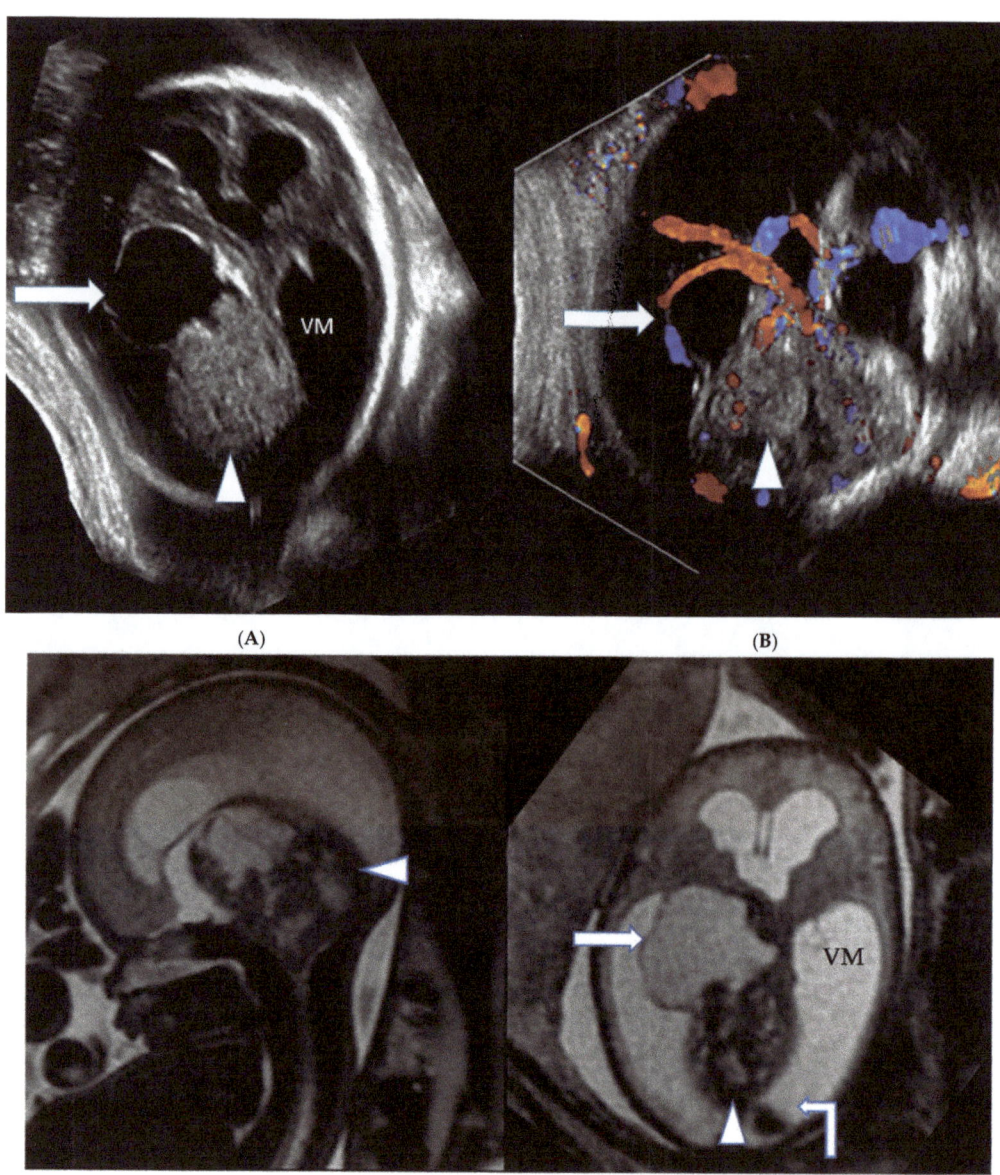

Figure 3. (**A**,**B**): Gray scale and color-coded Doppler sonography US shows a large heterogeneous hyperechogenic solid (arrowhead), partially hypoechogenic cystic (arrow) mass lesion filling out the posterior fossa with compression of the brainstem, cerebellum and vermis. A cystic component herniates through the tentorial incisura into the supratentorial left lateral ventricle. The lesion appears well perfused on Doppler ultrasound. (**C**,**D**): Matching T2-weighted fetal MRI confirms the large posterior fossa mass lesion (arrowhead) with resultant high grade supratentorial ventriculomegaly (VM). A large compared to the cerebrospinal fluid slightly T2-hypointense cyst extends into the left lateral ventricle indicating a higher protein content, possibly hemorrhage within the cyst (arrow). A blood-cerebro-spinal fluid level is noted in the right lateral ventricle (angeled arrow).

Patient delivered two weeks later (38 weeks) by cesarean section after PROM. A male newborn, with a weight of 3090 g and Apgar scores of 5 and 6 at respectively 1 and 5 min of life was admitted to our neonatal intensive care unit (NICU). MRI performed on the first day of life showed a 50% increase in tumor size, measuring 7 cm in maximal diameter, compressing, and infiltrating nearly the complete cerebellum and vermis as well as much of the midbrain structures. High grade obstructive supratentorial ventriculomegaly with a cystic intraventricular tumor component was again observed. The cystic component appeared T1-hyperintense indicating the high proteinaceous content. The solid tumor component showed multiple serpiginous flow-related signal voids (Figure 4A–C).

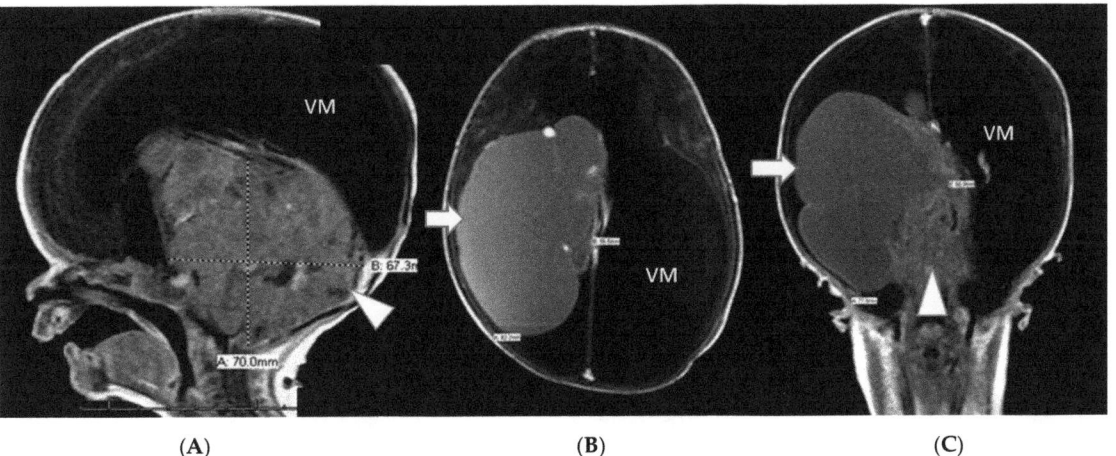

Figure 4. (A–C): Postnatal sagittal, axial and coronal T1-weighted contrast enhanced MRI showing an interval progression in tumor size in comparison to prenatal images, measuring 7 cm in diameter with near complete compression and infiltration of the cerebellum and brainstem (arrowhead). Large supratentorial, intraventricular protein rich tumor cyst similar to the prenatal imaging (arrow). Ventriculomegaly (VM).

After multiple multidisciplinary discussions, it was determined that the tumor was inoperable, and parents opted for comfort care. Baby died on the second day of life from respiratory insufficiency. Parents declined autopsy.

Case 3: A 35-year-old G3P2 pregnant patient was referred to our institution because of a suspected fetal brain tumor at 38 weeks of gestation after initial suspicion for this diagnosis at 34 weeks. Ultrasound and fetal MRI at referral revealed a well circumscribed T2-hypointense solid cortical/subcortical lesion in the left occipital lobe measuring 4.3 × 2.9 × 3.1 cm (Figure 5A,B), which appeared larger than on the imaging performed four weeks earlier.

The lesion exerted mild local mass effect on the left occipital horn without midline shift or hydrocephalus. On US, the lesion was mildly heterogeneously hyperechogenic and presented with an asymmetrically increased arterial flow in the left common carotid, middle cerebral and posterior cerebral arteries. There was no evidence for associated hemorrhage. Polyhydramnios was not observed. A neuroglial tumor with the differential diagnosis of cortical dysplasia was suspected. A female newborn was delivered via elective C-section. MRI and computer tomography (CT) scan performed on day one of life showed a 4.7 cm × 3 mm × 3.5 cm mass lesion in the left occipital lobe with T2-hypointense susceptibility related signal loss due to areas of microcalcification (Figure 6A–C).

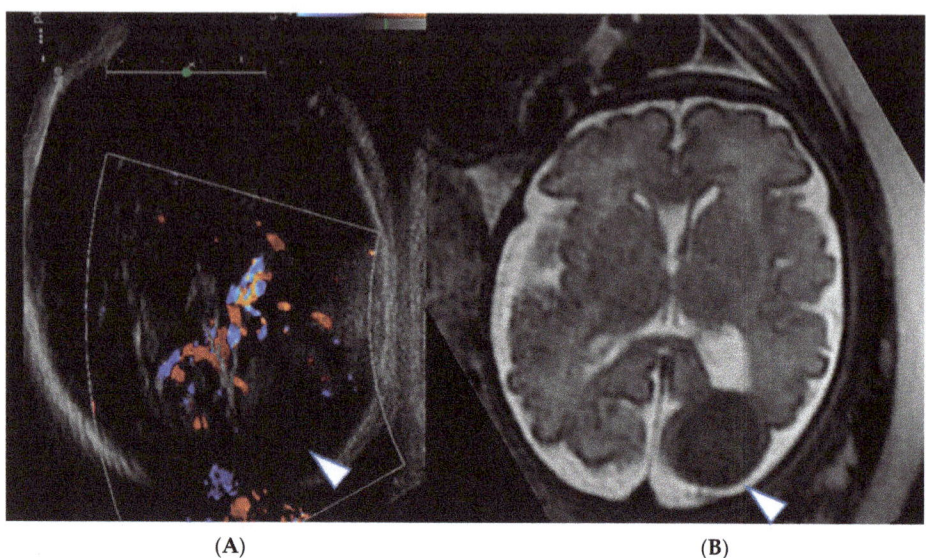

Figure 5. (**A,B**): Prenatal color coded axial US image and matching T2-weighted fetal MRI show a solid cortical/subcortical well circumscribed mass lesion within the left occipital lobe (arrowhead).

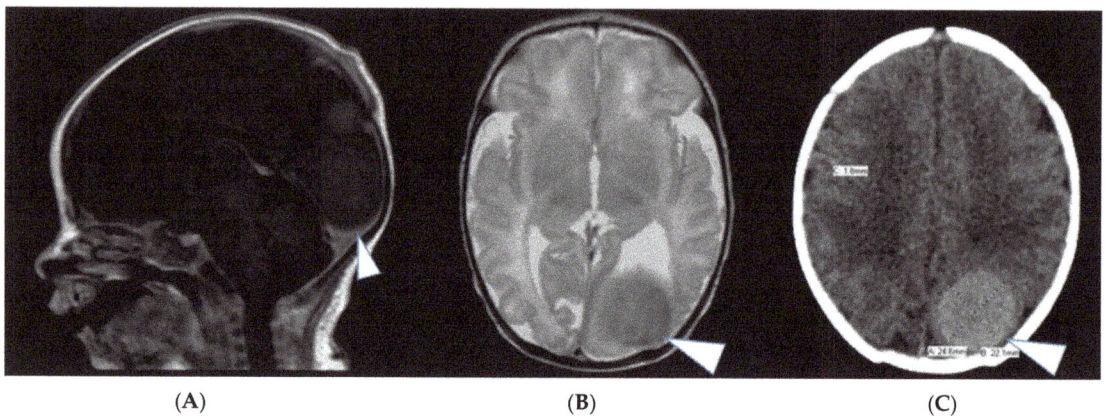

Figure 6. (**A–C**): Matching contrast enhanced sagittal contrast enhanced T1-weighted, axial T2-weighted and axial CT images confirm the left occipital lobe highly cellular (T2-hypointense), non-enhancing mass lesion with mild hyperdensity due to the high cellularity compatible with a neuroglial tumor (arrowhead).

Resection was performed on day 5 of life, followed by chemotherapy. Histopathology demonstrated a glioneural tumor with varying histomorphologies and anaplastic features. The patient successfully completed 12 months of chemotherapy with Cytoxan, Carboplatin, Etoposide and Vincristine following an individualized protocol. She is now 10 years old without tumor recurrence. Neuro-oncology follow-up was discontinued after 7 years without recurrence of disease. She is meeting normal neurodevelopment milestones.

Case 4: A 26 years old G2P1 patient presented at 28 weeks for further diagnostic work-up for ventriculomegaly in twin B in a dichorionic diamniotic twin pregnancy. Ultrasound at 31 weeks and 1 day showed a complex cystic-solid mass lesion in the left frontal lobe measuring 33 × 34 × 38 mm surrounded by echogenic brain parenchyma. Additionally, irregular echogenic borders of the third ventricle and lateral ventricles were observed suggesting intraventricular hemorrhage (Figure 7A). HC was within the normal range (73rd percentile), bilateral ventriculomegaly was noted (left and right atrial width measured 18 mm and 11 mm, respectively) (Figure 7A–C). Fetal MRI showed a heterogenous mass lesion predominately located within the left frontal lobe, containing a solid component with internal vascularity as well as a large hemorrhagic component. (Figure 7D). Image findings were considered most consistent with ATRT. Cesarean delivery was performed at 35.6 weeks because of preterm labor and the transverse position of twin B. Twin B, a female newborn with 2330 gr and Apgar score 8/8 at, respectively 1 and 5 min was delivered and transferred to the NICU on CPAP after delivery. MRI at the same day showed interval enlargement (5.6 cm × 6.5 cm × 4.7cm) of the left frontal lobe cystic-solid mass lesion extending into the suprasellar cisterna and ventricular system (Figure 7E). Multifocal hemorrhagic products with intralesional susceptibility effects were seen, the solid component of the tumor showed restricted diffusion and enhancement. The lesion was inseparable from the optic chiasm, optic nerves, and pituitary stalk. It incased the bilateral supraclinoid internal carotid arteries (ICAs), bilateral anterior cerebral arteries (ACAs), right proximal middle cerebral artery (MCA), distal basilar artery, and its branches. Biopsy and partial tumor resection were performed on day 5 of life, which confirmed an ATRT, WHO grade IV with heterogenic staining of the INI1 marker. Whole exome sequencing (WES) studies was negative for any known deleterious mutation. In the light of the very guarded prognosis and difficulties for radical neurosurgical tumor resection secondary to the encasement of much of the circle of Willis, parents opted for palliative care. The infant developed seizures during home care. To reassess the tumor and rule out progressing hydrocephalus, repeat MRI was done. Despite the expected poor prognosis, follow up MRI revealed a near complete involution of the solid tumor with multiple loculated cerebrospinal fluid (CSF) intensity fluid collections occupying much of the frontal lobe. There were no nodular areas of enhancement suggestive of residual tumor (Figure 7F) except for two non-enhancing angular areas of hemorrhagic material.

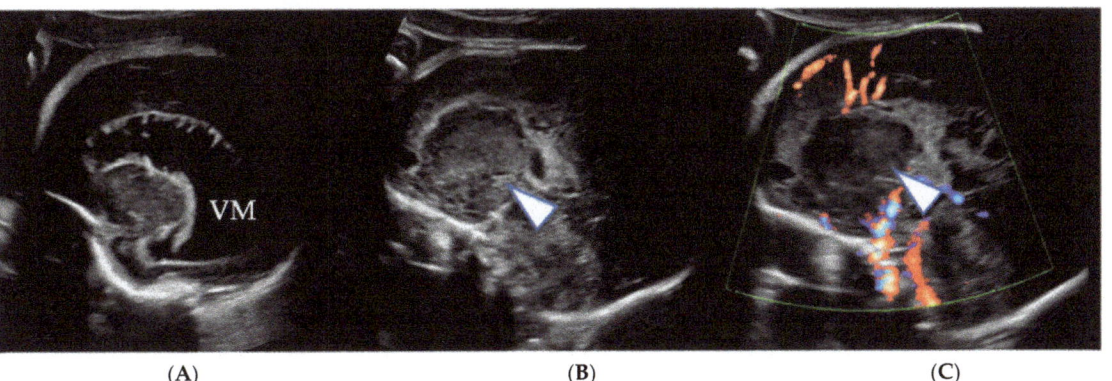

Figure 7. *Cont.*

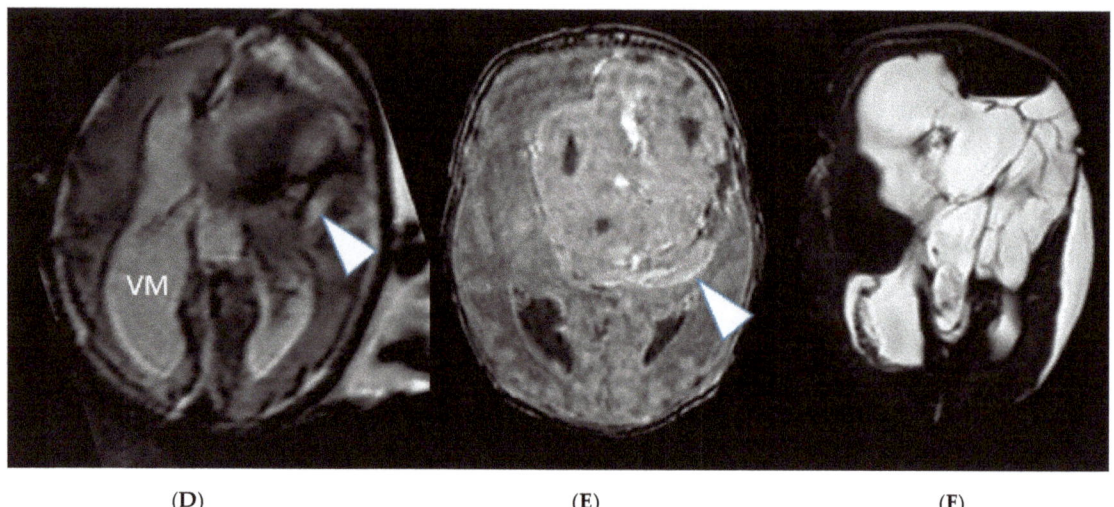

(D) (E) (F)

Figure 7. (**A–C**) Prenatal gray scale and color-coded Doppler US (**A–C**) and axial T2-weighted fetal MRI (**D**), postnatal contrast enhanced T1-weighted and postoperative follow up T2-weighted MRI show a large lobulated solid mass lesion in the left frontal lobe (arrowhead). Post-surgery the tumor has become T2-hyperintense cystic. Ventriculomegaly (VM) is secondary to compression of the foramina Monro (**E**,**F**).

Biopsy of the nodules, supratentorial ventriculostomy (ETV) with placement of an externally draining ventricular drain was performed. Pathology did not show viable tumor tissue. Subsequent need for the placement of a permanent ventriculoperitoneal (VP) shunt was indicated. This is a very unusual course, published and discussed by Peterson et al. [14]. The girl is currently 9-year-old. She suffers from global developmental delay, epilepsy, cerebral palsy and is mostly fed via a percutaneous G-tube.

3. Discussion

Our case series exemplifies various entities of FBT, the course of pregnancy and their postnatal outcome. Mortality is high and overall survival rate can be as low as 16%, depending on the histopathology, location and growth pattern of the tumor [10]. In our case series, two infants suffered neonatal demise (case 1 + 2). Autopsy and histopathological confirmation of prenatally suspected tumor was rejected in these cases, limiting diagnosis to pre- and postnatal imaging. This is in line with the current literature, showing that only 30–40% of parents agree to autopsy after the loss of their infant and highlights the need for alternative, less invasive options [15,16].

The gold standard for diagnosis of FBTs is histopathological examination. Molecular analysis can aid for further accurate classification [4]. Both can only be done safely after birth [7]. During gestation, diagnosis, counselling and treatment decisions primarily rely on prenatal imaging, clinical features and progression of disease [7]. FBTs are typically first suspected or identified on prenatal US screening. Findings like hydrocephalus, macrocephaly, and polyhydramnios are often the first sign and lead to further detailed imaging. Additional assessment by fetal MRI may improve diagnostic accuracy [2,3,7,10]. Depending on the gestational age, the diagnostic accuracy may increase up to 29% with a matching increase in the diagnostic confidence [3,13,17]. Differential diagnosis of FBT includes a focal intraparenchymal hemorrhage, which can mimic a mass lesion with or without hydrocephalus, or, possibly secondary to a vascular malformation [4,18].

Associated congenital anomalies can be present in 14–20% of cases, including anomalies of the corpus callosum in case of a pericallosal/midline lipoma and cleft lip and palate in case of teratoma [1]. Brain tumors can be part of a tumor predisposition syndrome or genetic disarrangement and genetic testing should be considered, even more in the presence of associated anomalies [4,5,13,18–20]. Different tumor types can be found before birth and exhibit a different prognosis for the fetus itself and the mother to be. The most common prenatal tumor types are teratoma, astrocytoma, craniopharyngioma, choroid plexus papilloma and embryonal tumors like medulloblastoma or ATRT [3,6,10,13,21]. However, reported frequencies of tumor types vary significantly in the existing literature [4,10,18,21]. With the advancing role of molecular diagnostics in tumor classification, implemented by the WHO classification of 2016 and updated in 2021, new tumor types are introduced, and former entities deleted. The reported frequencies of various congenital tumor types may consequently change in the future [4,22–24].

In our case series, we observed one case with suspected teratoma, one case with confirmed and one with suspected ATRT and one case with a glioneural tumor. Unfortunately, in 2/4 cases we do not have histopathological confirmation of the tumor histology. The differential diagnosis was based on pre- and postnatal MRI (case 1 + 2). Even though, post mortem autopsy is the gold standard, in case of parental decline, high quality prenatal imaging, and also postnatal or postmortem MRI add important information and can help to narrow down differential diagnosis [25,26]. A universal algorithm for follow-up and delivery planning after diagnosis of a FBT does currently not exist and sonographic follow-up may vary between several times a week to every 4 weeks [7].

In our experience, diagnosis of teratomas occurred early in pregnancy at 18 weeks GA (case 1). This is in accordance with the current literature, reporting that tumors found before 22 weeks GA are most often teratomas with an average age at diagnosis of 27 weeks, while gliomas and other entities are usually diagnosed after 32 weeks of pregnancy [7,13]. The primary tumor location or epicenter of the mass lesion may allow to narrow down the differential diagnosis but the invasive nature and frequently observed rapid growth may prevent or limit correct diagnosis.

Macrocephaly and obstructive, tumor related ventriculomegaly was present in 2/4 cases and are frequent concomitant findings [10,19]. They can lead to cephalopelvic disproportion and halt labor progression and delay delivery [27]. Rarely a spontaneous rupture of the fetal head or uterine rupture during delivery can happen [13]. Anomalous fetal position is frequently encountered [10]. Depending on the gestational age, head circumference and tumor characteristics, Cesarean-section is frequently advised [1,3,5,28]. When palliative care is elected at the time of delivery and there is significant hydrocephalus, a cephalocentesis can be considered to allow for a vaginal birth [29].

Maternal mirror syndrome is described in extremely severe cases of high-cardiac output failure leading to fetal hydrops [13,30].

Polyhydramnios is a well described finding in FBT. It occurs in up to one third of all cases and was seen in 2/4 cases of our series [10,18]. One of the etiologies can be related to high cardiac output status, as seen in case one, which also presumably led to PPROM and preterm delivery. Polyhydramnios may also result from impaired fetal swallowing due to brainstem dysfunction.

Prognosis is generally poor and worsens with increasing tumor size and decreasing gestational age at diagnosis [10]. Demise may occur in utero or after delivery. The options for prenatal therapy are very limited and mostly restricted to the treatment of concomitant symptoms, such as drainage of the polyhydramnios or cephalocentesis in case of severe tumor associated hydrocephalus/macrocephaly before birth. Recently, prenatal treatment of subependymal giant cell astrocytomas in fetuses with tuberous sclerosis with mTOR inhibitors has been reported [31]. Postnatal therapeutic options vary between palliation/comfort care and complete tumor resection with or without shunt placement and chemotherapy with a curative intent [27].

4. Conclusions

FBTs are a very rare entity. Prenatal counselling using high quality prenatal ultrasound, fetal MRI and clinical features should be multidisciplinary. In the light of the generally guarded fetal prognosis, associated increased risk of maternal morbidity and mortality during ongoing pregnancy and delivery, early termination of pregnancy may be discussed. However, as exemplified by case four, fetal prognosis, tumor development and life expectancy may be different than previously thought and readjustment of treatment plan may be necessary after birth. Histopathological confirmation of the prenatally suspected diagnosis is the gold standard and molecular analysis is increasingly used to further classify the tumor. Because of the rarity of FBTs, most conclusions and recommendations are based on case series. Larger multicenter studies are needed to provide better information on prenatal treatment options, pregnancy monitoring, and postnatal outcome in terms of survival and neurodevelopment.

Author Contributions: Conceptualization, M.S.C. and I.A.B.; methodology, I.A.B. and M.S.C.; data curation, I.A.B., M.S.C., W.W. and T.A.G.M.H.; writing—original draft preparation, I.A.B.; writing—review and editing, M.S.C., W.W., T.A.G.M.H., R.A.-F. and M.B.; supervision, M.S.C. All authors have read and agreed to the published version of the manuscript.

Funding: This research received no external funding.

Institutional Review Board Statement: The study was conducted in accordance with the Declaration of Helsinki and approved by the Baylor college of Medicine retrospective IRB protocol (protocol number H-37494).

Informed Consent Statement: Patient consent was waived as publication is covered by the retrospective IRB protocol.

Data Availability Statement: The analyzed data sets generated during the study are available from the corresponding author on reasonable request.

Conflicts of Interest: The authors declare no conflict of interest.

References

1. Woodward, P.J.; Sohaey, R.; Kennedy, A.; Koeller, K.K. From the Archives of the AFIP: A Comprehensive Review of Fetal Tumors with Pathologic Correlation. *RadioGraphics* **2005**, *25*, 215–242. [CrossRef] [PubMed]
2. Cassart, M.; Bosson, N.; Garel, C.; Eurin, D.; Avni, F. Fetal intracranial tumors: A review of 27 cases. *Eur. Radiol.* **2008**, *18*, 2060–2066. [CrossRef] [PubMed]
3. Feygin, T.; Khalek, N.; Moldenhauer, J.S. Fetal brain, head, and neck tumors: Prenatal imaging and management. *Prenat Diagn.* **2020**, *40*, 1203–1219. [CrossRef] [PubMed]
4. Viaene, A.N.; Pu, C.; Perry, A.; Li, M.M.; Luo, M.; Santi, M. Congenital tumors of the central nervous system: An institutional review of 64 cases with emphasis on tumors with unique histologic and molecular characteristics. *Brain Pathol.* **2021**, *31*, 45–60. [CrossRef]
5. Milani, H.J. Fetal brain tumors: Prenatal diagnosis by ultrasound and magnetic resonance imaging. *World J. Radiol.* **2015**, *7*, 17. [CrossRef]
6. Isaacs, H., Jr. I. Perinatal brain tumors: A review of 250 cases. *Pediatr. Neurol.* **2002**, *27*, 249–261. [CrossRef]
7. Sugimoto, M.; Kurishima, C.; Masutani, S.; Tamura, M.; Senzaki, H. Congenital Brain Tumor within the First 2 Months of Life. *Pediatr. Neonatol.* **2015**, *56*, 369–375. [CrossRef]
8. Stiller, C.A.; Bunch, K.J. Brain and spinal tumours in children aged under two years: Incidence and survival in Britain, 1971–1985. *Br. J. Cancer Suppl.* **1992**, *18*, S50–S53.
9. Rickert, C.H. Neuropathology and prognosis of foetal brain tumours. *Acta Neuropathol.* **1999**, *98*, 567–576. [CrossRef]
10. Isaacs, H. Fetal Brain Tumors: A Review of 154 Cases. *Am. J. Perinatol.* **2009**, *26*, 453–466. [CrossRef]
11. Ostrom, Q.T.; Cioffi, G.; Gittleman, H.; Patil, N.; Waite, K.; Kruchko, C.; Barnholtz-Sloan, J.S. CBTRUS Statistical Report: Primary Brain and Other Central Nervous System Tumors Diagnosed in the United States in 2012–2016. *Neuro Oncol.* **2019**, *21* (Suppl. S5), v1–v100. [CrossRef] [PubMed]
12. Wells, E.M.; Packer, R.J. Pediatric Brain Tumors. *Contin Lifelong Learn. Neurol.* **2015**, *21*, 373–396. [CrossRef] [PubMed]
13. Cornejo, P.; Feygin, T.; Vaughn, J.; Pfeifer, C.M.; Korostyshevska, A.; Patel, M.; Bardo, D.M.E.; Miller, J.; Goncalves, L.F. Imaging of fetal brain tumors. *Pediatr. Radiol.* **2020**, *50*, 1959–1973. [CrossRef] [PubMed]

14. Peterson, J.E.G.; Bavle, A.; Mehta, V.P.; Rauch, R.A.; Whitehead, W.E.; Mohila, C.A.; Su, J.M.; Adesina, A.M. Spontaneous Regression of Atypical Teratoid Rhabdoid Tumor Without Therapy in a Patient With Uncommon Regional Inactivation of SMARCB1 (hSNF5/INI1). *Pediatr. Dev. Pathol.* **2019**, *22*, 161–165. [CrossRef]
15. Shelmerdine, S.C.; Hutchinson, J.C.; Arthurs, O.J.; Sebire, N.J. Latest developments in post-mortem foetal imaging. *Prenat. Diagn.* **2020**, *40*, 28–37. [CrossRef]
16. Shelmerdine, S.C.; Arthurs, O.J. Post-mortem perinatal imaging: What is the evidence? *Br. J. Radiol.* **2022**, *2021*, 1078. [CrossRef]
17. Griffiths, P.D.; Bradburn, M.; Campbell, M.J.; Cooper, C.L.; Graham, R.; Jarvis, D.; Kilby, M.D.; Mason, G.; Mooney, C.; Robson, S.C.; et al. Use of MRI in the diagnosis of fetal brain abnormalities in utero (MERIDIAN): A multicentre, prospective cohort study. *Lancet* **2017**, *389*, 538–546. [CrossRef]
18. Severino, M.; Schwartz, E.S.; Thurnher, M.M.; Rydland, J.; Nikas, I.; Rossi, A. Congenital tumors of the central nervous system. *Neuroradiology* **2010**, *52*, 531–548. [CrossRef]
19. Vazquez, E.; Castellote, A.; Mayolas, N.; Carreras, E.; Peiro, J.L.; Enríquez, G. Congenital tumours involving the head, neck and central nervous system. *Pediatr. Radiol.* **2009**, *39*, 1158–1172. [CrossRef]
20. Sun, L.; Wu, Q.; Pei, Y.; Li, J.; Ye, J.; Zhi, W.; Liu, Y.; Zhang, P. Prenatal diagnosis and genetic discoveries of an intracranial mixed neuronal-glial tumor: A case report and literature review. *Medicine* **2016**, *95*, e5378. [CrossRef]
21. Isaacs, H., Jr. II. Perinatal brain tumors: A review of 250 cases. *Pediatr. Neurol.* **2002**, *27*, 333–342. [CrossRef] [PubMed]
22. Louis, D.N.; Perry, A.; Wesseling, P.; Brat, D.J.; Cree, I.A.; Figarella-Branger, D.; Hawkins, C.; Ng, H.K.; Pfister, S.M.; Reifenberger, G.; et al. The 2021 WHO Classification of Tumors of the Central Nervous System: A summary. *Neuro Oncol.* **2021**, *23*, 1231–1251. [CrossRef] [PubMed]
23. Louis, D.N.; Perry, A.; Reifenberger, G.; Von Deimling, A.; Figarella-Branger, D.; Cavenee, W.K.; Ohgaki, H.; Wiestler, O.D.; Kleihues, P.; Ellison, D.W. The 2016 World Health Organization Classification of Tumors of the Central Nervous System: A summary. *Acta Neuropathol.* **2016**, *131*, 803–820. [CrossRef] [PubMed]
24. Wen, P.Y.; Packer, R.J. The 2021 WHO Classification of Tumors of the Central Nervous System: Clinical implications. *Neuro Oncol.* **2021**, *23*, 1215–1217. [CrossRef] [PubMed]
25. Pérez-Serrano, C.; Bartolomé, Á.; Bargalló, N.; Sebastià, C.; Nadal, A.; Gómez, O.; Oleaga, L. Perinatal post-mortem magnetic resonance imaging (MRI) of the central nervous system (CNS): A pictorial review. *Insights Imaging* **2021**, *12*, 104. [CrossRef]
26. Sonnemans, L.J.P.; On Behalf of The Dutch Post-Mortem Imaging Guideline Group; Vester, M.E.M.; Kolsteren, E.E.M.; Erwich, J.J.H.M.; Nikkels, P.G.J.; Kint, P.A.M.; van Rijn, R.R.; Klein, W.M. Dutch guideline for clinical foetal-neonatal and paediatric post-mortem radiology, including a review of literature. *Eur. J. Pediatr.* **2018**, *177*, 791–803. [CrossRef]
27. Hwang, S.W.; Su, J.M.; Jea, A. Diagnosis and management of brain and spinal cord tumors in the neonate. *Semin. Fetal. Neonatal. Med.* **2012**, *17*, 202–206. [CrossRef]
28. Cavalheiro, S.; Moron, A.F.; Hisaba, W.; Dastoli, P.; Silva, N.S. Fetal brain tumors. *Childs Nerv. Syst.* **2003**, *19*, 529–536. [CrossRef]
29. Swetha, P.; Dhananjaya, S.; Ananda Rao, A.; Suresh, A.; Nadig, C. A Needle in the Fetal Brain: The Rare Role of Transabdominal Cephalocentesis in Fetal Hydrocephalus. *Cureus* **2021**, *13*, e14337. Available online: https://www.cureus.com/articles/52037-a-needle-in-the-fetal-brain-the-rare-role-of-transabdominal-cephalocentesis-in-fetal-hydrocephalus (accessed on 12 June 2022). [CrossRef]
30. Braun, T.; Brauer, M.; Fuchs, I.; Czernik, C.; Dudenhausen, J.W.; Henrich, W.; Sarioglu, N. Mirror syndrome: A systematic review of fetal associated conditions, maternal presentation and perinatal outcome. *Fetal. Diagn. Ther.* **2010**, *27*, 191–203. [CrossRef]
31. Cavalheiro, S.; da Costa, M.D.S.; Richtmann, R. Everolimus as a possible prenatal treatment of in utero diagnosed subependymal lesions in tuberous sclerosis complex: A case report. *Childs Nerv. Syst.* **2021**, *37*, 3897–3899. [CrossRef] [PubMed]

Disclaimer/Publisher's Note: The statements, opinions and data contained in all publications are solely those of the individual author(s) and contributor(s) and not of MDPI and/or the editor(s). MDPI and/or the editor(s) disclaim responsibility for any injury to people or property resulting from any ideas, methods, instructions or products referred to in the content.

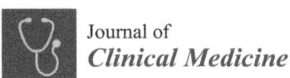

Article

The Value of Delta Middle Cerebral Artery Peak Systolic Velocity for the Prediction of Twin Anemia-Polycythemia Sequence—Analysis of a Heterogenous Cohort of Monochorionic Twins

Anthea de Sainte Fare [1,*], Ivonne Bedei [1], Aline Wolter [1], Johanna Schenk [1], Ellydda Widriani [1], Corinna Keil [2], Siegmund Koehler [2], Franz Bahlmann [3], Brigitte Strizek [4], Ulrich Gembruch [4], Christoph Berg [4,5] and Roland Axt-Fliedner [1,2]

1. Department of Prenatal Medicine and Fetal Therapy, University Hospital Giessen, 35392 Giessen, Germany
2. Department of Prenatal Medicine and Fetal Therapy, University Hospital Marburg, 35041 Marburg, Germany
3. Department of Ultrasound Diagnostics and Prenatal Medicine, Buergerhospital Frankfurt, 60318 Frankfurt, Germany
4. Department of Obstetrics and Prenatal Medicine, University Hospital Bonn, 53127 Bonn, Germany
5. Department of Prenatal Medicine and Gynaecological Ultrasound, University Hospital Cologne, 50937 Cologne, Germany
* Correspondence: thea-dsf@web.de; Tel.: +49-17-68458-5617

Abstract: Introduction: Twin anemia-polycythemia sequence (TAPS) is a complication in monochorionic-diamniotic (MCDA) twin pregnancies. This study analyzes whether the prenatal diagnosis using delta middle cerebral artery-peak systolic velocity (MCA-PSV) > 0.5 multiples of the median (MoM) (delta group) detects more TAPS cases than the guideline-based diagnosis using the MCA-PSV cut off levels of >1.5 and <1.0 MoM (cut-off group), in a heterogenous group of MCDA twins. Methods: A retrospective analysis of 348 live-born MCDA twin pregnancies from 2010 to 2021 with available information on MCA-PSV within one week before delivery and hemoglobin-values within 24 h postnatally were considered eligible. Results: Among postnatal confirmed twin pairs with TAPS, the cut-off group showed lower sensitivity than the delta group (33% vs. 82%). Specificity proved higher in the cut-off group with 97% than in the delta group at 86%. The risk that a TAPS is mistakenly not recognized prenatally is higher in the cut-off group than in the delta group (52% vs. 18%). Conclusions: Our data shows that delta MCA-PSV > 0.5 MoM detects more cases of TAPS, which would not have been diagnosed prenatally according to the current guidelines. In the collective examined in the present study, TAPS diagnostics using delta MCA-PSV proved to be a more robust method.

Keywords: monochorionic-twins; twin-anemia-polycythemia sequence; twin-to-twin transfusion syndrome; delta MCA-PSV

1. Introduction

Monochorionic diamniotic (MCDA) pregnancies represent the most common subgroup of monogynous twins, with approximately 65% [1]. A specific risk in MCDA pregnancies is the presence of vascular anastomoses across the common placenta. In 10% of MCDA fetuses, pregnancy is complicated by a twin-to-twin transfusion syndrome (TTTS), in 5% by a twin anemia-polycythemia sequence (TAPS) [2,3].

TAPS is a subtype of TTTS in MCDA twin pregnancies. The pathophysiological precondition of TAPS are tiny arterio-venous (AV) anastomoses (<1 mm) in the placenta, which connect the blood circulation between the twins [4]. This clinical picture can arise spontaneously or as a result of TTTS laser therapy (13%) after incomplete laser coagulation, as well as through recanalization of the coagulated anastomoses [5]. In contrast to classical TTTS, in which hypervolemia and hypovolemia dominate pathophysiologically due to a strong unbalanced net blood flow, in TAPS tiny anastomoses enable only a minimal but continuous unbalanced net intertwin flow of blood. This results in a large intertwin hemoglobin difference, but not in relevant hyper and hypovolemia [5]. Similar to the TTTS, there is a donor and a recipient twin. The donor twin shows anemia due to the loss of red blood cells to the recipient, whereas the recipient twin shows polycythemia due to the excessive transmission in red blood cells [6]. For the antenatal diagnosis of TAPS, the peak systolic velocity of the middle cerebral artery (MCA-PSV) is determined by Doppler measurements [7]. The criteria previously used to indicate a antenatal TAPS diagnosis according to the guidelines were the recipients MCA-PSV < 1.0 multiples of the median (MoM) and the donors MCA-PSV > 1.5 MoM, as well as the absence of amniotic fluid abnormalities [8]. Postnatal diagnostic criteria for TAPS are an intertwin hemoglobin difference >80 g/L, evidence of intertwin anastomoses in the placenta or a reticulocyte index of over 1.7 [8,9].

Various researchers recently proposed new cut-off values for MCA in TAPS diagnostics. This shows the urgency of revising the currently valid MCA cut-off values in TAPS diagnostics. After a retrospective data analysis with 154 monochorial-diamniotic twin pairs, Tavares de Sousa et al. even advocated setting the cut-off value of the delta MCA-PSV at 0.373 MoM [10].

Khalil et al. proposed that the best TAPS diagnosis can be made if the cut-off values are set at MCA-PSV > 1.5 MoM for the donor twin and <0.8 MoM for the recipient or delta MCV-PSV > 0.8 MoM [11].

Fishel-Bartal et al. [12] already observed the positive correlation between a high difference in the flow velocity of the middle cerebral artery (delta MCA-PSV) in the twins and a high hemoglobin difference measured postnatally. This hypothesis was tested by the University of Leiden in 2019 and confirmed with the same result [13]. It was also considered that this investigation method represents a better indicator for the antenatal detection of TAPS. A delta MCA-PSV value of more than 0.5 MoM was concluded to be pathological [13].

However, both studies were only carried out on a small group of patients. The aim of our study was to analyze the diagnostic potential of delta MCA-PSV > 0.5 MoM in a large group of heterogenous MCDA twin pairs.

2. Methods

This study is a retrospective data analysis in five tertiary referral centers in Germany attending a high number of twin pregnancies. All MCDA twin pregnancies from January 2010 to January 2021 were considered. Both antenatal and postnatal values were taken into account. The study included 348 MCDA twin pregnancies from the following German prenatal diagnostic centers: Justus Liebig University Giessen, Philipps University Marburg, Buergerhospital Frankfurt, Rheinische Friedrich-Wilhelm's University Bonn, and University of Cologne.

All perinatal medicine specialists participating were informed whether therapeutic interventions such as laser treatment were performed on the fetuses.

Every twin pair underwent detailed anomaly survey including sequential fetal echocardiography at the 18th–22nd weeks of gestation by experienced level 3 operators according to the DEGUM (Deutsche Gesellschaft fuer Ultraschall in der Medizin) guidelines [7]. Cardiac findings in TAPS twins included atrioventricular valve regurgitation, and/or functional pulmonary stenosis or atresia and/or a cardiothoracic ratio ≥ 0.5.

The confidence interval (CI) was determined to check the precision of the result.

Cases in which antenatal Doppler measurements of the MCA of both twins were available, as well as postnatal information about the hemoglobin values, were considered eligible. Cases with MCA Doppler longer than one week prior to delivery and those in which the postnatal hemoglobin value was not determined within 24 h of the time of birth were excluded. The postnatal diagnosis of TAPS was based on an intertwin hemoglobin difference >80 g/L. Postnatally, the twin pairs were divided into two groups:

1. Control group—without TAPS (postnatal hemoglobin difference of <79 g/L);
2. TAPS (hemoglobin-difference of >80 g/L).

The antenatal TAPS diagnosis was determined by ultrasound Doppler measuring MCA-PSV and divided into three groups:
1. Control group—with normal MCA-PSV values;
2. Twins who exceeded the cut-off values MCA-PSV > 1.5 and <1.0 MoM;
3. Twins with delta MCA-PSV > 0.5 MoM.

Statistical analysis was performed using SSPS-21 (IBM, Armonk, NY, USA). Multiples of median (MoM) were determined in dependence on the gestational age using the "Perinatology calculator" [14]. The nominal and ordinal scaled data were examined using the chi-square test and the differences between the two groups were shown in a cross table. In case the chi-square test could not be used to check the significance due to a rule violation, the Fisher test (exact chi-square test) was used. The statistical quality criteria sensitivity, specificity, positive and negative predictive values were calculated using a 2×2 table in order to determine the value of the respective tests. The confidence intervals were set to refine the results.

To test the strength of the correlation, a Pearson test was performed on the normally distributed data. Spearman's correlation coefficient was used to check the correlation of the metrically distributed data.

As a secondary question, it was checked if there was a more accurate prenatal delta MCA-PSV cut-off than the one used of 0.5 MoM by using a receiver operating statistics curve (ROC). The significance level of the p-value was set at 0.05 (5%). The Bonferroni correction was used to neutralize alpha accumulation in multiple tests [15].

The work was approved by the Ethics Committee Giessen (ID: 254/19).

3. Results

This study includes 348 live-born MCDA twin pairs. Of the 348 twin pairs, 95 were recruited at the University Hospital Giessen, 91 at the University Hospital Marburg, 73 at the Buergerhospital Frankfurt, 53 at the University Hospital Cologne, and 36 at the University Hospital Bonn.

A total of 288 twin pairs in the control group (83%) had a hemoglobin difference of less than 79 g/L postnatally; 60 twin pairs indicated a TAPS with a postnatal hemoglobin difference >80 g/L.

TAPS is a known complication after laser coagulation for TTTS. Data analysis shows that 45% ($n = 27$) of TAPS cases emerged after laser coagulation for TTTS. In 55% ($n = 33$) of the TAPS cases, the clinical picture emerged spontaneously. The mean maternal age of the study participants was 32 years (range 17 to 45 years).

A total of 258 twin pairs showed no abnormalities in MCA-PSV (control group). 29 twin pairs had an MCA-PSV > 1.5 MoM in one twin and <1.0 MoM in the other twin, and thus fulfilled the conditions of an antenatally diagnosed TAPS according to the current criteria. Of the cases, 90 showed a delta MCA-PSV > 0.5 MoM. The 90 twin pairs were composed of the 29 twin pairs detected by MCA-PSV cut-off level of >1.5 and <1.0 MoM method and 61 additional twin pairs detected as TAPS by the delta method only.

Both Figure 1 and Table 1 show the relationship between the hemoglobin difference and the MCA-PSV. The diagnostic criteria delta MCA-PSV > 0.5 MoM vs. MCA-PSV cut-off level of >1.5 and <1.0 MoM were analyzed regarding to the postnatal hemoglobin difference. Of 29 twin pairs diagnosed antenatally as TAPS based on the current criteria (MCA-PSV cut-off level of >1.5 and <1.0 MoM), 20 of the twin pairs (69%) were confirmed postnatally by an intertwin hemoglobin difference of >80 g/L. Of the 90 twin pairs diagnosed antenatally as TAPS due to delta MCA-PSV > 0.5 MoM, in 49 (54%) cases the diagnosis of TAPS was postnatally confirmed. Among the 61 additional TAPS cases suspected by the delta method, 29 (48%) showed postnatally a TAPS. A total of 11 twin pairs with TAPS were not detected prenatally neither by one nor the other diagnostic method. Of 60 TAPS cases, which were confirmed postnatally, the delta MCA-PSV > 0.5 MoM method would have detected 29 twin pairs that exceeded the cut off values of MCA-PSV cut-off level of >1.5 and <1.0 MoM, and 20 additional cases that would not have been diagnosed by using MCA-PSV cut-off level of >1.5 and <1.0 MoM. In total, 49 of the 60 cases would have been discovered by delta MCA-PSV > 0.5 MoM prenatally. Diagnosis by using MCA-PSV cut-off level of >1.5 and <1.0 MoM would have detected 29 of the 60 TAPS cases prenatally. A proportion of 46% (41 of 90) of cases discovered by delta MCA-PSV > 0.5 MoM were incorrectly diagnosed prenatally as TAPS (vs. 31%, 9 of 29) cases by MCA-PSV cut-off level of >1.5 and <1.0 MoM). A positive correlation between the hemoglobin difference and the MCA-PSV could be shown, both measured in delta MCA-PSV > 0.5 MoM and in the absolute MCA-PSV cut-off level of >1.5 and <1.0 MoM. This relationship turned out to be significant ($p \ll 0.001$).

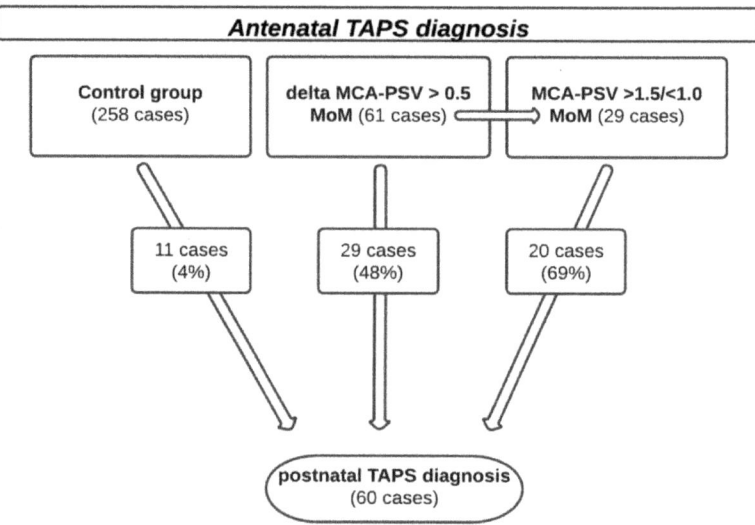

Figure 1. Shows the prenatal distribution of cases among the three diagnostic groups: the control group, the cases diagnosed as TAPS according to the criteria delta MCA-PSV > 0.5 MoM, and the cases that correspond to the diagnosis of TAPS according to the current guidelines (MCA-PSV >1.5/<1.0 MoM).

Table 1. Correlation between prenatal TAPS diagnosis and postnatal TAPS confirmation.

		Postnatal Diagnosis of TAPS (Hb diff. >80 g/L)			
		Yes	No	Total	p-Value
Prenatal	Delta MCA-PSV >0.5 MoM	49 (48%)	41 (52%)	90 (100%)	<<0.001
	MCA-PSV > 1.5/<1.0 MoM	20 (69%)	9 (31%)	29 (100%)	<<0.001
	undetected TAPS cases	11 (4%)	247 (96%)	258 (100%)	<<0.001

A p-value < 0.05 was assumed to be statistically significant. MoM, multiples of the median; Hb diff, Hemoglobin difference; MCA-PSV, middle cerebral artery peak systolic velocity.

The diagnostic quality of both antenatal TAPS diagnostic procedures is illustrated in Table 2.

Table 2. Quality of antenatal diagnostic procedures.

	Antenatal TAPS Diagnostic	
	Delta MCA-PSV > 0.5 MoM (n = 90)	MCA-PSV >1.5/<1.0 MoM (n = 29)
Sensitivity	(49/60), 82%	(20/60), 33%
Confidence interval (CI)	78–86%	28–37.9%
Specificity	(247/288), 86%	(279/288), 97%
Confidence interval (CI)	82.3–89.6%	95.2–98.8%
Positive predictive value	(49/90), 54%	(20/29), 69%
Confidence interval (CI)	48.7–59.2%	64.1–73.9%
Negative predictive value	(234/245), 96%	(279/319), 87%
Confidence interval (CI)	94–98%	83.5–90.5%
False positive rate	(41/90), 46%	(9/29), 31%
False negative rate	(11/60), 18%	(31/60), 52%

MoM, multiples of the median; MCA-PSV, middle cerebral artery peak systolic velocity.

Of the twin pairs actually suffering from TAPS, 49 of 60 (82%) were also diagnosed as well by using delta MCA-PSV > 0.5 MoM (sensitivity). The CI was set at 95%, which in the case of the sensitivity means that with a certainty of 95% the real values of the sensitivity are within the interval of 78% and 86%. In contrast, 86% (95% CI: 82–90%) of the MCDA pregnancies were correctly detected as not affected (specificity). In 54% (95% CI: 49–59%) of the cases, the twin pairs diagnosed antenatally as TAPS were also confirmed postnatal as TAPS (positive predictive value, PPV). The negative predictive value for diagnostics using delta MCA-PSV > 0.5 MoM is 96% (95% CI: 94–98%). In total, 49 of the 60 TAPS cases, which were confirmed postpartum would have also been detected antenatally with this diagnostic method. However, 11 cases still remained undetected antenatally, even with this method.

The diagnostic quality of the MCA-PSV cut-off level of >1.5 and <1.0 MoM, which is currently used in antenatal TAPS diagnostics according to the guidelines, is also shown in Table 2 [8,10]. The sensitivity of these current valid diagnostic criteria is 33% (95% CI: 28–38%) and the specificity is 97% (95% CI: 95–99%). In 69% (95% CI: 64–74%) of the cases, the TAPS twins diagnosed by means of MCA-PSV cut-off level of > 1.5 and < 1.0 MoM actually had TAPS (PPV). The negative predictive value for this method of antenatal diagnosis is 87% (95% CI: 84–91%).

Table 3 analyzes whether various fetal and neonatal characteristics are present or reduced for the respective diagnostic criterion. In this presentation, the delta MCA-PSV > 0.5 MoM considered only those 61 cases which would not have been detected by MCA-PSV cut-off level of >1.5 and <1.0 MoM. A total of 11 TAPS cases remained undetected prenatally with both methods. The data analysis shows that the twins who were diagnosed antenatally as TAPS due to MCA-PSV cut-off level of >1.5 and <1.0 MoM, were born earlier on average than those who were diagnosed using delta MCA-PSV > 0.5 MoM (29th vs. 32nd week of gestational age at birth). Furthermore, the data indicate a connection between the causality of TAPS (spontaneous vs. post-laser TAPS) and the TAPS diagnostic procedure. The post-laser TAPS cases, which were diagnosed as TAPS due to the absolute cut-off values (MCA-PSV cut-off level of >1.5 and <1.0 MoM), represent a larger proportion with 48% (15 twin pairs) than the TAPS cases, which were diagnosed using delta MCA-PSV > 0.5 MoM (15 twin pairs, 25%).

Table 3. Presentation of various fetal and neonatal characteristics in TAPS twins in relation to the different diagnostic criteria (delta MCA-PSV > 0.5 MoM, MCA-PSV >1.5/<1.0 MoM, and undiscovered TAPS cases prenatally).

Characteristic	Antenatal TAPS Diagnostic			p-Value
	delta MCA-PSV >0.5 MoM (n = 61)	MCA-PSV >1.5/<1.0 MoM (n = 29)	Undiscoverd TAPS (n = 11)	
Sex of twin pairs (f/m)	31/30	14/15	4/7	0.896
Gestational age at birth (weeks)	32	29	34	<0.001
Birth-weight discordance (g)	361	332	433	0.6
Type of TAPS:				
- Spontaneous	46 (75%)	14 (52%)	8 (78%)	
- Post-laser	15 (25%)	15 (48%)	3 (27%)	0.003
Intertwin Hb discordance (g/L)	75	108	110	<<0.001
Hk discordance	0.2	0.32	0.34	<<0.001
Delta MCA-PSV (MoM)	0.57	1.01	0.3	<<0.001
Amniotic fluid anomalies	17 (28%)	5 (17%)	1 (18%)	0.345
Cardiac findings	26 (42%)	21 (72%)	3 (27%)	<0.001

A p-Value < 0.05 was assumed to be statistically significant. The p-values refer to the association between the delta MCA-PSV and the MCA-PSV >1.5/<1.0 MoM Group. MoM, multiples of the median; MCA-PSV, middle cerebral artery peak systolic velocity; f/m, female/male; Hb, Hemoglobin.

The eleven undetected TAPS cases had an average hemoglobin difference of 110 g/L postnatally. The gestational age of 34 weeks was higher than in the prenatally diagnosed TAPS cases. The average delta MCA-PSV in this group was 0.3 MoM. The difference in birth weight of the twins in this group was 433 g (22%) on average, higher than that of the prenatally diagnosed TAPS cases.

Cardiac findings typical of TAPS occurred more frequently in the TAPS cases, which were diagnosed due to the absolute cut-off values, than in the cases which were diagnosed due to delta MCA-PSV > 0.5 MoM (72% vs. 42%). There was no association between postnatal diagnosis of TAPS and either amniotic fluid abnormalities or weight discrepancies of the twin pairs. The significantly higher intertwin hemoglobin difference of 108 g/L (vs. 75 g/L) in the twins diagnosed antenatally with MCA-PSV cut-off level of >1.5 and <1.0 MoM is noticeable ($p << 0.001$). All these data refer to cases that were prenatally indicative of TAPS and not to postnatally confirmed TAPS cases.

In this study the precision of the delta MCA-PSV value of 0.5 MoM is evaluated by using a ROC curve as a secondary question, which is shown in Figure 2.

To detect an optimal delta MCA-PSV cut-off value, the Youden index (sensitivity + specificity-1) was used. The optimal cut-off value is defined at a maximum high sensitivity and a lowest possible false positive value (1-specificity) [16]. With a sensitivity of 0.817 (81.7%) and a 1-specificity of 0.142 (14.2%), the most accurate delta MCA-PSV cut-off value in this collective was detected at 0.45 MOM. The area under the curve (AUC) is 0.889 (95% CI: 0.936–0.843).

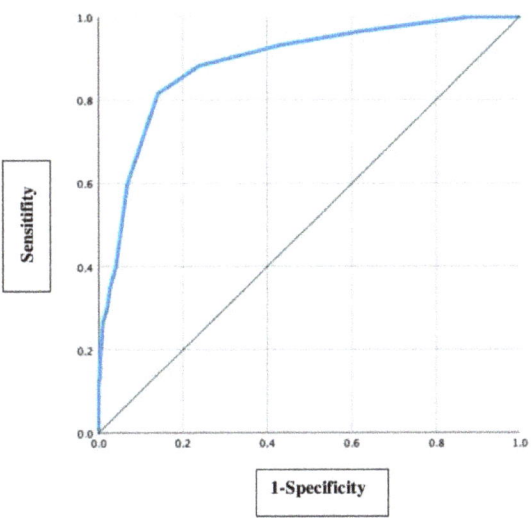

Figure 2. ROC curve to find the optimal MCA-PSV cut-off value.

4. Discussion/Conclusions

This study was conducted to evaluate the diagnostic accuracy of delta MCA-PSV in a heterogenous group of MCDA twin gestations regarding the presence of twin anemia polycythemia sequence (TAPS) postnatally. In 49 confirmed cases of TAPS twin pairs in this study delta MCV-PSV > 0.5 MoM turned out to be a higher diagnostic accuracy in terms of sensitivity and comparable specificity compared to the currently implemented MCA-PSV cut-off level of >1.5 and <1.0 MoM for diagnosis of antenatal TAPS in MCDA twin gestations.

The parameter delta MCA-PSV > 0.5 MoM achieved satisfactorily high sensitivity and specificity for the prediction of TAPS. Particularly noteworthy is the high negative predictive value of 96% for this criterion. In contrast, the standard definition of TAPS with MCA-PSV cut-off level of >1.5 and <1.0 MoM was shown to have an inferior sensitivity. Based on the delta MCA-PSV > 0.5 MoM cut-off, only 18% (11/60) of confirmed postnatal TAPS cases were missed, in contrast to 52% (31/60) with MCA-PSV cut-off level of >1.5 and <1.0 MoM.

In summary, Table 2 shows that the two methods are completely adjacent and significantly different in terms of sensitivity, specificity, positive and negative predictive value. The delta MCA-PSV method is far better at spotting those that are actually healthy, and the MCA-PSV absolute value method is far more effective at finding cases affected by TAPS. This means that the value of these methods mainly depends on the research question. If the primary goal is to filter out the affected cases precisely and with the lowest possible false positive rate, the absolute MCA-PSV method should be chosen. However, one should be aware that some cases remain undetected, so that appropriate diagnostics and therapy are not carried out and the children may grow up with permanent damage. However, if as many cases as possible are to be detected prenatally, even with the risk of a higher false positive rate, the delta MCA-PSV method must be chosen. It is certainly more important to detect cases that are very likely to be affected as early as possible, in order to observe further diagnosis in small steps and to be able to intervene as quickly as possible in event of aggravation.

Thus, the use of delta MCA-PSV > 0.5 MoM could clarify prenatal TAPS diagnosis and help affected twins benefit from more intensive prenatal surveillance and intervention, if appropriate.

The present results are consistent with the recently reported results of Tollenaar et al. [13], who presented results on the improved prediction of TAPS by delta MCA-PSV in a selected group of MCDA twin pregnancies with a confirmed diagnosis of TAPS postnatally. They reported in a series of 35 twin pairs with postnatally confirmed TAPS a sensitivity of 46% and 100% specificity for MCA-PSV cut-off level of >1.5 and <1.0 MoM compared to an 83% sensitivity and 100% specificity for delta MCA-PSV > 0.5 MoM. Of note, they reported on 13 twin pairs of the 35 confirmed TAPS cases postnatally with a delta MCA-PSV > 0.5 MoM but not reaching the MCA-PSV cut-off level of >1.5 and <1.0 MoM criterion; nine donors and four recipients of these 13 TAPS cases presented with normal MCA-PSV values. These results were considered in our study. Of the 60 TAPS cases, confirmed postnatally, 20 cases were prenatally discovered only by using delta MCA-PSV > 0.5 MoM. Diagnosis by MCA-PSV cut-off level of >1.5 and <1.0 MoM would have left these cases undetected prenatally. Previous reports found higher hemoglobin level sensitivity values for MCA-PSV cut-off values of >1.5 and <1.0 MoM in a general population of MCDA pregnant woman. However, this does not apply in a specific subgroup of TAPS twin pairs [12]. Specifically, this study and the recent study of Tollenaar et al. did not examine postnatal hemoglobin levels as the primary outcome, but rather the hemoglobin difference between the twins, which is the basis of a postnatal TAPS diagnosis [13].

With regard to perinatal outcomes, TAPS twins diagnosed by MCA-PSV cut-off level of >1.5 and <1.0 MoM were born at a significantly lower gestational age compared to those diagnosed by delta MCA-PSV > 0.5 MoM (29 weeks vs. 32 weeks, respectively, $p < 0.001$). In the group of MCA-PSV cut-off level of >1.5 and <1.0 MoM there were more intrauterine interventions compared to the delta MCA-PSV > 0.5 MoM twin pairs, with a statistical difference. It might be argued that since this was a retrospective analysis, the latter group was considered to be mildly or moderately affected TAPS pairs and therefore the decision to deliver was a conscious one. Consistent with this argument, in our study, twin pairs diagnosed by using delta MCA-PSV showed a lower Hb difference (75 g/L vs. 108 g/L) and thus lower expression of TAPS than the twin pairs diagnosed by cut-off MCA-PSV. This statement seems to contradict the data of Tollenaar et al., who found no significant differences in gestational ages at delivery between both groups, however, they also reported later gestational ages in the group of delta MCA-PSV > 0.5 MoM compared to MCA-PSV cut-off level of >1.5 and <1.0 MoM (34 weeks vs. 31 weeks of gestation). Moreover, in our study we reported a high proportion of cardiac findings in both groups (42% and 72%, respectively), probably reflecting a more advanced stage of disease (Stage $\geq$ 2 according to the current guidelines [8]), and therefore a lower gestational ages might be attributed to the fact of more severe stage of disease. Tollenaar et al. did not report on cardiac disease in their study.

An important finding of our analysis is the significantly lower hemoglobin and hematocrit difference in the twins detected prenatally as TAPS by the delta MCA-PSV > 0.5 MoM compared with those detected by MCA-PSV >1.5 and <1.0 MoM. This may indicate that the cut-off group primarily captures the cases with severe TAPS. This translates into significantly higher delta MCA-PSV values in the group of MCA-PSV cut-off level of >1.5 and <1.0 MoM.

Tollenaar et al. have established a modified antenatal TAPS staging. According to this classification, no stage 1 TAPS was detected by the guideline-based prenatal diagnosis with MCA-PSV cut-off level of >1.5 and <1.0 MoM. With TAPS diagnostics using delta MCA-PSV > 0.5 MoM, 50% were already diagnosed at stage 1. Intervention such as intrauterine transfusion should be considered from stage 2. However, it should be mentioned at this point that up to now there is no standard and verified therapy after the 28th week of gestation for TAPS twins. The indication for delivery is a pregnancy beyond the 32nd week, plus the presence of a stage $\geq$ 3. In conclusion, prenatal TAPS diagnosis using delta MCA-PSV > 0.5 MoM seems to detect earlier TAPS stages than MCA-PSV cut-off level of >1.5 and <1.0 MoM [17].

Neither a significant discrepancy in birth weight nor differences in amniotic fluid was found between both groups, arguing that selective intrauterine growth restriction had no impact on the intertwin hemoglobin difference observed in our cohort. The Leiden group, however, reported on a higher birth-weight discordance in the TAPS group with delta MCA-PSV > 0.5 MoM, however both birthweight discordance in % and the rate of birth-weight discordance > 20% was not reported to be statistically different in this report [13].

In this study, it was found that the ideal delta MCA-PSV value is 0.45 MoM (Figure 2). Beyond this value, the number of incorrectly diagnoses increases more rapidly than the sensitivity, so that a further reduction of the cut-off value would not bring any positive benefit. Thus, according to our data, delta MCA-PSV of 0.45 MoM represents the value at which the diagnosis of TAPS should be considered. It was decided to set 0.5 MoM as cut-off value despite the small deviation from the calculated optimal MCA-PSV value (0.45 MoM), as this keeps this study comparable to the study by Tollenaar et al. on this topic [13]. Furthermore, the analysis with the modified delta value of 0.45 MoM showed no difference in data interpretation; both with a cut-off at 0.45 and at 0.5 MoM, 90 TAPS cases were diagnosed prenatally. Hence, with this dataset we were able to further support the previously used delta value of 0.5 MoM [13] and add another study that demonstrates the accuracy of this value. Additional studies attempted to identify an optimal delta cut-off value. In a study, Liu et al. compared the available prenatal diagnostic methods in terms of incidence, progression, and intervention rates in the presence of TAPS [18]. Considered were the currently valid criteria (>1.5/<1.0 MoM), the value of 0.373 MoM recommended by Tavares De Sousa, the values established by a Delphi procedure (>1.5/>0.8 MoM or delta MCA-PSV > 1.0 MoM), and the delta MCA-PSV value > 0.5 MoM advocated by Tollenaar et al. in 2019 It was found that the different diagnostic criteria revealed significant differences in the incidence of TAPS, severity, and prenatal intervention. The TAPS cases identified by the Delphi method, as well as the TAPS cases detected by the currently valid criteria, diagnosed prenatally mainly the cases with the highest rates of progression and intervention, showing the lowest incidence. Delta MCA-PSV > 0.373 MoM had the highest incidence and revealed mainly low-grade TAPS cases with a low rate of progression.

The question is which value represents the optimal diagnostic value. This depends, as mentioned above, on what is important for the investigator. If the aim is to filter out as many cases as possible prenatally at the risk of overdiagnosis, the delta values of <0.5 MoM should be applied. If the focus is on the most precise prenatal diagnosis with a high specificity, the currently valid criteria or those from the Delphi method should be used.

According to Liu et al., this comparison of the currently available prenatal TAPS diagnostic options does not allow a definitive statement or standardization of the prenatal TAPS diagnostic criteria [18]. Further large studies are needed to determine the best possible cut-off value to achieve the highest possible diagnostic accuracy with the best possible neonatal outcomes.

A limitation of this retrospective study is the lack of histopathological studies on placental anastomosis, due to the inclusion of five different centers. An advantage of this study is that we analyzed a heterogenous group of MCDA twin pregnancies and not just a group of MCDA twins with postnatally confirmed diagnosis of TAPS. It is clear from our data that a prospective evaluation of MCDA twin pregnancies is warranted and intervention criteria and outcome parameters must be addressed. Another limitation is the definition of TAPS based on the postnatal hemoglobin difference. Different techniques of cord section, sometimes even consciously with a known diagnosis of TAPS, fluid applications, and different timings of postnatal blood sampling can lead to changes in hemoglobin concentrations and thus the intertwin hemoglobin difference.

In conclusion, from our data in a heterogenous group of MCDA twin pregnancies delta MCA-PSV > 0.5 MoM has a greater diagnostic accuracy for predicting TAPS compared to the MCA-PSV cut-off level of >1.5 and <1.0 MoM. Likewise, the earlier diagnosis of TAPS by delta MCA-PSV could lead to a more intense surveillance including fetal interventions, if indicated, of these pregnancies. Physicians involved in care of these high-risk twin pregnancies should be aware of these findings.

Finally, the question arises to what extent prenatal TAPS diagnostics can benefit from the results obtained. By diagnosing TAPS early and adjusting the prenatal observation accordingly, the progression of the disease can be detected as early as possible and, if necessary, mediated. Delta MCA-PSV does not imply any additional diagnostic effort and no diagnostic investments for the examiner. Only the evaluation differs from the currently used diagnostic method based on the absolute flow velocity of the ACM. An earlier diagnosis does not necessarily mean an earlier intervention but can sensitize the examiner and the patient to recognize a deterioration as early as possible.

The extent to which the outcome of the twins could improve if delta MCA-PSV > 0.5 MoM was diagnosed earlier needs to be controlled in further studies, preferably prospective studies. This cannot be adequately assessed in this study, since the prenatal diagnosis of TAPS disease with delta MCA-PSV > 0.5 MoM was not recognized by the prenatal diagnostician in most cases.

Author Contributions: Conceptualization and methodology designed by, A.d.S.F., R.A.-F. and J.S.; software, A.d.S.F. with the support of statisticians from the University of Giessen; validation, R.A.-F.; formal analysis, A.d.S.F., R.A.-F.; investigation, I.B., A.W., E.W., and J.S. were significantly involved in the data curation at the University Hospital Giessen, C.K. and S.K. at the University Hospital Marburg, R.A.-F. was involved in Giessen and Marburg, U.G. and B.S. collected data used in this study at the University Hospital Bonn, C.B. was instrumental in both the diagnosis and data collection at the University Hospital Cologne and the University Hospital Bonn, F.B. collected and provided the data from the Buergerhospital Frankfurt.; resources, A.d.S.F., R.A.-F.; data curation, A.d.S.F.; writing—original draft preparation, A.d.S.F.; writing—review and editing especially R.A.-F.; visualization A.d.S.F.; supervision and project administration by R.A.-F. The final product of this work was made in unified consultation and cooperation with all authors of this work. All authors have read and agreed to the published version of the manuscript.

Funding: This research received no external funding.

Institutional Review Board Statement: The work is a purely retrospective data analysis and is approved by the Ethics Committee Giessen (ID: 254/19). The study was conducted ethically in accordance with the Declaration of Helsinki of the World Medical Association.

Informed Consent Statement: Written informed consent was obtained from participants to participate in the study.

Data Availability Statement: All data generated or analyzed as part of this study are included in the long version of this paper. This article provides a compilation of the main results and findings. The long version of this work has not yet been published. If required, the complete work can be consulted at any time. If you have any questions, please contact the main authors de Sainte Fare or Axt-Fliedner.

Acknowledgments: We would like to thank the five institutes (University Hospitals of Giessen, Marburg, Cologne and Bonn and the Buergerhospital Frankfurt) who provided us with their data on monochorial-diamniotic twins over the last 10 years. We would also like to thank all the accompanying sonographers for their precise prenatal recording and diagnostics. In addition to Axt-Fliedner, Gembruch, Berg, and Bahlmann deserve special gratitude. We are also grateful for the work of Bedei, Wolter, Schenk, Strizek, Widrani, Keil, and Koehler who contributed to the prenatal diagnostics and data documentation. We would also like to thank all authors for their contribution to the writing of this manuscript. Special thanks also go to Helge Hudel and Anita Windhorst from the Institute for Medical Statistics of the Justus-Liebig University of Giessen, who were instrumental in assisting us in the development of the statistics.

Conflicts of Interest: The authors declare no conflict of interest.

References

1. Krampl-Bettelheim, E. Mehrlinge. In *Die Geburtshilfe*, 4th ed.; Springer: Berlin/Heidelberg, Germany, 2011; pp. 923–940.
2. Diehl, W.; Hecher, K. Mehrlingsschwangerschaft. In *Ultraschalldiagnostik in Geburtshilfe und Gynäkologie*; Gembruch, U., Hecher, K., Steiner, H., Eds.; Springer: Berlin/Heidelberg, Germany, 2017; pp. 567–591.
3. Slaghekke, F.; Kist, W.J.; Oepkes, D.; Pasman, S.A.; Middeldorp, J.M.; Klumper, F.J.; Walther, F.J.; Vandenbussche, F.P.H.A.; Lopriore, E. Twin anemia-polycythemia sequence: Diagnostic criteria, classification, perinatal management and outcome. *Fetal Diagn Ther.* **2010**, *27*, 181–190. [CrossRef] [PubMed]
4. Lopriore, E.; Middeldorp, J.M.; Oepkes, D.; Kanhai, H.H.; Walther, F.J.; Vandenbussche, F.P.H.A. Twin anemia-polycythemia sequence in two monochorionic twin pairs without oligo-polyhydramnios sequence. *Placenta* **2007**, *28*, 47–51. [CrossRef] [PubMed]
5. Robyr, R.; Lewi, L.; Salomon, L.J.; Yamamoto, M.; Bernard, J.P.; Deprest, J.; Ville, Y. Prevalence and management of late fetal complications following successful selective laser coagulation of chorionic plate anastomoses in twin-to-twin transfusion syndrome. *Am. J. Obstet. Gynecol.* **2006**, *194*, 796–803. [CrossRef] [PubMed]
6. Tchirikov, M. Monochorionic twin pregnancy: Screening, pathogenesis of complications and management in the era of microinvasive fetal surgery. *J. Perinat. Med.* **2010**, *38*, 451–459. [CrossRef] [PubMed]
7. Faber, R.; Heling, K.S.; Steiner, H.; Gembruch, U. Doppler Sonography during Pregnancy—DEGUM Quality Standards and Clinical Applications (Part 1). *Ultraschall Med.-Eur. J. Ultrasound* **2019**, *40*, 319–325. [CrossRef] [PubMed]
8. vonKaisenberg, C.; Klaritsch, P.; Ochsenbein-Kölble, N.; Hodel, M.; Nothacker, M.; Hecher, K. AWMF LL 015-087 S24 Überwachung und Betreuung von Zwillingsschwangerschaften. 2020. Available online: https://www.awmf.org/uploads/tx_szleitlinien/015-087l_S2e_Ueberwachung-Betreuung-Zwillingsschwangerschaften_2020-05.pdf (accessed on 25 September 2022).
9. Diehl, W.; Glosemeyer, P.; Tavares De Sousa, M.; Hollwitz, B.; Ortmeyer, G.; Hecher, K. Twin anemia-polycythemia sequence in a case of monoamniotic twins: Twin anemia-polycythemia sequence in monoamniotic twins. *Ultrasound Obstet. Gynecol.* **2013**, *42*, 108–111. [CrossRef] [PubMed]
10. Tavares de Sousa, M.; Fonseca, A.; Hecher, K. Role of fetal intertwin difference in middle cerebral artery peak systolic velocity in predicting neonatal twin anemia-polycythemia sequence. *Ultrasound Obstet. Gynecol. Off. J. Int. Soc. Ultrasound Obstet. Gynecol.* **2019**, *53*, 794–797. [CrossRef] [PubMed]
11. Khalil, A.; Gordijn, S.; Ganzevoort, W.; Thilaganathan, B.; Johnson, A.; Baschat, A.A.; Hecher, K.; Reed, K.; Lewi, L.; Deprest, J.; et al. Consensus diagnostic criteria and monitoring of twin anemia–polycythemia sequence: Delphi procedure. *Ultrasound Obstet. Gynecol.* **2020**, *56*, 388–394. [CrossRef] [PubMed]
12. Fishel-Bartal, M.; Weisz, B.; Mazaki-Tovi, S.; Ashwal, E.; Chayen, B.; Lipitz, S.; Yinon, Y. Can middle cerebral artery peak systolic velocity predict polycythemia in monochorionic-diamniotic twins? Evidence from a prospective cohort study: MCA and polycythemia in MCDA twins. *Ultrasound Obstet. Gynecol.* **2016**, *48*, 470–475. [CrossRef] [PubMed]
13. Tollenaar, L.; Lopriore, E.; Middeldorp, J.M.; Haak, M.C.; Klumper, F.J.; Oepkes, D.; Slaghekke, F. Improved prediction of twin anemia-polycythemia sequence by delta middle cerebral artery peak systolic velocity: New antenatal classification system. *Ultrasound Obstet. Gynecol. Off. J. Int. Soc. Ultrasound Obstet. Gynecol.* **2019**, *53*, 788–793. [CrossRef] [PubMed]
14. Perinatology.com. Available online: http://www.perinatology.com/calculators/MCA.htm (accessed on 10 June 2022).
15. Bonferroni, C. *Teoria Statistica delle Classi e Calcolo delle Probabilità*; Pubblicazioni del R Istituto Superiore di Scienze Economiche e Commericiali di Firenze: Florenz, Italy, 1936; 62p.
16. Moosbrugger, H.; Kelava, A. *Testtheorie und Fragebogenkonstruktion. 2. Aktualisierte und Überarbeitete Auflage*; Testtheorie und Fragebogenkonstruktion; Springer: Berlin/Heidelberg, Germany, 2012.
17. Tollenaar, L.; Slaghekke, F.; Middeldorp, J.M.; Klumper, F.J.; Haak, M.C.; Oepkes, D.; Lopriore, E. Twin Anemia Polycythemia Sequence: Current Views on Pathogenesis, Diagnostic Criteria, Perinatal Management, and Outcome. *Twin Res. Hum. Genet. Off. J. Int. Soc. Twin Stud.* **2016**, *19*, 222–233. [CrossRef] [PubMed]
18. Liu, B.; Kalafat, E.; Bhide, A.; Thilaganathan, B.; Khalil, A. Performance of Antenatal Diagnostic Criteria of Twin-Anemia-Polycythemia Sequence. *J. Clin. Med.* **2020**, *9*, 2754. [CrossRef] [PubMed]

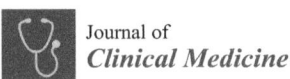

Article

Are Cervical Length and Fibronectin Predictors of Preterm Birth after Fetal Spina Bifida Repair? A Single Center Cohort Study

Ladina Vonzun [1,2,3,4,*,†], Ladina Rüegg [1,4,†], Julia Zepf [1,4], Ueli Moehrlen [2,3,4,5,6], Martin Meuli [2,3,4,5,6] and Nicole Ochsenbein-Kölble [2,3,4]

[1] Department of Obstetrics, University Hospital Zurich, Rämistrasse 100, 8091 Zurich, Switzerland
[2] Faculty of Medicine, University of Zurich, Rämistrasse 71, 8091 Zurich, Switzerland
[3] The Zurich Center for Fetal Diagnosis and Therapy, University of Zurich, 8091 Zurich, Switzerland
[4] Spina Bifida Academy, University Children's Hospital Zurich, Steinwiesstrasse 75, 8032 Zurich, Switzerland
[5] Spina Bifida Center, University Children's Hospital Zurich, Steinwiesstrasse 75, 8032 Zurich, Switzerland
[6] Department of Pediatric Surgery, University Children's Hospital Zurich, Steinwiesstrasse 75, 8032 Zurich, Switzerland
* Correspondence: ladina.vonzun@usz.ch; Tel.: +41-44-255-11-11; Fax: +41-44-255-44-48
† These authors contributed equally to this work.

Abstract: Background: A remaining risk of fetal spina bifida (fSB) repair is preterm delivery. This study assessed the value of preoperative cervical length (CL), CL dynamics (ΔCL) and fetal fibronectin (fFN) tests to predict obstetric complications and length of stay (LOS) around fSB repair. Methods: 134 patients were included in this study. All patients had CL measurement and fFN testing before fSB repair. ΔCL within the first 14 days after intervention and until discharge after fSB repair were compared in groups (ΔCL ≥ 10 mm/<10 mm; ≥20 mm/<20 mm). CL before surgery, ΔCL's, and positive fFN tests were correlated to obstetric complications and LOS. Results: Mean CL before surgery was 41 ± 7 mm. Mean GA at birth was 35.4 ± 2.2 weeks. In the group of ΔCL ≥ 10 mm within the first 14 days after intervention, LOS was significantly longer ($p = 0.02$). ΔCL ≥ 10 mm until discharge after fSB was associated with a significantly higher rate of GA at birth <34 weeks ($p = 0.03$). The 3 positive fFN tests before fSB repair showed no correlation with GA at birth. Conclusion: Perioperative ΔCL influences LOS after fetal surgery. ΔCL ≥ 10 mm until discharge after fSB repair has a 3-times higher rate of preterm delivery before 34 weeks. Preoperative fFN testing showed no predictive value for preterm birth after fSB repair and was stopped.

Keywords: fetal surgery; spina bifida; cervical length; fibronectin test; preterm birth; PPROM

1. Introduction

About 1 in 3000 pregnancies is affected by spina bifida aperta (SB), which is the most common neural tube defect [1,2]. Nowadays, the intrauterine repair of a SB is a valid therapeutic option for selected cases [3–5]. It has been shown to reduce the need for ventriculoperitoneal shunt placement and to improve long-term neurological function [3,5]. Even though fetal spina bifida (fSB) repair is a standard therapy in several centers, especially in the US and Europe, there are risks for mother and fetus to be considered [6,7]. Intrauterine surgery is associated with obstetrical complications such as preterm prelabour rupture of the membranes (PPROM), chorioamniotic membrane separation (CMS), and subsequently preterm birth with its adverse consequences for the newborn [7–11]. Preterm birth is, independently from fSB repair, the most frequent cause of perinatal mortality and severe perinatal morbidity in the Western world [12].

A short cervical length (CL) is known to be a good predictor of preterm birth [13,14]. Especially in high-risk pregnancies, measuring CL is valuable and helpful for further management [15]. For fetal interventions, such as laser therapies in twin pregnancies, CL measurement before surgery is the most important predictor for preterm birth [16].

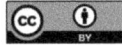

A further potential marker for preterm delivery is the fetal fibronectin (fFN) test [17]. fFN is a glycoprotein found in placental tissue, the extracellular substance of the decidua, and in the amniotic fluid. Through inflammatory or mechanical damage to the membranes before birth, it is thought to be released. A fFN test showing positive results indicates a high likelihood of preterm delivery within the next 7–10 days [18]. In the context of fSB repair, the value of CL measurements or fFN tests for the risk assessment of complications has never been evaluated.

Therefore, the goal of this study was to assess whether the preoperative CL measurements and its dynamics (ΔCL) and/or a positive fFN test before surgery is associated with preterm birth, PPROM, or CMS. An additional aim was to evaluate whether short CL measurements have an impact on the length of stay (LOS) after fSB repair.

2. Materials and Methods

2.1. Patients and Study Design

Between December 2010 and April 2020, 136 women underwent fSB repair at the Zurich Center for Fetal Diagnosis and Therapy (www.swissfetus.ch, accessed on 20 November 2022). Two patients were excluded from this study due to withdrawn consent. Data were collected prospectively and entered into our RedCap database. If available, missing data was completed by retrospective analysis of the ultrasound reports and images.

Eligibility criteria, the peri- and postoperative management, and the open surgical technique have been published previously in detail [4,5,7,19,20].

All patients received CL measurement before surgery. Postoperative CL measurements performed within the first 14 days after fetal surgery were considered for perioperative ΔCL assessment. CL measurements before discharge were considered for the assessment of CL dynamic until discharge after fSB repair. Analysis of ΔCL within the first 14 days after fetal surgery and until the end of hospitalization were performed in subgroups ($\Delta C \geq 10$ mm or <10 mm and $\Delta C \geq 20$ mm or <20 mm). Cut-offs were chosen in 10 mm steps as smaller changes likely underlie higher interobserver variability. All findings were correlated to the GA at birth, obstetric complications such as CMS and PPROM, and LOS. Ultrasound examination was performed by one of our senior consultants, specialist in prenatal ultrasound. A GE Voluson E8 or E10 system (GE Healthcare Austria GmbH & CO OG, Zipf, Austria) transvaginal transducer was used. CL was measured longitudinally, from the inner to the outer uterine orifice taking into account the natural curve of the cervix, and with an empty bladder, as recommended by the ISUOG Guidelines [21]. In case of preoperative CL below the 5th percentile according to the nomogram by Papastefanou et al. [22], a pessary (Arabin® Cerclage Pessar) was placed during fetal surgery. After placement of a pessary, no more routine CL measurements took place throughout the further course of pregnancy.

Furthermore, fFN test (QuickCheck fFN, Hologic Inc., Marlborough, MA, USA) was performed routinely before surgery. Swabs were taken from the ectocervix, or the posterior vaginal fornix and an enzyme linked immunosorbent assay (ELISA) with FDC6 monoclonal antibody was used to detect. The perioperative management did not differ in women with positive or negative fFN tests.

All patients received perioperative tocolysis as described previously [23]. After fSB repair, all women were monitored in an intensive care unit for 2 days where contractions were continuously monitored by tocography (IntelliSpace, Perinatal information system, Philips AG Healthcare, Horgen, Switzerland). Ultrasound was performed twice daily to check for amniotic fluid, CMS, hematoma formation, and fetal perfusion. After transferring the patient to our prenatal unit, contractions were monitored by tocography twice a day, and ultrasound was performed once a week. This regimen has been previously published in detail [23]. If clinically stable and in the absence of complications such as, e.g., PPROM, discharge was possible 2–3 weeks after fSB repair with planned preventative re-hospitalization at 34 weeks and elective C-section at 37 weeks.

2.2. Data Analysis

Descriptive statistics were performed with SPSS version 25.0 (IBM, SPSS Inc., Armonk, NY, USA). Quantitative data are presented as mean +/− standard deviation (SD) or median with interquartile range (IQR) depending on the distribution of the data. Categorical data were compared using chi square test and provided as percentages. For comparison of continuous data, a *t*-test or non-parametric analysis using Mann–Whitney U test was performed as appropriate. The Pearson correlations coefficient was used to measure the strength of relationship between variables. Statistical significance was given with $p < 0.05$.

This study was conducted with the principles of the Declaration of Helsinki and International Conference on Harmonisation E6 (Good Clinical Practice) guidelines. Written informed consent was obtained from all included women. The study was conducted in accordance with the approval of the local Ethic Commission (KEK-ZH. Nr. 2021-01101).

3. Results

Detailed patient's characteristics are shown in Table 1. The mean gestational age (GA) at birth was 35.4 ± 2.2 weeks with a total preterm birth rate of 66% and 20% before 34 weeks.

Table 1. Maternal and fetal characteristics of the Zurich study cohort.

Demographics	n = 134
Maternal age (years), mean ± SD	31.9 ± 5
Nulliparous, no. (%)	58 (43)
Body mass index (kg/m^2), mean ± SD	25.8 ± 4.8
Previous uterine surgeries, incl. cesarean, no. (%)	21 (16)
GA at surgery (weeks), mean ± SD	25.0 ± 0.8
GA at birth (weeks), mean ± SD	35.4 ± 2.2
extreme preterm (≤28 0/7 weeks), no. (%)	2 (1.5%)
very preterm (28 0/7–31 6/7 weeks), no. (%)	8 (5.9%)
moderately preterm (32 0/7–33 6/7 weeks), no. (%)	17 (12.5%)
late preterm (34 0/7–36 6/7 weeks), no. (%)	61 (45.5%)
term (≥37 0/7 weeks), no. (%)	47 (34.5%)
Birthweight (grams), mean ± SD	2565 ± 518
PPROM, no. (%)	44 (33%)
CMS, no. (%)	22 (16%)
LOS (days), median (IQR)	23 (19–38)

3.1. Cervical Length (CL) Measurements

An overview on perioperative CL measurements and fFN test results is given in Table 2.

Table 2. Results of cervical length (CL) before surgery and the fetal Fibronectin tests (fFN).

Evaluation before Surgery	n = 134
CL before surgery (mm), mean ± SD	41 ± 7
<25 mm, no. (%)	2 (1.5%)
≥25 mm, no. (%)	132 (99%)
fFN	
Positive, no (%)	3 (2%)
Negative, no. (%)	116 (87%)
No test results, no. (%)	15 (11%)

CL measurements before and after fSB repair are shown in Figure 1 on the nomogram by Papastefanou et al. [22].

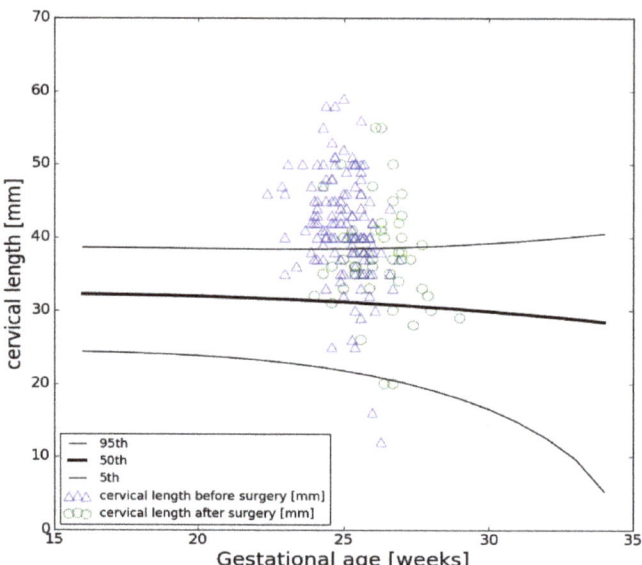

Figure 1. Overview of cervical length measurements before and after surgery on the nomogram by Papastefanou et al. [22].

Mean CL before surgery was 41 ± 7 mm. In 88 (65%) cases, the CL was ≥40 mm. Two (1.5%) women had a preoperative CL < 25 mm, of which both were below the 5th percentile, and thus a pessary was placed during fetal intervention.

In two further cases (1.5%) postoperative CL measurement was below the 5th percentile with a dynamic of 18 mm in one and 10 mm in the other case. Consequently, a pessary was placed upon diagnosis. In these four women presenting CL measurements below the 5th percentile, the LOS was comparable to the other cases (21 (18–23) vs. 23 (19–38)) ($p = 0.7$) and they all delivered between 35 and 37 weeks.

There was no significant correlation between the CL before surgery and GA at birth ($p = 0.83$). Preoperative CL measurements showed no significant correlation with the obstetrical complications as CMS ($p = 0.28$) and PPROM ($p = 1.0$), but a trend was seen for the LOS ($p = 0.06$) showing a slightly longer hospitalization when CL was shorter.

Further, there was no significant correlation between the overall ΔCL within 14 days after the intervention nor until the end of hospitalization and GA at delivery, CMS, PPROM and duration of hospitalization (Table 3).

Table 3. Overview of the missing correlation between the overall cervical length dynamics (ΔCL) within 14 days after fetal spina bifida repair and the ΔCL until the end of hospitalization, respectively, and GA at birth, chorioamniotic membrane separation (CMS), premature preterm prelabour rupture of the membranes (PPROM), and length of stay (LOS).

	ΔCL within 14 d		ΔCL until End of Hospitalisation	
	corr.coeff.	p-Value	corr.coeff.	p-Value
GA at birth	0.04	0.79	0.02	0.86
CMS	−0.12	0.42	−0.2	0.09
PPROM	−0.06	0.69	0.15	0.23
LOS	0.15	0.24	0.16	0.21

Subgroup analysis of the perioperative results with the ones of the first 14 days after fetal intervention showed a significant difference in GA at delivery for ΔCL ≥ 20 mm ($n = 2$)

(Table 4). No significant correlation with the analyzed obstetrical complications CMS and PPROM were observed within the subgroups of ΔCL ≥ 20 mm or <20 mm. In the group of perioperative ΔCL ≥ 10 mm, a significantly shorter hospitalization was observed ($p = 0.02$) (Table 4).

Table 4. Comparison of the groups with cervical length dynamics (ΔCL) ≥10 mm or <10 mm and ≥20 mm or <20 mm within the first 14 days after fetal spina bifida repair.

	ΔCL ≥ 10 mm (n = 10)	ΔCL < 10 mm (n = 40)	p-Value	ΔCL ≥ 20 mm (n = 2)	ΔCL < 20 mm (n = 48)	p-Value
CL preoperative, mm (mean ± SD)	46 ± 9	40 ± 6	0.03	57 ± 2	40 ± 7	0.001
GA at delivery, weeks (mean ± SD)	35.2 ± 2.3	35.1 ± 2.6	0.9	32.0 ± 0.5	35.3 ± 2.5	0.03
GA at delivery, n (%)						
<28 weeks	0 (0%)	1 (2.5%)	0.8	0 (0%)	1 (2%)	0.96
28 + 0–31 + 6 weeks	1 (10%)	5 (12.5%)	0.66	1 (50%)	5 (10%)	0.23
32 + 0–33 + 6 weeks	2 (20%)	3 (7.5%)	0.26	1 (50%)	4 (8%)	0.19
34 + 0–36 + 6 weeks	3 (30%)	19 (47.5%)	0.26	0 (0%)	22 (46%)	0.31
≥37 + 0 weeks	4 (40%)	12 (30%)	0.40	0 (0%)	16 (34%)	0.46
GA at delivery < 34 weeks, n (%)	3 (30%)	9 (23%)	0.45	2 (100%)	10 (21%)	0.05
CMS, n (%)	1 (10%)	7 (18%)	0.45	1 (50%)	7 (15%)	0.3
PPROM, n (%)	3 (30%)	13 (33%)	0.6	1 (50%)	15 (31%)	0.54
LOS, days (median, IQR)	19 (17–24)	30 (21–40)	0.02	22 (19–23)	28 (20–39)	0.49

Analysis of ΔCL until the end of hospitalization after fSB repair showed a significantly (3-times) higher rate of preterm birth before 34 weeks ($p = 0.03$), if ΔCL was ≥10 mm ($n = 9$) in comparison to the group of ΔCL < 10 mm ($n = 3$) (Table 5). In the group with ΔCL ≥ 10 mm, the mean GA at delivery was still 35.1 weeks and the rate of extremely and very preterm born infants was not significantly different between the two groups (Table 5). In the group of ΔCL > 10 mm a nearly 4-times higher rate of CMS was found ($p = 0.045$) (Table 5). Using the higher cut-off of ΔCL ≥ 20 mm, these differences could not be reproduced (Table 5).

Table 5. Comparison of the groups with cervical length dynamics (ΔCL) ≥10 mm or <10 mm and ≥20 mm or <20 mm until discharge after fetal spina bifida repair.

	ΔCL ≥ 10 mm (n = 30)	ΔCL < 10 mm (n = 34)	p-Value	ΔCL ≥ 20 mm (n = 11)	ΔCL < 20 mm (n = 53)	p-Value
CL preoperative, mm (mean ± SD)	44 ± 10	40 ± 5	0.02	47 ± 12	41 ± 7	0.02
GA at delivery, weeks (mean ± SD)	35.1 ± 2.7	36.0 ± 1.8	0.12	35.3 ± 2.1	35.6 ± 2.3	0.35
GA at delivery, n (%)						
<28 weeks	1 (3%)	0 (0%)	0.46	0 (0%)	1 (2%)	0.82
28 + 0–31 + 6 weeks	3 (10%)	1 (3%)	0.33	2 (18%)	2 (4%)	0.14
32 + 0–33 + 6 weeks	5 (17%)	2 (6%)	0.23	1 (9%)	6 (11%)	0.64
34 + 0–36 + 6 weeks	13 (43%)	17 (48%)	0.67	5 (46%)	24 (45%)	0.62
≥37 + 0 weeks	8 (27%)	15 (43%)	0.17	3 (27%)	20 (38%)	0.4
GA at delivery < 34 weeks, n (%)	9 (30%)	3 (9%)	0.03	3 (27%)	9 (17%)	0.36
CMS, n (%)	7 (23%)	2 (6%)	0.05	2 (18%)	7 (13%)	0.5
PPROM, n (%)	9 (30%)	6 (17%)	0.22	4 (36%)	11 (21%)	0.25
LOS, days (media, IQR)	30 (19–40)	26 (20–38)	1.0	29 (19–36)	31 (18–39)	0.86

3.2. Fetal Fibronectin (fFN) Test

Out of the 134 patients, fFN testing was performed in 121 (89%) cases. It was positive in 3 (2%) of these cases (GA 24–25 weeks) (Table 2). In all 3 cases, the preoperative CL was >35 mm (37–51 mm). Two of these women delivered at 37 weeks, one at 35 weeks, thus not showing an obvious correlation between the positive fFN test and GA at birth. Due to the low numbers, no statistical analysis was performed.

4. Discussion

CMS, PPROM, and ultimately preterm delivery are known risks after fetal surgery. In our study cohort, neither preoperative CL measurements nor perioperative ΔCL showed any correlation with preterm birth, CMS, or PPROM. However, perioperative ΔCL seems to influence LOS and a $\Delta CL \geq 10$ mm until the end of hospitalization is associated with a 3-times higher rate of preterm delivery before 34 weeks.

4.1. Cervical Length and Preterm Delivery

Independent from fetal surgery, CL is a known predictor for preterm delivery in asymptomatic women at increased risk for preterm birth [24]. Rottenstreich et al. [25] observed in a case–control study that a CL dynamic of $\geq$4 mm between 24 and 34 weeks had a higher rate of preterm deliveries compared to women matched for the maximal cervical length (<35 weeks: 15.9 vs. 5.3%, $p = 0.013$). The rates were comparable to women matched according to the minimal CL [25]. We did not find a difference in rate of preterm deliveries, CMS, or PPROM with CL dynamics.

For fetal interventions, such as laser therapies in twin pregnancies, a CL < 25 mm before surgery is associated with a lower GA at birth and worse outcomes at 6 months of age [16]. It therefore plays a crucial role in selecting candidates and for parental counseling [16]. Other studies on fSB repair even excluded patients with a high risk for preterm delivery (previous preterm delivery or short CL) from eligibility [26]. In light of the above considerations, it seemed logical that CL measurements before, or even more, CL dynamics around fetal surgery, might influence preterm birth rates. Thus, in our cohort, a high perioperative ΔCL of $\geq$20 mm showed a five-time higher preterm birth rate <34 weeks, very close to statistical significance ($p = 0.054$). However, we found that a cut-off of $\Delta CL \geq 10$ mm until the end of hospitalization was significantly associated with preterm birth before 34 weeks ($p = 0.03$), but not with a higher rate of extreme or very preterm births.

Our results (open repair!) are also in line with the results of an open fSB repair cohort published by Da Rocha et al. [27] who observed that CL before surgery was comparable between women who delivered before 34 ($n = 22$) and after 34 gestational weeks ($n = 17$). He further described a PPROM rate of 46% and a rate of preterm delivery of 77%, with chorioamnionitis being the only associated risk factor for preterm delivery and/or PPROM. Their mean GA at delivery was 33.2 ± 3.7 GW [27].

Several studies report their numbers of preterm deliveries, CMS, and PPROM rates [26,28,29]. CL measurements, however, were rarely taken into account. Retrospectively, we assume our strict pre- and postoperative management, as well as our rigorous rule of 'zero tolerance for contractions' might have prevented an association between short cervix and premature birth. Additionally, women with a short CL (<5th P) pre- or postoperatively received a cervical pessary possibly contributing to fewer preterm deliveries.

Taken together our results and the above considerations, independent factors such as CMS, PPROM and contractions definitely seem to play a more important role in prediction of preterm birth than preoperative CL measurements or perioperative ΔCL. The authors therefore conclude that neither preoperative CL measurements nor perioperative ΔCL, in the absence of other symptoms and unless CL measurement is <5th P, must result in a different care management of patients that undergo or underwent fSB repair.

4.2. Fetal Fibronectin (fFN) Testing

The prediction of preterm birth using fFN tests remains controversial. Honest et al. [18] published a systematic review and found impending that fFN testing is most accurate in predicting spontaneous preterm birth within the next 7–10 days in symptomatic women [18]. On the other hand, a systematic review and metaanalysis of randomized controlled trials from Berghella et al. [30] showed that fFN testing in singleton pregnancies with imminent or impending preterm labor is associated with higher cost, but does not prevent preterm birth nor improve in perinatal outcome [30].

Pinheiro et al. [31] performed a risk assessment for preterm delivery using fFN and CL measurement in symptomatic women. They concluded that a positive fFN and CL < 25 mm indicate an increased risk for preterm delivery within the next 14 days. In our cohort, we did not have any such cases.

Interestingly, a study by Chon et al. [32] looked at the quantitative fetal fibronectin (qfFN) and its association with spontaneous preterm birth after laser surgery for twin-to-twin transfusion syndrome. They collected qfFN 24 h before and after surgery. The qfFN level was not altered after surgery in their cohort. However, they reported that patients with a qfFN levels > 10 ng/mL were 19 times more likely to have spontaneous preterm delivery before 28 GW. During open fSB repair manipulation on fetal membranes is inevitably stronger. Assumed to be less sensitive, postoperative FN testing was therefore not in our protocol and thus not evaluated in our collective. Yet, our study could not detect women at risk for preterm birth after fSB by preoperative fFN testing. Consequently, considering cost-effectiveness its use was stopped.

4.3. Strengths and Weaknesses

Positively, to our knowledge, this is the first study on a large cohort to examine preoperative CL measurements and different ΔCL around fSB repair. We show that preoperative CL measurements and short-term perioperative ΔCL do not influence GA at birth. However, long-term ΔCL of $\geq$10 mm may help predicting preterm delivery <34 weeks. Additionally, this is the first study to examine preoperative fFN tests in the context of fetal surgery.

Negatively, the numbers of women with short CL and positive fFN tests were too small to allow statistical analyses. No qfFN analysis was made and consequently, since we did not perform postoperative fFN testing, no statement regarding an eventual postoperative predictive validity can be made.

Further, in cases with CL below the 5th percentile, a prompt pessary treatment was installed, potentially leading to a positive bias concerning the correlation between shortened CL and preterm birth.

5. Conclusions

Perioperative ΔCL seems to influence the LOS after fetal surgery. Further, a ΔCL $\geq$ 10 mm until discharge after fSB repair has a 3-times higher rate of preterm delivery before 34 weeks.

Preoperative fFN testing showed no predictive value for preterm birth after fSB repair and was consequently stopped.

Author Contributions: The initial study outline was designed by L.V., N.O.-K. and L.R. collected data. L.V. and N.O.-K. performed the quality control of the data. L.V. and L.R. performed the statistical analyses. L.V. and L.R. wrote the first draft of the manuscript. All authors, including J.Z., U.M. and M.M. participated in the drafting and/or revising of the manuscript and contributed to its intellectual content. All authors have read and agreed to the published version of the manuscript.

Funding: This research received no external funding.

Institutional Review Board Statement: This study was conducted in accord with the principles of the Declaration of Helsinki and International Conference on Harmonisation E6 (Good Clinical Practice) guidelines. All participants gave their written informed consent to participate in this study.

This study was approved by the Medical Ethics Commission of the Canton Zurich, Switzerland (KEK-ZH, Nr. 2021-01101).

Informed Consent Statement: Written informed consent was obtained from all included women.

Conflicts of Interest: The authors declare no conflict of interest.

References

1. Adzick, N.S. Fetal surgery for spina bifida: Past, present, future. *Semin. Pediatr. Surg.* **2013**, *22*, 10–17. [CrossRef]
2. Copp, A.J.; Stanier, P.; Greene, N.D. Neural tube defects: Recent advances, unsolved questions, and controversies. *Lancet Neurol.* **2013**, *12*, 799–810. [CrossRef] [PubMed]
3. Adzick, N.S.; Thom, E.A.; Spong, C.Y.; Brock, J.W.; Burrows, P.K.; Johnson, M.P.; Howell, L.J.; Farrell, J.A.; Dabrowiak, M.E.; Sutton, L.N.; et al. A randomized trial of prenatal versus postnatal repair of myelomeningocele. *N. Engl. J. Med.* **2011**, *364*, 993–1004. [CrossRef] [PubMed]
4. Mohrlen, U.; Ochsenbein-Kolble, N.; Mazzone, L.; Kraehenmann, F.; Husler, M.; Casanova, B.; Biro, P.; Wille, D.; Latal, B.; Scheer, I.; et al. Benchmarking against the MOMS Trial: Zurich Results of Open Fetal Surgery for Spina Bifida. *Fetal Diagn. Ther.* **2020**, *47*, 91–97. [CrossRef] [PubMed]
5. Moehrlen, U.; Ochsenbein, N.; Vonzun, L.; Mazzone, L.; Horst, M.; Schauer, S.; Wille, D.A.; Hagmann, C.; Kottke, R.; Grehten, P.; et al. Fetal surgery for spina bifida in Zurich: Results from 150 cases. *Pediatr. Surg. Int.* **2021**, *37*, 311–316. [CrossRef] [PubMed]
6. Vonzun, L.; Kahr, M.K.; Noll, F.; Mazzone, L.; Moehrlen, U.; Meuli, M.; Husler, M.; Krahenmann, F.; Zimmermann, R.; Ochsenbein-Kolble, N. Systematic classification of maternal and fetal intervention-related complications following open fetal myelomeningocele repair—Results from a large prospective cohort. *BJOG* **2021**, *128*, 1184–1191. [CrossRef]
7. Winder, F.M.; Vonzun, L.; Meuli, M.; Moehrlen, U.; Mazzone, L.; Krahenmann, F.; Husler, M.; Zimmermann, R.; Ochsenbein-Kolble, N. Maternal Complications following Open Fetal Myelomeningocele Repair at the Zurich Center for Fetal Diagnosis and Therapy. *Fetal Diagn. Ther.* **2019**, *46*, 153–158. [CrossRef]
8. Moldenhauer, J.S.; Soni, S.; Rintoul, N.E.; Spinner, S.S.; Khalek, N.; Martinez-Poyer, J.; Flake, A.W.; Hedrick, H.L.; Peranteau, W.H.; Rendon, N.; et al. Fetal myelomeningocele repair: The post-MOMS experience at the Children's Hospital of Philadelphia. *Fetal Diagn. Ther.* **2015**, *37*, 235–240. [CrossRef]
9. Soni, S.; Moldenhauer, J.S.; Spinner, S.S.; Rendon, N.; Khalek, N.; Martinez-Poyer, J.; Johnson, M.P.; Adzick, N.S. Chorioamniotic membrane separation and preterm premature rupture of membranes complicating in utero myelomeningocele repair. *Am. J. Obstet. Gynecol.* **2016**, *214*, e641–e647. [CrossRef]
10. Zamłyński, J.; Olejek, A.; Koszutski, T.; Ziomek, G.; Horzelska, E.; Gajewska-Kucharek, A.; Maruniak-Chudek, I.; Herman-Sucharska, I.; Kluczewska, E.; Horak, S.; et al. Comparison of prenatal and postnatal treatments of spina bifida in Poland—A non-randomized, single-center study. *J. Matern. Fetal Neonatal Med.* **2014**, *27*, 1409–1417. [CrossRef]
11. Belfort, M.; Deprest, J.; Hecher, K. Current controversies in prenatal diagnosis 1: In utero therapy for spina bifida is ready for endoscopic repair. *Prenat Diagn* **2016**, *36*, 1161–1166. [CrossRef]
12. Slattery, M.M.; Morrison, J.J. Preterm delivery. *Lancet* **2002**, *360*, 1489–1497. [CrossRef] [PubMed]
13. Navathe, R.; Saccone, G.; Villani, M.; Knapp, J.; Cruz, Y.; Boelig, R.; Roman, A.; Berghella, V. Decrease in the incidence of threatened preterm labor after implementation of transvaginal ultrasound cervical length universal screening. *J. Matern. Fetal Neonatal Med.* **2019**, *32*, 1853–1858. [CrossRef] [PubMed]
14. Berghella, V.; Saccone, G. Cervical assessment by ultrasound for preventing preterm delivery. *Cochrane Database Syst. Rev.* **2019**, *9*, CD007235. [CrossRef] [PubMed]
15. Guzman, E.R.; Walters, C.; Ananth, C.V.; O'Reilly-Green, C.; Benito, C.W.; Palermo, A.; Vintzileos, A.M. A comparison of sonographic cervical parameters in predicting spontaneous preterm birth in high-risk singleton gestations. *Ultrasound Obstet. Gynecol.* **2001**, *18*, 204–210. [CrossRef] [PubMed]
16. Rüegg, L.; Hüsler, M.; Krähenmann, F.; Natalucci, G.; Zimmermann, R.; Ochsenbein-Kölble, N. Outcome after fetoscopic laser coagulation in twin-twin transfusion syndrome—Is the survival rate of at least one child at 6 months of age dependent on preoperative cervical length and preterm prelabour rupture of fetal membranes? *J. Matern. Fetal Neonatal Med.* **2020**, *33*, 852–860. [CrossRef] [PubMed]
17. Bulletins–Obstetrics, A.C.o.P. ACOG practice bulletin. Management of preterm labor. Number 43, May 2003. *Int. J. Gynaecol. Obstet.* **2003**, *82*, 127–135.
18. Honest, H.; Bachmann, L.M.; Gupta, J.K.; Kleijnen, J.; Khan, K.S. Accuracy of cervicovaginal fetal fibronectin test in predicting risk of spontaneous preterm birth: Systematic review. *BMJ* **2002**, *325*, 301. [CrossRef]
19. Mazzone, L.; Moehrlen, U.; Casanova, B.; Ryf, S.; Ochsenbein-Kölble, N.; Zimmermann, R.; Kraehenmann, F.; Meuli, M. Open Spina Bifida: Why Not Fetal Surgery? *Fetal Diagn. Ther.* **2019**, *45*, 430–434. [CrossRef]
20. Meuli, M.; Meuli-Simmen, C.; Mazzone, L.; Tharakan, S.J.; Zimmermann, R.; Ochsenbein, N.; Moehrlen, U. In utero Plastic Surgery in Zurich: Successful Use of Distally Pedicled Random Pattern Transposition Flaps for Definitive Skin Closure during Open Fetal Spina Bifida Repair. *Fetal Diagn. Ther.* **2018**, *44*, 173–178. [CrossRef]
21. Kagan, K.O.; Sonek, J. How to measure cervical length. *Ultrasound Obstet. Gynecol.* **2015**, *45*, 358–362. [CrossRef] [PubMed]

22. Papastefanou, I.; Pilalis, A.; Kappou, D.; Souka, A.P. Cervical length at 11-40 weeks: Unconditional and conditional longitudinal reference ranges. *Acta Obstet. Gynecol. Scand.* **2016**, *95*, 1376–1382. [CrossRef] [PubMed]
23. Ochsenbein-Kölble, N.; Krähenmann, F.; Hüsler, M.; Meuli, M.; Moehrlen, U.; Mazzone, L.; Biro, P.; Zimmermann, R. Tocolysis for in utero Surgery: Atosiban Performs Distinctly Better than Magnesium Sulfate. *Fetal Diagn. Ther.* **2018**, *44*, 59–64. [CrossRef] [PubMed]
24. Crane, J.M.; Hutchens, D. Transvaginal sonographic measurement of cervical length to predict preterm birth in asymptomatic women at increased risk: A systematic review. *Ultrasound Obstet. Gynecol.* **2008**, *31*, 579–587. [CrossRef] [PubMed]
25. Rottenstreich, A.; Gochman, N.; Kleinstern, G.; Levin, G.; Sompolinsky, Y.; Rottenstreich, M.; Sela, H.Y.; Yagel, S.; Porat, S. Is real-time dynamic cervical shortening predictive of preterm birth?—A case control study. *J. Matern. Fetal Neonatal Med.* **2020**, *35*, 4687–4694. [CrossRef]
26. Guilbaud, L.; Maurice, P.; Lallemant, P.; De Saint-Denis, T.; Maisonneuve, E.; Dhombres, F.; Friszer, S.; Di Rocco, F.; Garel, C.; Moutard, M.L.; et al. Open fetal surgery for myelomeningocele repair in France. *J. Gynecol. Obstet. Hum. Reprod.* **2021**, *50*, 102155. [CrossRef]
27. Da Rocha, L.S.N.; Bunduki, V.; de Amorim Filho, A.G.; Cardeal, D.D.; Matushita, H.; Fernandes, H.S.; Nani, F.S.; de Francisco, R.P.V.; de Carvalho, M.H.B. Open fetal myelomeningocele repair at a university hospital: Surgery and pregnancy outcomes. *Arch. Gynecol. Obstet.* **2021**, *304*, 1443–1454. [CrossRef]
28. Corroenne, R.; Yepez, M.; Barth, J.; Pan, E.; Whitehead, W.E.; Espinoza, J.; Shamshirsaz, A.A.; Nassr, A.A.; Belfort, M.A.; Sanz Cortes, M. Chorioamniotic membrane separation following fetal myelomeningocele repair: Incidence, risk factors and impact on perinatal outcome. *Ultrasound Obstet. Gynecol.* **2020**, *56*, 684–693. [CrossRef]
29. Kahr, M.K.; Winder, F.; Vonzun, L.; Meuli, M.; Mazzone, L.; Moehrlen, U.; Krähenmann, F.; Hüsler, M.; Zimmermann, R.; Ochsenbein-Kölble, N. Risk Factors for Preterm Birth following Open Fetal Myelomeningocele Repair: Results from a Prospective Cohort. *Fetal Diagn. Ther.* **2020**, *47*, 15–23. [CrossRef]
30. Berghella, V.; Saccone, G. Fetal fibronectin testing for prevention of preterm birth in singleton pregnancies with threatened preterm labor: A systematic review and metaanalysis of randomized controlled trials. *Am. J. Obstet. Gynecol.* **2016**, *215*, 431–438. [CrossRef]
31. Pinheiro Filho, T.R.C.; Pessoa, V.R.; Lima, T.S.; Castro, M.M.; Linhares, J.J. Risk Assessment for Preterm Delivery using the Fetal Fibronectin Test Associated with the Measurement of Uterine Cervix Length in Symptomatic Pregnant Women. *Rev. Bras. Ginecol. Obstet.* **2018**, *40*, 507–512. [CrossRef] [PubMed]
32. Chon, A.H.; Chan, Y.; Korst, L.M.; Llanes, A.; Abdel-Sattar, M.; Chmait, R.H. Quantitative fetal fibronectin to predict spontaneous preterm delivery after laser surgery for twin-twin transfusion syndrome. *Sci. Rep.* **2019**, *9*, 4438. [CrossRef] [PubMed]

Disclaimer/Publisher's Note: The statements, opinions and data contained in all publications are solely those of the individual author(s) and contributor(s) and not of MDPI and/or the editor(s). MDPI and/or the editor(s) disclaim responsibility for any injury to people or property resulting from any ideas, methods, instructions or products referred to in the content.

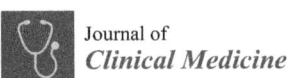

Article

Stage 2: The Vaginal Flora in Women Undergoing Fetal Spina Bifida Repair and Its Potential Association with Preterm Rupture of Membranes and Preterm Birth

Fanny Tevaearai [1,2,*], Maike Katja Sachs [1,2], Samia El-Hadad [1,2], Ladina Vonzun [1,2,3], Ueli Moehrlen [2,3,4], Luca Mazzone [2,3,4], Martin Meuli [2,3,4], Franziska Krähenmann [1,2,3] and Nicole Ochsenbein-Kölble [1,2,3,*]

1. Department of Obstetrics, University Hospital Zurich, 8091 Zurich, Switzerland
2. Department of Obstetrics, Faculty of Medicine, University of Zurich, 8006 Zurich, Switzerland
3. Zurich Center for Fetal Diagnosis and Therapy, 8091 Zurich, Switzerland
4. Department of Pediatric Surgery, University Children's Hospital Zurich, 8032 Zurich, Switzerland
* Correspondence: fanny.tevaearai@chuv.ch (F.T.); nicole.ochsenbein@usz.ch (N.O.-K.); Tel.: +41-79-595-4295 (F.T.); +41-43-253-9712 (N.O.-K.)

Abstract: Introduction: Vaginal dysbiosis affects pregnancy outcomes, however, the relevance of abnormal findings on pre/post-surgical vaginal culture in women undergoing fetal spina bifida (fSB) repair is unknown. Objectives: To describe the incidence of normal and abnormal pre- and post-surgical vaginal microorganisms in fSB patients and to investigate potential associations between the type of vaginal flora and the occurrence of preterm prelabour rupture of membranes (PPROM) and preterm birth (PTB). Methods: 99 women undergoing fSB repair were eligible (2010–2019). Pre-surgical vaginal culture was routinely taken before surgery. Post-surgical cultures were taken on indication. Vaginal flora was categorized into four categories: healthy vaginal flora (HVF), bacterial vaginosis (BV), desquamative inflammatory vaginitis (DIV), and yeast infection. Results: The incidence of HVF, BV, DIV, or yeast infections was not statistically different between the pre- and postoperative patients. Furthermore, an abnormal pre/post-surgical vaginal flora was not associated with PPROM (OR 1.57 (0.74–3.32), $p = 0.213$)/OR 1.26 (0.62–2.55), $p = 0.515$), or with PTB (OR 1.19 (0.82–1.73), $p = 0.315$)/(OR 0.86 (0.60–1.24), $p = 0.425$). Conclusions: Abnormal vaginal microbiome was not associated with PPROM and PTB when appropriate treatment was performed.

Keywords: fetal spina bifida (fSB) repair; preterm prelabour rupture of the membranes (PPROM); preterm birth (PTB); vaginal flora

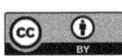

1. Introduction

The vaginal microbiome is a complex combination of multiple bacteria and is known to undergo natural variation during pregnancy [1–4]. Large studies have shown that vaginal dysbiosis is associated with an increased risk for preterm prelabour rupture of membranes (PPROM) and preterm birth (PTB) [5–7]. After open fetal spina bifida (fSB) repair, PPROM and PTB occur in approximately 30–50% and 60–80% [8–10], however, no previous study has yet focused on the prevalence of vaginal dysbiosis and its association with PPROM and PTB in the fSB repair population. This study explores the incidence of normal and abnormal pre- and post-surgical vaginal flora and its possible association with PPROM and PTB in fSB patients.

Healthy vaginal flora (HVF) is composed mostly by *Lactobacillus*, which is absent in bacterial vaginosis (BV) and desquamative inflammatory vaginitis (DIV). The flora in BV is dominated by *Gardnerella vaginalis*, whereas in DIV, vaginal inflammation is combined with the presence of *Escherichia coli*, group B streptococcus, *Staphylococcus aureus*, or *Enterococcus faecalis* [4].

2. Material and Methods

2.1. Patient Population and Study Design

One hundred and one pregnant women undergoing open fSB repair from 01/2010-12/2019 at the Zurich Center for Fetal Diagnosis and Therapy were included in this study. Inclusion and exclusion criteria have been adapted from the MOMS (Management of Myelomeningocele Study) criteria and have been described previously [10]. Prenatal closure of the fSB defect was carried out using open fetal surgery. Informed consent was obtained from every patient undergoing fSB repair during pre-operative counseling. Two patients were excluded from the study due to missing informed consent. A total of ninety-nine patients were, therefore, eligible for this study.

Our study was approved by the ethics committee of Canton Zurich (KEK-ZH.Nr. 2015-0172).

The detailed standard admission process on the prenatal ward, as well as intra- and postoperative care at our center, has been described previously [8]. We included the following demographic variables to describe our patient population: maternal age, ethnicity, BMI, smoking, parity, gestational age (GA) at surgery, delivery and birth, cervical length at surgery, fetal gender, and birthweight (Table 1). All patients undergoing open fSB operation received prophylactic antibiotic therapy intraoperative: 1 g of Cefazoline was given iv and 900 mg of Clindamycine was given directly in the amniotic fluid during the operation. In cases of allergy, 500 mg of Vancomycine was given. In the immediate postoperative period, patients were given 1 g of Cefazoline iv 4×/day during 1 day and Clindamycine in cases of allergies.

Table 1. Demographic and Clinical Variables.

Demographic and Clinical Variables (n = 99)	
Maternal age (years)	32 (26; 35)
Body mass index (kg/m^2)	25.4 (23; 30)
Smoking	1 (1%)
Nullipara	56 (57%)
Race/Ethnicity (N; %)	
White	93 (94%)
African–American	2 (2%)
Hispanic	2 (2%)
Others	2 (2%)
Cervical length at surgery (mm)	40 (32; 43)
Gestational age at surgery (weeks)	25.0 (24; 26)
Gestational age at delivery (weeks)	36.1 (35; 37)
PPROM	33 (33%)
Preterm birth	65 (66%)
Birthweight (grams)	2650 (2300; 2870)
Female fetal gender	52 (52%)

Data presented as n (%) or median (interquartile range).

2.2. Vaginal Flora and Treatment

In our cohort, at least three vaginal swabs were taken routinely from all patients before fSB repair at admission to the prenatal ward at 24 + 3/7 GA (20 + 6/7 GA–25 + 5/7 GA).

A wet mount microscopic test was carried out bedside and analyzed by skilled physicians. The vaginal flora was categorized into four adapted categories. Three have recently been established by Paavonen et al. [4]: HVF, BV, and DIV. To these, we added a fourth category, vaginal candidiasis.

A control swab was taken on indication: a control swab in women with a prior abnormal swab after antibiotic therapy, vaginal swabs in case of common clinical symptoms of vaginal infection, and directly after PPROM. These were sent to the laboratory for culture analyses. Whenever the result from the laboratory did not match the diagnosis made by wet mount microscopy, the laboratory results were used.

A third vaginal swab was taken for direct group B streptococcus (GBS)-PCR (GeneXpert, Baden, Switzerland), providing a result of GBS infection status within about 45 min.

Only women with abnormal vaginal bedside swabs were treated promptly with adequate antibiotics before undergoing surgery. If necessary, the antibiotic treatment was adjusted after receipt of the microbiology results.

Postoperatively, vaginal swabs were taken on specific indication: a control swab was repeated in women with a prior abnormal swab after antibiotic therapy to monitor the success of treatment. Vaginal swabs were also performed in case of common clinical symptoms of vaginal infection and directly after PPROM. In the case of PPROM without proof of vaginal dysbiosis, empiric antibiotic treatment was started with erythromycin orally for 7 days and adapted if necessary once culture results were available. After PPROM, a vaginal swab was routinely repeated all 2–3 weeks. In cases with pathological findings, antibiotic treatment was adjusted (or given) according to microbiology results.

BV was treated with dequaliniumchlorid (10 mg vaginally for 6 days), an antimicrobial agent covering Gram-positive and Gram-negative bacteria, anaerobic bacteria, protozoa, and candida. The same treatment was given to women with DIV if no colonization with a resistant germ was found that required other specific treatment. Vaginal candidiasis was treated with fluconazole (150 mg orally, single dose).

3. Statistical Analysis

Statistical analysis was performed using the statistical software package SPSS (version 24, IBM, New York, NY, USA). Variables were tested by Kolmogorov–Smirnov test for normal distribution. Quantitative data are presented as mean +/− standard deviation (SD) or medians with IQR. The results of categorical variables are given as percentages.

Odds ratios and 95% confidence intervals were calculated for PPROM and PTB. A p-value < 0.05 was considered significant.

4. Results

Relevant demographics and clinical variables of the study cohort are shown in Table 1.

Pre-surgical vaginal swabs were taken routinely from all 99 women: 69 women (69.7%) had a HVF and 30 women revealed an abnormal vaginal flora (30.4%), consisting of 7.1% BV, 16.2% DIV, 1% DIV and BV, and 6.1% yeast infection (see Figure 1A). The relation between these different groups and women ending up having a PPROM vs. PTB is shown in Figure 2A.

Post-surgical cultures were taken in 53 cases on indication: control swab in women with a prior abnormal swab after antibiotic therapy, vaginal swabs in case of common clinical symptoms of vaginal infection and directly after PPROM, while in some women, indications were overlapping. A total of 24 women had a HVF (45.3%), while 29 (54.7%) women showed abnormal vaginal colonization: 3 women with BV (5.7%), 19 women with DIV (35.8%), and 7 women with a yeast infection (13.2%) (see Figure 1B). Once again, the relation between these groups and PPROM vs. PTB is shown in Figure 2B.

An abnormal pre-surgical vaginal flora was not associated with PPROM (OR 1.57 (0.74–3.32), p = 0.213) or with PTB (OR 1.19 (0.82–1.73), p = 0.315). The same was true for a post-surgical culture where neither PPROM (OR 1.26 (0.62–2.55), p = 0.515) nor PTB (OR 0.86 (0.60–1.24), p = 0.425) was associated with BV, DIV, or yeast infections.

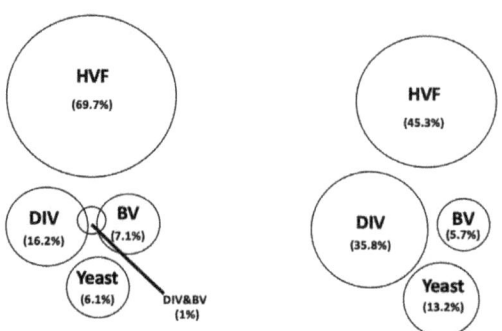

Figure 1. Results of vaginal swabs pre-surgical (**A**) and post-surgical (**B**); HVF—healthy vaginal flora, DIV—desquamative inflammatory vaginitis, BV—bacterial vaginosis.

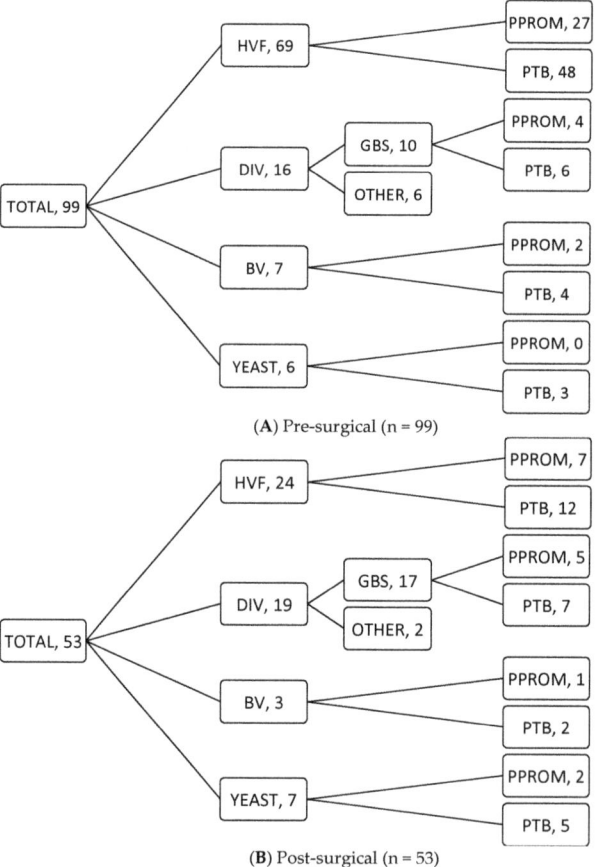

Figure 2. Results of vaginal swabs pre-surgical (**A**) and post-surgical (**B**) and their relation with PPROM and PTB; HVF—healthy vaginal flora, DIV—desquamative inflammatory vaginitis, BV—bacterial vaginosis.

5. Discussion

In our cohort of ninety-nine patients undergoing open fSB repair, there was no association found between abnormal vaginal flora before and after surgery and PPROM or PTB. We found that about two-thirds of women had a HVF before undergoing fSB repair. This is in line with MacIntyre's study regarding the vaginal microbiome during pregnancy in the general European population, where HVF was found in 66% during pregnancy [3].

As seen in Figure 2, discrepancies appear between the pre- and post-surgical groups. This is probably explained by the fact that post-surgical swabs were only taken on indication. There is, therefore, a selection bias as these indications include women with a prior abnormal swab after antibiotic therapy, women with common clinical symptoms of vaginal infection and directly after PPROM, thus explaining the differences between the two groups. This difference is also explained by the fact that not every infection led to PPROM and/or PTB.

According to previous data [11,12] and in line with this present study, in-utero surgery itself seems to be the major factor causing PTB, most likely as a consequence of direct mechanical membrane damage [13]. Similar to other in utero procedures (i.e., placenta laser [14]), it is presumed that this mechanism is directly linked to PPROM and, therefore, PTB in this population [11,12]. The direct mechanical damage of the membranes puts the woman at a higher risk for chorioamniotic membrane separation and PPROM [15], especially with the earlier timing of surgery [12,16]. Summing up, these studies suggest that PPROM may more likely be due to an iatrogenic effect than it may be induced by an abnormal vaginal flora. However, we cannot exclude that BV, DIV, and yeast infections still represent a risk factor for PPROM and PTB in the fSB repair population as other studies have already shown evidence that vaginal dysbiosis is associated with a higher risk for PPROM and PTB [5,17]. For instance, according to the ACOGs (American College of Obstetricians and Gynecologists) practice bulletin from March 2020, intraamniotic infection was diagnosed in 15–35% of women with PPROM, the incidence being higher in early GA [18]. Although systematic screening and treatment is not recommended in the general low-risk population with asymptomatic BV [19–21], studies recommend treating pregnant women with symptomatic BV in order to resolve symptoms [20,22,23]. Regarding pregnant women with BV and a high risk for PTB (i.e., previous PTB or late miscarriage), multiple studies have shown benefits regarding PPROM and PTB when treating BV [24,25]. In Yudin's study, for instance, treating women with increased risk for PTB was, therefore, recommended [23]. Furthermore, the Oracle I study has shown that an antibiotic treatment in cases of PPROM is evidence-based, hence, decreasing the amount of PTB [26]. In summary, there is evidence that prompt treatment of BV in high-risk situations, such as fSB repair, reduce PTB and PRROM rates.

In cases of vaginal candidiasis, a recent systematic review found no association between asymptomatic vaginal candidiasis and PTB [27]. In other studies, however, treatment of asymptomatic candidiasis is advised in order to prevent PTB [28,29]. As shown in Schusters systematic review, this effect is more likely due to the anti-inflammatory effect of the treatment rather than its anti-fungal treatment [27].

According to the study by Bennett et al., it is assumed that antibiotic treatment destroys the HVF by targeting Lactobacillus and therefore leading to an increased risk for vaginal dysbiosis [5]. This might explain the doubling in yeast infections in our cohort.

As none of these studies focuses on the fSB population, we still think that an appropriate treatment for women with or without symptoms of vaginal dysbiosis or candidiasis may have helped prevent PPROM and PTB in this specific population.

We would like to address a number of limitations and strengths of this study. Our study did not include a control group with patients who were not treated in case of an abnormal vaginal flora. Therefore, we cannot draw any conclusions about whether antibiotic treatment of an abnormal vaginal flora reduced PPROM or PTB.

Another interesting fact to discuss is the antibiotic treatment provided. As described earlier, all women undergoing fSB repair routinely received a prophylactic perioperative antibiotic treatment and no amniotic fluid was collected during the fetal spina bifida repair for bacteriological examination. Recommended treatments for BV include Metronidazole or Clindamycine. Treatments for DIV include Clindamycine or topical glucocorticoid [4]. It is, hence, unknown whether protocol prophylactic antibiotic treatments given to the patients have influenced our results or not. In fact, postoperative vaginal swabs were carried out in the same amount of time, suggesting a possible bias.

A strength of this investigation is the high number of patients of this rather unique study population. In fact, almost all women with PPROM or PTB came back to our center, leading to excellent data quality and completeness. Another interesting aspect of this study is the fact that an evaluation of the vaginal flora was standardized in all patients with an internal control of microscopic diagnosis with the help of an additional swab that was analyzed in the microbiology lab. To our knowledge, other centers do not routinely screen for abnormal vaginal flora and patients are often admitted for delivery to other hospitals than the one that performed the perioperative care.

6. Conclusions

In our fSB repair cohort, we found a normal pre-operative distribution of a HVF and there was no association between an abnormal vaginal flora treated antibiotically and PPROM and PTB.

Author Contributions: F.T. and M.K.S. wrote the manuscript. The initial study outline was designed by N.O.-K. and M.K.S.; F.T., M.K.S. and L.V. collected data and performed its quality control. S.E.-H. and M.K.S. performed the data analysis. F.T., M.K.S., N.O.-K., S.E.-H., L.V., U.M., L.M., M.M. and F.K. participated in the drafting and/or revising of the manuscript and contributed to its intellectual content. The final version of the manuscript was approved by all authors prior to publication. All authors have read and agreed to the published version of the manuscript.

Funding: There are no funding sources for this study.

Institutional Review Board Statement: The study was conducted in accordance with the Declaration of Helsinki, and approved by the Ethics Committee of Canton Zurich (KEK-ZH.Nr.2015-0172).

Informed Consent Statement: Informed consent was obtained from all subjects involved in the study.

Data Availability Statement: All data generated or analyzed during this study are included in this article. Further enquiries can be directed to the corresponding author.

Conflicts of Interest: The authors have no conflict of interest to declare.

References

1. Gupta, P.; Singh, M.P.; Goyal, K. Diversity of Vaginal Microbiome in Pregnancy: Deciphering the Obscurity. *Front. Public Health.* **2020**, *8*, 326. [CrossRef] [PubMed]
2. Freitas, A.C.; Chaban, B.; Bocking, A.; Rocco, M.; Yang, S.; Hill, J.E.; Money, D.M. The vaginal microbiome of pregnant women is less rich and diverse, with lower prevalence of Mollicutes, compared to non-pregnant women. *Sci. Rep.* **2017**, *7*, 9212. [CrossRef] [PubMed]
3. MacIntyre, D.A.; Chandiramani, M.; Lee, Y.S.; Kindinger, L.; Smith, A.; Angelopoulos, N.; Lehne, B.; Arulkumaran, S.; Brown, R.; Teoh, T.G.; et al. The vaginal microbiome during pregnancy and the postpartum period in a European population. *Sci. Rep.* **2015**, *5*, 8988. [CrossRef] [PubMed]
4. Paavonen, J.; Brunham, R.C. Bacterial Vaginosis and Desquamative Inflammatory Vaginitis. *N. Engl. J. Med.* **2018**, *379*, 2246–2254. [CrossRef] [PubMed]
5. Bennett, P.R.; Brown, R.G.; MacIntyre, D.A. Vaginal Microbiome in Preterm Rupture of Membranes. *Obstet. Gynecol. Clin. N. Am.* **2020**, *47*, 503–521. [CrossRef]
6. Hillier, S.L.; Nugent, R.P.; Eschenbach, D.A.; Krohn, M.A.; Gibbs, R.S.; Martin, D.H.; Cotch, M.F.; Edelman, R.; Pastorek, J.G.; Rao, A.V.; et al. Association between bacterial vaginosis and preterm delivery of a low-birth-weight infant. The Vaginal Infections and Prematurity Study Group. *N. Engl. J. Med.* **1995**, *333*, 1737–1742. [CrossRef]
7. Chu, D.M.; Seferovic, M.; Pace, R.M.; Aagaard, K.M. The microbiome in preterm birth. *Best Pract. Res. Clin. Obstet. Gynaecol.* **2018**, *52*, 103–113. [CrossRef]
8. Kahr, M.K. Risk Factors for Preterm Birth following Open Fetal Myelomeningocele Repair: Results from a Prospective Cohort—PubMed. Available online: https://pubmed.ncbi.nlm.nih.gov/31104051/ (accessed on 4 August 2021).

9. Moldenhauer, J.S.; Adzick, N.S. Fetal surgery for myelomeningocele: After the Management of Myelomeningocele Study (MOMS). *Semin. Fetal Neonatal Med.* **2017**, *22*, 360–366. [CrossRef]
10. Vonzun, L.; Kahr, M.K.; Noll, F.; Mazzone, L.; Moehrlen, U.; Meuli, M.; Hüsler, M.; Krähenmann, F.; Zimmermann, R.; Ochsenbein-Kölble, N. Systematic classification of maternal and fetal intervention-related complications following open fetal myelomeningocele repair—Results from a large prospective cohort. *BJOG Int. J. Obstet. Gynaecol.* **2021**, *128*, 1184–1191. [CrossRef]
11. Beck, V.; Lewi, P.; Gucciardo, L.; Devlieger, R. Preterm prelabor rupture of membranes and fetal survival after minimally invasive fetal surgery: A systematic review of the literature. *Fetal Diagn. Ther.* **2012**, *31*, 1–9. [CrossRef]
12. Soni, S.; Moldenhauer, J.S.; Spinner, S.S.; Rendon, N.; Khalek, N.; Martinez-Poyer, J.; Johnson, M.P.; Adzick, N.S. Chorioamniotic membrane separation and preterm premature rupture of membranes complicating in utero myelomeningocele repair. *Am. J. Obstet. Gynecol.* **2016**, *214*, e1–e7. [CrossRef] [PubMed]
13. Saadai, P.; Lee, T.H.; Bautista, G.; Gonzales, K.D.; Nijagal, A.; Busch, M.P.; Kim, C.J.; Romero, R.; Lee, H.; Hirose, S.; et al. Alterations in maternal-fetal cellular trafficking after fetal surgery. *J. Pediatr. Surg.* **2012**, *47*, 1089–1094. [CrossRef] [PubMed]
14. Rüegg, L.; Hüsler, M.; Krähenmann, F.; Natalucci, G.; Zimmermann, R.; Ochsenbein-Kölble, N. Outcome after fetoscopic laser coagulation in twin-twin transfusion syndrome—Is the survival rate of at least one child at 6 months of age dependent on preoperative cervical length and preterm prelabour rupture of fetal membranes? *J. Matern. Fetal Neonatal Med.* **2020**, *33*, 852–860. [CrossRef] [PubMed]
15. Adzick, N.S.; Thom, E.A.; Spong, C.Y.; Brock, I.I.I.J.W.; Burrows, P.K.; Johnson, M.P.; Howell, L.J.; Farrell, J.A.; Dabrowiak, M.E.; Sutton, L.N.; et al. A randomized trial of prenatal versus postnatal repair of myelomeningocele. *N. Engl. J. Med.* **2011**, *364*, 993–1004. [CrossRef] [PubMed]
16. Wilson, R.D.; Johnson, M.P.; Crombleholme, T.M.; Flake, A.W.; Hedrick, H.L.; King, M.; Howell, L.J.; Adzick, N.S. Chorioamniotic membrane separation following open fetal surgery: Pregnancy outcome. *Fetal Diagn. Ther.* **2003**, *18*, 314–320. [CrossRef]
17. Seo, K.; McGregor, J.A.; French, J.I. Preterm birth is associated with increased risk of maternal and neonatal infection. *Obstet. Gynecol.* **1992**, *79*, 75–80.
18. Prelabor Rupture of Membranes: ACOG Practice Bulletin, Number 217. *Obstet. Gynecol.* **2020**, *135*, e80–e97. [CrossRef]
19. Tebes, C.C.; Lynch, C.; Sinnott, J. The effect of treating bacterial vaginosis on preterm labor. *Infect. Dis. Obstet. Gynecol.* **2003**, *11*, 123–129. [CrossRef]
20. Brabant, G. [Bacterial vaginosis and spontaneous preterm birth]. *J. Gynecol. Obstet. Biol. Reprod.* **2016**, *45*, 1247–1260. [CrossRef]
21. Subtil, D.; Brabant, G.; Tilloy, E.; Devos, P.; Canis, F.; Fruchart, A.; Bissinger, M.C.; Dugimont, J.C.; Nolf, C.; Hacot, C.; et al. Early clindamycin for bacterial vaginosis in pregnancy (PREMEVA): A multicentre, double-blind, randomised controlled trial. *Lancet* **2018**, *392*, 2171–2179. [CrossRef]
22. Bacterial Vaginosis—STI Treatment Guidelines. 2021. Available online: https://www.cdc.gov/std/treatment-guidelines/bv.htm (accessed on 4 August 2021).
23. Yudin, M.H.; Money, D.M. No. 211-Screening and Management of Bacterial Vaginosis in Pregnancy. *J. Obstet. Gynaecol. Can.* **2017**, *39*, e184–e191. [CrossRef] [PubMed]
24. McDonald, H.M.; O'Loughlin, J.A.; Vigneswaran, R.; Jolley, P.T.; McDonald, P.J. Bacterial vaginosis in pregnancy and efficacy of short-course oral metronidazole treatment: A randomized controlled trial. *Obstet. Gynecol.* **1994**, *84*, 343–348. [PubMed]
25. McDonald, H.M.; Brocklehurst, P.; Gordon, A. Antibiotics for treating bacterial vaginosis in pregnancy. *Cochrane Database Syst. Rev.* **2007**, CD000262. Available online: https://www.ncbi.nlm.nih.gov/pmc/articles/PMC4164464/ (accessed on 24 September 2006).
26. Kenyon, S.L.; Taylor, D.J.; Tarnow-Mordi, W.; ORACLE Collaborative Group. Broad-spectrum antibiotics for preterm, prelabour rupture of fetal membranes: The ORACLE I randomised trial. ORACLE Collaborative Group. *Lancet* **2001**, *357*, 979–988. [CrossRef] [PubMed]
27. Schuster, H.J.; de Jonghe, B.A.; Limpens, J.; Budding, A.E.; Painter, R.C. Asymptomatic vaginal Candida colonization and adverse pregnancy outcomes including preterm birth: A systematic review and meta-analysis. *Am. J. Obstet. Gynecol MFM* **2020**, *2*, 100163. [CrossRef] [PubMed]
28. Roberts, C.L.; Rickard, K.; Kotsiou, G.; Morris, J.M. Treatment of asymptomatic vaginal candidiasis in pregnancy to prevent preterm birth: An open-label pilot randomized controlled trial. *BMC Pregnancy Childbirth* **2011**, *11*, 18. [CrossRef] [PubMed]
29. Farr, A.; Kiss, H.; Holzer, I.; Husslein, P.; Hagmann, M.; Petricevic, L. Effect of asymptomatic vaginal colonization with Candida albicans on pregnancy outcome. *Acta Obstet. Gynecol. Scand.* **2015**, *94*, 989–996. [CrossRef]

Review

The Evolution and Developing Importance of Fetal Magnetic Resonance Imaging in the Diagnosis of Congenital Cardiac Anomalies: A Systematic Review

Marios Mamalis [1], Ivonne Bedei [1], Bjoern Schoennagel [2], Fabian Kording [3], Justus G. Reitz [4], Aline Wolter [1], Johanna Schenk [1] and Roland Axt-Fliedner [1,*]

1. Division of Prenatal Medicine & Fetal Therapy, Department of Obstetrics & Gynecology, Justus-Liebig-University Giessen, 35390 Giessen, Germany
2. Diagnostic and Interventional Radiology and Nuclear Medicine, University Medical Centre Hamburg-Eppendorf, 20246 Hamburg, Germany
3. Northh Medical GmbH, 22335 Hamburg, Germany
4. Department of Cardiovascular Surgery, Justus-Liebig-University Giessen, 35390 Giessen, Germany
* Correspondence: roland.axt-fliedner@gyn.med.uni-giessen.de

Abstract: Magnetic Resonance Imaging (MRI) is a reliable method, with a complementary role to Ultrasound (US) Echocardiography, that can be used to fully comprehend and precisely diagnose congenital cardiac malformations. Besides the anatomical study of the fetal cardiovascular system, it allows us to study the function of the fetal heart, remaining, at the same time, a safe adjunct to the classic fetal echocardiography. MRI also allows for the investigation of cardiac and placental diseases by providing information about hematocrit, oxygen saturation, and blood flow in fetal vessels. It is crucial for fetal medicine specialists and pediatric cardiologists to closely follow the advances of fetal cardiac MRI in order to provide the best possible care. In this review, we summarize the advance in techniques and their practical utility to date.

Keywords: fetal cardiac magnetic resonance; congenital heart abnormalities

1. Introduction

Fetal cardiac abnormalities represent the subgroup of prenatally diagnosed abnormalities with the highest incidence (9:1000). Fetal echocardiography to date is the gold standard in fetal cardiology. Recently, reports on fetal cardiac MRI using different techniques have been published. Cardiac MRI is able to precisely demonstrate the cardiac anatomy and abnormal heart morphology in case of congenital heart disease (CHD). Furthermore, by applying the knowledge gained on fetal lambs, it can provide information about the impact of CHD on human fetal hemodynamic status by quantifying blood flow in fetal vessels [1–3] and provides details about fetal oxygenation [1]. In this setting, MRI has been applied to define the effect of CHD and fetal growth restriction (FGR) on brain development in fetal life [1,2] in recent studies.

In this review, the established techniques and the clinical utility of cardiac MRI in daily clinical practice will be discussed.

2. Fetal Cardiac MRI Techniques

Several authors refer to the utility of single-shot balanced Steady State Free Precession (bSSFP) and Fast Spin Echo sequences (SS-FSE) for detecting fetal defects [4–11]. Their contribution in providing multislice protocols is the result of a combination of high-resolution 2D static images in short time (1.0 to 1.5 mm in-plane and ≥500 ms). Although they cannot resolve fetal cardiac motion, resulting in the blurring of dynamic structures, they contribute to identify gross anatomical defects. Although bSSFP cannot preclude blurring resulting from fetal motion, it can be used for the assessment of the intracardiac anatomy as a stack of a single slice cine or 2D slices and it is capable to provide information about tissue when it is combined with SS-FE. SS-FE produces "black blood" images, useful for examining the extracardiac vasculature [11].

Furthermore, the repeated acquisition of bSSFP images in the same anatomical location over time has been used to provide a dynamic "real-time" assessment of the fetal heart including measurements of cardiac function [4,6–8,12–14].

Cine imaging requires the synchronization of use of high spatial and temporal resolution images to the patient's heart rate (cardiac gating) in order to provide assessment of both cardiac anatomy and function [15]. In order to overcome the limitation of long reconstruction times, devices are developed to monitor fetal heart rate during MRI data acquisition. The most mature device for this purpose uses an MRI-compatible Doppler ultrasound gating (DUS) probe placed over the maternal abdomen [16,17]. This device monitors the blood flow and cardiac contraction based on Doppler waveform (Figure 1). The disadvantages of this method are the equipment procurement, preparation time, and monitoring of fetal lie ensuring that it is within the detection range.

The need of acceleration of acquisition led several studies to investigate the use of compressed sensing to achieve highly accelerated fetal acquisitions using either Cartesian [18,19] or radial sequences [20–22].

In order to limit the artifacts from maternal respiration, it has been attempted to either acquire data under maternal breath hold or apply free breathing methods using motion correction. The latter allows for multislice acquisition, in contrast to the method under maternal breath hold, which limits the number of slices [21–23].

With the aid of 2D, real imaging motions are recognized and data acquired during those periods are discarded. The latest fully automated methods are implied; previously used for the fetal brain volumetric reconstruction. The outlier rejection, results in better quality images by estimating the probability of each voxel and real-time image frame, classifying them as in- or outlier, and, finally, rejecting the outlier voxels and frames from the final CINE reconstruction [23–25].

To achieve a 3D demonstration of the fetal heart and extracardiac vasculature [26], and a 4D whole-heart visualization [23], the combination of 2D images and multi-planar acquisition using volumetric reconstruction methods has been applied. For instance, a 4D flow cine MRI reconstruction was achieved by exploiting the velocity-sensitive information inherent to the phase of dynamic bSSFP acquisitions in combination with signal-to-voice ratio (SVR). Multiple non-coplanar bSSFP stacks were used to reconstruct spatially identical, temporally resolved, motion-corrected magnitudes and vector flow volumes [24]. The advantages of this method represent the robustness in motion, the capability of both in-plane and through-plane motion to be corrected, and the full coverage of the fetal heart.

In 2010, an artificial cardiac triggering, or self-gating system, was proposed to the so-called Metric Optimized Gating (MOG). It detects mis gating artifact through evaluation of image metrics while images are retrospectively analyzed. Whereas this method was first developed for time-resolved phase-contrast measurements of fetal blood flow, it has since been applied to both Cartesian and radial bSSFP acquisitions and was the first method to demonstrate dynamic CINE MRI of the human fetal cardiovascular system [27,28]. MOG, however, does not address fetal or maternal body motion.

To achieve multidimensional flow in fetuses, a golden-angle radial phase-contrast cardiovascular magnetic resonance has been applied with real-time reconstructions; first performed for retrospective motion correction and cardiac gating using MOG [29].

Another approach to fetal cardiac gating is MRI self-gating, where a periodic gating signal is extracted from the MRI data itself and it is used to sort the data retrospectively [30].

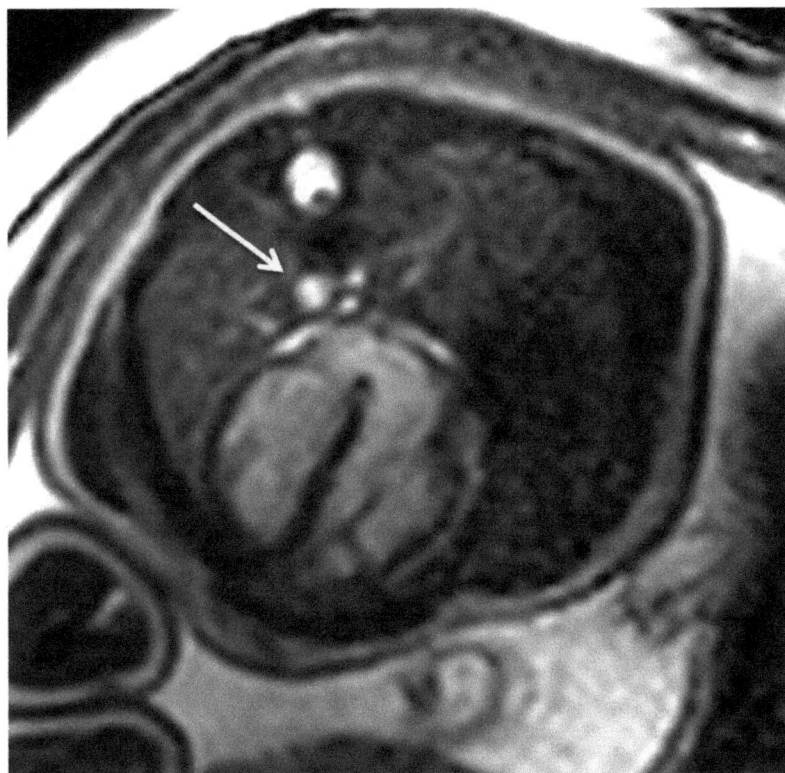

Figure 1. Fetal cardiac MRI using Doppler ultrasound gating at 3 Tesla: The applied rapid gradient-recalled echo (GRE) steady-state free-precession (SSFP) sequence (TR = 3.9 ms, TE = 1.9 ms, field of view = 246 × 246 mm, flip angle = 60°, slice thickness = 6 mm, matrix size 164 × 164) is adopted from standard adult cardiac MRI protocols. SSFP sequences have short acquisition times and provide high myocardium-blood contrast (composed of both T1 and T2 contributions). Fetal cardiac gating using a Doppler ultrasound sensor enables dynamic/cine imaging by acquisition of multiple images (i.e., heart phases) over the cardiac cycle. The example illustrates an end-diastolic four-chamber SSFP image and reveals physiological situs, cardiac chambers, and left descending aorta (arrow) in a healthy late term fetus (gestational age: 35 + 0 weeks). Morphometry: LCD = 441 mm, TCD = 387 mm, LVmidtransverse = 152 mm, LVlongitudinal = 261 mm, RVmidtransverse = 158 mm, RVlongitudinal = 247 mm, mitral valve plane = 86 mm, tricuspidal valve plane = 91 mm.

3. Current Potential and Clinical Application of Fetal Cardiac MRI

A cardiovascular fetal MRI was first attempted in 2005 when applying real-time sequences with the aim of estimating the ventricular volume. Small case series of investigating the normal heart anatomy and congenital heart defects (CHD) followed and although some reviews have attempted to establish protocols [31], there is no consensus on which are the indications of a cardiovascular MRI. Manganaro et al. performed fetal MRI in 32 fetuses with a mean gestational age of 30 weeks from January 2007 to March 2008 with a US-assessed CHD. All the morpho-volumetric abnormalities of the heart, cardiac axis abnormal rotation, ventricular septal defects (VSDs) as well as cases with abnormal origin and course of the great vessels (GV) could be confirmed by MRI using SSFP sequences. In Figure 2, a hypoplastic right heart and a VSD in 4CV are illustrated utilizing cine SSFP in a late-term fetus in the overdiagnosis of two VSDs, the restricted evaluation of atrial septum (AS) due to the presence of foramen ovale (FO) and its low thickness, the restricted evaluation of the size of GV due to MRI spatial resolution and SNR, and the insufficient evaluation of valves have proven that although MRI is a useful adjunct, improvements in gating, speed of sequences, and signal-to-noise improvement were necessary at that time.

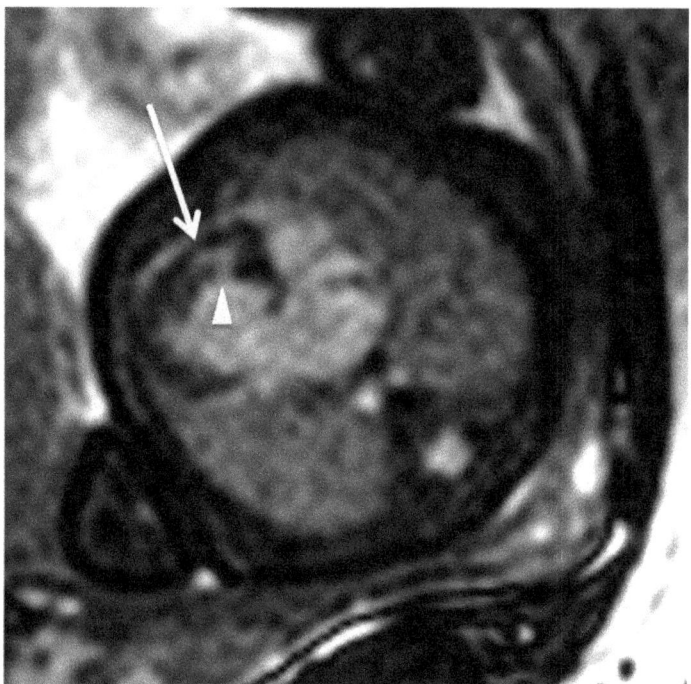

Figure 2. Fetal cardiac MRI using Doppler ultrasound gating for assessment of dynamic/cine steady-state free-precession (SSFP) sequences (TR = 3.3 ms, TE = 1.6 ms, field of view = 300 × 300 mm, flip angle = 60°, slice thickness = 5 mm, matrix size 288 × 288) at 1.5 Tesla: The end-diastolic four-chamber SSFP image illustrates hypoplastic right heart (arrow) and ventricular septal defect (arrowhead) in a late term fetus (gestational age: 30 + 5 weeks). Postnatal diagnosis revealed atresia of the tricuspid valve, malposition of the great arteries, and interrupted aortic arch (not visualized in the presented four-chamber view).

Over next years, some of the improvements have been achieved and cardiac MRI is able to detect the patency of the interatrial septum that is crucial information for the delivery and treatment plan for Transposition of Great Arteries (TGA) fetuses [32,33]. In a large study of Su-Zhen Dong et al., MRI was applied as an adjunct to classic fetal US, when the latter was not able, due to common known difficulties, to make a conclusive diagnosis [34]. Over 14 years, 71 cases with confirmed CHD have been reviewed applying a multi-planar reformatting reconstruction 2D SSFP technique to reconstruct the fetal cardiovascular MR images. In 60.6% of cases, MRI put a conclusive correct diagnosis and only 4.2% of cases were correct but incomplete. However, the author considers some types of defect, such as unclosed Ductus Arteriosus (DA), at birth or secundum Septal Defect (SD) as impossible to diagnose prenatally. For complex CHD, such as Pulmonary Atresia with intact ventricular septum (PA/IVS), severe Tetralogy of Fallot (TOF), Double Outlet Right Ventricle (DORV), or Transposition of Great Arteries (TGA) a definitive diagnosis could not be made by use of MRI. Finally, mild Pulmonary Stenosis (PS) and small Ventricular Septal Defect (VSD) are missed by cardiac MRI.

CMR is a useful adjunct for the evaluation of the cardiac vascular anatomy and several attempts have been made to study the aortic arch, its branches, and its anatomical position in relation to the trachea; in particular when vascular rings are suspected. Similarly, as regards the blood supply of the lungs challenging for echocardiography cases, such as pulmonary atresia with MAPCAs or pulmonary trunk can be elucidated with the aid of MRI. The drainage of both pairs of pulmonary veins is feasible to be demonstrated by MRI as well.

Su-Zhen Dong et al., in their in 2020 review, using data from 71 cases with confirmed CHD over 14 years, concluded that the Coarctation of Aorta (CoA) prenatal diagnosis was unreliable due to both the technical difficulty of imaging this region and the obligatory patency of the arterial duct in fetal life and physiologic changes of the DA after birth [34]. Su-Zhen Dong concluded in a previous study in 2018, after having examined six fetuses of mean gestational age (26.5 weeks) with Aortic Arch (AoA) abnormality using bSSFP and SSFE techniques, that fetal cardiac MRI is a useful complementary tool to assess fetuses with right aortic arch and right ductus arteriosus. In half of the cases, the aortic arch laterality abnormality was missed in prenatal US [35]. In the same line, the same author reported that MRI was able to demonstrate the abnormal course of left brachiocephalic vein in nine fetuses in a retrospective review of 7282 fetuses from June 2006 to March 2017 [36] and a LPSVC in 49 fetuses in a retrospective review from January 2010 to October 2015 [37]. A recent study of Ryd et al. has proven, after having investigated 31 fetuses at a median age of 31 weeks, that CMR had clinical utility affecting patient management and/or parental counselling in 26 cases (84%) [38]. For assessment of univentricular vs. biventricular outcome in borderline left ventricle, unbalanced atrioventricular septal defect and pulmonary atresia with intact ventricular septum (15 fetuses) fetal CMR visualized intracardiac anatomy and ventricular function, allowing assessment of outcome in 13 cases (87%). In four fetuses with hypoplastic left heart syndrome, it helped delivery planning in three of those cases (75%). For aortic arch anatomy including signs of coarctation (20 fetuses), CMR added diagnostic information in 16 cases (80%), which is not in line with the previously mentioned study of Su-Zhen Dong et al. [34]

Loyd et al., by applying novel MRI with high-resolution motion-corrected three-dimensional volumes of the fetal heart and phase-contrast flow sequences gated with metric-optimized gating on 51 fetuses with suspected CoA, concluded that MRI with the aid of a multivariate logistic regression model, including aortic flow and isthmic displacement, may have an important role in predicting severe neonatal CoA outcome and need for intervention in 93% of cases [39]. In the same line is another prospective single-center cohort study of Lyod et al. in which 85 fetuses with suspected CHD have been examined from October 2015 to June 2017 using MRI with motion-corrected slice-volume registration. The data as overlapping stacks of 2D images were processed with a bespoke open-source reconstruction algorithm to produce a super-resolution 3D volume of the fetal thorax. Vascular measurements, although showed good overall agreement with 2D echocardiography in 51 cases, fetal vascular structures have been more effectively visualized with 3D MRI and have had a higher diagnostic quality score [27]. Finally, Xu Li et al. compared the accuracy in correct diagnoses of aortic arch anomalies of both fetal US and CMR using SSFP and SSFSE in 600 pregnant women from January 2013 to 22 December 2015 of them with aortic arch anomalies. MRI revealed a 95.6% accuracy misdiagnosing only one case of right aortic arch with aberrant left subclavian artery as a double aortic arch. The same case has been misdiagnosed by US, which showed an accuracy of 60.8% [40].

Apart from cardiovascular features, the application of cardiac MRI can play an additive role on extracardiac anatomy, such as laterality disorders and lung parenchyma characterization in cases of pulmonary venous obstruction or intact interatrial septum in which lymphangiectasia is suspected [41,42]. Elisabeth Mlczoch et al. investigated fetal lung volume (TLV) in 105 fetuses with CHD and mean gestational age 26 + 6 weeks of gestation from January 2004 to December 2011 by applying fetal cardiac MRI SSFP and FSE only axial T2 sequences, concluding that fetuses with CHD had significantly smaller TLV in comparison with non-CHD fetuses and that small pulmonary arteries correlate with small TLV. A total of 17% of fetuses had TLV below normal indicating pulmonary hypoplasia [43].

Saul et al. investigated 44 fetuses with HLHS to identify which ones developed Lymphangiectasia described as nutmeg lung in MRI; the nutmeg lung MR appearance in HLHS fetuses is associated with increased mortality/OHT (100% in the first 5 months of life compared to 35% with HLHS alone). Not all patients with restrictive lesions develop nutmeg lung, and the outcome is not as poor when restriction is present in isolation. Dedicated evaluation for nutmeg lung pattern on fetal MR studies may be useful in guiding prognostication and aiding clinicians in counselling parents of fetuses with HLHS [44].

Investigations into the circulatory physiology of fetal sheep were undertaken in the 1930s by Sir Joseph Barcroft at Cambridge University. Sir Geoffrey Dawes conducted the first detailed studies of the fetal circulation. MRI spectroscopy at high field strengths and BOLD (Blood Oxygenation Level Dependent) signal allowed for information about blood and tissue oxygenation by relating the T2 and T2* transverse-relaxation time of blood and the oxygenation state of hemoglobin on erythrocytes. Although BOLD does not provide quantitative data about blood oxygen saturation, it is possible to estimate both hematocrit and oxygen saturation by combining T1 and T2 measurements of blood. Sun et al., by applying MOG for fetal triggering and using an accelerated version of the acquisition utilized by Wedergartner's fetal lambs, which incorporates a motion correction algorithm, were able to make reproducible measurements of T2 in the larger fetal vessels in 40 late-gestation human fetuses [45].

Moreover, the relationship of fetal hemodynamics to brain and lung development in cases of fetal growth restriction (FGR) and complex CHD could be demonstrated by several studies [2]. Successively, MRI plays a role in studying hemodynamics. In Figure 3, 2D phase-contrast MR angiography is illustrated using Doppler ultrasound gating at 1.5 Tesla in a late term fetus (gestational age: 30 + 4 weeks) for the assessment of blood flow hemodynamics. In the intrauterine peri-operational period in cases of CHD, such as HLHS, it can investigate the grade of pulmonary obstruction. Furthermore, it detects the patency of foramen ovale (FO) indirectly by estimating the higher oxygen saturation in the Left Ventricle (LV) resulting from the preferential streaming of oxygenated blood through FO.

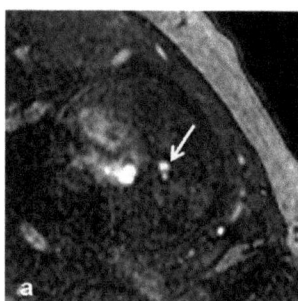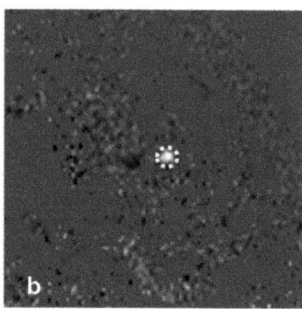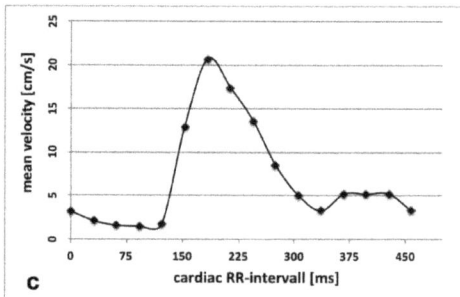

Figure 3. 2-D phase-contrast MR angiography (TR = 4.9 ms, TE = 3 ms, field of view = 250 mm, flip angle = 15°, slice thickness 5 mm, matrix size = 194 × 194 mm) using Doppler ultrasound gating at 1.5 Tesla for assessment of blood flow hemodynamics. Transversal orientation through the descending aorta (arrow in **a**) with resulting magnitude image (**a**) and phase image (**b**). Blood flow hemodynamics are assessed by placement of a region of interest (ROI; dotted circle in **b**) in the vessel lumen. Dynamic blood flow over the whole cardiac cycle is encoded by signal intensities within the ROI. (**c**) In this example of a late term fetus (gestational age: 30 + 4 weeks) resulting mean flow velocity illustrates typical arterial flow waveform over the cardiac cycle.

From 2010 to 2012, Bahiyah al Nafisi et al. investigated the fetal circulation distribution in 22 fetuses with left-sided CHD at a mean of 35 weeks of gestation using phase contrast MRI and compared them with twelve normal fetuses. Fetuses with left-sided CHD had a mean combined ventricular output (CVO) that was 19% lower than normal controls. In fetuses with left-sided CHD with pulmonary venous obstruction, pulmonary blood flow was significantly lower than in those with left-sided CHD without pulmonary venous obstruction. All 3 fetuses with pulmonary venous obstruction had pulmonary lymphangiectasia. Fetuses with small but apex-forming left ventricles with left ventricular outflow tract or aortic arch obstruction had reduced ascending aortic (AAo) and FO flow compared with normal [46]. The reference ranges of the blood flow in the GV of a fetus in the late gestation have been established with the aid of MRI [47]. Recently, Roberts et al. presented a novel method for in utero whole-heart fetal 4D cine quantitative blood flow imaging. A 4D flow cine MRI reconstruction was possible by utilizing the velocity-sensitive information inherent to the phase of dynamic bSSFP and SVR. Multiple non-coplanar bSSFP stacks were used to reconstruct spatially identical, temporally resolved, motion-corrected magnitude, and vector flow volumes [24].

4. Conclusions

Fetal cardiac MRI has been studied, has evolved and has an adjunctive role to fetal US, which has remained the gold standard over the last two decades. Its place, where the US cannot overcome its known limitations, has recently become of interest to several researchers. Its evolution will establish it as a necessary tool for the correct and complete diagnosis and comprehension of the anatomy and pathophysiology of CHD, the proper prenatal counselling for the outcome, and the postnatal or even prenatal operative preparation of individuals.

Funding: This research received no external funding.

Conflicts of Interest: The authors declare no conflict of interest.

References

1. Sun, L.; Macgowan, C.K.; Sled, J.G.; Yoo, S.-J.; Manlhiot, C.; Porayette, P.; Grosse-Wortmann, L.; Jaeggi, E.; McCrindle, B.W.; Kingdom, J.; et al. Reduced fetal cerebral oxygen consumption is associated with smaller brain size in fetuses with congenital heart disease. *Circulation* **2015**, *131*, 1313–1323. [CrossRef]
2. Zhu, M.Y.; Milligan, N.; Keating, S.; Windrim, R.; Keunen, J.; Thakur, V.; Ohman, A.; Portnoy, S.; Sled, J.G.; Kelly, E.; et al. The hemodynamics of late-onset intrauterine growth restriction by MRI. *Am. J. Obstet. Gynecol.* **2016**, *214*, 367.e1–367.e17. [CrossRef]
3. Limperopoulos, C.; Tworetzky, W.; McElhinney, D.B.; Newburger, J.W.; Brown, D.W.; Robertson, R.L.; Guizard, N.; McGrath, E.; Geva, J.; Annese, D.; et al. Brain volume and metabolism in fetuses with congenital heart disease: Evaluation with quantitative magnetic resonance imaging and spectroscopy. *Circulation* **2010**, *121*, 26–33. [CrossRef] [PubMed]
4. Gorincour, G.; Bourliere-Najean, B.; Bonello, B.; Fraisse, A.; Philip, N.; Potier, A.; Kreitmann, B.; Petit, P. Feasibility of fetal cardiacmmagnetic resonance imaging: Preliminary experience. *Ultrasound Obstret. Gynecol.* **2007**, *29*, 105–108. [CrossRef]
5. Saleem, S.N. Feasibility of MRI of the fetal heart with balanced steady-state free precession sequence along fetal body and cardiac planes. *Am. J. Roentgenol.* **2008**, *191*, 1208–1215. [CrossRef]
6. Manganaro, L.; Savelli, S.; Di Maurizio, M.; Perrone, A.; Tesei, J.; Francioso, A.; Angeletti, M.; Coratella, F.; Irimia, D.; Fierro, F.; et al. Potential role of fetal cardiac evaluation with magnetic resonance imaging: Preliminary experience. *Prenat. Diagn.* **2008**, *28*, 148–156. [CrossRef]
7. Votino, C.; Jani, J.; Damry, N.; Dessy, H.; Kang, X.; Cos, T.; Divano, L.; Foulon, W.; De Mey, J.; Cannie, M. Magnetic resonance imaging in the normal fetal heart and in congenital heart disease. *Ultrasound Obstet. Gynecol.* **2012**, *39*, 322–329. [CrossRef] [PubMed]
8. Dong, S.-Z.; Zhu, M.; Li, F. Preliminary experience with cardiovascular magnetic resonance in evaluation of fetal cardiovascular anomalies. *J. Cardiovasc. Magn. Reson.* **2013**, *15*, 40. [CrossRef] [PubMed]
9. Gaur, L.; Talemal, L.; Bulas, D.; Donofrio, M.T. Utility of fetal magnetic resonance imaging in assessing the fetus with cardiac malposition. *Prenat. Diagn.* **2016**, *36*, 752–759. [CrossRef] [PubMed]
10. Dong, S.-Z.; Zhu, M. MR imaging of fetal cardiac malposition and congenital cardiovascular anomalies on the four-chamber view. *Springerplus* **2016**, *5*, 1214. [CrossRef]
11. Lloyd, D.F.A.; van Amerom, J.F.P.; Pushparajah, K.; Simpson, J.M.; Zidere, V.; Miller, O.; Sharland, G.; Allsop, J.; Fox, M.; Lohezic, M.; et al. An exploration of the potential utility of fetal cardiovascular MRI as an adjunct to fetal echocardiography. *Prenat. Diagn.* **2016**, *36*, 916–925. [CrossRef]
12. Manganaro, L.; Savelli, S.; Di Maurizio, M.; Perrone, A.; Francioso, A.; La Barbera, L.; Totaro, P.; Fierro, F.; Tomei, A.; Coratella, F.; et al. Assessment of congenital heart disease (CHD): Is there a role for fetal magnetic resonance imaging (MRI)? *Eur. J. Radiol.* **2009**, *72*, 172–180. [CrossRef]

13. Fogel, M.A.; Wilson, R.D.; Flake, A.; Johnson, M.; Cohen, D.; McNeal, G.; Tian, Z.-Y.; Rychik, J. Preliminary investigations into a new method of functional assessment of the fetal heart using a novel application of "real-time" cardiac magnetic resonance imaging. *Fetal Diagn. Ther.* **2005**, *20*, 475–480. [CrossRef]
14. Tsuritani, M.; Morita, Y.; Miyoshi, T.; Kurosaki, K.; Yoshimatsu, J. Fetal cardiac functional assessment by fetal heart magnetic resonance imaging. *J. Comput. Assist. Tomogr.* **2019**, *43*, 104–108. [CrossRef]
15. Jansz, M.S.; Seed, M.; van Amerom, J.F.P.; Wong, D.; Grosse-Wortmann, L.; Yoo, S.-J.; Macgowan, C.K. Metric optimized gating for fetal cardiac MRI. *Magn. Reson. Med.* **2010**, *64*, 1304–1314. [CrossRef]
16. Kording, F.; Schoennagel, B.P.; de Sousa, M.T.; Fehrs, K.; Adam, G.; Yamamura, J.; Ruprecht, C. Evaluation of a portable doppler ultrasound gating device for fetal cardiac MR imaging: Initial results at 1.5T and 3T. *Magn. Reson. Med. Sci.* **2018**, *17*, 308–317. [CrossRef] [PubMed]
17. Kording, F.; Yamamura, J.; De Sousa, M.T.; Ruprecht, C.; Hedström, E.; Aletras, A.H.; Ellen Grant, P.; Powell, A.J.; Fehrs, K.; Adam, G. Dynamic fetal cardiovascular magnetic resonance imaging using Doppler ultrasound gating. *J. Cardiovasc. Magn. Reson.* **2018**, *20*, 17. [CrossRef]
18. Roy, C.W.; Seed, M.; Macgowan, C.K. Accelerated MRI of the fetal heart using compressed sensing and metric optimized gating. *Magn. Reson. Med.* **2017**, *77*, 2125–2135. [CrossRef] [PubMed]
19. Roy, C.W.; Seed, M.; Macgowan, C. Accelerated phase contrast measurements of fetal blood flow using compressed sensing. *J. Cardiovasc. Magn. Reson.* **2016**, *18*, 30. [CrossRef]
20. Haris, K.; Hedström, E.; Bidhult, S.; Testud, F.; Maglaveras, N.; Heiberg, E.; Hansson, S.R.; Arheden, H.; Aletras, A.H. Self-gated fetal cardiac MRI with tiny golden angle iGRASP: A feasibility study. *J. Magn. Reson. Imaging* **2017**, *46*, 207–217. [CrossRef]
21. Chaptinel, J.; Yerly, J.; Mivelaz, Y.; Prsa, M.; Alamo, L.; Vial, Y.; Berchier, G.; Rohner, C.; Gudinchet, F.; Stuber, M. Fetal cardiac cine magnetic resonance imaging in utero. *Sci. Rep.* **2017**, *7*, 15540. [CrossRef]
22. Roy, C.W.; Seed, M.; Macgowan, C.K. Motion compensated cine CMR of the fetal heart using radial undersampling and compressed sensing. *J. Cardiovasc. Magn. Reson.* **2017**, *19*, 29. [CrossRef] [PubMed]
23. van Amerom, J.F.; Lloyd, D.F.; Deprez, M.; Price, A.N.; Malik, S.J.; Pushparajah, K.; van Poppel, M.P.; Rutherford, M.A.; Razavi, R.; Hajnal, J.V. Fetal whole-heart 4D imaging using motion-corrected multi-planar real-time MRI. *Magn. Reson. Med.* **2019**, *82*, 1055–1072. [CrossRef] [PubMed]
24. Roberts, T.A.; van Amerom, J.F.P.; Uus, A.; Lloyd, D.F.A.; van Poppel, M.P.M.; Price, A.N.; Tournier, J.D.; Mohanadass, C.A.; Jackson, L.H.; Malik, S.J.; et al. Fetal whole heart blood flow imaging using 4D cine MRI. *Nat. Commun.* **2020**, *11*, 4992. [CrossRef] [PubMed]
25. Gholipour, A.; Estroff, J.A.; Warfield, S.K. Robust super-resolution volume reconstruction from slice acquisitions: Application to fetal brain MRI. *IEEE Trans. Med. Imaging* **2010**, *29*, 1739–1758. [CrossRef]
26. Kuklisova-Murgasova, M.; Quaghebeur, G.; Rutherford, M.; Hajnal, J.; Schnabel, J.A. Reconstruction of fetal brain MRI with intensity matching and complete outlier removal. *Med. Image Anal.* **2012**, *16*, 1550–1564. [CrossRef] [PubMed]
27. Lloyd, D.F.A.; Pushparajah, K.; Simpson, J.; van Amerom, J.; van Poppel, M.P.; Schulz, A.; Kainz, B.; Deprez, M.; Lohezic, M.; Allsop, J.; et al. Three-dimensional visualisation of the fetal heart using prenatal MRI with motion-corrected slicevolume registration: A prospective, single-centre cohort study. *Lancet* **2019**, *393*, 1619–1627. [CrossRef] [PubMed]
28. Roy, C.W.; Seed, M.; van Amerom, J.F.P.; Al Nafisi, B.; Grosse-Wortmann, L.; Yoo, S.-J.; Macgowan, C.K. Dynamic imaging of the fetal heart using metric optimized gating. *Magn. Reson. Med.* **2013**, *70*, 1598–1607. [CrossRef] [PubMed]
29. Goolaub, D.S.; Roy, C.W.; Schrauben, E.; Sussman, D.; Marini, D.; Seed, M.; Macgowan, C.K. Multidimension-al fetal flow imaging with cardiovascular magnetic resonance: A feasibility study. *J. Cardiovasc. Magn. Reson.* **2018**, *20*, 77. [CrossRef]
30. Spraggins, T.A. Wireless retrospective gating: Application to cine cardiac imaging. *Magn. Reson. Imaging* **1990**, *8*, 675–681. [CrossRef]
31. Manganaro, L.; Di Maurizio, M.; Savelli, S. Feasibility, Technique and Potential Role of Fetal Cardiovascular MRI: Evaluation of Normal Anatomical Structures and Assessment of Congenital Heart Disease. In *4D Fetal Echocardiography*; Bentham Science Publishers: Sharjah, United Arab Emirates, 2010; pp. 178–196.
32. Jouannic, J.M.; Gavard, L.; Fermont, L.; Le Bidois, J.; Parat, S.; Vouhé, P.R.; Dumez, Y.; Sidi, D.; Bonnet, D. Sensitivity and specificity of prenatal features of physiological shunts to predict neonatal clinical status in transposition of the great arteries. *Circulation* **2004**, *110*, 1743–1746. [CrossRef]
33. Mawad, W.; Chaturvedi, R.R.; Ryan, G.; Jaeggi, E. Percutaneous fetal atrial balloon septoplasty for simple transposition of the great arteries with an intact atrial septum. *Can. J. Cardiol.* **2018**, *34*, 342.e9–342.e11. [CrossRef]
34. Dong, S.-Z.; Zhu, M.; Ji, H.; Ren, J.Y.; Liu, K. Fetal cardiac MRI: A single center experience over 14-years on the potential utility as an adjunct to fetal technically inadequate echocardiography. *Sci. Rep.* **2020**, *10*, 12373. [CrossRef]
35. Dong, S.Z.; Zhu, M.J. Utility of fetal cardiac magnetic resonance imaging to assess fetuses with right aortic arch and right ductus arteriosus. *Matern. Fetal Neonatal Med.* **2018**, *31*, 1627–1631. [CrossRef] [PubMed]
36. Dong, S.Z.; Zhu, M. MR imaging of subaortic and retroesophageal anomalous courses of the left brachiocephalic vein in the fetus. *Sci. Rep.* **2018**, *8*, 14781. [CrossRef] [PubMed]
37. Dong, S.Z.; Zhu, M. Magnetic resonance imaging of fetal persistent left superior vena cava. *Sci. Rep.* **2017**, *7*, 4176. [CrossRef]
38. Ryd, D.; Fricke, K.; Bhat, M.; Arheden, H.; Liuba, P.; Hedström, E. Utility of Fetal Cardiovascular Magnetic Resonance for Prenatal Diagnosis of Complex Congenital Heart Defects. *JAMA Netw. Open* **2021**, *4*, e213538. [CrossRef]

39. Lloyd, D.F.; van Poppel, M.P.; Pushparajah, K.; Vigneswaran, T.V.; Zidere, V.; Steinweg, J.; van Amerom, J.F.; Roberts, T.A.; Schulz, A.; Charakida, M.; et al. Analysis of 3-Dimensional Arch Anatomy, Vascular Flow, and Postnatal Outcome in Cases of Suspected Coarctation of the Aorta Using Fetal Cardiac Magnetic Resonance Imaging. *Circ. Cardiovasc. Imaging* **2021**, *14*, e012411. [CrossRef] [PubMed]
40. Li, X.; Li, X.; Hu, K.; Yin, C. The value of cardiovascular magnetic resonance in the diagnosis of fetal aortic arch anomalies. *J. Matern. Fetal Neonatal Med.* **2017**, *30*, 1366–1371. [CrossRef] [PubMed]
41. Seed, M.; Bradley, T.; Bourgeois, J.; Jaeggi, E.; Yoo, S.J. Antenatal MR imaging of pulmonary lymphangiectasia secondary to hypoplastic left heartsyndrome. *Pediatr. Radiol.* **2009**, *39*, 747–749. [CrossRef] [PubMed]
42. Chaturvedi, R.; Ryan, G.; Seed, M.; van Arsdell, G.; Jaeggi, E. Fetal stenting of the atrial septum: Technique and initial results in cardiac lesions with left atrial hypertension. *Int. J. Cardiol.* **2013**, *168*, 2029–2036. [CrossRef]
43. Mlczoch, E.; Schmidt, L.; Schmid, M.; Kasprian, G.; Frantal, S.; Berger-Kulemann, V.; Prayer, D.; Michel-Behnke, I.; Salzer-Muhar, U. Fetal cardiac disease and fetal lung volume: An in utero MRI investigation. *Prenat. Diagn.* **2014**, *34*, 273–278. [CrossRef]
44. Saul, D.; Degenhardt, K.; Iyoob, S.D.; Surrey, L.F.; Johnson, A.M.; Johnson, M.P.; Rychik, J.; Victoria, T. Hypoplastic left heart syndrome and the nutmeg lung pattern in utero: A cause and effect relationship or prognostic indicator? *Pediatr. Radiol.* **2016**, *46*, 483–489. [CrossRef]
45. Sun, L.; Macgowan, C.K.; Portnoy, S.; Sled, J.G.; Yoo, S.-J.; Grosse-Wortmann, L.; Jaeggi, E.; Kingdom, J.; Seed, M. New advances in fetal cardiovascular magnetic resonance imaging for quantifying the distribution of blood flow and oxygen transport: Potential applications in fetal cardiovascular disease diagnosis and therapy. *Echocardiography* **2017**, *34*, 1799–1803. [CrossRef]
46. Al Nafisi, B.; Van Amerom, J.F.; Forsey, J.; Jaeggi, E.; Grosse-Wortmann, L.; Yoo, S.J.; Macgowan, C.K.; Seed, M. Fetal circulation in leftsided congenital heart disease measured by cardiovascular magnetic resonance: A case-control study. *J. Cardiovasc. Magn. Reson.* **2013**, *15*, 1. [CrossRef] [PubMed]
47. Prsa, M.; Sun, L.; Van Amerom, J.; Yoo, S.J.; Grosse-Wortmann, L.; Jaeggi, E.; Macgowan, C.; Seed, M. Reference ranges of blood flow in the major vessels of the normal human fetal circulation at term by phase-contrast magnetic resonance imaging. *Circ. Cardiovasc. Imaging* **2014**, *7*, 663–670. [CrossRef]

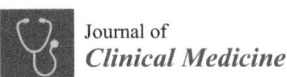

Article

Cord Blood Cardiovascular Biomarkers in Left-Sided Congenital Heart Disease

Iris Soveral [1,2], Laura Guirado [1], Maria C. Escobar-Diaz [3,4], María José Alcaide [5,6], Josep Maria Martínez [1,7,8,9], Víctor Rodríguez-Sureda [1,9], Bart Bijnens [8,10], Eugenia Antolin [6,11], Elisa Llurba [12,13], Jose L. Bartha [6,11], Olga Gómez [1,7,8,9,*] and Fàtima Crispi [1,7,8,9]

1. BCNatal, Fetal Medicine Research Center (Hospital Clínic and Hospital Sant Joan de Déu), 08028 Barcelona, Spain
2. Obstetrics Department, Hospital General de Hospitalet, 08906 Barcelona, Spain
3. Pediatric Cardiology Department, Sant Joan de Déu Hospital, Esplugues de Llobregat, 08950 Barcelona, Spain
4. Cardiovascular Research Group, Sant Joan de Deu Research Institute, Esplugues de Llobregat, 08028 Barcelona, Spain
5. Laboratory Medicine Department, Hospital Universitario La Paz, 28046 Madrid, Spain
6. Research Institute IdiPAZ, 28029 Madrid, Spain
7. Facultat de Medicina i Ciencies de la Salut, Universitat de Barcelona, 08007 Barcelona, Spain
8. Institut d'Investigacions Biomèdiques August Pi i Sunyer (IDIBAPS), 08036 Barcelona, Spain
9. Centre for Biomedical Research on Rare Diseases (CIBER-ER), 28029 Madrid, Spain
10. Catalan Institution for Research and Advanced Studies ICREA, 08010 Barcelona, Spain
11. Obstetrics and Gynecology Department, Hospital Universitario La Paz, 28046 Madrid, Spain
12. Obstetrics and Gynecology Department, Santa Creu i Sant Pau University Hospital, 08025 Barcelona, Spain
13. Facultat de Medicina, Universitat Autònoma de Barcelona, 08193 Barcelona, Spain
* Correspondence: ogomez@clinic.cat; Tel.: +34-932-27-9333

Abstract: Fetal echocardiography has limited prognostic ability in the evaluation of left-sided congenital heart defects (left heart defects). Cord blood cardiovascular biomarkers could improve the prognostic evaluation of left heart defects. A multicenter prospective cohort (2013–2019) including fetuses with left heart defects (aortic coarctation, aortic stenosis, hypoplastic left heart, and multilevel obstruction (complex left heart defects) subdivided according to their outcome (favorable vs. poor), and control fetuses were evaluated in the third trimester of pregnancy at three referral centers in Spain. Poor outcome was defined as univentricular palliation, heart transplant, or death. Cord blood concentrations of N-terminal precursor of B-type natriuretic peptide, Troponin I, transforming growth factor β, placental growth factor, and soluble fms-like tyrosine kinase-1 were determined. A total of 45 fetuses with left heart defects (29 favorable and 16 poor outcomes) and 35 normal fetuses were included, with a median follow-up of 3.1 years (interquartile range 1.4–3.9). Left heart defects with favorable outcome showed markedly increased cord blood transforming growth factor β (normal heart median 15.5 ng/mL (6.8–21.4) vs. favorable outcome 51.7 ng/mL (13.8–73.9) vs. poor outcome 25.1 ng/mL (6.9–39.0), $p = 0.001$) and decreased placental growth factor concentrations (normal heart 17.9 pg/mL (13.8–23.9) vs. favorable outcome 12.8 pg/mL (11.7–13.6) vs. poor outcome 11.0 pg/mL (8.8–15.4), $p < 0.001$). Poor outcome left heart defects had higher N-terminal precursor of B-type natriuretic peptide (normal heart 508.0 pg/mL (287.5–776.3) vs. favorable outcome 617.0 pg/mL (389.8–1087.8) vs. poor outcome 1450.0 pg/mL (919.0–1645.0), $p = 0.001$) and drastically reduced soluble fms-like tyrosine kinase-1 concentrations (normal heart 1929.7 pg/mL (1364.3–2715.8) vs. favorable outcome 1848.3 pg/mL (646.9–2313.6) vs. poor outcome 259.0 pg/mL (182.0–606.0), $p < 0.001$. Results showed that fetuses with left heart defects present a distinct cord blood biomarker profile according to their outcome.

Keywords: congenital heart defects; fetal echocardiography; B-type natriuretic peptide; transforming growth factor beta; aortic stenosis; aortic coarctation; hypoplastic left heart syndrome; angiogenic factors; fetal cardiac remodeling

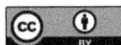

1. Introduction

Left-sided congenital heart defects (left-CHD) are the most common group of severe congenital heart defects and a major contributor to neonatal morbi-mortality [1]. In specialized settings, prenatal diagnosis is feasible in up to 90% of CHD [2]. Thus, fetal cardiology is now focused on predicting medium- and long-term cardiovascular outcomes. However, fetal echocardiography has shown limited prognostic ability, and therefore, new parameters are necessary to improve the prognostic evaluation of these anomalies in fetal life.

Several existing biomarkers are promising candidates. B-type natriuretic peptide (BNP) and its N-terminal precursor (NT-proBNP) have demonstrated utility in screening for CHD in newborns [3] and in predicting surgical outcomes in children with CHD [4]. Increased levels of Troponin, a specific marker of myocardial damage [5], have been found in the cord blood of neonates with single ventricle CHD and seem to relate to poorer prognosis [6]. Transforming growth factor beta (TGFβ), a cytokine implicated in different physiological and pathological responses [7,8], is expressed mainly by endothelial cells (at the cardiovascular level) and has been associated with fibrotic and hypertrophic remodeling (in heart failure and myocardial infarction), and extracellular matrix modulation in cardiac pressure overload [9–11]. However, it has never been studied in fetuses with CHD.

Additional biomarkers with a possible role in CHD are placental growth factor (PlGF) and its soluble receptor soluble fms-like tyrosine kinase-1 (sFlt1). PlGF regulates trophoblastic endothelial growth and is expressed by cardiomyocytes affecting ventricular remodeling in response to stress [12–14]. sFlt1 prevents the interaction of PlGF with cell receptors. An imbalance between PlGF and sFlt1 has been implicated in the pathogenesis of preeclampsia and intrauterine growth restriction [15]. Increased sFlt1 has also been detected in the cord blood of fetuses with CHD [16]. However, the role of PlGF and sFlt1 in CHD pathogenesis, associated cardiovascular remodeling, and/or prognosis has been insufficiently studied.

Thus, a differential expression profile of BNP, TGFβ, Troponin I, PlGF, and sFlt1 in cord blood could improve our understanding of cardiac remodeling in CDH and eventually help to identify those cases with poorer prognosis. We designed a prospective, multicenter study to measure cord blood biomarkers in fetuses with left-CHD and evaluate its association with disease severity.

2. Materials and Methods

2.1. Study Population

A prospective multicenter cohort study was conducted between 2013 and November 2019, including fetuses prenatally diagnosed with left-CHD. The cardiac outcome of these fetuses was regularly evaluated, and analysis was performed in terms of cardiac outcome. Fetuses with structurally normal hearts were also included as a non-exposed cohort. Pregnancies of women older than 18 years with accurate gestational age calculated by first-trimester crown–rump length [17] were considered eligible. Fetal standard ultrasound and echocardiography were performed in the third trimester, cord blood was obtained at delivery, and perinatal results and cardiac outcome data were collected.

Fetuses with left-CHD were recruited at the Fetal Cardiology Units from three tertiary Spanish referral centers: BCNatal (Hospitals Clinic and Sant Joan de Déu) and Hospital Vall d'Hebrón in Barcelona, and Hospital La Paz in Madrid. The group of left-CHD included aortic coarctation (CoA), aortic stenosis (AoS), hypoplastic left heart syndrome (HLHS), and complex left-CHD with multilevel left ventricular (LV) tract obstruction, including complete or incomplete Shone syndrome. Fetuses with CoA were included based on high prenatal echocardiographic suspicion (significant right dominance and aortic isthmus diameter < −2 z-score) [18] with postnatal diagnostic confirmation. AoS was defined based on fetal echocardiographic visualization of thickened aortic valve with abnormal Doppler flow and diastolic length of the left ventricle > −2 z-score at the time of evaluation [19]. HLHS was defined by an absent or small left ventricle (LV length < −2 or −3 z-score) with weak contractility with the absence of antegrade flow through the aortic valve and ascending aorta hypoplasia of variable degree [19]. This group included cases of mitral and/or aortic atresia and evolving HLHS secondary to severe aortic stenosis. Diagnosis of complex left-CHD was considered in fetuses with multilevel LV tract obstruction, including complete Shone syndrome (supravalvular mitral membrane, parachute mitral valve, muscular or membranous subvalvular aortic stenosis, and coarctation of aorta) and partial forms involving only two or three out of the four anomalies (incomplete Shone syndrome) [20]. Exclusion criteria in the left-CHD population included pre or postnatal diagnosis of additional major cardiac malformations, presence of major extracardiac malformations, or genetic anomalies. Minor cardiovascular anomalies (such as small ventricular septal defects, persistent left superior vena cava, or aberrant right subclavian artery) were not exclusion criteria. Clinical outcome was obtained from medical records at least one year after birth and reevaluated yearly if necessary. Prior to analysis, left-CHD cases were classified into favorable vs. poor cardiac outcome. Poor cardiac outcome was defined by the presence of at least one of the following: postnatal univentricular surgical palliation, need for heart transplant, or death related to CHD or its complications.

Control fetuses with structurally normal hearts were recruited from singleton uncomplicated and spontaneously conceived pregnancies attended at the Maternal-Fetal Medicine Department at BCNatal in Barcelona. They were matched for gestational age (± 2 weeks) at scan with left-CHD fetuses. Exclusion criteria in this group included pre or postnatal diagnosis of CHD, extracardiac malformations, genetic anomalies or conditions potentially affecting fetal cardiac function, or cord biomarkers such as intrauterine growth restriction [21–24], maternal diabetes [25,26], exposure to toxins [27], or macrosomia [26].

2.2. Fetal Standard Ultrasound and Echocardiography

Standard obstetric ultrasound and fetal echocardiography were performed using a Siemens Sonoline Antares (Siemens Medical Systems, Malvern, PA, USA) or Voluson E8 (General Electric, Zipf, Austria) using a curved-array 2–6 MHz transducer.

Fetal ultrasound was performed according to recommended guidelines and included calculation of estimated fetal weight [28] and centile [29], extracardiac and cardiac detailed examinations [30], and measurement of mean uterine artery, umbilical artery, and middle cerebral artery pulsatility indices [31]. The cerebroplacental ratio was calculated as the quotient between the median cerebral artery and umbilical artery pulsatility indices [32]. IUGR was defined as estimated fetal weight below the 3rd centile or below the 10th centile with abnormal maternal or fetal Doppler values [33].

The fetal cardiac morphometric assessment included cardiothoracic ratio [34,35], cardiac sphericity [35], atrial and ventricular-to-heart ratios [35], right-to-left ventricular ratio [35], and septal myocardium thickness [36,37]. Cardiac measurements were obtained in a two-dimensional apical or basal four-chamber view at end-diastole, except atrial areas, which were measured at end-systole.

Cardiac function evaluation included heart rate, right ventricular fractional area change [38], LV shortening fraction [39], and filling and ejection time fractions [40]. LV filling and ejection time fractions were only measured when LV inflow or outflow waves could be identified, thus excluding cases with mitral and aortic atresia.

2.3. Cord Blood Biomarkers

Cord blood samples were obtained from the umbilical vein after cord clamping at birth. Plasma was separated from ethylenediaminetetraacetic acid-treated blood using centrifugation at $1400\times g$ for 10 min at 4 °C. Serum was separated using centrifugation at $2000\times g$ for 10 min at room temperature. Sample aliquots were immediately stored at -80 °C until assayed.

N-terminal precursor of B-type natriuretic peptide (NT-proBNP) and Troponin I concentrations was measured in plasma by electrochemiluminescence immunoassay using Siemens Atellica IM NT-proBNP and High Sensitivity Troponin I, respectively (Siemens Healthcare, Erlangen, Germany). Transforming growth factor $\beta 1$ (TGFβ) was measured in serum by conventional ELISA assay Quantikine Human TGF-beta1 (R&D Systems, Minneapolis, MN, USA). Concentrations of placental growth factor (PlGF) and soluble fms-like tyrosine kinase-1 (sFlt1) were determined in serum by the fully automated Elecsys assays for sFlt-1 and PlGF on an electrochemiluminescence immunoassay platform Cobas analyzer (Roche Diagnostics, Mannheim, Germany). Concentrations of cord NT-proBNP, TGFβ, PlGF, and sFlt1 are presented as continuous variables (NT-proBNP, PlGF, and sFlt1 in pg/mL and TGFβ in ng/mL). Troponin I was treated as a dichotomous variable, and concentrations above the technical detection limit (>0.017 ng/mL) were considered positive [41].

2.4. Statistical Analysis

Data were analyzed using the IBM SPSS Statistics version 23 statistical package (IBM Corp., Armonk, NY, USA). The Shapiro–Wilk test of normality was performed for continuous variables. Continuous variables are presented as median (interquartile range) or mean ± standard deviation, as appropriate. For normally distributed variables, overall differences between study groups were examined using parametric analysis of variance (one-way ANOVA) followed by post hoc Bonferroni tests for pairwise comparison. Differences between study groups in non-normally distributed variables were analyzed using Kruskal–Wallis one-way ANOVA followed by post-hoc pairwise comparisons using the Dunn–Bonferroni approach. Categorical variables are presented as n (percentage %), and differences between the groups were compared using the appropriate chi-square test. When necessary and appropriate, Student's *t*-test or Mann–Whitney U-test was also used. A significance level of 0.05 was used throughout.

Analysis of baseline variables for possible confounders (included maternal age, maternal body mass index, nulliparity, smoking, pregestational diabetes, gestational diabetes, preeclampsia, gestational age at delivery, birth weight, gender, mode of delivery, and echocardiographic diagnosis), identified an association between cesarean section and increased levels of NT-proBNP (cesarean section median 547.0 pg/mL (interquartile range 304.0–996.0) vs. vaginal delivery 893.0 pg/mL (488.5–1523.8), $p = 0.026$); thus, NT-proBNP was analyzed separately according to delivery route. The remaining cord biomarkers were not affected by the delivery route, and no other confounders were identified.

Logistic regression analysis adjusted by cardiac anatomy and delivery mode was performed, and receiver–operating characteristics (ROC) curves were constructed for cord blood biomarkers in the form of areas under the curve to investigate the presence of a cutoff value that might be predictive of outcome in those fetuses with expected biventricular outcome.

3. Results

3.1. Study Populations

The study population consisted of 35 healthy control pregnancies and 45 fetuses with left-CHD divided into favorable ($n = 29$) and poor ($n = 16$) cardiac outcome (Figure 1). Left-CHD with favorable cardiac outcome included 19 fetuses with CoA, 5 with AoS, and 5 cases of complex left-CHD. The poor cardiac outcome group was formed by 1 fetus with CoA, 2 with AoS, 2 cases of complex left-CHD, and 11 fetuses with HLHS. Univentricular surgical palliation was performed in the 14 newborns in the poor cardiac outcome group (87.5%), and there were 5 postnatal deaths (31.3%), of which 4 corresponded to surgical complications of the univentricular palliation procedure. The remaining case corresponded to a 5-month-old infant with complex left-CHD that died from severe pulmonary hypertension after biventricular management. One 3-year-old infant with complex left-CHD and biventricular management is awaiting a heart transplant at the time of writing. The medium follow-up of left-CHD cases was 3.1 years (interquartile range 1.4–3.9).

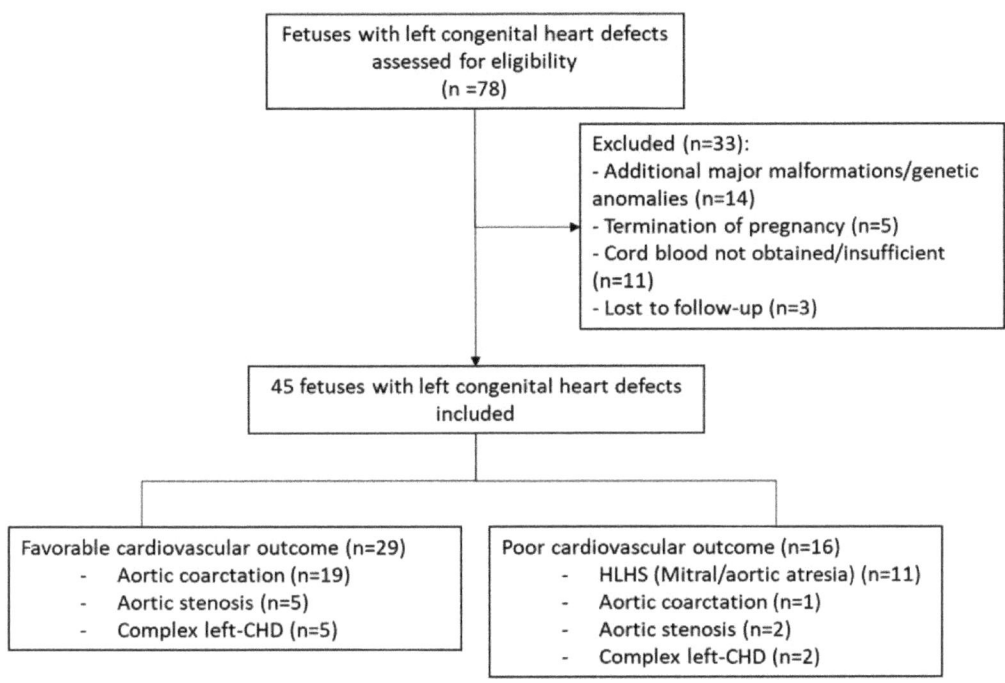

Figure 1. Flowchart of fetuses with left-side congenital heart defects included in the study.

Maternal baseline characteristics, standard obstetrical ultrasound results, and perinatal results are shown in Table 1. The three study populations were similar in terms of maternal characteristics, gestational age at scan, estimated fetal weight, and centile and fetal Doppler. The mean uterine artery pulsatility index was more frequently abnormal (>95th centile) in the favorable cardiac outcome left-CHD group as compared to the normal heart group. Gestational age at delivery was similar across groups, and only two fetuses were born prematurely (one control and one favorable cardiac outcome left-CHD). Cesarean section was more frequent in the poor cardiac outcome group. Prevalence of pregnancy complications was similar in the three groups, including gestational diabetes, preeclampsia, birthweight < 3rd centile, and macrosomia. Birthweight, Apgar score, and umbilical artery pH were also similar.

Table 1. Maternal baseline characteristics, standard ultrasound, and perinatal results in the study populations.

	Normal Heart (n = 35)	Favorable Outcome Left-CHD (n = 29)	Poor Outcome Left-CHD (n = 16)	p
	Maternal baseline characteristics			
Maternal age (years)	33.2 ± 5.2	31.9 ± 6.7	33.7 ± 5.6	0.567
Maternal body mass index	23.2 ± 3.2	25.6 ± 3.7	25.6 ± 5.4	0.095
Nulliparity	17 (48.6%)	15 (51.7%)	7 (43.8%)	0.877
Smoking	4 (11.4%)	4 (13.8%)	1 (6.3%)	0.745
Pregestational diabetes	0 (0%)	0 (0%)	0 (0%)	1.000

Table 1. Cont.

	Normal Heart (n = 35)	Favorable Outcome Left-CHD (n = 29)	Poor Outcome Left-CHD (n = 16)	p
	Standard Obstetrical Ultrasound			
Gestational age at scan (weeks)	33.1 (29.6–35.1)	33.1 (32.3–34.3)	33.1 (32.3–34.3)	0.646
Female fetus	14 (40%)	15 (51.7%)	6 (37.6%)	0.548
Estimated fetal weight (g)	2011 ± 681	2037 ± 560	1918 ± 680	0.933
Estimated fetal weight centile	58.0 (27.0–76.0)	32.5 (18.3–73.0)	84.0 (43.0–86.5)	0.132
Intrauterine growth restriction	0 (0%)	2 (6.9%)	0 (0%)	0.165
Umbilical artery PI	1.0 (0.9–1.1)	1.0 (0.8–1.3)	1.0 (0.8–1.3)	0.723
Umbilical artery PI >95th centile	0 (0%)	1 (3.4%)	0 (0%)	0.410
Median cerebral artery PI	2.0 ± 0.4	1.8 ± 0.3	1.7 ± 0.1	0.087
Median cerebral artery <5th centile	1 (2.9%)	1 (3.4%)	0 (0%)	0.765
Cerebro-placental ratio	2.0 ± 0.5	1.8 ± 0.4	1.8 ± 0.5	0.111
Cerebro-placental ratio <5th centile	2 (5.7%)	2 (6.7%)	0 (0%)	0.577
Mean Uterine Artery PI	0.7 (0.5–0.8)	0.9 (0.7–1.1)	0.7 (0.7–0.9)	0.074
Mean Uterine Artery PI >95th centile	1 (2.9%)	5 (17.2%)	0 (0%)	0.042
	Perinatal Results			
Gestational age delivery (weeks)	39.8 (38.6–40.5)	39.7 (38.4–40.3)	40.0 (39.5–40.0)	0.723
Cesarean section	8 (22.8%)	6 (21.4%)	7 (63.6%) *	0.019
Spontaneous preterm birth < 37 weeks	1 (2.9%)	1 (3.4%)	0 (0%)	0.765
Gestational diabetes	3 (8.6%)	3 (10.3%)	2 (12.5%)	0.907
Preeclampsia	0 (0%)	1 (3.4%)	1 (6.3%)	0.381
Birth weight (g)	3256 ± 416	3173 ± 525	3275 ± 415	0.660
Birth weight < 3rd centile	0 (0%)	2 (6.9%)	0 (0%)	0.165
Birth weight > 4000 g	0 (0%)	1 (3.4%)	0 (0%)	0.410
5-min Apgar score < 7	0 (0%)	1 (3.4%)	0 (0%)	0.410
Umbilical artery pH	7.22 (7.17–7.27)	7.25 (7.18–7.27)	7.26 (7.20–7.30)	0.416
	Cardiovascular outcome			
Follow-up (years)	—	3.1 (1.4–3.9)		—
Univentricular circulation	—	—	11 (68.8%)	—
Cardiac transplant	—	—	1 (6.3%)	—
Death	—	—	5 (31.3%)	—

Data are presented as mean ± standard deviation, median (interquartile range), or n (percentage %) as appropriate. Left-CHD: left-sided congenital heart disease. Poor outcome defined as postnatal univentricular surgical palliation, need for heart transplant, or death. PI: pulsatility index. Intrauterine growth restriction is defined as estimated fetal weight below the 3rd centile or below the 10th centile with abnormal maternal or fetal Doppler values. p is shown for the ANOVA between the 3 groups. * $p < 0.05$ in pairwise comparisons in ANOVA post hoc Bonferroni or Dunn–Bonferroni tests of favorable and poor outcome vs. normal heart.

Cardiac morphological and functional evaluation in control, left-CHD with favorable and poor cardiac outcome fetuses are shown in Table 2. The cardiothoracic ratio was higher in both left-CHD groups compared to the normal heart group. Left atrial-to-heart and left ventricular-to-heart ratios were significantly lower in left-CHD, more markedly so in the poor cardiac outcome group. Concerning the right side of the heart, right atrial-to-heart and right ventricular-to-heart ratios were significantly increased in the poor cardiac outcome left-CHD compared to the normal heart group but not in the favorable cardiac outcome group. Right-to-left ventricular ratio (basal transverse diameter) was significantly increased in both groups of left-CHD. Septal thickness tended to be higher in left-CHD with poor prognosis; however, in post hoc pairwise comparison, the difference was not statistically significant ($p = 0.068$). Heart rate was similar in the three groups. The left shortening fraction was increased in the favorable cardiac outcome group of left-CHD and decreased in the poor cardiac outcome left-CHD compared to the normal heart group. The remaining functional parameters evaluated did not show significant differences between the three study populations.

Table 2. Fetal echocardiographic results in the study populations.

Parameter	Normal Heart ($n = 35$)	Favorable Outcome Left-CHD ($n = 29$)	Poor Outcome Left-CHD ($n = 16$)	p
Cardiac morphometric parameters				
Gestational age at scan (weeks)	33.1 (29.6–35.1)	33.1 (32.3–34.3)	33.1 (32.3–34.3)	0.646
Cardio-thoracic ratio	0.28 ± 0.04	0.30 ± 0.05 *	0.32 ± 0.05 *	0.002
Cardiac sphericity index	1.2 (1.1–1.3)	1.2 (1.1–1.3)	1.1 (1.0–1.3)	0.087
Left atrial-to-heart ratio	0.15 ± 0.04	0.13 ± 0.03 *	0.10 ± 0.03 *	<0.001
Left ventricular-to-heart ratio †	0.23 (0.19–0.28)	0.15 (0.14–0.20) *	0.11 (0.03–0.14) *	<0.001
Right atria-to-heart ratio	0.17 ± 0.05	0.20 ± 0.03	0.23 ± 0.08 *	0.001
Right ventricle-to-heart ratio	0.23 (0.20–0.27)	0.24 (0.21–0.26)	0.29 (0.25–0.36) *	0.016
Right-to-left ventricular ratio (basal)	1.0 (0.9–1.1)	1.4 (1.3–1.7) *	2.1 (1.9–3.7) *	<0.001
Septal wall thickness (mm)	3.1 (2.6–3.7)	3.5 (3.0–4.1)	3.6 (3.4–3.9)	0.040
Cardiac function parameters				
Heart rate	141 (134–144)	137 (131–145)	140 (131–141)	0.693
Left ventricular Shortening Fraction ‡	36.7 ± 8.8	44.3 ± 12.9 *	21.0 ± 11.2 *	<0.001
Left filling time fraction ‡	43.2 ± 4.9	42.0 ± 3.6	41.2 ± 14.6	0.633
Left ejection time fraction ‡	41.0 (338.9–43.4)	42.1 (37.9–44.8)	45.1 (38.4–64.6)	0.282
Right ventricular Fractional Area Change	30.4 ± 8.4	30.7 ± 11.2	35.6 ± 10.6	0.371
Right filling time fraction	40.4 (37.6–43.9)	42.3 (38.4–44.2)	38.9 (35.4–43.4)	0.480
Right ejection time fraction	42.6 ± 3.3	41.8 ± 3.8	43.0 ± 4.1	0.577

Data are presented as mean ± standard deviation or median (interquartile range). Left-CHD: left-sided congenital heart disease. Poor cardiac outcome defined by the presence of postnatal univentricular circulation, need for heart transplant, or death. † Measured when the left ventricle was visible ($n = 10$ in the poor outcome group). ‡ Measured when left ventricular inflow/outflow was detectable ($n = 5$ in the poor outcome group). P is shown for the ANOVA between the 3 groups. * $p < 0.05$ in pairwise comparisons in ANOVA post hoc Bonferroni or Dunn–Bonferroni tests of favorable and poor outcome vs. normal heart.

3.2. Cord Blood Biomarkers Results

Results of cord blood biomarkers in left-CHD and normal heart groups are presented in Table 3 and Figure 2. Compared to the normal heart group, left-CHD cases with favorable cardiac outcome presented preserved NT-proBNP concentrations. Cord blood Troponin I seemed to be more frequently elevated in the favorable cardiac outcome group, but this was not statistically significant. Fetuses with a favorable outcome also presented a markedly increased cord blood concentration of TGFβ and lower PlGF with no significant changes in sFlt1. Conversely, poor outcome left-CHD cases presented increased concentrations of NT-proBNP, which was independent of delivery mode. Troponin I showed positive results in a similar proportion to the control group. In the poor prognosis group, TGFβ concentrations were not significantly higher than in the normal heart group. Finally, PlGF was slightly reduced, while cord blood sFlt1 concentrations were drastically reduced in this group. These findings were independent of the specific anatomy.

Table 3. Concentrations of N-terminal precursor of B-type natriuretic peptide (NT-Pro-BNP), Troponin I, transforming growth factor β (TGFβ), placental growth factor (PlGF), and soluble fms-like tyrosine kinase-1 (sFlt1) in the cord blood of control fetuses and fetuses with favorable versus poor outcome left congenital heart defects.

Cord Blood Cardiovascular Biomarkers	Normal Heart (n = 35)	Favorable Outcome Left-CHD (n = 29)	Poor Outcome Left-CHD (n = 16)	p
NT Pro-BNP (pg/mL)	508.0 (287.5–776.3)	617.0 (389.8–1087.8)	1450.0 (919.0–1645.0) *	0.001
TroponinI (% positive)	7/31 (22.6%)	9/19 (47.4%)	2/9 (22.2%)	0.153
TGFβ (ng/mL)	15.0 (6.8–21.4)	51.7 (13.8–73.9) *	25.1 (6.9–39.0)	0.001
PlGF (pg/mL)	17.9 (13.8–23.9)	12.8 (11.7–13.6) *	11.0 (8.8–15.4) *	<0.001
sFlt1 (pg/mL)	1929.7 (1364.3–2715.8)	1848.3 (646.9–2313.6)	259.0 (182.0–606.0) *	<0.001

Data are presented as median (interquartile range) or n (percentage). Left-CHD: left-sided congenital heart disease. Troponin I was considered positive when higher than 0.017 ng/mL. P is shown for the ANOVA or chi-square tests between the 3 groups. * $p < 0.05$ in pairwise comparisons in ANOVA post hoc Dunn–Bonferroni tests of favorable and poor outcome vs. normal heart.

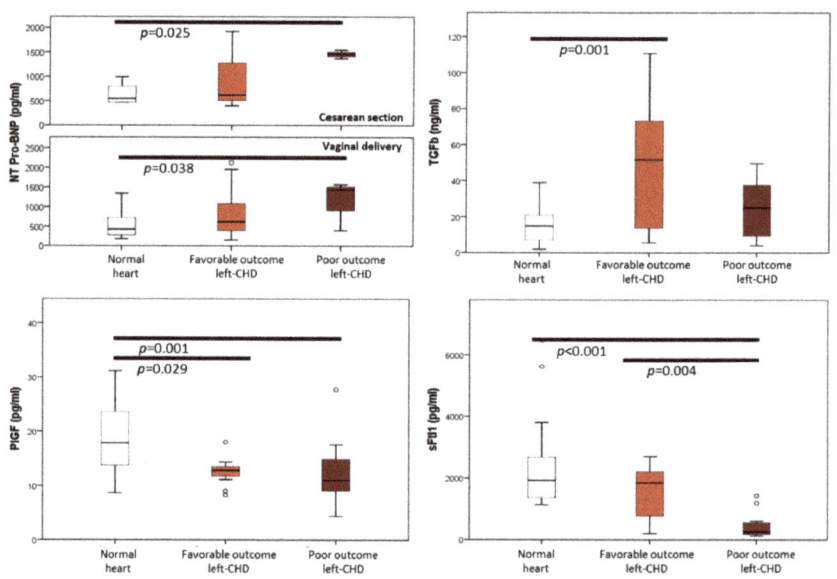

Figure 2. Concentrations of N-terminal precursor of B-type natriuretic peptide (NT-Pro-BNP), Troponin I, transforming growth factor β (TGFβ), placental growth factor (PlGF), and soluble fms-like tyrosine kinase-1 (sFlt1) in the cord blood of fetuses with normal heart and with favorable and poor outcome left congenital heart defects. Poor cardiac outcome is defined as univentricular circulation, heart transplant, or death. p-values are shown for significantly different ($p < 0.05$) comparisons.

Logistic regression analysis and evaluation of ROC curves of concentration of cord blood biomarkers for the prediction of outcome in fetuses with expected biventricular repair, adjusted for cardiac anatomy and cesarean section, found that only sFlt1 was useful as an outcome predictor. The sFlt1ROC curve had an AUC of 0.848 (95% confidence interval 0.706–0.991) with a cutoff value of 1520.7, having a specificity of 100% and a sensitivity of 72% for a favorable outcome (Figure 3).

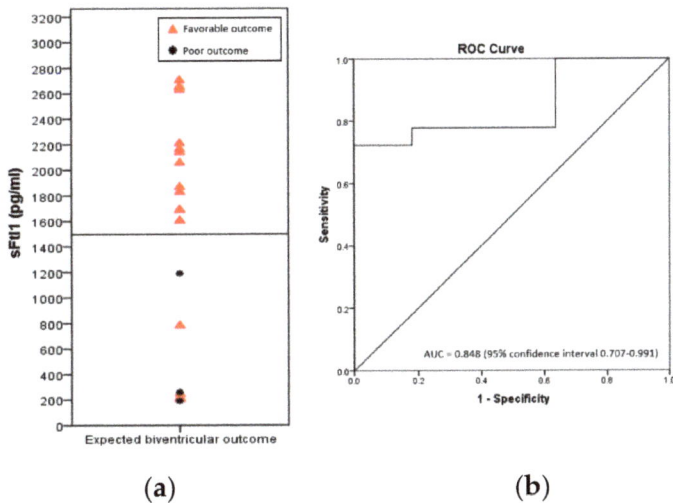

(a) (b)

Figure 3. (**a**) Concentrations of soluble fms-like tyrosine kinase-1 (sFlt1) in the cord blood of control fetuses and fetuses with expected biventricular repair, classified according to outcome (red triangle, favorable outcome; black star, poor outcome. Reference line set at 1520.7 pg/mL identified at (**b**) ROC curve for sFlt1 as a predictor of favorable outcome in fetuses with expected biventricular outcome.

4. Discussion

Cord blood cardiovascular biomarkers are differentially expressed according to the clinical outcome of left-CHD. Fetuses with left-CHD and favorable outcome showed an active cardiac remodeling biomarker profile, with an increase in TGFβ and Troponin I cord blood concentrations. Conversely, fetuses with left-CHD and poor outcome presented a compensatory and proangiogenic biomarker profile with increased NT-proBNP and decreased sFlt1 concentrations.

Prior studies reported increased NT-proBNP concentrations in children with systemic right ventricle and in single ventricle CHD before completion of staged palliation [42–44]. A different study evaluated cord blood NT-proBNP and Troponin T plus an echocardiographic score (including aortic size and cardiomegaly) to predict mortality in a variety of single ventricle CHD (approximately half were left-CHD) [6]. Both NT-proBNP and Troponin T were found to be useful predictors in this setting [6]. While obvious differences exist between both studies [6] in terms of CHD included and outcome definition, increased NT-proBNP seems to be reflecting fetal adaptation to ventricular stretching or hypoxia and correlate with the disease severity and outcome.

Positive cord blood Troponin I was more frequent in left-CHD with favorable cardiac outcome than in fetuses with normal hearts or fetuses with poor outcome. Differences were not statistically significant, and these results must be interpreted with caution as the normal heart group presented higher positive rates of Troponin I than previously reported in healthy fetuses [41,45,46]. In a prior study, Troponin I was detected more frequently in children with pressure overload CHD (CoA, AoS, and pulmonary stenosis) rather than volume overload CHD (atrial septal defect and patent ductus arteriosus) [45]. In the present study, most cases of pressure overload (AoS and complex left-CHD) presented a favorable outcome, while the poor outcome group included mostly fetuses with HLHS (right ventricular volume overload), which may explain our findings. Increased levels of Troponin I in cord blood might reflect endocardial hypoxia and myocardial damage secondary to increased end-diastolic ventricular pressure and wall stress [47].

To our knowledge, this is the first study to evaluate cord blood concentrations of TGFβ in fetuses with CHD, showing increased TGFβ concentrations in left-CHD with favorable outcome. High levels of circulating TGBβ are usually associated with increased endothelial shear stress, secondary to abnormal fluid dynamics within blood vessels [48,49]. All cases in the favorable outcome group presented anatomical impediments to normal blood flow and, thus, turbulent flow and increased endothelial shear stress that could stimulate the production of TGFβ by endothelial cells. In addition, increased TGFβ expression has been related to extracellular matrix deposition and fibrosis and arterial intima-media thickening and can be detected by immunohistochemistry at the coarctation site, especially in infants with a closed arterial duct [9,10,50]. On the other hand, TGFβ concentrations were not increased in the poor outcome group, which was mostly composed of fetuses with full cardiac output handled by the right heart and laminar flow through the pulmonary artery.

Cord blood concentrations of PlGF were found to be modestly decreased in left-CHD compared to normal heart fetuses. However, sFlt1 was markedly decreased in the poor outcome group conferring a proangiogenic profile of PlGF and sFlt1. Such low levels of sFlt1 had not been described previously in pregnancy, and their cause is unclear. However, sFlt1 is down-regulated by hypoxia [51], and therefore, our findings might be explained by the hypoxic damage of the left ventricular endocardium of fetuses with poor outcome left-CHD [52,53]. A previous study including a mixed group of CHDs, including atrioventricular septal defects (A-V defects), conotruncal anomalies, and left-CHD reported similar PlGF but increased sFlt1 cord blood levels in CHD [16]. This inconsistency might be explained by the different types of CHD included in both studies. The presence of a high proportion of A-V defects and conotruncal anomalies, as well as missing information in terms of left-CHD types and/or severity, precludes direct comparison between both studies.

Finally, cord blood sFlt1 was identified for the first time as a possible outcome predictor in fetuses with expected biventricular repair and may eventually help to identify cases at risk of an unexpectedly poor prognosis despite favorable anatomy. Naturally, due to the limited number of cases in this subgroup, confirmation in larger cohorts is required prior to clinical application. A larger number of cases might also demonstrate the utility of NT-proBNP or TGFβ in these patients in which a poor prognosis comes as a surprise.

Strengths and Limitations

To the best of our knowledge, this is the first study to evaluate cord blood biomarkers in a specific set of CHDs and to evaluate TGFβ in the cord blood of fetuses with CHDs. It is also the first study to identify TGFβ and specially sFlt1 as potentially useful cardiovascular biomarkers in left-CHD.

This is mainly an exploratory study, and therefore, the eventual clinical application of our findings will likely be distant. The main limitation of this (and other studies) is the limited number of cases that precludes the evaluation of these biomarkers in each specific type of CHD. Interpretation of results is also limited by the presence of mixed pathologies in the favorable and poor outcome left-CHD groups. Cord blood biomarker levels were analyzed after adjustment for possible confounders; however, additional confounders might exist. Additionally, levels of Troponin I in the cord blood of normal fetuses were higher than previously reported [41,45,46], which limits the interpretation of our results.

5. Conclusions

This study provides evidence of a differential biomarker profile in left-CHD according to its outcome. It opens new opportunities for improving prognosis prediction and potentially helping in prenatal monitoring, neonatal management, and parental counseling. If confirmed in future studies, these biomarkers could potentially be useful as a prognosis tool in prenatal or neonatal life. In addition, future studies are warranted to study cardiovascular biomarkers in different matrices such as amniotic fluid or maternal blood. Long-term multicenter studies might be able to include enough patients and allow specific evaluation and analysis of each individual type of left-CHD. Additionally, the investigation of these biomarkers in the cord blood of other CHDs might also yield interesting results.

Author Contributions: Conceptualization, I.S., O.G. and F.C.; methodology, I.S., O.G. and F.C.; software, I.S.; validation, I.S. and L.G.; formal analysis, I.S., O.G. and F.C.; investigation, I.S., O.G., L.G., M.C.E.-D., M.J.A., V.R.-S., J.M.M., E.A., E.L., J.L.B. and F.C.; resources I.S., O.G., L.G., M.C.E.-D., M.J.A., V.R.-S., J.M.M., B.B., E.A., E.L., J.L.B. and F.C.; data curation, I.S.; writing—original draft preparation, I.S.; writing—review and editing, I.S., O.G., M.C.E.-D., M.J.A., J.M.M., E.A., E.L., J.L.B. and F.C.; visualization, I.S.; supervision, O.G. and F.C.; project administration, O.G., B.B., E.A., E.L., J.L.B. and F.C.; funding acquisition, I.S., O.G., J.M.M., B.B., E.A., E.L., J.L.B. and F.C. All authors have read and agreed to the published version of the manuscript.

Funding: This research was funded by grants from Hospital Clinic de Barcelona (Ajut Josep Font 2015, Barcelona, Spain), Instituto de Salud Carlos III (PI15/00263, PI17/00675, PI20/00246, INT21/00027) within the Plan Nacional de I+D+I and co-financed by Instituto de Salud Carlos III-Subdirección General de Evaluación together with the Fondo Europeo de Desarrollo Regional (FEDER) "Una manera de hacer Europa", Fundación Jesús Serra, "LaCaixa" Foundation under grant agreements LCF/PR/GN14/10270005 and LCF/PR/GN18/10310003AS, Cerebra Foundation for the Brain Injured Child (Carmarthen, Wales, UK), Fundació La Marató de TV3 (Ref 202016-30-31), and Maternal and Child Health and Development Network (SAMID), RD16/0022/0015. This publication reflects the views of the authors only, and the Commission cannot be held responsible for any usage, which may be made of the information contained therein. No industry funding was used in the development of this work.

Institutional Review Board Statement: The study was conducted in accordance with the Declaration of Helsinki and approved by the Ethics Committee of BCNatal (Hospitals Clinic and Sant Joan de Déu. PR (AMI)317/2012, May 2013) and Hospital Vall d'Hebrón in Barcelona, and Hospital La Paz in Madrid.

Informed Consent Statement: Informed consent was obtained from all subjects involved in the study.

Acknowledgments: We would like to thank Biobanks of Clínic-IDIBAPS and Fundació Sant Joan de Déu for the valuable management of samples.

Conflicts of Interest: The authors declare no conflict of interest. The funders had no role in the design of the study; in the collection, analyses, or interpretation of data; in the writing of the manuscript; or in the decision to publish the results.

References

1. Wren, C.; Reinhardt, Z.; Khawaja, K. Twenty-Year Trends in Diagnosis of Life-Threatening Neonatal Cardiovascular Malformations. *Arch. Dis. Child. Fetal Neonatal Ed.* **2008**, *93*, F33–F35. [CrossRef]
2. Khoo, N.S.; Van Essen, P.; Richardson, M.; Robertson, T. Effectiveness of Prenatal Diagnosis of Congenital Heart Defects in South Australia: A Population Analysis 1999–2003. *Aust. N. Z. J. Obstet. Gynaecol.* **2008**, *48*, 559–563. [CrossRef]
3. Davlouros, P.A.; Karatza, A.A.; Xanthopoulou, I.; Dimitriou, G.; Georgiopoulou, A.; Mantagos, S.; Alexopoulos, D. Diagnostic Role of Plasma BNP Levels in Neonates with Signs of Congenital Heart Disease. *Int. J. Cardiol.* **2011**, *147*, 42–46. [CrossRef]
4. Cantinotti, M.; Giordano, R.; Scalese, M.; Molinaro, S.; Della Pina, F.; Storti, S.; Arcieri, L.; Murzi, B.; Marotta, M.; Pak, V.; et al. Prognostic Role of BNP in Children Undergoing Surgery for Congenital Heart Disease: Analysis of Prediction Models Incorporating Standard Risk Factors. *Clin. Chem. Lab. Med.* **2015**, *53*, 1839–1846. [CrossRef]
5. Agewall, S.; Giannitsis, E.; Jernberg, T.; Katus, H. Troponin Elevation in Coronary vs. Non-Coronary Disease. *Eur. Heart J.* **2011**, *32*, 404–411. [CrossRef]
6. Lee, S.M.; Kwon, J.E.; Song, S.H.; Kim, G.B.; Park, J.Y.; Kim, B.J.; Lee, J.H.; Park, C.W.; Park, J.S.; Jun, J.K. Prenatal Prediction of Neonatal Death in Single Ventricle Congenital Heart Disease. *Prenat. Diagn.* **2016**, *36*, 346–352. [CrossRef]
7. Dabek, J.; Kułach, A.; Monastyrska-Cup, B.; Gasior, Z. Transforming Growth Factor β and Cardiovascular Diseases: The Other Facet of the "Protective Cytokine". *Pharmacol. Rep.* **2006**, *58*, 799–805.
8. Clark, D.A.; Coker, R. Transforming Growth Factor-Beta (TGF-β). *Int. J. Biochem. Cell Biol.* **1998**, *30*, 293–298. [CrossRef]
9. Guerri-Guttenberg, R.A.; Castilla, R.; Francos, G.C.; Müller, A.; Ambrosio, G.; Milei, J. Transforming Growth Factor B1 and Coronary Intimal Hyperplasia in Pediatric Patients With Congenital Heart Disease. *Can. J. Cardiol.* **2013**, *29*, 849–857. [CrossRef]
10. Doetschman, T.; Barnett, J.V.; Runyan, R.B.; Camenisch, T.D.; Heimark, R.L.; Granzier, H.L.; Conway, S.J.; Azhar, M. Transforming Growth Factor Beta Signaling in Adult Cardiovascular Diseases and Repair. *Cell Tissue Res.* **2012**, *347*, 203–223.
11. Dobaczewski, M.; Chen, W.; Frangogiannis, N.G. Transforming Growth Factor (TGF)-β Signaling in Cardiac Remodeling. *J. Mol. Cell. Cardiol.* **2011**, *51*, 600–606. [CrossRef]
12. Iwama, H.; Uemura, S.; Naya, N.; Imagawa, K.I.; Takemoto, Y.; Asai, O.; Onoue, K.; Okayama, S.; Somekawa, S.; Kida, Y.; et al. Cardiac Expression of Placental Growth Factor Predicts the Improvement of Chronic Phase Left Ventricular Function in Patients With Acute Myocardial Infarction. *J. Am. Coll. Cardiol.* **2006**, *47*, 1559–1567. [CrossRef]

13. Nakamura, T.; Funayama, H.; Kubo, N.; Yasu, T.; Kawakami, M.; Momomura, S.I.; Ishikawa, S.E. Elevation of Plasma Placental Growth Factor in the Patients with Ischemic Cardiomyopathy. *Int. J. Cardiol.* **2009**, *131*, 186–191. [CrossRef]
14. Accornero, F.; Molkentin, J.D. Placental Growth Factor as a Protective Paracrine Effector in the Heart. *Trends Cardiovasc. Med.* **2011**, *21*, 220–224. [CrossRef]
15. Chau, K.; Hennessy, A.; Makris, A. Placental Growth Factor and Pre-Eclampsia. *J. Hum. Hypertens.* **2017**, *31*, 782–786. [CrossRef]
16. Llurba, E.; Sanchez, O.; Ferrer, Q.; Nicolaides, K.H.; Ruiz, A.; Dominguez, C.; Sanchez-de-Toledo, J.; Garcia-Garcia, B.; Soro, G.; Arevalo, S.; et al. Maternal and Foetal Angiogenic Imbalance in Congenital Heart Defects. *Eur. Heart J.* **2014**, *35*, 701–707. [CrossRef]
17. Robinson, H.P.; Sweet, E.M.; Adam, A.H. The Accuracy of Radiological Estimates of Gestational Age Using Early Fetal Crown-Rump Length Measurements by Ultrasound as a Basis for Comparison. *Br. J. Obstet. Gynaecol.* **1979**, *86*, 525–528. [CrossRef]
18. Familiari, A.; Morlando, M.; Khalil, A.; Sonesson, S.-E.; Scala, C.; Rizzo, G.; Del Sordo, G.; Vassallo, C.; Elena Flacco, M.; Manzoli, L.; et al. Risk Factors for Coarctation of the Aorta on Prenatal UltrasoundClinical Perspective. *Circulation* **2017**, *135*, 772–785. [CrossRef]
19. Schneider, C.; McCrindle, B.W.; Carvalho, J.S.; Hornberger, L.K.; McCarthy, K.P.; Daubeney, P.E.F. Development of Z-Scores for Fetal Cardiac Dimensions from Echocardiography. *Ultrasound Obstet. Gynecol.* **2005**, *26*, 599–605. [CrossRef]
20. Shone, J.D.; Sellers, R.D.; Anderson, R.C.; Adams, P.; Lillehei, C.W.; Edwards, J.E. The Developmental Complex of "Parachute Mitral Valve," Supravalvular Ring of Left Atrium, Subaortic Stenosis, and Coarctation of Aorta. *Am. J. Cardiol.* **1963**, *11*, 714–725. [CrossRef]
21. Rodríguez-López, M.; Cruz-Lemini, M.; Valenzuela-Alcaraz, B.; Garcia-Otero, L.; Sitges, M.; Bijnens, B.; Gratacos, E.; Crispi, F. Descriptive Analysis of the Different Phenotypes of Cardiac Remodeling in Fetal Growth Restriction. *Ultrasound Obstet. Gynecol.* **2017**, *50*, 207–214. [CrossRef] [PubMed]
22. Crispi, F.; Bijnens, B.; Figueras, F.; Bartrons, J.; Eixarch, E.; Le Noble, F.; Ahmed, A.; Gratacos, E. Fetal Growth Restriction Results in Remodeled and Less Efficient Hearts in Children. *Circulation* **2010**, *121*, 2427–2436. [CrossRef] [PubMed]
23. Barker, D.J.P. Adult Consequences of Fetal Growth Restriction. *Clin. Obstet. Gynecol.* **2006**, *49*, 270–283. [CrossRef]
24. Kocylowski, R.D.; Dubiel, M.; Gudmundsson, S.; Sieg, I.; Fritzer, E.; Alkasi, Ö.; Breborowicz, G.H.; von Kaisenberg, C.S. Biochemical Tissue-Specific Injury Markers of the Heart and Brain in Postpartum Cord Blood. *Am. J. Obstet. Gynecol.* **2009**, *200*, 273.e1–273.e25. [CrossRef]
25. Patey, O.; Carvalho, J.S.; Thilaganathan, B. Perinatal Changes in Fetal Cardiac Geometry and Function in Diabetic Pregnancy at Term. *Ultrasound Obstet. Gynecol.* **2019**, *54*, 634–642. [CrossRef]
26. Mert, M.K.; Satar, M.; Özbarlas, N.; Yaman, A.; Özgünen, F.T.; Asker, H.S.; Çekinmez, E.K.; Tetiker, T. Troponin T and NT ProBNP Levels in Gestational, Type 1 and Type 2 Diabetic Mothers and Macrosomic Infants. *Pediatr. Cardiol.* **2016**, *37*, 76–83. [CrossRef]
27. García-Otero, L.; López, M.; Gómez, O.; Goncé, A.; Bennasar, M.; Martínez, J.M.; Valenzuela-Alcaraz, B.; Rodriguez-López, M.; Sitges, M.; Loncà, M.; et al. Zidovudine Treatment in HIV-Infected Pregnant Women Is Associated with Fetal Cardiac Remodelling. *AIDS* **2016**, *30*, 1393–1401. [CrossRef]
28. Hadlock, F.P.; Harrist, R.B.; Shah, Y.P.; King, D.E.; Park, S.K.; Sharman, R.S. Estimating Fetal Age Using Multiple Parameters: A Prospective Evaluation in a Racially Mixed Population. *Am. J. Obstet. Gynecol.* **1987**, *156*, 955–957. [CrossRef]
29. Figueras, F.; Meler, E.; Iraola, A.; Eixarch, E.; Coll, O.; Figueras, J.; Francis, A.; Gratacos, E.; Gardosi, J. Customized Birthweight Standards for a Spanish Population. *Eur. J. Obstet. Gynecol. Reprod. Biol.* **2008**, *136*, 20–24. [CrossRef]
30. Carvalho, J.; Allan, L.; Chaoui, R.; Copel, J.; DeVore, G.; Hecher, K.; Lee, W.; Munoz, H.; Paladini, D.; Tutschek, B.; et al. ISUOG Practice Guidelines (Updated): Sonographic Screening Examination of the Fetal Heart. *Ultrasound Obstet. Gynecol.* **2013**, *41*, 348–359. [CrossRef]
31. Bhide, A.; Acharya, G.; Bilardo, C.M.; Brezinka, C.; Cafici, D.; Hernandez-Andrade, E.; Kalache, K.; Kingdom, J.; Kiserud, T.; Lee, W.; et al. ISUOG Practice Guidelines: Use of Doppler Ultrasonography in Obstetrics. *Ultrasound Obstet. Gynecol.* **2013**, *41*, 233–239. [CrossRef] [PubMed]
32. Baschat, A.A.; Gembruch, U. The Cerebroplacental Doppler Ratio Revisited. *Ultrasound Obstet. Gynecol.* **2003**, *21*, 124–127. [CrossRef] [PubMed]
33. Figueras, F.; Gratacós, E. Update on the Diagnosis and Classification of Fetal Growth Restriction and Proposal of a Stage-Based Management Protocol. *Fetal Diagn. Ther.* **2014**, *36*, 86–98. [CrossRef]
34. Paladini, D.; Chita, S.K.; Allan, L.D. Prenatal Measurement of Cardiothoracic Ratio in Evaluation of Heart Disease. *Arch. Dis. Child.* **1990**, *65*, 20–23. [CrossRef]
35. García-Otero, L.; Soveral, I.; Sepúlveda-Martínez, Á.; Rodriguez-lópez, M.; Torres, X.; Guirado, L.; Nogué, L.; Valenzuela-Alcaraz, B.; Martínez, J.M.; Gratacós, E.; et al. Reference Ranges for Fetal Cardiac, Ventricular and Atrial Relative Size, Sphericity, Ventricular Dominance, Wall Asymmetry and Relative Wall Thickness from 18 to 41 Weeks of Gestation. *Ultrasound Obstet. Gynecol.* **2020**, *58*, 388–397. [CrossRef]
36. Sepúlveda-Martínez, A.; García-Otero, L.; Soveral, I.; Guirado, L.; Valenzuela-Alcaraz, B.; Torres, X.; Rodriguez-Lopez, M.; Gratacos, E.; Gómez, O.; Crispi, F. Comparison of 2D versus M-Mode Echocardiography for Assessing Fetal Myocardial Wall Thickness. *J. Matern. Neonatal Med.* **2018**, *32*, 2319–2327. [CrossRef]

37. García-Otero, L.; Gómez, O.; Rodriguez-López, M.; Torres, X.; Soveral, I.; Sepúlveda-Martínez, Á.; Guirado, L.; Valenzuela-Alcaraz, B.; López, M.; Martínez, J.M.; et al. Nomograms of Fetal Cardiac Dimensions at 18–41 Weeks of Gestation. *Fetal Diagn. Ther.* **2020**, *47*, 387–398. [CrossRef]
38. Guirado, L.; Crispi, F.; Soveral, I.; Valenzuela-Alcaraz, B.; Rodriguez-López, M.; García-Otero, L.; Torres, X.; Sepúlveda-Martínez, Á.; Escobar-Diaz, M.C.; Martínez, J.M.; et al. Nomograms of Fetal Right Ventricular Fractional Area Change by 2D Echocardiography. *Fetal Diagn. Ther.* **2020**, *47*, 399–410. [CrossRef]
39. DeVore, G.R.; Siassi, B.; Platt, L.D. Fetal Echocardiography. *Am. J. Obstet. Gynecol.* **1984**, *150*, 981–988. [CrossRef]
40. Soveral, I.; Crispi, F.; Guirado, L.; García-Otero, L.; Torres, X.; Bennasar, M.; Sepúlveda-Martínez, Á.; Nogué, L.; Gratacós, E.; Martínez, J.M.; et al. Cardiac Filling and Ejection Time Fractions by Pulsed Doppler: Fetal Nomograms and Potential Clinical Application. *Ultrasound Obstet. Gynecol.* **2020**, *58*, 83–91. [CrossRef]
41. Trevisanuto, D.; Pitton, M.; Altinier, S.; Zaninotto, M.; Plebani, M.; Zanardo, V. Cardiac Troponin I, Cardiac Troponin T and Creatine Kinase MB Concentrations in Umbilical Cord Blood of Healthy Term Neonates. *Acta Paediatr. Int. J. Paediatr.* **2003**, *92*, 1463–1467. [CrossRef]
42. Eindhoven, J.A.; Van Den Bosch, A.E.; Jansen, P.R.; Boersma, E.; Roos-Hesselink, J.W. The Usefulness of Brain Natriuretic Peptide in Complex Congenital Heart Disease: A Systematic Review. *J. Am. Coll. Cardiol.* **2012**, *60*, 2140–2149. [CrossRef] [PubMed]
43. Holmgren, D.; Westerlind, A.; Berggren, H.; Lundberg, P.A.; Wåhlander, H. Increased Natriuretic Peptide Type B Level after the Second Palliative Step in Children with Univentricular Hearts with Right Ventricular Morphology but Not Left Ventricular Morphology. *Pediatr. Cardiol.* **2008**, *29*, 786–792. [CrossRef] [PubMed]
44. Wåhlander, H.; Westerlind, A.; Lindstedt, G.; Lundberg, P.A.; Holmgren, D. Increased Levels of Brain and Atrial Natriuretic Peptides after the First Palliative Operation, but Not after a Bidirectional Glenn Anastomosis, in Children with Functionally Univentricular Hearts. *Cardiol. Young* **2003**, *13*, 268–274. [CrossRef] [PubMed]
45. Eerola, A.; Jokinen, E.O.; Savukoski, T.I.; Pettersson, K.S.I.; Poutanen, T.; Pihkala, J.I. Cardiac Troponin I in Congenital Heart Defects with Pressure or Volume Overload. *Scand. Cardiovasc. J.* **2013**, *47*, 154–159. [CrossRef] [PubMed]
46. Sugimoto, M.; Ota, K.; Kajihama, A.; Nakau, K.; Manabe, H.; Kajino, H. Volume Overload and Pressure Overload Due to Left-to-Right Shunt-Induced Myocardial Injury: Evaluation Using a Highly Sensitive Cardiac Troponin-I Assay in Children with Congenital Heart Disease. *Circ. J.* **2011**, *75*, 2213–2219. [CrossRef]
47. Goodwill, A.G.; Dick, G.M.; Kiel, A.M.; Tune, J.D. Regulation of Coronary Blood Flow. *Compr. Physiol.* **2017**, *7*, 321–382. [CrossRef]
48. Briana, D.D.; Liosi, S.; Gourgiotis, D.; Boutsikou, M.; Marmarinos, A.; Baka, S.; Hassiakos, D.; Malamitsi-Puchner, A. Fetal Concentrations of the Growth Factors TGF-α and TGF-B1 in Relation to Normal and Restricted Fetal Growth at Term. *Cytokine* **2012**, *60*, 157–161. [CrossRef]
49. Walshe, T.E.; Dela Paz, N.G.; D'Amore, P.A. The Role of Shear-Induced Transforming Growth Factor-β Signaling in the Endothelium. *Arterioscler. Thromb. Vasc. Biol.* **2013**, *33*, 2608–2617. [CrossRef]
50. Swartz, M.F.; Morrow, D.; Atallah-Yunes, N.; Cholette, J.M.; Gensini, F.; Kavey, R.E.; Alfieris, G.M. Hypertensive Changes within the Aortic Arch of Infants and Children with Isolated Coarctation. *Ann. Thorac. Surg.* **2013**, *96*, 190–195. [CrossRef]
51. Ikeda, T.; Sun, L.; Tsuruoka, N.; Ishigaki, Y.; Yoshitomi, Y.; Yoshitake, Y.; Yonekura, H. Hypoxia Down-Regulates SFlt-1 (SVEGFR-1) Expression in Human Microvascular Endothelial Cells by a Mechanism Involving MRNA Alternative Processing. *Biochem. J.* **2011**, *436*, 399–407. [CrossRef] [PubMed]
52. Salhiyyah, K.; Sarathchandra, P.; Latif, N.; Yacoub, M.H.; Chester, A.H. Hypoxia-Mediated Regulation of the Secretory Properties of Mitral Valve Interstitial Cells. *Am. J. Physiol. Circ. Physiol.* **2017**, *313*, H14–H23. [CrossRef] [PubMed]
53. Lee, J.W.; Ko, J.; Ju, C.; Eltzschig, H.K. Hypoxia Signaling in Human Diseases and Therapeutic Targets. *Exp. Mol. Med.* **2019**, *51*, 1–13. [CrossRef] [PubMed]

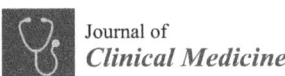

Journal of
Clinical Medicine

Communication

Longitudinal Surveillance of Fetal Heart Failure Using Speckle Tracking Analysis

Julia Murlewska [1,*], Oskar Sylwestrzak [1,2], Maria Respondek-Liberska [1,2], Mark Sklansky [3,4] and Greggory Devore [4,5]

1. Cardiology Department, Polish Mother's Memorial Hospital, Research Institute, 93-338 Lodz, Poland
2. Department for Fetal Malformations Diagnoses & Prevention, Medical University of Lodz, 93-338 Lodz, Poland
3. Division of Pediatric Cardiology, Department of Pediatrics, UCLA Mattel Children's Hospital, David Geffen School of Medicine at UCLA, Los Angeles, CA 90095, USA
4. Division of Maternal-Fetal Medicine, Department of Obstetrics and Gynecology, David Geffen School of Medicine at UCLA, Los Angeles, CA 90095, USA
5. Fetal Diagnostic Centers, Pasadena, CA 91105, USA
* Correspondence: juliamurlewska.jm@gmail.com

Abstract: Long-term monitoring of a fetus with heart failure is an undeniable challenge for prenatal cardiology. Echocardiography is constrained by many fetal and maternal factors, and it is difficult to maintain the reproducibility of the measured and analyzed parameters. In our study, we presented the possibilities of using modern speckle tracking technology in combination with standard echocardiography parameters that may be insufficient or less sensitive in the context of monitoring life-threatening fetal conditions. Our analysis shows the superiority of the parameters used to assess fetal cardiac architecture, such as the GSI Global sphericity Index, and fetal cardiac function, such as the FAC fractional area change and the EF ejection fraction, which temporal change may indicate a worsening condition of the fetus with heart failure. The significant increase in the parameters of fetal heart size in speckle tracking allows for an improved echocardiographic diagnosis and monitoring of the fetus with heart failure and the prognostic conclusions about the clinical condition after birth. Significant decreases in FAC for the left and right ventricles and EF for the left ventricle may indicate an unfavourable prognosis for the monitored fetus due to heart failure.

Keywords: fetal echocardiography; fetal strain; fetal speckle tracking; fetal heart failure

1. Introduction

For longitudinal echocardiographic monitoring during fetal life, there is no consensus on the best approach to evaluate fetal cardiovascular function. Compared to postnatal echocardiographic evaluation, fetal evaluations may be complicated by various fetal positions and orientations, making serial assessment with a single measurement more challenging. Therefore, we compared conventional echocardiographic measurements with speckle-tracking derived assessments [1] (Figure 1) to determine which approach, in a single fetus with progressive heart failure, may be most useful to predict fetal well-being.

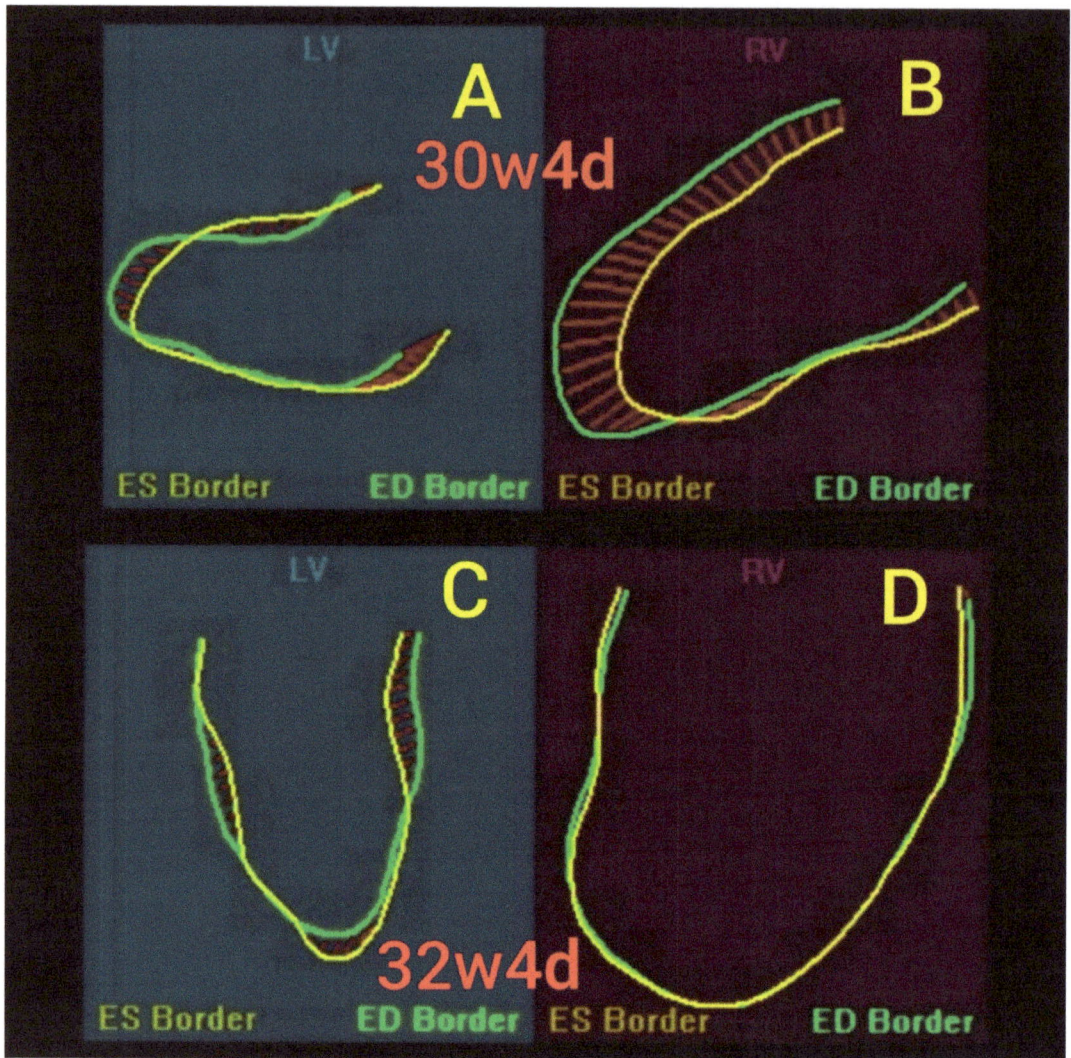

Figure 1. (**A,B**) Fetal strain at 30 weeks 4 days. (**C,D**) Fetal strain at 32 weeks 4 days. End-Systolic/End-Diastolic Borders of LV-left ventricle and RV-right ventricle displacement.

2. Materials and Methods

During the first pregnancy of a 26-year-old woman, the first trimester evaluation demonstrated active herpes labialis and shingles, which were treated with Aciclovir. New onset of ascites, hydrops testis, and ductus venosus reversal flow was seen at 30 weeks of gestation. With the subsequent development of fetal cardiomegaly, cardiac hypertrophy, pericardial effusion, mitral, tricuspid, and pulmonary valve regurgitation, and fetal heart failure, transplacental digoxin treatment was initiated, along with dexamethasone and cefuroxime. The standard echo-sonographic findings are presented in Table 1. Speckle tracking analysis (Table 2, video S1) has been demonstrated to provide both qualitative and quantitative assessments of fetal size, shape, and function, as recently described by DeVore [1–4]. Speckle tracking forms a characteristic pattern of spots and kernels on the irregular surfaces of fetal myocardium to measure longitudinal, radial, and circumferential regional strain [5]. Pregnancy was maintained for over two more weeks, but was then complicated by polyhydramnios, maternal hypertension, and premature rapture of membrane. Due to abnormal fetal tracings, an emergency CS was performed at 32 weeks of gestation. The newborn baby boy had a birth weight of 2500 g, Apgars 5/6/6, and was admitted to the ICU. Following aggressive postnatal medical management, as well as PDA-patent ductus arteriosus ligation at 1 month of age, he was discharged home after 79 days with a diagnosis of congestive herpetic cardiomyopathy.

Table 1. Standard selected echocardiographic parameters analyzed in the present case indicating the progression of fetal heart failure.

GA	30 Weeks 4 Days	32 Weeks 4 Days
Cardiomegaly/HA/CA	0.4	0.4
Tei RV	0.9	0.9
Tei LV	0.7	0.7
RV SF	18%	16%
LV SF	24%	17%
CVPS	5	5

GA: gestational age; HA/CA: heart area/chest area; RV/Tei LV: MPI-myocardial performance index for right and left ventricle; RV/LV SF: shortening fraction for right and left ventricle; CVPS: cardiovascular profile score.

Table 2. Advanced echocardiographic parameters of the fetal heart using speckle tracking technology.

	30 Weeks 4 Days		32 Weeks 4 Days		
	Measurement	Z-Score	Measurement	Z-Score	
Global Sphericity Index (BAL/TL)	1.46	2.38	1.21	−0.22	↓
BAL-Basal–Apical Length (mm)	63.10	8.12	57.00	4.76	↓
TL-Transverse Length (mm)	43.20	5.02	47.00	5.19	↑
Area	1929.00	8.51	2177.00	6.23	↑
Circumference	164.00	7.60	171.00	5.39	↑
Left Ventricular Area (mm^2)	3.22	2.89	3.60	2.91	↑
Right Ventricular Area (mm^2)	4.59	8.28	4.43	6.06	
Right Ventricular Fractional Area Change (%)	5.68	−6.65	−16.22	−10.78	↓
Left Ventricular Fractional Area Change (%)	28.89	−2.97	12.97	−6.29	↓
Left Ventricular Ejection Fraction (%)	41.61	−2.93	24.61	−5.69	↓

3. Results

Our analysis and interpretation of the standard and advanced echocardiographic parameters using speckle tracking technology allowed us to evaluate the efficacy of prenatal treatment with digoxin. Digoxin was administered from week 30 to week 32. Standard size of the HA/CA (heart area/chest area) was constant, and a detailed speckle tracking analysis revealed a significant prolongation of the TL transverse length dimension and a shortening of the BAL-basal–apical length dimension, thereby reducing the GSI-global Sphericity Index GSI = BAL/TL) [2]. We also observed an increase in the following parameters: the area and circumference of the heart and the area for the left and right ventricles. Standard cardiovascular parameters, such as the Tei index or MPI, for the left and right ventricles increased without significant difference over a two-week period (values between 0.7 and 0.9), and the CVPS cardiovascular profile score remained unchanged at level 5. Fetal global cardiac contractility was also analyzed using the parameters FAC-fractional area change (%) and EF-ejection fraction (%) [3,4], which significantly decreased over time (Tables 1 and 2 show the analyzed echocardiographic parameters). The tables contain selected parameters that allow the analysis of fetal heart failure.

4. Discussion

Fetal circulatory failure may have various causes and, therefore, it is very difficult to assess the effectiveness of any treatment [6]. So far, cardiovascular profile score has been considered a very useful diagnostic tool to quantify the severity of heart failure, which is a composite score based on five different echocardiographic parameters [7]. Our long-term analysis presents a modern approach of monitoring a fetus with circulatory failure. We tried to show the superiority of speckle tracking analysis, which is a more detailed method; although it is more involved and time-consuming, it can have a very important place precisely for the studies of fetuses with the most severe cardiovascular and non-cardiovascular conditions that lead to circulatory failure and fetal death. Speckle tracking may indicate some changes in fetal cardiac architectonics not seen by standard echocardiography, and may also have superiority over standard fetal cardiac function exponents, which may be less sensitive than FAC and EF; we have highlighted these findings which seem very promising in the context of monitoring a fetus with circulatory failure. The pattern of speckles within a defined region, known as a kernel, can be conceptualized as an 'acoustic fingerprint'. The spatial movement of multiple kernels can be used to measure longitudinal, radial, and circumferential regional strain. Changes in myocardial strain precede the changes in ejection fraction in patients with cardiomyopathy. STE is less dependent on the angle of insonation than conventional echocardiography, allowing more flexibility in image acquisition than Doppler-based techniques. STE is less susceptible to fetal and maternal movements. The accuracy of STE has been confirmed in postnatal life in animal models [5].

FAC should generally take values $\geq 35\%$ [3], while EF should be $>50\%$ [4]. In our case, these values corresponded to <-2.93 Z-score and significantly decreased over a two-weeks below the mean, the CVPS was constant, and its analysis made it difficult to predict an impending premature birth. M-mode analysis of the myocardial shortening fraction can also be made more accurate using speckle tracking and 24-segment examination [8] Finally, a HA/CA analysis associated with fetal cardiomegaly may not be adequate for serious cases of fetuses with heart failure, in which more demanding and more sensitive parameters to the deterioration of circulatory performance, such as GSI, LV Area, or RV Area, could be used.

5. Conclusions

The speckle tracking analysis performed in our case allows a detailed monitoring of a fetus with heart failure.

Author Contributions: Conceptualization: J.M.; methodology: J.M. and O.S.; software: G.D.; validation,: O.S., M.R.-L. and M.S., formal analysis: J.M. and O.S.; investigation: J.M.; resources: J.M. and M.R.-L.; data curation: J.M.; writing—original draft preparation: J.M.; writing—review and editing: J.M., G.D. and M.S.; visualization: J.M.; supervision: M.S., M.R.-L. and G.D.; project administration: J.M. and G.D.; funding acquisition: none. All authors have read and agreed to the published version of the manuscript.

Funding: This research received no external funding.

Institutional Review Board Statement: Ethical review and approval were waived for this study, due to the retrospective analysis.

Informed Consent Statement: Written informed consent was obtained from the patient to publish this paper.

Data Availability Statement: Not applicable.

Conflicts of Interest: The authors declare no conflict of interest.

References

1. Devore, G.R.; Polanco, B. Two-Dimensional Speckle Tracking of the Fetal Heart. *J. Ultrasound Med.* **2016**, *35*, 1765–1781. [CrossRef] [PubMed]
2. Devore, G.R.; Satou, G. Abnormal Fetal Findings Associated With a Global Sphericity Index of the 4-Chamber View Below the 5th Centile. *J. Ultrasound Med.* **2017**, *36*, 2309–2318. [CrossRef] [PubMed]
3. Devore, G.R.; Klas, B.; Satou, G.; Sklansky, M. Quantitative evaluation of fetal right and left ventricular fractional area change using speckle-tracking technology. *Ultrasound Obstet. Gynecol.* **2019**, *53*, 219–228. [CrossRef] [PubMed]
4. Messing, B.; Cohen, S.M.; Valsky, D.V.; Rosenak, D.; Hochner-Celnikier, D.; Savchev, S.; Yagel, S. Fetal cardiac ventricle volumetry in the second half of gestation assessed by 4D ultrasound using STIC combined with inversion mode. *Ultrasound Obstet. Gynecol.* **2007**, *30*, 142–151. [CrossRef] [PubMed]
5. Day, T.G.; Charakida, M.; Simpson, J.M. Using speckle-tracking echocardiography to assess fetal myocardial deformation: Are we there yet? *Ultrasound Obs. Gynecol.* **2019**, *54*, 575–581. [CrossRef] [PubMed]
6. Strzelecka, I.; Respondek-Liberska, M.; Słodki, M.; Zych-Krekora, K.; Cuneo, B. Transplacental digoxin treatment in prenatal cardiac problems in singleton pregnancies-meta analysis (based on literature: 1992–2015). *Prenat. Cardiol.* **2016**, *6*, 67–74. [CrossRef]
7. Huhta, J.C. Fetal congestive heart failure. *Semin. Fetal Neonatal Med.* **2005**, *10*, 542–552. [CrossRef]
8. Devore, G.R.; Klas, B. Twenty-four Segment Transverse Ventricular Fractional Shortening: A New Technique to Evaluate Fetal Cardiac Function. *J. Ultrasound Med.* **2018**, *37*, 1129–1141. [CrossRef]

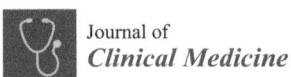

Article

ABO Incompatibility between the Mother and Fetus Does Not Protect against Anti-Human Platelet Antigen-1a Immunization by Pregnancy

Laila Miserre [1,†], Sandra Wienzek-Lischka [1,2,†], Andreas Mann [1], Nina Cooper [1,2], Sentot Santoso [1], Harald Ehrhardt [3], Ulrich J. Sachs [1,2,4] and Gregor Bein [1,2,*]

1. Institute for Clinical Immunology, Transfusion Medicine and Hemostasis, Justus-Liebig-University, Langhansstr. 7, 35392 Giessen, Germany
2. German Centre for Feto-Maternal Incompatibility, University Hospital Giessen and Marburg, Campus Giessen, Langhansstr. 7, 35392 Giessen, Germany
3. Department of General Pediatrics and Neonatology, Justus-Liebig-University, Feulgenstr. 10-12, 35392 Giessen, Germany
4. Department of Thrombosis and Haemostasis, University Hospital Giessen and Marburg, Campus Giessen, Langhansstr. 2, 35392 Giessen, Germany
* Correspondence: gregor.bein@immunologie.med.uni-giessen.de
† These authors contributed equally to this work.

Abstract: (1) Background: ABO blood group incompatibility between the mother and fetus protects against anti-D immunization by pregnancy. The possible role of ABO incompatibility in protecting against anti-human platelet antigen-1a immunization is unclear. (2) Methods: This study retrospectively screened 817 families (mother-father-neonate trios) of suspected fetal and neonatal alloimmune thrombocytopenia for inclusion. ABO genotypes were determined in 118 mother-child pairs with confirmed alloimmune thrombocytopenia due to anti-HPA-1a antibodies, and 522 mother-child pairs served as the control group. The expression of blood group antigen A on platelets was determined in 199 consecutive newborns by flow cytometry and compared with adult controls. (3) Results: ABO incompatibility between mother and fetus did not protect against anti-human platelet antigen-1a immunization by pregnancy. ABO blood groups of mothers and/or fetuses were not associated with the severity of fetal and neonatal alloimmune thrombocytopenia. The expression pattern of blood group A antigens on the platelets of newborns mirrored that of adults, albeit on a lower level. Blood group A antigen was detected on a subpopulation of neonatal platelets, and some newborns revealed high platelet expression of A determinants on all platelets (type II high-expressers). (4) Conclusion: The lack of a protective effect of ABO incompatibility between mother and fetus against anti-human platelet antigen-1a immunization by pregnancy may indicate that fetal platelets are not the cellular source by which the mother is immunized.

Keywords: fetal and neonatal alloimmune thrombocytopenia; ABO blood group; anti-human platelet antigen-1a

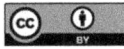

1. Introduction

Fetal and neonatal alloimmune thrombocytopenia (FNAIT) is caused by maternal antibodies against fetal platelet antigens inherited from the father. Placental transport of immunoglobulin G class antibodies from the maternal to the fetal circulation may lead to opsonization of fetal platelets resulting in thrombocytopenia and bleeding complications (for review see [1]). In Caucasian populations, most cases of severe FNAIT are caused by antibodies directed at human platelet antigen (HPA)-1a [2]. The incidence of FNAIT is 1 in 1000 pregnancies and the incidence of its most severe complication, intracranial hemorrhage (ICH) leading to intrauterine death or long-term neurologic sequelae, occurs in 1 of 10,000 pregnancies [3].

The etiology of FNAIT equals those of hemolytic disease of the fetus and newborn (HDFN), where maternal antibodies against fetal blood group antigens may lead to fetal red blood cell opsonization resulting in fetal anemia, in severe cases, hydrops, and fetal demise. HDFN is most frequently caused by maternal anti-D antibodies. An RhD-negative mother is immunized by fetal transplacental hemorrhage of D-positive red blood cells during pregnancy and a larger volume at delivery (for review see [4]). Levine was the first to observe that in matings of RhD-negative mothers with HDFN, the incidence of incompatible ABO blood group matings was lower than expected [5]. The protective action of ABO incompatibility on anti-D immunization was confirmed in subsequent studies [6]. Recently, Zwiers et al. corroborated that ABO incompatibility protects against non-D red blood cell alloimmunization by pregnancy [7].

A small study of 25 FNAIT cases suggested that ABO incompatibility between the mother and fetus protects similarly against HPA-1a immunization by pregnancy [8]. In all 25 FNAIT cases, the mother and child were ABO compatible. The authors of this study concluded that fetal platelets must express ABO antigens, and fetal platelets may be cleared from the maternal circulation in cases of ABO-incompatible pregnancies before immunization of the mother occurs. Two studies investigated the possible association of the maternal ABO blood group with FNAIT severity [9,10]. Both studies reported a similar maternal ABO blood group distribution in FNAIT cases and controls. However, the possible protective role of ABO incompatibility between the mother and fetus on the incidence of anti-HPA-1a immunization by pregnancy was not investigated in either study. Ahlen et al. observed an association of severe FNAIT (neonatal platelet count $<50 \times 10^9/\text{L}$) with maternal blood group A [10].

Given these conflicting findings, we investigated (1) whether ABO incompatibility between the mother and fetus protects against anti-HPA-1a immunization by pregnancy and (2) whether ABO blood groups of the mother and/or the fetus are associated with FNAIT severity in a cohort of 817 families of suspected FNAIT. Furthermore, we investigated the expression of the blood group A antigen on platelets of 199 consecutive newborns. This is the first systematic study on blood group A antigen expression on platelets in neonates.

2. Materials and Methods

2.1. Patients and Case Definitions

This study retrospectively screened 817 families (mother-father-neonate trios) of suspected FNAIT, referred to our Centre for Feto-maternal Incompatibility between January 2000 and April 2016 for inclusion (Figure 1). Confirmed FNAIT cases were HPA-1bb mothers who had serological detection of anti-HPA-1a antibodies and were delivered by an HPA-1ab neonate. FNAIT cases with antibodies other than anti-HPA-1a (e.g., anti-HPA-5b) were excluded from the study group because of differences in clinical FNAIT presentation, such as higher neonatal platelet counts in FNAIT cases due to anti-HPA-5b compared with FNAIT cases due to anti-HPA-1a [2]. Mothers with additional anti-HPA-antibodies (mainly anti-HPA-5b) besides anti-HPA-1a were also excluded. Controls included mothers without detection of anti-HPA antibodies. Furthermore, possible FNAIT cases of HPA-1bb mothers without detectable HPA-1a antibodies at the time of post-partum blood sampling were excluded from controls. Finally, restricted by lack of material, we included 118 mother-child pairs with FNAIT due to anti-HPA-1a antibodies. Additionally, 522 mother-child pairs of suspected FNAIT where FNAIT was excluded served as the control group. Clinical data were retrieved from the in-house laboratory information system and medical records, including the referring physician's letter.

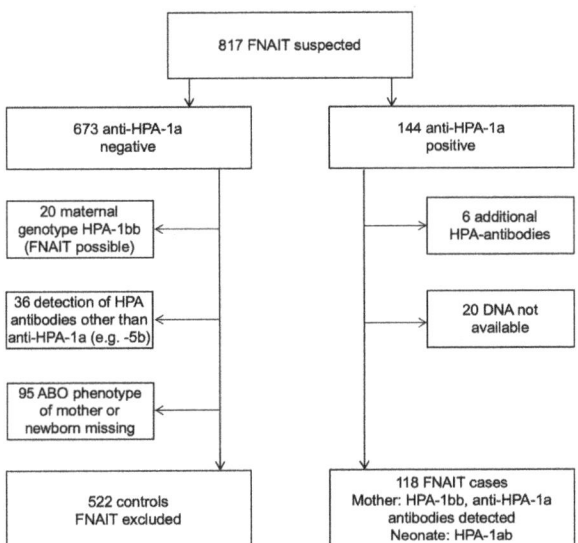

Figure 1. Screening of 817 families of suspected FNAIT. Definition of controls and cases.

2.2. Work-Up of FNAIT Families

Platelet counts were determined in ethylenediaminetetraacetic acid (EDTA)-anticoagulated whole blood using a hematology analyzer (KX-21N, Sysmex Corporation, Kobe, Japan). Platelet counts <10 × 10^9/L were controlled microscopically in a counting chamber. ABO blood groups of all suspected cases were determined following routine standards for adult and neonatal pretransfusion testing. The diagnosis of HPA genotypes and detection of anti-HPA antibodies are described elsewhere [11].

2.3. ABO Genotyping in FNAIT Cases (Mother and Newborn)

ABO*A1 and *ABO*A2* alleles and hetero- and homozygosity of major *ABO* alleles were discriminated by performing genotyping with in-house TaqMan real-time PCR assays (TaqMan; applied biosystems/ThermoFisher Scientific, Waltham, MA, USA), to detect the major *ABO* alleles *ABO*A1.01*, *ABO*A2.01*, *ABO*B.01*, *ABO*O.01*, and *ABO*O.02* according to the International Society of Blood Transfusion blood group allele database (*ABO* blood group alleles v1.1 171023; Supplementary Table S1). Inconclusive genotyping results were resolved using PCR with sequence-specific primers (PCR-SSP; inno-train, Kronberg, Germany).

2.4. Flow Cytometric Measurement of A Antigens on Adult and Neonatal Platelets

The following procedure was used for flow cytometric measurement of A antigens on adult and neonatal platelets. First, 5 mL of EDTA anticoagulated cord blood samples (newborns) or blood samples (adults) was added to 6 mL 0.5 g% EDTA/NaCl buffer and centrifuged for 16 min. at 250× *g* (w/o brake). Next, 3 mL of platelet-rich plasma was harvested and mixed with 4 mL NaCl (pH 6.5), followed by 2 washing steps (1200× *g*, 10 min). The final pellet was carefully resuspended in 1 mL phosphate-buffered-saline (PBS)-EDTA (supplemented with prostaglandin E1), and the concentration of platelets was measured (hematology analyzer KX-21N, Sysmex Corporation, Kobe, Japan) and adjusted to 5 × 10^7/mL. Then, 10 μL of this suspension was added to 30 μL PBS and stained with anti-CD41a (final concentration 0.25 μg/mL) and anti-A or isotype control antibody, respectively (final concentration 1 μg/mL), in a final volume of 50 μL for 30 min. at room temperature. Without further centrifugation, staining was adjourned by adding 700 μL PBS, and flow cytometric analysis was conducted within 2 h. Stained platelets were analyzed by flow cytometry (FACS Canto II, BD Biosciences, Franklin Lakes, NJ,

USA; FACSDiva software version 8.01). Finally, 30,000 events were counted, and platelets were gated by forward/side scatter and staining for CD41a. The distribution of the anti-A signal (median fluorescence intensity) on CD41a positive cells was statistically evaluated. A cut-off for positive anti-A staining was defined by a window that included $\leq$1% positive events within the specimen stained in parallel with irrelevant isotype control antibody. We did not investigate the expression of B antigen since the phenotype of blood group B is only 12% in this population (Table 1). Furthermore, the expression pattern of A and B antigens on adult platelets is similar [12]. Newborns with known HDFN were excluded. All adult and newborn cohort samples were analyzed prospectively on alternating days within 4 months.

Table 1. The ABO phenotype distribution between FNAIT cases (mothers or neonates) and controls did not differ (Chi-square test, $p > 0.05$).

ABO Phenotype	Cases (Mothers) ($n = 118$)	Cases (Neonates) ($n = 118$)	First Time Blood Donors ($n = 45,295$)
0	35%	39%	41%
A	47%	44%	42%
B	13%	10%	12%
AB	5%	7%	5%

2.5. Antibodies

The antibodies used in this study were mouse anti-A: IgG1, kappa, phycoerythrin-conjugated; Clone: BRIC 145; International Blood Group Reference Laboratory, Bristol, UK. Mouse isotype control: IgG1, kappa, phycoerythrin-conjugated; Clone MOPC-21; BioLegend, San Diego, CA, USA. Mouse anti-human CD41a: IgG1, kappa, APC conjugated; Clone HIP8; ThermoFisher Scientific, Waltham, MA, USA.

2.6. Statistical Analysis

Data were managed using Excel (Microsoft Office 365; Microsoft Corporation, Redmond, WA, USA) and analyzed using IBM SPSS Statistics Version 25 for Windows (IBM, Armonk, NY, USA). The graphical illustration was performed with the Prism 8 software package (GraphPad Software, Inc., San Diego, CA, USA). Groups' characteristics are presented as medians and interquartile ranges (IQRs).

ABO phenotype frequencies were compared between FNAIT cases and 45,295 first-time blood donors using a Chi-square test. Proportions of ABO-compatible pregnancies were compared between 118 FNAIT cases and 522 controls. The effect of ABO phenotypes on the occurrence of ICH, magnitude of thrombocytopenia, and birth weight was assessed using a two-sided Fisher's exact test and Pearson Chi-square test, Kruskal–Wallis test, and Welch-ANOVA, respectively. Effects of hetero-or homozygosity for alleles $ABO*A1.01$, $ABO*O.01/O.02$, and fetomaternal ABO compatibility on the occurrence of ICH, the magnitude of thrombocytopenia, and birth weight were evaluated using the two-sided Fisher's exact test, Mann–Whitney test, and t-test, respectively. A p value < 0.05 was considered significant. Missing values are depicted in each figure, if applicable.

3. Results

3.1. ABO Phenotype Frequencies Do Not Differ between FNAIT Cases and Controls

ABO phenotype frequencies of cases (mothers and neonates) were compared with the ABO phenotype frequencies among 45,295 first-time blood donors to test the hypothesis that the maternal propensity for alloimmunization against HPA-1a is associated with blood groups (Table 1). The differences were not statistically significant.

3.2. ABO Incompatibility between the Mother and Fetus Does Not Protect against Anti-HPA-1a Immunization by Pregnancy

The proportion of ABO-incompatible pregnancies did not differ between cases and controls (Figure 2). Thus, we did not confirm the hypothesis that ABO incompatibility protects against anti-HPA-1a immunization by pregnancy. In this case, the proportion of incompatible pregnancies would be lower in FNAIT cases.

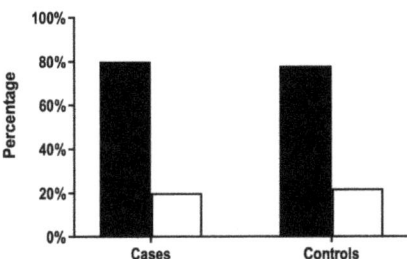

Figure 2. Distribution of ABO-compatible (black bars) and ABO-incompatible (white bars) pregnancies among cases (n = 118) and controls (n = 522) (Chi-square test, p > 0.05).

3.3. Maternal ABO Phenotypes Are Not Associated with FNAIT Severity

We tested the hypothesis that maternal blood groups may affect the neonatal outcome in cases of FNAIT. The comparison of maternal ABO phenotypes and the occurrence of neonatal ICH revealed no significant associations (Figure 3a). There were no significant associations between the neonatal platelet count (Figure 3b), neonatal birth weight (Figure 3c), and the maternal ABO phenotype. The cases with maternal blood group AB were excluded due to the low number of individuals.

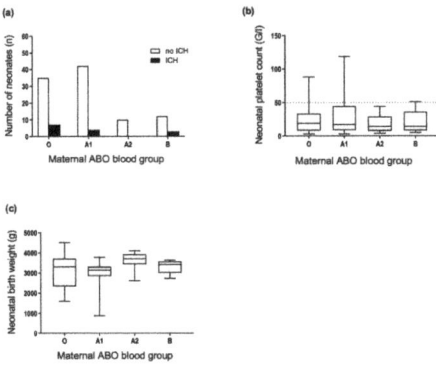

Figure 3. Distribution of maternal ABO phenotypes and the occurrence of (**a**) ICH, (**b**) platelet count nadir, and (**c**) birth weight in neonates of anti-HPA-1a immunized mothers. Dotted line in (**b**) threshold of severe thrombocytopenia, platelet count <50 × 10^9/L. (**a**) n = 113, two-sided Fisher's exact test, p = 0.35; (**b**) n = 110, Kruskal–Wallis test, p = 0.85; (**c**) n = 64, Welch-ANOVA test, p = 0.066.

3.4. Maternal Gene Dose of the ABO*A1.01 Allele Is Not Associated with FNAIT Severity

According to a study by Ahlen et al. [10], the gene dose of the *ABO*A1.01* allele was associated with FNAIT severity. Among blood group A mothers, the frequency of newborns with severe FNAIT (neonatal platelet count <50 × 10^9/L) was lower in pregnancies where the mother carried only one *ABO*A1.01* allele and higher where mothers carried two *ABO*A1.01* alleles. Mothers were stratified according to zygosity for A and O alleles (*ABO*A1.01* and *ABO*O.01* alleles) to analyze the possible association between maternal ABO genotype and neonatal outcomes. For alleles *ABO*A2.01*, *ABO*O.02* and *ABO*B.01*, the number of homozygous mothers was too small for valid statistics. There was no significant difference in the incidence of ICH in neonates suffering from FNAIT born to mothers that were hetero- or homozygous for *ABO*A1.01* (Figure 4a) or *ABO*O.01* (data not shown). Similarly, we observed no significant difference in the platelet count nadir (Figure 4b) in neonates suffering from FNAIT born to mothers that were hetero- or homozygous for *ABO*A1.01* or *ABO*O.01* (data not shown).

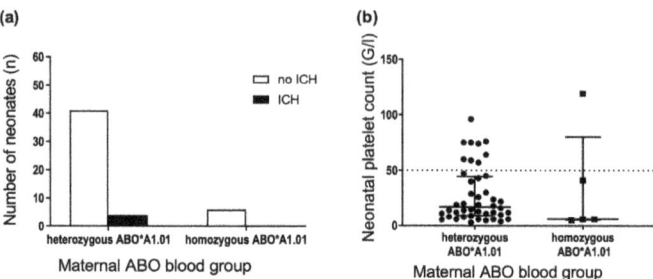

Figure 4. Comparison of maternal *ABO*A1.01* hetero- or homozygosity and the occurrence of (**a**) ICH and (**b**) platelet count nadir in neonates of anti-HPA-1a immunised mothers. Dotted line in (**b**) threshold of severe thrombocytopenia, platelet count $<50 \times 10^9$/L. (**a**) $n = 51$, two-sided Fisher's exact test, $p = 1.000$; (**b**) Mann–Whitney test, $p = 0.536$, median and interquartile range displayed.

3.5. Neonatal ABO Phenotypes Are Not Associated with FNAIT Severity

We analyzed the possible association between neonatal ABO phenotype and neonatal outcomes. Results showed a significant difference in the incidence of ICH in newborns stratified according to ABO phenotype. Further tests revealed that ICH occurred significantly more often in neonates with phenotype O than phenotype A (Chi-square test, $p = 0.035$) (Figure 5a). Ten of 47 neonates with blood group O suffered from ICH, compared with 2 of 51 neonates with blood group A. To replicate this association, we evaluated an independent cohort of suspected FNAIT cases with the following inclusion criteria: period 1991–1999; ICH of the fetus or newborn; mother HPA-1bb; maternal anti-HPA-1a antibody detected (no other HPA antibodies); newborn HPA-1ab; ABO blood group determined. 4 of 10 (40%) newborns were blood group O. Thus, the association of blood group O with ICH in the initial cohort could be due to a type 1 error. There were no significant differences in the platelet count nadir and birth weight (Figure 5b,c) between newborns grouped according to ABO phenotype.

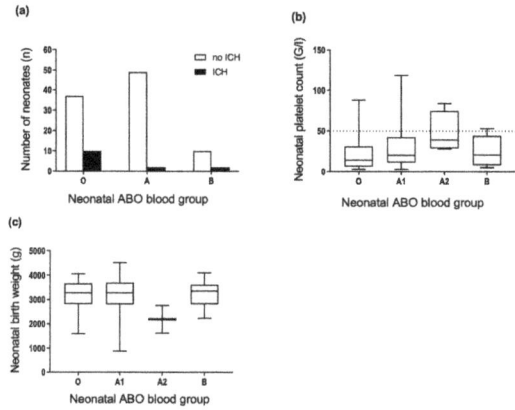

Figure 5. Comparison of neonatal ABO phenotypes and the occurrence of (**a**) ICH, (**b**) platelet count nadir, and (**c**) birth weight. Dotted line in (**b**) threshold of severe thrombocytopenia, platelet

count <50 × 10^9/L. (**a**) n = 110, Chi-square test, p = 0.035; (**b**) n = 107, Kruskal–Wallis test (4) p = 0.067, median and interquartile range displayed; (**c**) n = 64, Welch-ANOVA, p = 0.55, median and interquartile range displayed.

3.6. ABO Incompatibility between the Mother and Fetus Is Not Associated with FNAIT Severity

ABO incompatibility between the mother and fetus was not associated with the occurrence of ICH (Figure 6a) and neonatal platelet count (Figure 6b). The possible association of ABO incompatibility with birth weight was not analyzed because of the small sample size. This analysis was repeated with a stricter definition of ABO incompatibility: mother, predicted blood group O, and neonate, predicted blood group A_1. Employing this strict definition of ABO incompatibility, no association between ABO incompatibility and the occurrence of ICH or neonatal platelet count was found (data not shown).

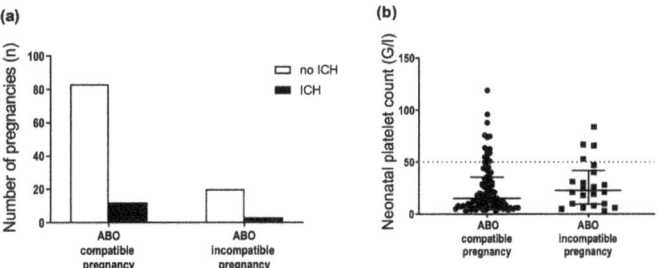

Figure 6. Comparison of fetomaternal ABO compatible and incompatible pregnancies and occurrence of (**a**) ICH, and (**b**) platelet count nadir in neonates. Dotted line in (**b**) threshold of severe thrombocytopenia, platelet count <50 × 10^9/L. (**a**) n = 118, two-sided Fisher's exact test, p = 1.00; (**b**) n = 115, Mann–Whitney test, p = 0.40, median and interquartile range displayed.

3.7. Blood Group A Antigens Are Weakly Expressed on Newborn Platelets but Strongly Expressed on Platelets of Some Newborns

First, we replicated the findings of Curtis et al. [12] and others regarding A antigen expression on adult platelets (Figure 7). The binding of the monoclonal anti-A antibody BRIC 145 on adult blood group A_2 platelets could not be distinguished from binding on adult blood group O platelets. An analysis of anti-A-stained platelets of adult blood group A_1 donors by flow cytometry demonstrated broad histograms that overlapped the histograms of blood group O and blood group A_2 platelets. According to the definition of Ogasawara et al. [13] 7 of 169 (4.14%) donors were categorized as high-expresser phenotypes (mean of median fluorescence intensities +2 SD). Platelets from one of these 7 donors demonstrated a sharp histogram peak with high A antigen expression on all platelets (type II high-expresser phenotype).

The expression level of blood group A antigens on neonatal platelets was significantly lower compared with adult platelets of blood group A_1 (Figure 7). The median fluorescence intensity (MFI) of adult blood group A_1 platelets was 486.0 (95% CI of median 417.0–569.0, n = 169) compared with 94.0 (95% CI of median 84.0–112.0, n = 199) of neonatal blood group A platelets (p < 0.0001, Mann–Whitney test). All but three newborns demonstrated an MFI of anti-A staining below the median MFI of anti-A staining of adult platelets. The histograms of neonatal blood group A platelets broadly overlapped the histograms of neonatal group O platelets. Three newborns were categorized as high-expressers (mean of median fluorescence intensities +2 SD); two demonstrated a sharp histogram peak with high A expression on all platelets (type II high-expresser phenotype). ABO expressor traits influence quantitative ABO(H) expression on platelets, red blood cells and soluble plasma proteins [14]. Due to the blinded design of our study, information about platelet count or signs of hemolysis in the newborns with high-expresser phenotype was not available.

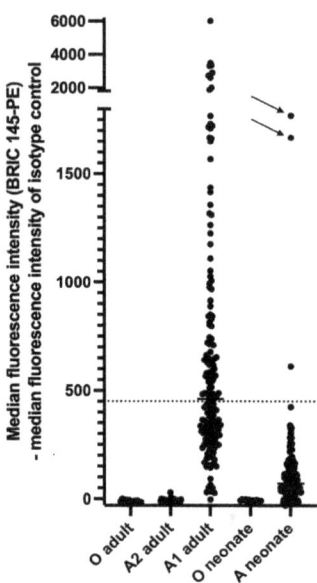

Figure 7. Flow cytometric analysis of blood group A antigen expression by binding of phycoerythrin (PE)-conjugated moAb BRIC 145 on adult blood group O platelets ($n = 13$), adult blood group A_2 platelets ($n = 31$), adult blood group A_1 platelets ($n = 181$), neonatal blood group O platelets ($n = 13$), and neonatal blood group A platelets ($n = 199$). Y-axis: median fluorescence intensity (MFI) (BRIC 145-PE)–MFI of isotype control. The dotted line represents the mean fluorescence intensity of neonatal blood group A platelets + 2 SD. Arrows: neonatal type II high-expressers.

We compared the proportion of adult and neonatal platelets that exhibited anti-A antibody binding above the pre-defined cut-off (see material and methods). Of these, 40.9% (median, 95% CI of median 37.1–44.0; $n = 169$) of adult blood group A_1 platelets and 15.5% (median, 95% CI of median 13.2–16.5; $n = 199$) of neonatal blood group A platelets were blood group A antigen-positive. The proportion of adult platelets exhibiting anti-A antibody binding did not differ between blood group O and A_2 platelets.

4. Discussion

In a large cohort of well-characterized FNAIT cases, we did not confirm the initial observation by Gratwohl and Shulman [8] that ABO incompatibility between the mother and fetus protects against anti-HPA-1a immunization by pregnancy. Furthermore, ABO blood groups of mothers and/or fetuses were not associated with FNAIT severity. The propensity for the mother to develop anti-HPA-1a antibodies is closely linked to the expression of HLA-DRB3*01:01. Since almost all mothers in this cohort were HLA-DRB3*01:01 positive [15], we did not stratify the groups of this study according to the presence or absence of HLA-DRB3*01:01.

Adult platelets express A and B blood group antigens [16], which are synthesized within the platelet or platelet precursor and are passively absorbed to a minor extent [17,18]. Blood group A and B determinants are expressed on platelet glycoproteins (GP) IIa, IIIa, Ib [19], IIb [20], IV, V, [21], CD109, PECAM [22] and various glycolipids [23,24]. Platelets of adult blood group A_2 individuals demonstrate minimal expression of A determinants [25], and adults of blood group A_1 display a broad spectrum from low to high platelet A antigen expression. Strong expression of A and B antigens on platelets of some individuals was first described by Ogasawara et al. [13] and confirmed by others [12,26–28]. The expression of A determinants is associated with the gene dose and genetic variants [14,29,30]. Representative fluorescence histograms of adult and neonatal platelets are shown in supplemental Figure S1.

In this study, we systematically investigated the expression of blood group A antigens on platelets of newborns. We demonstrated that the expression pattern mirrors that of adults, albeit on a lower level. In most newborns of blood group A, binding of monoclonal anti-A was detected on a subpopulation of platelets. Some newborns revealed high platelet expression of A determinants on all platelets (type II high-expressers). This phenotype was associated with neonatal thrombocytopenia in on case report [31]. We conclude that maternal anti-A (and/or anti-B) antibodies should also bind in vivo to a subset of antigen-positive fetal platelets in cases of fetal transplacental hemorrhage.

In HDFN, ABO incompatibility between the mother and fetus protects against primary D and non-D red blood cell alloimmunization by pregnancy (for review see [7]). D sensitization in RhD-negative women results from the passage of D-positive fetal red blood cells across the placenta into maternal circulation (for review see [32]). Chown was the first to demonstrate fetomaternal (macro) transfusion in an RhD-negative woman who had given birth to a baby with severe normoblastic anemia by detecting D-positive red blood cells in her circulation. She developed anti-D within three weeks of delivery [33]. Later, it was shown that transplacental (micro) hemorrhage is a regular phenomenon in pregnancy. In one study, the incidence of fetal transplacental hemorrhage was 3% in the first trimester, 12.1% in the second trimester, 45.5% in the third trimester, and 63.6% after delivery [34]. In this study, the amount of fetal transplacental hemorrhage ranged from 0.01 mL to 0.06 mL of fetal red blood cells already in the first and second trimesters, and the amount increased during the third trimester. In post-delivery samples, approximately 50% of women demonstrated ≥ 0.15 mL of circulating fetal red blood cells [34]. However, anti-D is rarely found in blood samples taken after delivery in RhD-negative primiparae giving birth to ABO-compatible RhD-positive babies [35]. The incidence of anti-D six months after delivery of an ABO-compatible RhD-positive baby is estimated to be 8.5%, and there is a direct relation between the amount of fetal red blood cells in the maternal circulation after delivery and the risk of immunization. A further 8.5% of mothers develop anti-D by the end of the second pregnancy, and it is postulated that these mothers had been primed by the first pregnancy (The incidence of anti-D six months after delivery of an ABO-incompatible RhD-positive baby in this study was 1%) [35]. Thus, the first pregnancy is usually not affected by HDFN, and immunization of pregnant women by fetal D-positive red blood cells occurs late in pregnancy and at delivery.

The protective effect of ABO incompatibility between the mother and child on anti-D immunization by pregnancy prompted Finn to suggest that it might be possible to destroy fetal red blood cells in the maternal circulation using a suitable antibody. This would prevent immunization mimicking the natural protection afforded by ABO incompatibility [5]. This suggestion led to the development of one of the most successful immunoprophylaxis therapies today, anti-D immunoglobulin: immunization of RhD-negative mothers was suppressed when gamma-globulin containing a high titer of incomplete anti-D was injected i.m. soon after delivery [36]. Today, anti-D immunoglobulin is the standard of care to prevent D immunization in pregnant women at risk.

The natural history of maternal immunization against D and HPA-1a exhibits two striking differences: (a) ABO incompatibility between the mother and fetus protects against immunization to red blood cell antigens (D and non-D antigens) but not against HPA-1a immunization by pregnancy (this study). (b) Primigravidae are immunized during pregnancy or at delivery against D without any consequences for the firstborn baby in most cases. Usually, clinically overt HDFN occurs only in a subsequent pregnancy (see above). In contrast, clinically overt FNAIT due to maternal anti-HPA-1a antibodies occurs regularly in primigravidae [37,38] and the fetuses of primigravidae can be severely affected by ICH. In a case series of 21 FNAIT cases with ICH, 71% ($n = 15$) occurred during the first-affected pregnancies as early as 18 weeks gestational age [38].

In the case of fetal transplacental hemorrhage, whole fetal blood, including platelets and leukocytes, is transferred to the maternal circulation [39]. Why does ABO incompatibility not protect against maternal anti-HPA-1a immunization? The expression of A and B blood group antigens on fetal platelets may be too low compared with the expression on red blood cells. However, A antigen expression on red blood cells of newborns is also weak compared with adult cells [40]. In one study, only 26% (median, $n = 13$) of newborn red blood cells of blood group A were agglutinated by Dolichos biflorus lectin compared with 94% (median) of adult A_1 red blood cells [41]. Thus, the expression pattern of blood group A antigens on platelets and red blood cells of newborns is similar: the expression is weak compared with adult cells and absent or nearly absent on subpopulations.

To our knowledge, the mechanism of action of the protective effect of ABO incompatibility against anti-D immunization by pregnancy is unknown. Fetal red blood cells are also detectable at delivery in ABO-incompatible pregnancies, albeit at a lower incidence than in compatible pregnancies (in one series in 19% versus 50% of post-partum samples [42]). This result may be due to the absence of A and/or B antigens on a subpopulation of fetal red blood cells [41], which survive in the maternal circulation despite the presence of anti-A and/or anti-B antibodies. This finding makes it unlikely that all incompatible fetal red blood cells are destroyed by maternal IgM and/or IgG anti-A and/or anti-B antibodies, preventing their recognition by the immune system. In consequence, in ABO incompatibility, antibody-mediated immune suppression (AMIS; for review see [43]), mediated by maternal anti-A and/or anti-B IgG antibodies, may be causative of the protective effect. In animal models of AMIS, immunosuppressive IgG does not necessarily mask all epitopes, and red blood cell clearance does not mediate the immunosuppressive effect [43]. Furthermore, several animal models have shown that injection of presensitized (IgG coated) platelets could prevent alloimmunization (for review see [44]). If fetal platelets are the cellular source of HPA-1a antigens immunizing the mother via fetal transplacental hemorrhage,-like red blood cells in HDFN -, we would expect sensitization by maternal A and/or B antibodies and a protective effect of ABO incompatibility since at least a subpopulation of neonatal platelets expresses blood group A antigens. However, the research on the mechanism of action of AMIS in murine models came to different conclusions, and murine models of AMIS cannot be inevitably extrapolated to humans.

An alternative hypothesis is that the cellular source immunizing the pregnant mother against HPA-1a antigens are fetal cells that do not express A and/or B antigens, e.g., leukocytes or trophoblast cells. The entry of fetal trophoblast cells, lymphocytes, hematopoietic stem cells, and other fetal cells into the maternal circulation is a physiological phenomenon that occurs as early as 4–6 weeks in pregnancy (for review see [45]). Trophoblast cells express β3 integrin [46], carrying the HPA-1a/1b polymorphism, and lack A and B blood group antigen expression [47,48]. The early confrontation of primigravidae with an alloantigen on trophoblast cells or trophoblast cell debris may cause immunization against HPA-1a and FNAIT during the first pregnancy. The lack of A and B blood group antigens on trophoblast cells may explain the absence of protection against HPA-1a immunization by ABO incompatibility between the mother and fetus. The striking differences in the natural history of maternal immunization against D and HPA-1a should be considered in the development of anti-HPA-1a immunoprophylaxis in pregnant women at risk [49].

Supplementary Materials: The following supporting information can be downloaded at: https://www.mdpi.com/article/10.3390/jcm11226811/s1, Table S1: Analysis of *ABO* genotyping TaqMan probes for redundancy. Figure S1: Fluorescence histograms of adult and neonatal platelets.

Author Contributions: S.W.-L., U.J.S. and G.B. designed the study. L.M., S.W.-L. and N.C. retrieved data from the in-house laboratory information system and performed retrospective analysis of clinical data. L.M. and S.W.-L. performed and interpreted ABO genotyping. A.M. designed and performed the analysis of A antigen expression on neonatal platelets by flow cytometry. L.M., S.W.-L. and G.B. contributed to the first draft of the manuscript. S.S., H.E. and U.J.S. interpreted the data and critically revised the manuscript. G.B. assumed the final responsibility to submit the manuscript for publication. All authors had full access to all data, carefully reviewed the manuscript and approved the final version. All authors have read and agreed to the published version of the manuscript.

Funding: This research received no external funding.

Institutional Review Board Statement: The study was conducted in accordance with the Declaration of Helsinki and approved by the Ethics Committee of the Medical Faculty, Justus-Liebig University, Giessen, Germany (file no. 82/09 and file no. 18/20).

Informed Consent Statement: Patient consent was waived due to deidentified analysis of retrospective data or deidentified analysis of blood samples.

Data Availability Statement: Requests for the deidentified data used in this study can be sent to the corresponding author, ending 24 months after publication of this article. The study protocol will be made available upon reasonable request to the corresponding author.

Acknowledgments: We are indebted to Carlheinz Mueller, University of Ulm, Germany, who analyzed the set of *ABO* genotyping TaqMan probes for redundancy employing the MinProb algorithm.

Conflicts of Interest: U.J.S. is principal investigator, and S.W.L. and G.B. are sub-investigators in a study to evaluate the safety, efficacy, pharmacokinetics and pharmacodynamics of Nipocalimab administered to pregnant women at high risk for early onset severe hemolytic disease of the fetus and newborn, sponsored by Janssen Pharmaceuticals. G.B. reports consultancy fees from Janssen Pharmaceuticals for participating on the advisory board on FNAIT.

References

1. De Vos, T.W.; Winkelhorst, D.; de Haas, M.; Lopriore, E.; Oepkes, D. Epidemiology and management of fetal and neonatal alloimmune thrombocytopenia. *Transfus. Apher. Sci.* **2020**, *59*, 102704. [CrossRef] [PubMed]
2. Alm, J.; Duong, Y.; Wienzek-Lischka, S.; Cooper, N.; Santoso, S.; Sachs, U.J.; Kiefel, V.; Bein, G. Anti-human platelet antigen-5b antibodies and fetal and neonatal alloimmune thrombocytopenia; incidental association or cause and effect? *Br. J. Haematol.* **2022**, *198*, 14–23. [CrossRef]
3. Kamphuis, M.M.; Paridaans, N.P.; Porcelijn, L.; Lopriore, E.; Oepkes, D. Incidence and consequences of neonatal alloimmune thrombocytopenia: A systematic review. *Pediatrics* **2014**, *133*, 715–721. [CrossRef]
4. Urbaniak, S.J.; Greiss, M.A. RhD haemolytic disease of the fetus and the newborn. *Blood Rev.* **2000**, *14*, 44–61. [CrossRef] [PubMed]
5. Liverpool medical institution. *Lancet* **1960**, *275*, 526–527. [CrossRef]
6. Levine, P. The protective action of ABO Incompatibility on Rh isoimmunization and Rh hemolytic disease-theoretical and clinical implications. *Am. J. Hum. Genet.* **1959**, *11*, 418.
7. Zwiers, C.; Koelewijn, J.M.; Vermij, L.; van Sambeeck, J.; Oepkes, D.; de Haas, M.; van der Schoot, C.E. ABO incompatibility and RhIG immunoprophylaxis protect against non-D alloimmunization by pregnancy. *Transfusion* **2018**, *58*, 1611–1617. [CrossRef]
8. Gratwohl, A.A.; Shulman, N.R. ABO-Kompatibilität und isoimmune neonatale Thrombopenie. *Schweiz. Med. Wochenschr.* **1977**, *107*, 1464.
9. Bertrand, G.; Drame, M.; Martageix, C.; Kaplan, C. Prediction of the fetal status in noninvasive management of alloimmune thrombocytopenia. *Blood* **2011**, *117*, 3209–3213. [CrossRef]
10. Ahlen, M.T.; Husebekk, A.; Killie, M.K.; Kjeldsen-Kragh, J.; Olsson, M.L.; Skogen, B. The development of severe neonatal alloimmune thrombocytopenia due to anti-HPA-1a antibodies is correlated to maternal ABO genotypes. *Clin. Dev. Immunol.* **2012**, *2012*, 156867. [CrossRef]
11. Sachs, U.J.; Wienzek-Lischka, S.; Duong, Y.; Qiu, D.; Hinrichs, W.; Cooper, N.; Santoso, S.; Bayat, B.; Bein, G. Maternal antibodies against paternal class I human leukocyte antigens are not associated with foetal and neonatal alloimmune thrombocytopenia. *Br. J. Haematol.* **2020**, *189*, 751–759. [CrossRef] [PubMed]
12. Curtis, B.R.; Edwards, J.T.; Hessner, M.J.; Klein, J.P.; Aster, R.H. Blood group A and B antigens are strongly expressed on platelets of some individuals. *Blood* **2000**, *96*, 1574–1581. [CrossRef] [PubMed]
13. Ogasawara, K.; Ueki, J.; Takenaka, M.; Furihata, K. Study on the expression of ABH antigens on platelets. *Blood* **1993**, *82*, 993–999. [CrossRef]
14. O'Donghaile, D.; Jenkins, P.V.; McGrath, R.T.; Preston, L.; Field, S.P.; Ward, S.E.; O'Sullivan, J.M.; O'Donnell, J.S. Expresser phenotype determines ABO(H) blood group antigen loading on platelets and von Willebrand factor. *Sci. Rep.* **2020**, *10*, 18366. [CrossRef] [PubMed]
15. Wienzek-Lischka, S.; König, I.R.; Papenkort, E.-M.; Hackstein, H.; Santoso, S.; Sachs, U.J.; Bein, G. HLA-DRB3*01:01 is a predictor of immunization against human platelet antigen-1a but not of the severity of fetal and neonatal alloimmune thrombocytopenia. *Transfusion* **2017**, *57*, 533–540. [CrossRef] [PubMed]
16. Moureau, P.; Andre, A. Blood groups of human blood platelets. *Nature* **1954**, *174*, 88. [CrossRef]

17. Dunstan, R.A.; Simpson, M.B.; Knowles, R.W.; Rosse, W.F. The origin of ABH antigens on human platelets. *Blood* **1985**, *65*, 615–619. [CrossRef]
18. Mollicone, R.; Caillard, T.; Le Pendu, J.; François, A.; Sansonetti, N.; Villarroya, H.; Oriol, R. Expression of ABH and X (Lex) antigens on platelets and lymphocytes. *Blood* **1988**, *71*, 1113–1119. [CrossRef]
19. Santoso, S.; Kiefel, V.; Mueller-Eckhardt, C. Blood group A and B determinants are expressed on platelet glycoproteins IIa, IIIa, and Ib. *Thromb. Haemost.* **1991**, *65*, 196–201. [CrossRef]
20. Hou, M.; Stockelberg, D.; Rydberg, L.; Kutti, J.; Wadenvik, H. Blood group A antigen expression in platelets is prominently associated with glycoprotein Ib and IIb. Evidence for an A1/A2 difference. *Transfus. Med.* **1996**, *6*, 51–59. [CrossRef]
21. Stockelberg, D.; Hou, M.; Rydberg, L.; Kutti, J.; Wadenvik, H. Evidence for an expression of blood group A antigen on platelet glycoproteins IV and V. *Transfus. Med.* **1996**, *6*, 243–248. [CrossRef] [PubMed]
22. Kelton, J.G.; Smith, J.W.; Horsewood, P.; Warner, M.N.; Warkentin, T.E.; Finberg, R.W.; Hayward, C.P. ABH antigens on human platelets: Expression on the glycosyl phosphatidylinositol-anchored protein CD109. *J. Lab. Clin. Med.* **1998**, *132*, 142–148. [CrossRef]
23. Holgersson, J.; Breimer, M.E.; Jacobsson, A.; Svensson, L.; Ulfvin, A.; Samuelsson, B.E. Glycolipid- and glycoprotein-based blood group A antigen expression in human thrombocytes. A1/A2 difference. *Glycoconj. J.* **1990**, *7*, 601–608. [CrossRef]
24. Cooling, L.L.; Zhang, D.; Koerner, T.A. Human platelets express gangliosides with LKE activity and ABH blood group activity. *Transfusion* **2001**, *41*, 504–516. [CrossRef] [PubMed]
25. Skogen, B.; Rossebø Hansen, B.; Husebekk, A.; Havnes, T.; Hannestad, K. Minimal expression of blood group A antigen on thrombocytes from A2 individuals. *Transfusion* **1988**, *28*, 456–459. [CrossRef]
26. Julmy, F.; Achermann, F.; Schulzki, T.; Carrel, T.; Nydegger, U. PLTs of blood group A1 donors express increased surface A antigen owing to apheresis and prolonged storage. *Transfusion* **2003**, *43*, 1378–1385. [CrossRef]
27. Cooling, L.L.W.; Kelly, K.; Barton, J.; Hwang, D.; Koerner, T.A.W.; Olson, J.D. Determinants of ABH expression on human blood platelets. *Blood* **2005**, *105*, 3356–3364. [CrossRef]
28. Sant'Anna Gomes, B.M.; Estalote, A.C.; Palatnik, M.; Pimenta, G.; Pereira, B.d.B.; Do Nascimento, E.M. Prevalence, serologic and genetic studies of high expressers of the blood group A antigen on platelets. *Transfus. Med.* **2010**, *20*, 303–314. [CrossRef]
29. DeLelys, M.E.; Ochoa, G.; Cserti-Gazdewich, C.M.; Vietz, C.; Preffer, F.I.; Dzik, W. Relationship between ABO genotype and A antigen expression on platelets. *Transfusion* **2013**, *53*, 1763–1771. [CrossRef]
30. Xu, X.; Xu, F.; Ying, Y.; Hong, X.; Liu, Y.; Chen, S.; He, J.; Zhu, F.; Hu, W. ABO antigen levels on platelets of normal and variant ABO blood group individuals. *Platelets* **2019**, *30*, 854–860. [CrossRef]
31. Curtis, B.R.; Fick, A.; Lochowicz, A.J.; McFarland, J.G.; Ball, R.H.; Peterson, J.; Aster, R.H. Neonatal alloimmune thrombocytopenia associated with maternal-fetal incompatibility for blood group B. *Transfusion* **2008**, *48*, 358–364. [CrossRef] [PubMed]
32. Zipursky, A.; Pollock, J.; Neelands, P.; Chown, B.; Israels, L. The transplacental passage of foetal red blood cells and the pathogenesis of Rh immunisation during pregnancy. *Lancet* **1963**, *282*, 489–493. [CrossRef]
33. Chown, B. Anaemia from bleeding of the fetus into the mother's circulation. *Lancet* **1954**, *266*, 1213–1215. [CrossRef]
34. Bowman, J.M.; Pollock, J.M.; Penston, L.E. Fetomaternal transplacental hemorrhage during pregnancy and after delivery. *Vox Sang.* **1986**, *51*, 117–121. [CrossRef] [PubMed]
35. Woodrow, J.C.; Donohoe, W.T. Rh-immunization by pregnancy: Results of a survey and their relevance to prophylactic therapy. *Br. Med. J.* **1968**, *4*, 139–144. [CrossRef]
36. Prevention of Rh-haemolytic disease: Results of the clinical trial. A combined study from centres in England and Baltimore. *Br. Med. J.* **1966**, *2*, 907–914. [CrossRef]
37. Mueller-Eckhardt, C.; Kiefel, V.; Grubert, A.; Kroll, H.; Weisheit, M.; Schmidt, S.; Mueller-Eckhardt, G.; Santoso, S. 348 cases of suspected neonatal alloimmune thrombocytopenia. *Lancet* **1989**, *333*, 363–366. [CrossRef]
38. Jin, J.C.; Lakkaraja, M.M.; Ferd, P.; Manotas, K.; Gabor, J.; Wissert, M.; Berkowitz, R.L.; McFarland, J.G.; Bussel, J.B. Maternal sensitization occurs before delivery in severe cases of fetal alloimmune thrombocytopenia. *Am. J. Hematol.* **2019**, *94*, E213–E215. [CrossRef]
39. Desai, R.G.; McCutcheon, E.; Little, B.; Driscoll, S.G. Fetomaternal passage of leukocytes and platelets in erythroblastosis fetalis. *Blood* **1966**, *27*, 858–862. [CrossRef]
40. Habibi, B.; Bretagne, M.; Bretagne, Y.; Forestier, F.; Daffos, F. Blood group antigens on fetal red cells obtained by umbilical vein puncture under ultrasound guidance: A rapid hemagglutination test to check for contamination with maternal blood. *Pediatr. Res.* **1986**, *20*, 1082–1084. [CrossRef]
41. Fischer, K. *Morbus Haemolyticus Neonatorum im AB0-System*; Georg Thieme Verlag: Stuttgart, Germany, 1961.
42. Cohen, F.; Zuelzer, W.W. Mechanisms of isoimmunization. II. Transplacental passage and postnatal survival of fetal erythrocytes in heterospecific pregnancies. *Blood* **1967**, *30*, 796–804. [CrossRef] [PubMed]
43. Brinc, D.; Lazarus, A.H. Mechanisms of anti-D action in the prevention of hemolytic disease of the fetus and newborn. *Hematology Am. Soc. Hematol. Educ. Program* **2009**, *2009*, 185–191. [CrossRef] [PubMed]
44. Crow, A.R.; Freedman, J.; Hannach, B.; Lazarus, A.H. Monoclonal antibody-mediated inhibition of the human HLA alloimmune response to platelet transfusion is antigen specific and independent of Fcgamma receptor-mediated immune suppression. *Br. J. Haematol.* **2000**, *110*, 481–487. [CrossRef] [PubMed]

45. Sabbatinelli, G.; Fantasia, D.; Palka, C.; Morizio, E.; Alfonsi, M.; Calabrese, G. Isolation and enrichment of circulating fetal cells for NIPD: An overview. *Diagnostics* **2021**, *11*, 2239. [CrossRef]
46. Kumpel, B.M.; Sibley, K.; Jackson, D.J.; White, G.; Soothill, P.W. Ultrastructural localization of glycoprotein IIIa (GPIIIa, beta 3 integrin) on placental syncytiotrophoblast microvilli: Implications for platelet alloimmunization during pregnancy. *Transfusion* **2008**, *48*, 2077–2086. [CrossRef]
47. Thiede, H.A.; Choate, J.W.; Gardner, H.H.; Santhay, H. Immunofluorescent examination of the human chorionic villus for blood group A and B substance. *J. Exp. Med.* **1965**, *121*, 1039–1050. [CrossRef]
48. Goto, S.; Hoshino, M.; Tomoda, Y.; Ishizuka, N. Innumoelectron microscopy of the human chorionic villus in search of blood group A and B antigens. *Lab. Investig.* **1976**, *35*, 530–536.
49. Kjær, M.; Geisen, C.; Akkök, Ç.A.; Wikman, A.; Sachs, U.; Bussel, J.B.; Nielsen, K.; Walles, K.; Curtis, B.R.; Vidarsson, G.; et al. Strategies to develop a prophylaxis for the prevention of HPA-1a immunization and fetal and neonatal alloimmune thrombocytopenia. *Transfus. Apher. Sci.* **2020**, *59*, 102712. [CrossRef]

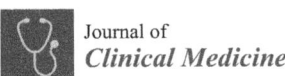

Case Report

Enlarged Abdominal Lymph Node as a Cause of Polyhydramnios in the Course of Congenital Neonatal Leukaemia: A Case Report and Review of the Literature on Foetal Abdominal Tumours with Coexisting Polyhydramnios

Daria Salloum *, Paweł Jan Stanirowski, Aleksandra Symonides, Paweł Krajewski, Dorota Bomba-Opoń and Mirosław Wielgoś

1st Department of Obstetrics and Gynecology, Medical University of Warsaw, Starynkiewicza Sq. 1/3, 02-015 Warsaw, Poland
* Correspondence: dariasalloum@gmail.com

Abstract: Polyhydramnios represents a complication found in 0.2–2% of pregnancies, and it is usually diagnosed between 31 and 36 weeks of pregnancy. Although most cases of polyhydramnios are idiopathic, maternal diabetes or foetal malformations constitute frequent causes of the excessive accumulation of the amniotic fluid. Considering the latter, polyhydramnios may rarely be caused by foetal abdominal tumours, with the incidence rate of 2–14 cases per 100,000 live births. Congenital neonatal leukaemia (CNL) is a rare disease with a reported incidence rate of 5–8.6 cases per million live births. In the prenatal period, the ultrasound abnormalities associated with CNL include hepatomegaly and splenomegaly. In this paper, we presented a case of polyhydramnios caused by mechanical pressure on the foetal gastrointestinal tract by an enlarged lymph node in the course of CNL, as well as reviewing the available literature on foetal abdominal tumours with concurrent polyhydramnios.

Keywords: polyhydramnios; congenital neonatal leukaemia; abdominal tumour; lymph node

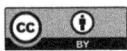

1. Introduction

Polyhydramnios represents a complication found in 0.2–2% of pregnancies, and it is usually diagnosed between 31 and 36 weeks of pregnancy [1]. Although most cases of polyhydramnios are idiopathic, maternal diabetes or foetal malformations constitute frequent causes of the excessive accumulation of the amniotic fluid [2]. Considering the latter, polyhydramnios may rarely be caused by foetal abdominal tumours, with the incidence rate of 2–14 cases per 100,000 live births [3]. The abdominal tumours most frequently diagnosed in the prenatal period include teratomas, neuroblastomas and hepatic tumours [4]. The mechanism responsible for the occurrence of polyhydramnios in the case of abdominal tumours may be twofold—the mechanical pressure on the gastrointestinal tract or hyperdynamic circulation leading to excessive foetal urination. Interestingly, the vast majority of described cases of abdominal tumours coexisting with excessive amniotic fluid volume concern solid, neoplastic lesions, and no case of polyhydramnios caused by reactive tumours in the course of myeloproliferative disorders has been published to date. Congenital neonatal leukaemia (CNL) is a rare disease with a reported incidence rate of 5–8.6 cases per million live births [5]. The characteristic changes found in a neonate include abnormal blood count (hyperleukocytosis, thrombocytopenia and anaemia), enlargement of internal organs, such as liver and spleen, and skin infiltration [6,7]. In the prenatal period, the ultrasound abnormalities associated with CNL include hepatomegaly and splenomegaly, as well as generalised foetal oedema [8,9]. The prognosis in most cases of CNL is unfavourable, with a 23% survival rate at 24 months [10].

This paper presents a review of the literature on foetal abdominal tumours coexisting with polyhydramnios. The analysis is based on a rare case of polyhydramnios diagnosed in the third trimester of pregnancy and caused by mechanical pressure on the gastrointestinal tract by an enlarged lymph node in the course of CNL. The above-mentioned observation emphasizes the need to differentiate between abdominal tumours of different aetiology, including myeloproliferative neoplasms, as potential causes of abnormal amniotic fluid volume.

2. Materials and Methods

A review of the English and Polish literature was undertaken for articles published between January 1980 and September 2022 to identify case reports and case series related to foetal abdominal tumours coexisting with polyhydramnios. Studies were identified via PubMed, Scopus, EMBASE and Web of Science database searching using the key words: "polyhydramnios"; "abdominal tumour" and "congenital neonatal leukaemia" by two authors independently (DS, PJS). The reference lists of retrieved articles were reviewed to locate additional studies. Reviews and articles written in language other than English and Polish, as well as cases of foetal tumours without concomitant polyhydramnios, were excluded from further analysis.

After the initial literature search, publications were analysed by title and abstract to exclude studies that did not meet the inclusion criteria. Following abstract selection, the remaining full-text articles were screened for eligibility. The following data were collected by two investigators independently: tumour type, gestational age at diagnosis, ultrasound findings, pregnancy management and neonatal outcome.

3. Case Presentation

A 38-year-old patient (gravida VII, para IV) was admitted to the clinic at 34 + 6 gestational weeks due to the observed increase in the abdominal circumference for several days and dyspnoea. The course of the pregnancy was uncomplicated so far, and the only maternal co-morbidity observed at the admission was moderate obesity (BMI 38 kg/m^2). The result of a combined test performed at 12 weeks of pregnancy indicated a high risk of trisomy 21 (1:65). Nonetheless, the patient did not follow up with further diagnostics, including invasive procedures, as well as did not report for ultrasound examinations for the assessment of foetal anatomy between 18–22 and 28–32 weeks of pregnancy, as recommended by the Polish Society of Gynaecologists and Obstetricians [11].

The physical examination at admission did not reveal any abnormalities, both blood pressure and heart rate were normal. The CTG recording was reactive, with normal variability and a short-term variability of 8.7 ms. Laboratory tests revealed haemoglobin, leukocyte and platelet concentrations of 12.6 g/dL; 10,700/μL and 292,000/μL, respectively. The foetal ultrasound demonstrated severe polyhydramnios, with amniotic fluid index (AFI) of 37.63 cm, and small stomach (Figure 1A,B). Doppler indices in both the umbilical artery and middle cerebral artery were normal (MCA PSV 60.8 cm/s = 1.206 MoM). Due to difficulties in visualization associated with the patient's obesity and polyhydramnios, a precise anatomy assessment of the foetus was not performed during initial ultrasound examination. Due to the excessive accumulation of amniotic fluid, resulting in clinical symptoms as well as high risk of chromosomal aberration in the foetus, an amnioreduction was performed following the patient's consent, and amniotic fluid was collected for the determination of foetal karyotype (result: 46 XX). The procedure was uncomplicated, and 1600 mL of clear amniotic fluid was collected. After two days, the patient again reported dyspnoea. A second amnioreduction was performed, and 1700 mL of amniotic fluid was collected. Three days later, the last amnioreduction was conducted, resulting in the collection of 1700 mL of clear fluid. During the procedure, the ultrasound examination revealed the presence of a solid tumour in the hepatic hilum area, measuring 55.6 × 24.12 mm, without signs of increased vascularisation (Figure 1B). Due to the presence of the tumour, the patient was qualified for elective Caesarean section. At 35 + 6 gestational weeks a female foetus was born, weighing 3400 g, in moderately good general condition (6-6-6-7 Apgar points).

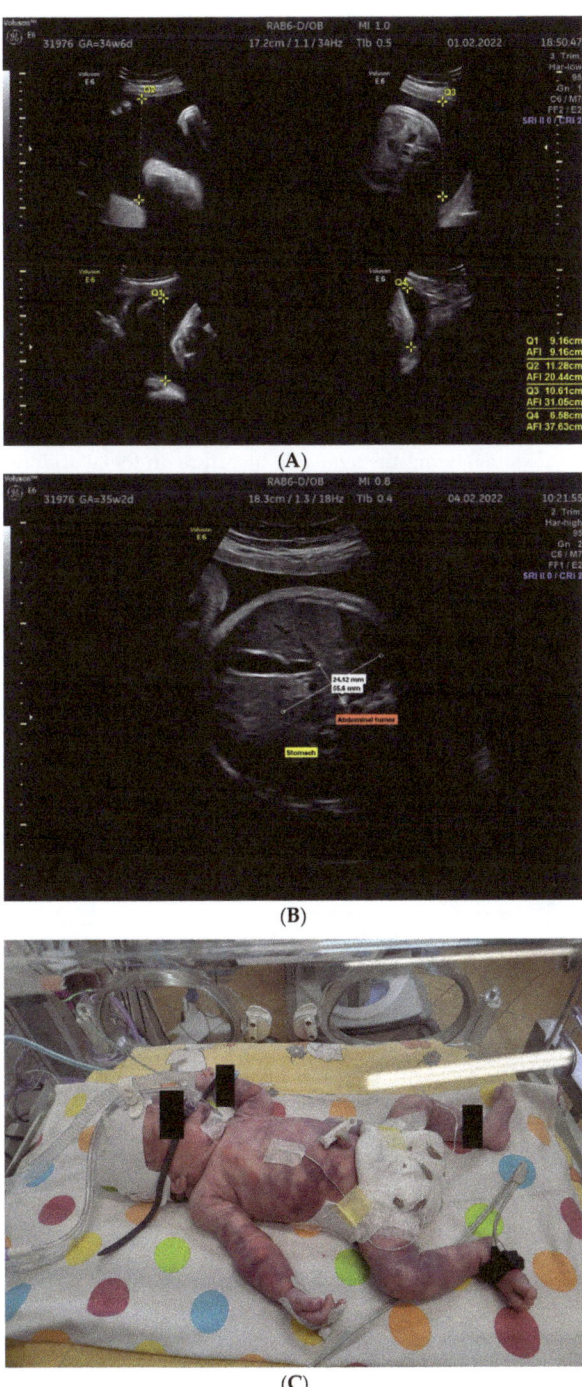

Figure 1. (**A**) Ultrasound image presenting amniotic fluid index measurement. (**B**) Ultrasound image presenting foetal abdomen and tumour in the hepatic hilum area. (**C**) Bruisings and nodular lesions on the skin of the neonate with congenital neonatal leukaemia.

The physical examination of the neonate revealed numerous bruisings and nodular lesions on the skin (Figure 1C). Laboratory tests revealed thrombocytopenia (25,000 μ/L), leukocytosis (33,400 μ/L), anaemia (Hg 8.3 g/dL) and abnormalities in the coagulation profile (APTT 107 s, INR 4.59). A total of 98% of the cells found in the manual blood smear were blast cells. The ultrasound of the neonate's abdomen confirmed presence of a tumour measuring 58.5 × 25.1 mm localized in the hepatic hilum area. Due to the severe general condition, subdural haemorrhage and suspected CNL, the neonate was transferred to the Department of Neonatology, Pathology and Intensive Therapy at the Children's Memorial Health Institute. Two days after the birth, the neonate died. The histopathological examination of the neonate confirmed the diagnosis of a diffuse neoplastic process in the course of CNL and the presence of an enlarged abdominal lymph node. At the same time the histopathological examination of the placenta did not reveal any abnormalities.

4. Results and Discussion

In this study we presented a case of polyhydramnios caused by mechanical pressure on the foetal gastrointestinal tract by an enlarged lymph node in the course of CNL, as well as reviewing the available literature on foetal abdominal tumours with concurrent polyhydramnios. A total of 263 articles were identified through a database search, of which 120 were duplicates (Figure 2). Following abstract screening, 102 articles were determined to be outside the scope of the investigation and a further 14 full-text articles described cases of abdominal tumours without concomitant polyhydramnios. The remaining 27 publications describing 32 cases constituted the basis of this review (Supplementary Table S1), [12–38].

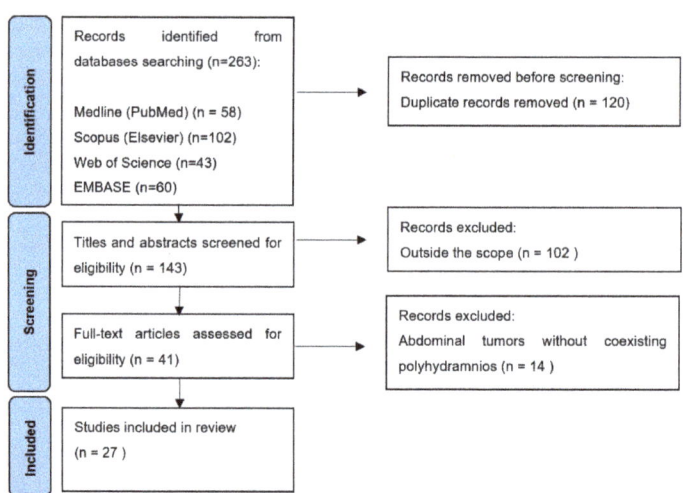

Figure 2. Flow chart displaying the selection process.

In the prenatal period, leukaemia is found much less frequently than in childhood [39]. A higher risk of leukaemia has been identified in patients with Down syndrome [40]. In the presented case, despite a high risk of trisomy 21 in the combined test, we did not demonstrate any abnormalities in the foetal karyotype. Only one case of pregnancy complicated by polyhydramnios in the course of CNL was described in the available literature [41]. According to the authors' suggestion, the excessive volume of the amniotic fluid could result from the neoplastic invasion of the placental villi, which was confirmed in their histopathological examination. In our case, however, no neoplastic lesions were found in the placental tissue, and the most probable cause of the polyhydramnios was the mechanical pressure on the gastrointestinal tract by an enlarged lymph node localized in the hepatic hilum area.

The analysis of the literature revealed that the mean gestational age in which an abdominal tumour coexisting with polyhydramnios was diagnosed is 34 weeks (18–36) (Supplementary Table S1). In 9 out of 32 cases (28.1%) an amnioreduction was performed, and in 8 cases (25%) the premature rupture of membranes occurred (in 4 cases following amnioreduction). The preferred mode of delivery was Caesarean section (62.5%; 20/32), including four cases (20%) classified as an emergency CS. The mean gestational age at the delivery was 35 weeks (25–40). In only one case a decision was made to terminate the pregnancy [37].

Half of the analysed cases of abdominal tumours concurrent with polyhydramnios were represented by mesoblastic nephroma (50%, 16/32), a rare tumour of mesenchymal origin, accounting for 3% of the renal tumours diagnosed in children [42]. The majority of mesoblastic nephroma cases (90%) are diagnosed in the first year of life [43]. Regarding the prenatal period, the mean gestational age at the diagnosis was 31 weeks (22–36). Importantly, in over half (9/16) of the ultrasound examinations a renal mass was detected. In 56% of cases a Caesarean section was performed, and the mean gestational age at delivery was 36 weeks (25–38). The preferred method of treatment of mesoblastic nephroma is surgery—depending on its histological type, only the tumour is excised, or nephrectomy or nephroureterectomy is conducted [44]. In most cases the prognosis is favourable [22]. In the analysed group of children, only two neonates died soon after birth, while in the remaining patients no disease recurrence was found during a follow-up period of 6 to 36 months.

In the available literature, the second most common abdominal tumour coexisting with polyhydramnios is immature gastric teratoma (9.4%, 3/32) (Supplementary Table S1). It is a very rare tumour, accounting for less than 2% of abdominal tumours diagnosed in neonates. In three reported cases of immature gastric teratoma, ultrasound studies revealed not only polyhydramnios, but also placentomegaly, ascites and intraperitoneal calcifications [34–36,45]. Treatment of a tumour in the post-partum period involves removal of the lesion, sometimes combined with a partial gastric resection. All the presented cases of pregnancies with immature gastric teratomas were delivered by Caesarean section.

Similarly to immature gastric teratoma, congenital neuroblastoma is a rare tumour, accounting for 5% of neuroblastomas diagnosed in children [46]. It originates from the neural crest cells which, in normal conditions, form sympathetic ganglia and adrenal medullas [47]. Due to the presence of characteristic "blueberry muffin" skin lesions in neonates, neuroblastoma is frequently considered in differential diagnosis of CNL [48]. Congenital neuroblastoma is most frequently diagnosed in the 3rd trimester of pregnancy, and apart from the presence of tumour lesions in the abdomen, the most common ultrasound findings include generalised foetal oedema, placentomegaly and placental metastases (Supplementary Table S1) [49]. The 10-year survival rate is approximately 49% [35], and the preferred method of treatment is chemotherapy [50]. In the analysed literature, pregnancies complicated by polyhydramnios and congenital neuroblastoma were delivered via Caesarean section, and the treatment method of choice was chemotherapy, as mentioned before.

Nephroblastoma, also known as Wilms' tumour, is the most common kidney tumour diagnosed in children [51]. It is frequently associated with congenital defects or genetic syndromes, such as Beckwith–Wiedemann syndrome [35]. Ultrasound findings include foetal oedema, ascites and nephromegaly (Supplementary Table S1). The preferred method of treatment in most cases is laparotomy and nephrectomy, without the need for adjuvant chemotherapy [52]. Despite the favourable prognosis—the overall survival rate is approximately 90%—in the reported cases associated with polyhydramnios, one of the neonates died shortly after the delivery, while the other one demonstrated developmental delay one year after the delivery and laparotomy.

5. Conclusions

In the course of pregnancy, abdominal tumours constitute rare causes of polyhydramnios. During the ultrasound examination of excessive amniotic fluid volume, attention should be paid to potential abnormal masses in the foetal abdomen. In rare cases, the mechanical pressure on the foetal gastrointestinal tract may be caused not only by neoplastic tumours, but also by a reactive lymph node in the course of a myeloproliferative diseases.

Supplementary Materials: The following supporting information can be downloaded at: https://www.mdpi.com/article/10.3390/jcm11216598/s1, Table S1: Foetal Abdominal Tumours with Coexisting Polyhydramnios.

Author Contributions: Conceptualization, P.J.S. and D.S.; methodology, D.S. and P.J.S.; investigation, D.S., P.J.S., P.K, A.S. and M.W.; data curation, D.S., P.J.S. and A.S.; writing—original draft preparation, D.S.; writing—review and editing, P.J.S., P.K., D.B.-O. and M.W.; supervision, P.J.S. and M.W. All authors have read and agreed to the published version of the manuscript.

Funding: This research received no external funding.

Institutional Review Board Statement: Ethical review and approval were waived for this study.

Informed Consent Statement: Informed consent for publication of this case report was obtained from the newborn's parents.

Data Availability Statement: The data that support the findings of this study are available from the corresponding author on reasonable request. The data are not publicly available due to privacy or ethical restrictions.

Conflicts of Interest: The authors declare no conflict of interest.

References

1. Panting-Kemp, A.; Nguyen, T.; Chang, E.; Quillen, E.; Castro, L. Idiopathic polyhydramnios and perinatal outcome. *Am. J. Obstet. Gynecol.* **1999**, *181*, 1079–1082. [CrossRef]
2. Phelan, J.P.; Smith, C.V.; Broussard, P.; Small, M. Amniotic fluid volume assessment with the four-quadrant technique at 36-42 weeks' gestation. *J. Reprod. Med.* **1987**, *32*, 540–542. [PubMed]
3. Peiro, J.L.; Sbragia, L.; Scorletti, F.; Lim, F.Y. Perinatal Management of Fetal Tumors. *Curr. Pediatr. Rev.* **2015**, *11*, 151–163. [CrossRef] [PubMed]
4. Bruny, J.; Crombleholme, T.M. Perinatal management of infant tumors and the promise of fetal surgery. *Curr. Opin. Pediatr.* **2013**, *25*, 31–39. [CrossRef] [PubMed]
5. Bajwa, R.P.S. Demographic study of leukaemia presenting within the first 3 months of life in the Northern Health Region of England. *J. Clin. Pathol.* **2004**, *57*, 186–188. [CrossRef]
6. Zhang, Q.; Ren, Z.; Yang, J.; Yin, A. Analysis of 59 cases of congenital leukemia reported between 2001 and 2016. *J. Int. Med. Res.* **2019**, *47*, 4235–4625. [CrossRef] [PubMed]
7. Isaacs, H. Fetal and Neonatal Leukemia. *J. Pediatr. Hematol. Oncol.* **2003**, *25*, 348–361. [CrossRef]
8. Robertson, M.; de Jong, G.; Mansvelt, E. Prenatal diagnosis of congenital leukemia in a fetus at 25 weeks' gestation with Down syndrome: Case report and review of the literature. *Ultrasound Obstet. Gynecol.* **2003**, *21*, 486–489. [CrossRef]
9. Isaacs, H. Fetal Hydrops Associated with Tumors. *Am. J. Perinatol.* **2008**, *25*, 43–68. [CrossRef]
10. Bresters, D.; Reus, A.C.W.; Veerman, A.J.P.; van Wering, E.R.; van der Does-van den Berg, A.; Kaspers, G.J.L. Congenital leukaemia: The Dutch experience and review of the literature. *Br. J. Haematol.* **2002**, *117*, 513–524. [CrossRef]
11. Borowski, D.; Pietryga, M.; Basta, P.; Cnota, W.; Czuba, B.; Dubiel, M.; Fuchs, T.; Huras, H.; Iciek, R.; Jaczynska, R.; et al. Practice guidelines of the Polish Society of Gynecologists and Obstetricians—Ultrasound Section for ultrasound screening in uncomplicated pregnancy—2020. *Ginekol. Pol.* **2020**, *91*, 490–501. [CrossRef] [PubMed]
12. ben David, Y.; Sela, N.; ben David, C.; Dujovni, T. Case of fetal ovarian juvenile granulosa cell tumor: Complications and management. *J. Obstet. Gynaecol. Res.* **2021**, *47*, 2220–2224. [CrossRef] [PubMed]
13. Schurr, P.; Moulsdale, W. Infantile myofibroma: A case report and review of the literature. *Adv. Neonatal. Care* **2008**, *8*, 13–20. [CrossRef] [PubMed]
14. Küpeli, S.; Guliyev, A.; Varan, A.; Akata, D.; Büyüpamukçu, M. Neuroblastoma presented with polyhydramniosis. *Pediatr. Hematol. Oncol.* **2011**, *28*, 159–163. [CrossRef]
15. Chapa, H.O.; Geddie, S.G.; Flores, R. Metastatic neuroblastoma diagnosed on prenatal sonographic examination performed for decreased fetal movement. *J. Clin. Ultrasound* **2017**, *45*, 502–506. [CrossRef]
16. Izbizky, G.; Elias, D.; Gallo, A.; Farias, P.; Sod, R. Prenatal diagnosis of fetal bilateral adrenal carcinoma. *Ultrasound Obstet. Gynecol.* **2005**, *26*, 669–671. [CrossRef]

17. Cornette, J.; Festen, S.; van den Hoonaard, T.L.; Steegers, E.A. Mesenchymal hamartoma of the liver: A benign tumor with deceptive prognosis in the perinatal period. Case report and review of the literature. *Fetal Diagn Ther.* **2009**, *25*, 196–202. [CrossRef]
18. van de Bor, M.; Verwey, R.A.; van Pel, R. Acute polyhydramnios associated with fetal hepatoblastoma. *Eur. J. Obstet. Gynecol. Reprod. Biol.* **1985**, *20*, 65–69. [CrossRef]
19. Vadeyar, S.; Ramsay, M.; James, D.; O'Neill, D. Prenatal diagnosis of congenital Wilms' tumor (nephroblastoma) presenting as fetal hydrops. *Ultrasound Obstet. Gynecol.* **2000**, *16*, 80–83. [CrossRef]
20. Holzgreve, W.; Winde, B.; Willital, G.H.; Beller, F.K. Prenatal diagnosis and perinatal management of a fetal ovarian cyst. *Prenat Diagn* **1985**, *5*, 155–158. [CrossRef]
21. Shima, Y.; Ikegami, E.; Takechi, N.; Migita, M.; Hayashi, Z.; Araki, T.; Tanaka, Y.; Sugiyama, M.; Hashizume, K. Congenital fibrosarcoma of the jejunum in a premature infant with meconium peritonitis. *Eur. J. Pediatr. Surg.* **2003**, *13*, 134–136. [CrossRef] [PubMed]
22. Do, A.Y.; Kim, J.S.; Choi, S.J.; Oh, S.Y.; Roh, C.R.; Kim, J.H. Prenatal diagnosis of congenital mesoblastic nephroma. *Obstet. Gynecol. Sci.* **2015**, *58*, 405–408. [CrossRef] [PubMed]
23. Kato, H.; Mitani, Y.; Goda, T.; Yamaue, H. Neonatal congenital mesoblastic nephroma that caused respiratory oncologic emergency early after birth: A case report. *BMC Pediatr.* **2022**, *22*, 139. [CrossRef] [PubMed]
24. Al-Turkistani, H.K. Congenital mesoblastic nephroma: A case report. *J. Family Community Med.* **2008**, *15*, 91–93.
25. Daskas, N.; Argyropoulou, M.; Pavlou, M.; Andronikou, S. Congenital mesoblastic nephroma associated with polyhydramnios and hypercalcemia. *Pediatr. Nephrol.* **2002**, *17*, 187–189. [CrossRef]
26. Che, M.; Yang, F.; Huang, H.; Zhang, H.; Han, C.; Sun, N. Prenatal diagnosis of fetal congenital mesoblastic nephroma by ultrasonography combined with MR imaging. *Medicine* **2021**, *100*, e24034. [CrossRef]
27. Mata, R.P.; Alves, T.; Figueiredo, A.; Santos, A. Prenatal diagnosis of congenital mesoblastic nephroma: A case with poor prognosis. *BMJ Case Rep.* **2019**, *12*, e230297. [CrossRef]
28. Chen, W.Y.; Lin, C.N.; Chao, C.S.; Yan-Sheng Lin, M.; Mak, C.W.; Chuang, S.S.; Tzeng, C.C.; Huang, K.F. Prenatal diagnosis of congenital mesoblastic nephroma in mid-second trimester by sonography and magnetic resonance imaging. *Prenat. Diagn.* **2003**, *23*, 927–931. [CrossRef]
29. Chen, Y.X.; Huang, C.; He, Q.M.; Wang, Z.; Huang, L.; Wang, H.Y.; Mei, S.S.; Chai, C.W.; Zhang, G.L.; Zhong, W.; et al. Prenatal diagnosis and postnatal management of congenital mesoblastic nephroma: Experience at a single center in China. *Prenat. Diagn.* **2021**, *41*, 766–771. [CrossRef]
30. Blank, E.; Neerhout, R.C.; Burry, K.A. Congenital mesoblastic nephroma and polyhydramnios. *JAMA* **1978**, *240*, 1504–1505. [CrossRef]
31. Kimani, W.; Ashiundu, E.; Saula, P.W.; Kimondo, M.; Keitany, K. Congenital mesoblastic nephroma: Case study. *J. Pediatr. Surg. Case Rep.* **2020**, *55*, 101336. [CrossRef]
32. Robertson-Bell, T.; Newberry, D.M.; Jnah, A.J.; DeMeo, S.D. Congenital Mesoblastic Nephroma Presenting with Refractory Hypertension in a Premature Neonate: A Case Study. *Neonatal Netw.* **2017**, *36*, 32–39. [CrossRef]
33. Allen, L.M.; Williams, K.D. Prenatal Diagnosis of a Cyst of the Canal of Nuck Associated with an Ovarian Cyst and Acute Polyhydramnios. *J. Diagn. Med. Sonogr.* **2020**, *36*, 277–286. [CrossRef]
34. Caballes, A.B.; Dungca, L.B.P.; Uy, M.E.V.; Torralba, M.G.C.; Embuscado, C.M.G. Hydrops fetalis and neonatal abdominal compartment syndrome continuum from immature gastric teratoma: A case report. *BMC Pediatr.* **2020**, *20*, 186. [CrossRef] [PubMed]
35. Falikborenstein, T.C.; Korenberg, J.R.; Davos, I.; Platt, L.D.; Gans, S.; Goodman, B.; Schreck, R.; Graham, J.M. Congenital gastric teratoma in Wiedemann-Beckwith syndrome. *Am. J. Med. Genet.* **1991**, *38*, 52–57. [CrossRef] [PubMed]
36. Jeong, H.C.; Cha, S.J.; Kim, G.J. Rapidly grown congenital fetal immature gastric teratoma causing severe neonatal respiratory distress. *J. Obstet. Gynaecol. Res.* **2012**, *38*, 449–451. [CrossRef]
37. Arora, A.; Gupta, M. Beckwith-Wiedemann syndrome—A rare case report. *JK Sci.* **2019**, *21*, 193–194.
38. Greenberg, F.; Stein, F.; Gresik, M.V.; Finegold, M.J.; Carpenter, R.J.; Riccardi, V.M.; Beaudet, A.L.; Opitz, J.M.; Reynolds, J.F. The Perlman familial nephroblastomatosis syndrome. *Am. J. Med. Genet.* **1986**, *24*, 101–110. [CrossRef]
39. Sande, J.E.; Arceci, R.J.; Lampkin, B.C. Congenital and neonatal leukemia. *Semin. Perinatol.* **1999**, *23*, 274–285. [CrossRef]
40. Lange, B.J.; Kobrinsky, N.; Barnard, D.R.; Arthur, D.C.; Buckley, J.D.; Howells, W.B.; Gold, S.; Sanders, J.; Neudorf, S.; Smith, F.O.; et al. Distinctive demography, biology, and outcome of acute myeloid leukemia and myelodysplastic syndrome in children with Down syndrome: Children's Cancer Group Studies 2861 and 2891. *Blood* **1998**, *91*, 608–615.
41. Sato, Y.; Izumi, Y.; Minegishi, K.; Komada, M.; Yamada, S.; Kakui, K.; Tatsumi, K.; Mikami, Y.; Fujiwara, H.; Konishi, I. Prenatal Findings in Congenital Leukemia: A Case Report. *Fetal Diagn Ther.* **2011**, *29*, 325–330. [CrossRef] [PubMed]
42. Pettinato, G.; Carlos Manivel, J.; Wick, M.R.; Dehner, L.P. Classical and cellular (atypical) congenital mesoblastic nephroma: A clinicopathologic, ultrastructural, immunohistochemical, and flow cytometric study. *Hum. Pathol.* **1989**, *20*, 682–690. [CrossRef]
43. Jones, V.S.; Cohen, R.C. Atypical congenital mesoblastic nephroma presenting in the perinatal period. *Pediatr. Surg. Int.* **2007**, *23*, 205–209. [CrossRef] [PubMed]
44. Powis, M. Neonatal renal tumours. *Early Hum. Dev.* **2010**, *86*, 607–612. [CrossRef]
45. Minakova, E.; Lang, J. Congenital neuroblastoma. *Neoreviews* **2020**, *21*, e716–e727. [CrossRef]
46. Handler, M.Z.; Schwartz, R.A. Neonatal leukaemia cutis. *J. Eur. Acad. Dermatol. Venereol.* **2015**, *29*, 1884–1889. [CrossRef]

47. Heling, K.S.; Chaoui, R.; Hartung, J.; Kirchmair, F.; Bollmann, R. Prenatal diagnosis of congenital neuroblastoma. Analysis of 4 cases and review of the literature. *Fetal Diagn Ther.* **1999**, *14*, 47–52. [CrossRef]
48. Crombleholme, T.M.; Murray, T.A.; Harris, B.H. Diagnosis and management of fetal neuroblastoma. *Curr. Opin. Obstet. Gynecol.* **1994**, *6*, 199–202. [CrossRef]
49. Isaacs, H. Fetal and neonatal neuroblastoma: Retrospective review of 271 cases. *Fetal. Pediatr. Pathol.* **2007**, *26*, 177–184. [CrossRef]
50. Martínez, C.H.; Dave, S.; Izawa, J. Wilms' tumor. *Adv. Exp. Med. Biol.* **2010**, *685*, 196–209.
51. Cass, D.L. Fetal abdominal tumors and cysts. *Translational Pediatrics.* **2021**, *10*, 1530. [CrossRef] [PubMed]
52. Servaes, S.E.; Hoffer, F.A.; Smith, E.A.; Khanna, G. Imaging of Wilms tumor: An update. *Pediatr. Radiol.* **2019**, *49*, 1441–1452. [CrossRef] [PubMed]

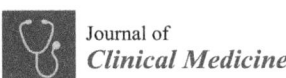

Systematic Review

Analysis of Circulating C19MC MicroRNA as an Early Marker of Hypertension and Preeclampsia in Pregnant Patients: A Systematic Review

Adrianna Kondracka [1], Ilona Jaszczuk [2], Dorota Koczkodaj [2], Bartosz Kondracki [3,*], Karolina Frąszczak [4], Anna Oniszczuk [5], Magda Rybak-Krzyszkowska [6], Jakub Staniczek [7], Agata Filip [2] and Anna Kwaśniewska [1]

1. Department of Obstetrics and Pathology of Pregnancy, Medical University of Lublin, 20-059 Lublin, Poland
2. Department of Cancer Genetics with Cytogenetic Laboratory, Medical University of Lublin, 20-059 Lublin, Poland
3. Department of Cardiology, Medical University of Lublin, 20-059 Lublin, Poland
4. Department of Oncological Gynecology and Gynecology, Medical University of Lublin, 20-059 Lublin, Poland
5. Department of Inorganic Chemistry, Medical University of Lublin, 20-059 Lublin, Poland
6. Department of Obstetrics and Perinatology, University Hospital, 31-501 Krakow, Poland
7. Department of Gynecology, Obstetrics and Gynecologic Oncology, Medical University of Silesia, 40-055 Katowice, Poland
* Correspondence: kondracki.bartosz@gmail.com

Abstract: Preeclampsia and hypertension complicate several pregnancies. Identifying women at risk of developing these conditions is essential to establish potential treatment modalities. Biomarkers such as C19MC microRNA in pregnant patients wopuld assist in defining pregnancy surveillance and implementing interventions. This study sought to analyze circulating C19MC microRNA as an early marker of hypertension and preeclampsia in pregnant patients. A systematic review was undertaken using the following registers: disease registries, pregnancy registries, and pregnancy exposure registries, and the following databases: PubMed, CINAHL, Web of Science, Scopus, and EMBASE. The risk of bias was assessed using the Cochrane technique. From the 45 publications retrieved from the registers and databases, only 21 were included in the review after the removal of duplicates, screening, and eligibility evaluation. All 210 publications had a low risk of bias and illuminated the potential use of circulating C19MC microRNA as an early marker of hypertension and preeclampsia in pregnant patients. Therefore, it was concluded that C19MC microRNA can be used as an early marker of gestational preeclampsia and hypertension.

Keywords: C19MC microRNA; early pregnancy biomarkers; hypertension; preeclampsia

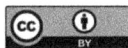

1. Introduction

MicroRNAs have been suggested as possible hypertension and pre-eclampsia indicators since they are crucial cell process regulators. Most investigations have conducted the primate-specific microRNA cluster on chromosome 19 (C19MC microRNA) profiling analysis on total serum samples or maternal plasma to treat the later incidence of pregnancy-related problems, such as gestational pre-eclampsia, hypertension, and fetal growth restriction. Exosomal nanoparticles released into the blood and extracellular space include microRNAs [1]. They allow communication between close-by and far-off cells. Over the past decade, interest in forming non-invasive modes of cell-free nucleic acid detection has been on an upward trajectory. They include microRNAs during maternal circulation [2]. The ability to diagnose via given molecular biomarkers alongside amalgamating them into current prognosis algorithms for issues linked to pregnancy is vital [2]. Small non-coding RNAs (sncRNAs) guide post-transcriptional gene expression by blocking messenger RNA targets from translation. This systematic literature review analyzes findings from different sources on circulating C19MC microRNA as an early marker of hypertension and pre-eclampsia in pregnant patients. It establishes that circulating C19MC microRNAs may contribute to developing pre-eclampsia and prenatal hypertension in early pregnancy.

2. Materials and Methods

The review followed the PRISMA rule to report the stepwise procedure used to retrieve information from various databases and registers. The PRISMA guidelines were also adhered to strictly to eliminate bias and ensure the successful completion of the systematic literature review. Figure 1 below shows the PRISMA chart demonstrating various phases of the review.

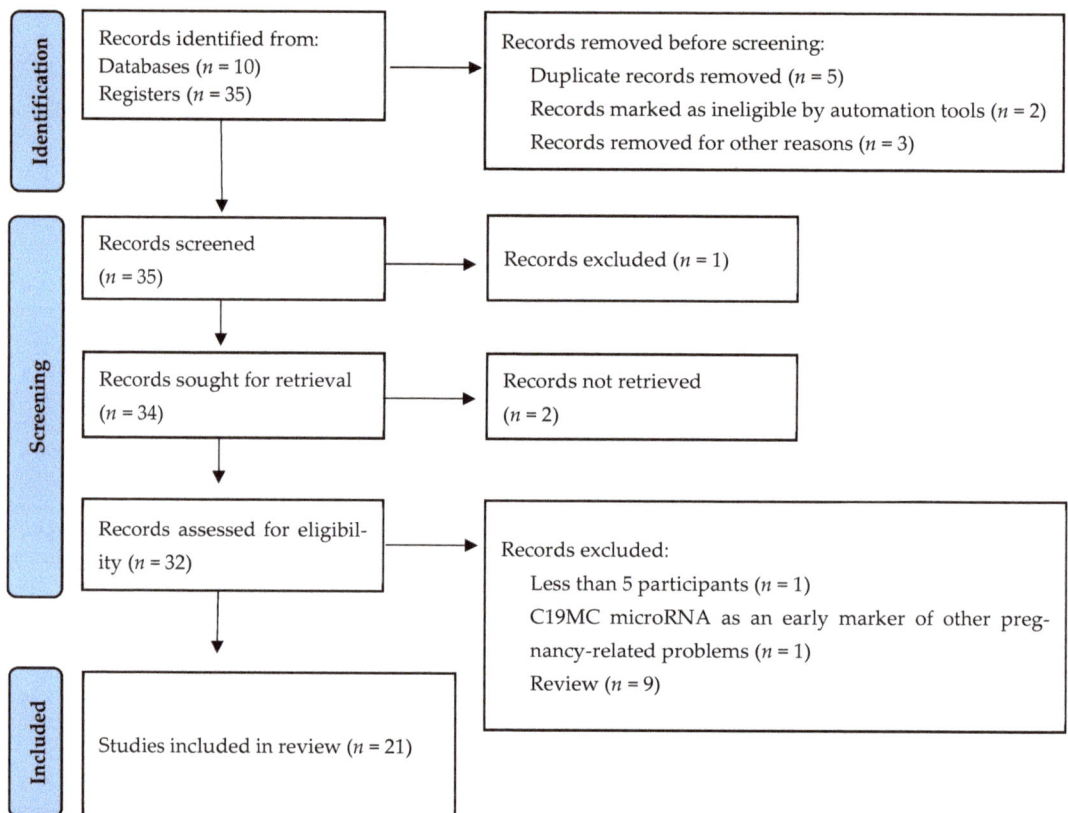

Figure 1. PRISMA chart showing the different stages of the systematic literature review. Ten records were retrieved from databases: PubMed, CINAHL, Web of Science, Scopus, and EMBASE. Thirty-five records were retrieved from registers: disease registries, pregnancy registries, and pregnancy exposure registries. Before the screening, 5 duplicate records were removed, 2 were marked as ineligible using RobotAnalyst, and 3 records were removed because they were written in languages other than English. Thirty-five records were screened, and one was excluded, as its abstract did not include all the crucial keywords required. Thirty-four records were sought for retrieval and only thirty-two were retrieved. Two records could not be retrieved. The 32 records were assessed for eligibility and 2 records were excluded because 1 had less than five participants, while the other focused on C19MC microRNA as an early marker of pregnancy-related problems other than pre-eclampsia and hypertension and nine were review. Therefore, 21 records were included in the review.

The inclusion criterion required using systematic reviews investigating circulating C19MC microRNA as an early marker of hypertension and pre-eclampsia in pregnant patients. Other inclusion requirements included any study, be it experimental, cohort, or case study, articles published in English between 1 January 2013, and 5 August 2022, and original research undertaken in any region of the world with a sample size of at least five participants. The exclusion criteria were papers with fewer than 5 cases, papers published before 2013, and review papers except for systematic reviews. The exclusion criteria required the removal of studies from the review, encompassing articles published in languages other than English and materials that did not concentrate on investigating circulating C19MC microRNA as an early marker of hypertension and pre-eclampsia in pregnant patients.

2.1. Information Sources

The databases used in the review included PubMed, CINAHL, Web of Science, Scopus, and EMBASE. These databases were consulted simultaneously within one month (May 2022) to identify studies that could be included in the review. Similarly, registers such disease registries, pregnancy registries, and pregnancy exposure registries were also searched to identify publications aligned with the topic of interest. These registers were also searched simultaneously within one month (June 2022). The reference lists of the articles obtained from the databases and registers were also used to identify studies that focused on investigating various aspects of the topic of interest, circulating C19MC microRNA as an early marker of hypertension and pre-eclampsia in pregnant patients. The studies were also retrieved from the abovementioned databases and stored for subsequent processes and steps.

2.2. Search Strategy

The scholarly materials retrieved from the databases and registers mentioned above were limited to those published between 1 January 2013, and 5 August 2022. The keywords included C19MC microRNA, early hypertension markers, early pre-eclampsia markers, hypertension in pregnant patients, pre-eclampsia in pregnant patients, and C19MC microRNA in pregnant patients. A manual search was conducted by reading the bibliographies of the review articles or materials that were retrieved from the reference lists, and frequently mentioned publications on gestational hypertension and pre-eclampsia were used to uncover papers that were not identified by the electronic search.

2.3. Selection Process

The selection process was undertaken using three crucial steps. First, reviewers who worked independently selected all articles that were retrieved from the databases and registers to reduce the chances of bias. Second, all the randomly selected publications were reviewed to determine their eligibility. Their abstracts and titles were screened against the eligibility criteria to determine whether the articles that met the inclusion criterion. RobotAnalyst was used as an automation tool during the eligibility screening. This second step enabled the removal of duplicate publications and ushered in the last phase of the selection criterion, which mainly handled the articles with titles and abstracts that did not give sufficient information regarding the study. The last step involved a full-content evaluation by the reviewer to assert whether those particular publications could be included in the review. This three-step process was undertaken independently to ensure that only the necessary publications were included in the review.

2.4. Data Collection Process

The search yielded thirty articles about circulating C19MC microRNA, gestational hypertension, or pre-eclampsia. The threshold index was assessed before synthesizing the data. The diagnostic index tests, including summary receiver operating characteristic

(SROC), diagnostic odds ratio (DOR), negative or positive likelihood ratio (NLR or PLR), specificity (Spe), and sensitivity (Sen), were measured with a confidence interval of 95%.

2.5. Data Items

The data items were manually extracted from the publications included in the review. The essential information from the selected reports was amassed and recorded in a table. Since this review focused on analyzing the circulating C19MC microRNA as an early marker of hypertension and pre-eclampsia in pregnant patients, the data collected from the selected articles included the author(s), titles, years of publication, and outcomes of the reports. The results segment of the chosen publications provided information concerning circulating C19MC microRNA as an early marker of gestational pre-eclampsia and hypertension. For all statistical studies, the statistical analysis tool or technique used and the statistical results were recorded under the data item and outcomes of the reports.

2.6. Study Risk of Bias Assessment

The Cochrane technique was used to assess the risk of bias in all the publications included in the review. Cochrane is a standard risk appraisal instrument that uses judgments of unclear risks (?), high risk (-), and low risk (+) on different axes for studies such as systematic reviews, which may have biases in their decisions, results, strategies, and other aspects of interest. One reviewer independently assessed the risk of bias in each study using the Cochrane tool.

2.7. Synthesis Method

The data in this review were synthesized using thematic analysis and grouping similar information, all presented in Table 1. The four columns included the publications' author(s), titles, publication years, and outcomes. Under the outcomes column, the studies' results were thematically presented, focusing on whether C19MC microRNA can be used as an early marker of gestational hypertension and pre-eclampsia. The rows comprised the heading row and the thirty studies included in the review.

2.8. Reporting Bias Assessment

The bias risk assessment performed using the Cochrane technique was reported using the Cochrane bias risk assessment, as shown in Table 2, which has eight columns and thirty-one rows. The columns included the study of interest, selection bias (random sequence generation), selection bias (allocation concealment), performance bias, detention bias, attrition bias, reporting bias, and other biases. The first row provides the heading information, while the other thirty comprise the publications included in the review.

Table 1. Study Characteristics.

Author(s)	Title	Year	Sample Size	Source	Method	Outcomes
Ali, Asghar et al. [3]	MicroRNA–mRNA Networks in Pregnancy Complications: A Comprehensive Downstream Analysis of Potential Biomarkers	2021	127	Maternal circulation/Placenta	Real-time PCR	Upregulation of microRNAs appears only in the maternal circulation in pre-eclampsia cases
Cronqvist Tina et al. [4]	Syncytiotrophoblast Derived Extracellular Vesicles Transfer Functional Placental Mirnas to Primary Human Endothelial Cells	2017	10	Placental cotyledons	Real-time PCR	Circulating syncytiotrophoblast debris contributes to some of the symptoms of maternal inflammation. Pre-eclampsia (PE), hypertension, and other diseases' clinical characteristics may be explained by an increase in inflammation-related symptoms that are reportedly present in healthy pregnancies at term
Demirer, Selin et al [5]	Expression Profiles of Candidate MicroRNAs in the Peripheral Blood Leukocytes of Patients with Early- and Late-Onset Preeclampsia versus Normal Pregnancies	2020	148	Maternal blood samples	Real-time PCR	The pilot study involved six pregnant women who had one early IUGR, four late pre-eclampsias, and one early pre-eclampsia
He, Xin, and Dan-Ni Ding [6]	Expression and Clinical Significance of Mir-204 in Patients with Hypertensive Disorder Complicating Pregnancy	2022	196	Maternal peripheral blood	Real-time PCR	Preeclampsia often appears after 20 weeks of pregnancy and is characterized by proteinuria and gestational or chronic hypertension
Hromadnikova, Ilona et al. [1]	Circulating C19MC microRNAs in Preeclampsia, Gestational Hypertension, and Fetal Growth Restriction	2013	113	Maternal peripheral blood	Real-time PCR	No correlation exists between microRNA and a history of hypertension among individuals with pre-eclampsia that had already developed
Jelena, Munjas et al. [7]	Placenta-Specific Plasma miR518b is a Potential Biomarker for Preeclampsia	2020	36	Maternal peripheral blood	Digital droplet PCR	Circulating C19MC microRNAs have a role in the etiology of pre-eclampsia
Jin, Yan et al. [8]	The Predictive Value of microRNA in Early Hypertensive Disorder Complicating Pregnancy (HDCP)	2021	136	Maternal peripheral blood	Fluorescence quantitative PCR	Pre-eclampsia with a clinically confirmed diagnosis is linked to changes in extracellular microRNA expression
Jing, Jia et al. [9]	Maternal Obesity alters C19MC microRNAs Expression Profile In Fetal Umbilical Cord Blood	2020	66	Fetal umbilical cord blood samples	Real-time PCR	According to miRNA profiling using the high-throughput Open Array TM technology, seven microRNAs have a distinct abundance profile in early pre-eclampsia

Table 1. Cont.

Author(s)	Title	Year	Sample Size	Source	Method	Outcomes
Légaré, Cécilia et al. [10]	First Trimester Plasma microRNAs Levels Predict Matsuda Index-Estimated Insulin Sensitivity Between 24th And 29th Week of Pregnancy	2022	421	Plasma samples	PCR	Up-regulation of circulating C19MC microRNAs is a hallmark of early pregnancy, which is predisposed to developing issues linked to gestational hypertension and placental insufficiency Elevated plasmatic levels of miR-516-5p, miR-518b, and miR-520h in the first trimester alone are strong indicators of future gestational hypertension
Li, Hui et al. [11]	Unique MicroRNA Signals In Plasma Exosomes from Pregnancies Complicated By Preeclampsia	2020	60	Maternal peripheral blood	Real-time PCR	Females who subsequently had severe pre-eclampsia had upregulated placental-specific miR-520a in their sera at 12–14 weeks of pregnancy
Lv, Yan et al. [12]	Roles of microRNAs in Preeclampsia	2019	No information	Various	Various	Circulating C19MC microRNAs have a role in pre-eclampsia
Miura, Kiyonori et al. [13]	Circulating Chromosome 19 miRNA Cluster microRNAs In Pregnant Women with Severe Pre-Eclampsia	2015	40	Maternal peripheral blood	Real-time PCR	Changes in extracellular microRNA expression are linked to clinically confirmed hypertension and pre-eclampsia
Munjas, Jelena et al. [14]	Non-Coding RNAs in Preeclampsia—Molecular Mechanisms and Diagnostic Potential	2021	No information	Various	Various	Females who subsequently had severe pre-eclampsia had upregulated placental-specific microRNAs in their sera at 12–14 weeks of pregnancy
Murakami, Yuko et al. [15]	Reference Values For Circulating Pregnancy-Associated Micrornas in Maternal Plasma and their Clinical Usefulness in Uncomplicated Pregnancy and Hypertensive Disorder of Pregnancy	2018	33	Maternal peripheral blood	Real-time PCR	Four of the fifteen of the C19MC microRNAs that were examined showed down-regulation in placental tissues when gestational hypertension patients were present
Oostdam, Herrera-Van et al. [16]	Placental Exosomes Isolated from the Urine of Patients with Gestational Diabetes Exhibit a Differential Profile Expression of microRNAs across Gestation	2020	61	Maternal urine samples	Real-time PCR	Pregnancy-related difficulties are caused by several pathological and physiological processes in which microRNAs play a vital role
Qin, Shiting et al. [17]	The Value of Circulating microRNAs for Diagnosis and Prediction of Pre-eclampsia: A Meta-analysis and Systematic Review	2021	4727	Various	Various	The up-regulation of the C19MC microRNAs is a defining feature of pre-eclampsia that has already developed

Table 1. *Cont.*

Author(s)	Title	Year	Sample Size	Source	Method	Outcomes
Špačková, Kamila [2]	First-trimester Screening of Pregnancy-Related Complications Using Plasma Exosomal C19MC microRNAs	2019	97	Maternal peripheral blood	Real-time PCR	Several hypoxia-regulated microRNAs were complicated by extremely preterm fetal growth restriction
Srinivasan, Srimeenakshi et al. [18]	Discovery and Verification of Extracellular miRNA Biomarkers for Non-Invasive Prediction of Pre-Eclampsia in Asymptomatic Women	2020	1097	Various	Various	Used microarray analysis to find 19 mature miRNAs that were differentially expressed in the blood of pregnant women who later had acute pre-eclampsia. Extracellular C19MC microRNAs are capable of distinguishing between individuals at risk of later developing placental sufficiency-related issues and normal pregnancies at the onset of gestation
Ura, Blendi et al. [19]	Potential Role of Circulating Micrornas as Early Markers of Pre-eclampsia	2014	48	Maternal peripheral blood	Real-time PCR	Circulating C19MC microRNAs may contribute to developing pre-eclampsia and prenatal hypertension in early pregnancy
Whigham, Carole-Anne et al. [20]	MicroRNAs 363 and 149 are Differentially Expressed in the Maternal Circulation Preceding a Diagnosis of Pre-eclampsia	2020	46	Maternal peripheral blood	Real-time PCR	Elevated plasma levels of microRNAs were seen in the group of participants with developed pre-eclampsia
Wommack, Joel C., et al. [21]	Micro RNA Clusters in Maternal Plasma are Associated with Preterm Birth and Infant Outcomes	2018	42	Maternal peripheral blood	Real-time PCR	miRNAs act as signaling molecules that coordinate infant outcomes and length of gestation

Table 2. Cochrane Bias Risk Assessment.

Study	(1)	(2)	(3)	(4)	(5)	(6)	(7)
Ali, Asghar et al. [3]	+	+	-	-	?	+	+
Cronqvist, Tina et al. [4]	+	+	-	+	+	+	?
Demirer, Selin et al. [5]	+	+	-	+	+	+	+
He, Xin, and Dan-Ni Ding [6]	+	+	-	-	?	+	+
Hromadnikova, Ilona et al. [1]	+	+	-	-	+	+	?
Jelena, Munjas et al. [7]	+	+	-	+	+	+	+
Jin, Yan et al. [8]	+	+	-	+	+	+	?
Jing, Jia et al. [9]	+	+	-	-	?	+	+
Légaré, Cécilia et al. [10]	+	+	+	+	+	+	+
Li, Hui et al. [11]	+	+	+	+	+	+	+
Lv, Yan et al. [12]	+	+	+	+	+	+	+
Miura, Kiyonori et al. [13]	+	+	+	+	?	+	+
Munjas, Jelena et al. [14]	+	+	-	-	+	+	?
Murakami, Yuko et al. [15]	+	+	+	-	+	+	+
Oostdam, Herrera-Van et al. [16]	+	+	-	+	+	+	+
Qin, Shiting et al. [17]	+	+	-	-	+	+	+
Špačková, Kamila [2]	+	+	-	+	?	+	?
Srinivasan, Srimeenakshi et al. [18]	+	+	+	+	+	+	?
Ura, Blendi et al. [19]	+	+	+	-	+	+	+
Whigham, Carole-Anne et al. [20]	+	+	-	+	+	+	+
Wommack, Joel C., et al. [21]	+	+	-	+	+	+	+

(1) Selection Bias (Random Sequence Generation); (2) Selection Bias (Allocation Concealment); (3) Performance Bias; (4) Detention Bias; (5) Attrition Bias; (6) Reporting Bias; and (7) Other Bias. Symbols: unclear risks (?), high risk (-), and low risk (+).

3. Results

3.1. Study Selection

The results of this review can be categorized according to PRISMA guidelines. The search, identification, and retrieval of articles resulted in a collection of fifty-five publications; ten were retrieved from the databases, and forty-five were from the registers. The fifty-five publications were then checked, and five duplicates were removed. Two articles were removed because of their ineligibility, as marked by RobotAnalyst. Three publications were also removed because they were written in languages other than English. Only thirty-five remaining reports were subjected to screening. The screening process involved checking and evaluating their abstracts and titles to determine their suitability to be included in the review. One publication was excluded because its abstract did not include all the crucial keywords required. The remaining thirty-four articles were sought for retrieval, but only thirty-two were obtained because two publications were inaccessible. The thirty-two reports were assessed for eligibility. Two did not meet the eligibility criteria because one had less than five participants, while the other focused on C19MC microRNA as an early marker of pregnancy-related problems other than pre-eclampsia and hypertension. The remaining thirty publications met the eligibility criteria and were included in the review.

3.2. Study Characteristics

The study characteristics obtained in this review were divided into four groups: author(s), title, year of publication, and outcomes of the reports, as evident in Table 1.

Table 1 shows that only one article was published by one author [2]. All other twenty-nine studies were published by two or more authors. All the publications had different titles directly associated with the research topic. Furthermore, they were published during different periods, as evident via their years of publication. Regarding year of publication, 3.33% of the articles were published in 2013 [1], 2014 [19], or 2015 [13], and 6.67% of the reports were published in 2016 [22,23] and 2019 [2,12]. In addition, 10% of the studies were published in 2017 [4,24,25] and 2018 [15,21,26], while 13.33% of the articles were published in 2021 [3,8,14,17] and 2022 [6,10,27,28]. Finally, 30% of the studies were published in 2020 [5,7,9,11,16,18,20,29,30]. This statistic shows the diversity of the documents' retrieval where their publication years are concerned.

3.3. Risk of Bias in Studies

The results of the Cochrane bias risk assessment are evident in Table 2, which illuminates that all the materials have low reporting and selection bias risks and a high-performance bias risk. A significant number of the other Cochrane method measures underscored low bias risk. These results suggest that all the publications were of good quality and deserved to be included in the review.

3.4. Results of Individual Studies

3.4.1. miRNAs of Different Stages of Preeclampsia

This review discovered informative facts about the role of C19MC microRNA as an early marker of gestational hypertension and pre-eclampsia. For instance, clinically confirmed hypertension and pre-eclampsia have been linked to changes in extracellular microRNA expression [13]. No distinction between fetal and normal pregnancies could be made on the basis of the levels of circulating microRNA expression. Furthermore, according to He and Ding, pre-eclampsia often appears after 20 weeks of pregnancy and is characterized by proteinuria and gestational or chronic hypertension [6]. The condition arises from a problem with placentation, which leads to insufficient uteroplacental blood perfusion and ischemia. Pre-eclampsia is an implantation condition, and its reasons are yet unclear. Its fundamental etiological theory assumes that placentation and insufficient trophoblast invasion are related to a poor adaptation of the local maternal immune system to extra-villous cytotrophoblast produced at the fetal–maternal interface [19].

Czernek and Duchler examined the C19MC microRNA gene expression in simple and complex pregnancies. According to their assertion, there are 56 microRNA genes in the chromosome 19 microRNA cluster. The research focused primarily on microRNAs previously indicated to be substantially present in placental tissues and those reported to be uniquely expressed in them. The research examined C19MC microRNA gene expression in connection with established risk factors for worse perinatal results. Analysis of C19MC microRNA gene expression connected to the degree of clinical symptoms, the doppler ultrasonography parameters, and the delivery date was conducted to determine the severe condition. Complex pregnancies and controls generally have distinct expression profiles for C19MC microRNAs. Pre-eclampsia patients had down-regulation of C19MC microRNAs more often in specific subgroups of pregnancy-related disorders. Further results demonstrated that one C19MC microRNA (miR-517-5p) was changed in pre-eclampsia, necessitating abortion before the nine month gestation period, while five C19MC microRNAs (miR-26b-5p, miR-7-5p, miR-181a-5p, hsa-miR-486-1-5p, and hsa-miR-486-2-5p) in severe preeclamptic pregnancies were dysregulated. The findings imply that the microRNAs have a role in pre-eclampsia's pathophysiology [29].

Additionally, moderate pre-eclampsia that lasted for a few weeks and was closely followed from the time of diagnosis to birth was shown to have a similar expression pattern of placental-specific microRNAs [22]. However, the down-regulation of placental-specific microRNAs seemed to be more profound the longer the pregnancy-related illness persisted. This implies that certain C19MC microRNA dysregulation may represent a compensatory strategy rather than the disease process itself. In another study, Whigham et al. discovered maternal plasma C19MC microRNAs that distinguish between healthy pregnancies and non-pregnancies [20]. More recent research has shown that established pre-eclampsia is characterized by an increase in the circulating miR-526a, miR-525, miR-520a-5p, miR-517-5p, and miR-516-5p genes. While the group of patients with hypertension alongside the control did not have different plasma levels of microRNAs, elevated levels were seen in the group of participants with developed pre-eclampsia [20].

Whigham et al. also note the capacity of extracellular C19MC microRNAs to distinguish between complicated and normal pregnancies at the beginning of pre-eclampsia with or without fetal growth restriction, which was verified using both relative and absolute quantification methods. Unfortunately, there is a lack of information comparing extracellular C19MC microRNA levels in abnormal and normal pregnancies [20]. The study's findings disagree with MacDonald et al., who noted an increase of extracellular miR-520h in four pre-eclampsia patients. The findings prompted an additional investigation into the relationships between circulating C19MC microRNAs and illness severity concerning the degree of delivery needs and clinical symptoms [28].

Furthermore, no correlation among the gene, plasmatic expression, and risk factors for lower C19MC microRNA neonatal levels was found in the association investigation. In both pregnancies with moderate and severe pre-eclampsia, the microRNA plasmatic and gene expression levels were comparable. According to the study's findings, many pathological and physiological processes depend heavily on microRNAs and are to blame for pregnancy-related problems. Consequently, circulating C19MC microRNAs may have a role in the etiology of pre-eclampsia [7]. The research involved increased circulating C19MC microRNAs that characterize the intriguing discovery that developed pre-eclampsia.

miRNAs in the Normal and Abnormal Pregnancies

Even though C19MC microRNAs appear to be down-regulated in the placental tissues in response to a variety of pregnancy-related disorders, including pre-eclampsia and hypertension, as noted above, upregulation of the specific microRNAs appears only in the maternal circulation in pre-eclampsia cases [3]. The contradictory result may be interpreted in several different ways. This recent research by Ali et al. showed that, compared with gestation-matched controls, numerous microRNAs regulated by hypoxia were upregulated in pregnancies affected by significant preterm fetal growth limitation [3]. However, most studies focused on examining pregnancy-related microRNAs whose genes are not found in the miRNA clusters on the chromosome.

A large number of the physiological changes that occur during a typical pregnancy are caused by an acute-phase reaction that is triggered by an inflammatory response. The proximal source of the issues is the placenta [4]. Apoptotic bodies or syncytiotrophoblast microparticles, which include fetus and placenta extracellular nucleic acids, are released by the placenta while it undergoes continuous remodeling throughout normal pregnancy. Cronqvist et al. contended that circulating syncytiotrophoblast exosomes contribute to some syndrome symptoms and maternal inflammation. Pre-eclampsia (PE), hypertension, and other diseases' clinical characteristics may be explained by increased inflammation-related symptoms that are reportedly present in healthy pregnancies at term [4].

According to Jin et al., pre-eclampsia with a clinically confirmed diagnosis is linked to changes in extracellular microRNA expression. However, after the evaluation of circulating microRNA, there was no difference between normal and abnormal pregnancies [8]. Špačková found that several hypoxia-regulated microRNAs were complicated by extremely preterm fetal growth restriction [2]. Nonetheless, most researchers concentrated on investigating microRNAs connected with pregnancy whose genes are not included in the chromosome 19 miRNA clusters or C14MC.

Additionally, Qin et al. further discovered that C19MC microRNAs are present in maternal plasma and have been shown to distinguish between healthy pregnancies and non-pregnancies. They observed increased extracellular C19MC microRNA levels in regularly developing pregnancies. The findings of a follow-up study demonstrated that the up-regulation of the C19MC microRNAs is a defining feature of pre-eclampsia that has already developed [17]. Srinivasan et al. indicated the ability of extracellular C19MC microRNAs to distinguish between individuals at risk of later developing placental-sufficiency-related issues and normal pregnancies at the onset of gestation. The findings emphasized the necessity for further investigation of extracellular microRNAs in maternal circulation with the goal of regular evaluation in daily practice and identification as possible indicators for pregnancy complications linked to placental insufficiency [18].

In addition, Jing et al. asserted that even though fetal growth restriction and pre-eclampsia may be detected using separate serum indicators or maternal plasma, combination screening tests are presently employed in clinical settings to determine the likelihood of developing pre-eclampsia. Pregnancy-associated plasma protein-A, placental growth factor, and, together with maternal blood biomarkers, uterine artery Doppler and maternal risk factors may detect roughly 95% of patients with early-onset pre-eclampsia with a 10% false-positive rate. [9] To enhance the prediction of problems associated with placental insufficiency, additional studies are required to find additional biomarkers with higher diagnostic performance. Jing et al. examined 754 miRNAs and found no predictive value for early pre-eclampsia in first-trimester maternal blood miRNA evaluation. According to miRNA profiling using the high-throughput Open Array TM technology, seven microRNAs have a distinct abundance profile in early pre-eclampsia. Hence, there were no discernible changes between pre-eclampsia and controls after validation by real-time quantitative analysis [9].

3.4.2. miRNA as a Biomarker of Gestational Hypertension

To determine whether a combination of miR-518b and miR-520h biomarkers or a single plasmatic miR-520h biomarker offers valuable tools in the risk assessment for gestational hypertension, several large-scale, multi-center studies, including individuals from various demographics, are required [25]. The rise in extracellular C19MC microRNAs during the first trimester of pregnancy may be related to the down-regulation of various hormones and proteins studied as potential early markers for pre-eclampsia and hypertension. Various diseases, such as gestational hypertension, are associated with placental exosomes' content during pregnancy [27]. Wommack et al. focused on examining the role of miRNAs as signaling molecules. The authors discovered that miRNAs operate as co-regulated groups of signaling molecules to coordinate infant outcomes and gestation length [21].

However, using quantitative RT-PCR to test 30 non-placental microRNAs in maternal mononuclear cells from peripheral blood, Mavreli et al. accurately predicted late pre-eclampsia and miscarriage during the first trimester of pregnancy. The results were assessed with the help of a designed system, awarding points to each participant whose microRNA quantification outcome fell within the top eight. Findings were arranged from the highest to the lowest Ct value for each microRNA. Each patient's unique pregnancy risk score was calculated once the findings of all microRNAs were added together. Four microRNAs had very low values; therefore, they were deemed technically unfit for analysis and were not included in the score [26]. Similarly, Špačková used microarray analysis to find 19 mature miRNAs that were differentially expressed in the blood of pregnant women who later had acute pre-eclampsia. Of them, 12 were upregulated, and 7 were down-regulated during the early gestational phases. In the blood of women who eventually experienced acute pre-eclampsia, mir-1233 was the most overexpressed [2].

In addition, to identify C19MC microRNAs with extracellular placental specificity in maternal circulation as possible biomarkers for problems associated with placental insufficiency, Li et al. suggested the necessity for a more thorough investigation of the microRNAs. Using the absolute and relative quantification methods, the ability of extracellular C19MC microRNAs to distinguish between normal pregnancies and people predisposed to develop intrauterine growth restrictions and pre-eclampsia in early pregnancy was described [11]. The pilot study involved six pregnant women with one early IUGR, four late pre-eclampsias, and one early pre-eclampsia [5]. As the findings revealed that the females who subsequently had severe pre-eclampsia had upregulated placental-specific miR-520a in their sera at 12–14 weeks of pregnancy, Li et al. considerably contributed to validating the findings by Munjas et al. [14]. From the stem-loop and miR-520a* combined, mir-520a (miR-520a-3p) is produced. Akin as well as Li et al. and Hornakova et al. found that circulating miR-517* was upregulated in preeclampsia-prone early pregnancy [11,14,30].

Consequently, subsequent large-scale investigations are required to evaluate the positive predictive value, specificity, and sensitivity of C19MC microRNAs for hypertension or pre-eclampsia. The effectiveness of placental-specific microRNAs for diagnosing disease severity should be assessed in connection with Doppler ultrasonography characteristics, delivery needs, and clinical symptoms [10]. The research produced intriguing results, showing that up-regulation of circulating C19MC microRNAs is a hallmark of early pregnancy, which is predisposed to developing issues linked to gestational hypertension and placental insufficiency. In addition, elevated plasmatic levels of miR-516-5p, miR-518b, and miR-520h in the first trimester alone are strong indicators of future gestational hypertension. One C19MC placental-specific microRNA biomarker may be used to screen for the start of hypertension in the first trimester of pregnancy [23]. Alternately, miR-518b and miR-520h, both placental-specific C19MC microRNA prediction biomarkers, may be combined to forecast the incidence of prenatal hypertension.

3.4.3. Possibilities of Using miRNA in Clinical Diagnostics

Although combinations of second-trimester biochemical indicators, markers, and ultrasonography have been proposed, none has yet shown findings that are sound enough to be used in a therapeutic setting [19]. In the first trimester of maternal serum/plasma samples collected from patients with hypertension or pre-eclampsia, a number of the hypothesized targets of C19MC microRNAs in which the current study was interested were previously shown to be enhanced [10]. Several miRNAs may control the same gene. It is feasible to fully pinpoint the ones responsible for regulating specific genes of interest. Unfortunately, it is difficult to directly interpret experimental outcomes since complex networks typically govern the routes. Most of them target many genes for repression and collectively control them [16]. Hence, as mentioned earlier, pregnancy-related difficulties are caused by several pathological and physiological processes in which microRNAs play a vital role. The literature shows that circulating C19MC microRNAs may contribute to developing pre-eclampsia and prenatal hypertension in early pregnancy.

Furthermore, a different study by Légaré et al. did not find any information about "C19MC microRNA profiling in maternal plasma exosomes during the first trimester of pregnancy" [10]. Instead, it discovered that placental tissues generated from individuals with gestational hypertension and pre-eclampsia after childbirth had the same C19MC microRNA expression profile as first-trimester circulating plasma exosomes. Four of the fifteen C19MC microRNAs that were examined showed down-regulation in placental tissues when GH patients were present [15]. It is similar to the results in placental tissues taken from individuals with gestational hypertension at birth in patients with subsequent occurrences of hypertension. It was discovered after examining the first-trimester maternal plasma exosome C19MC microRNA expression profile of pregnancy, with the selection of only those with diagnostic potential.

In addition, eleven of the fifteen C19MC microRNAs evaluated showed down-regulation in pre-eclampsia patients. Légaré et al. discovered lower levels of miR-525-5p, miR-520a-5p, and miR-517-5p in individuals who subsequently developed pre-eclampsia, broadly matching the expression patterns reported in afflicted placental tissues [10]. The finding are in line with what was revealed in the researcher's previous study. The microRNAs were tested for their diagnostic potential during the first trimester in maternal plasma exosomes of pregnancy. However, the findings are at odds with those of He and Ding, which showed that circulating C19MC microRNAs in maternal plasma were upregulated in the first trimester and accurately predicted the eventual onset of pre-eclampsia or gestational hypertension [6]. From 12 to 14 weeks of pregnancy, other researchers noticed elevated levels of several C19MC microRNAs in sera of women who eventually had severe preeclampsia [10]. Hence, a combination of variables, including those resulting from several different circumstances, may affect the different expression patterns of C19MC microRNAs between maternal plasma and their exosomes. At the very least, a representation of a specific C19MC microRNA expression in maternal plasma can be seen in placental cells from different regions undergoing apoptosis [24]. It releases placental debris into the mother's bloodstream and actively secretes exosomes that promote intercellular communication.

4. Discussion

Research by Hromadnikova et al. revealed no correlation between microRNA and a history of hypertension among individuals with pre-eclampsia that had already developed. The expression of microRNA genes in placental tissues did not alter Doppler ultrasonography parameters linked to worse outcomes in pre-eclampsia. The elevation of pertinent proteins involved in the direction of critical biological processes, including hemocoagulation, apoptosis, stress response, and angiogenesis, may result from the lowered amounts of C19MC microRNAs in placental tissues [1]. Lv et al. further argued that ischemia, hypoxia, insufficient uteroplacental blood perfusion, and defective placental angiogenesis may all lead to blood coagulation–fibrinolysis system failure, aberrant placental trophoblast apoptosis, and, lastly, the emergence of a widespread maternal inflammatory response. Predicted targets of C19MC microRNAs are elevated in placental tissue samples from women who had problems during pregnancy [12].

However, the observed down-regulation of C19MC microRNAs is at odds with the lower levels of several proteins found in the tissue of the placenta in patients with problems in their pregnancies. According to Miura et al., the microRNAs are anticipated to be targeted. There exist modes of fully identifying miRNAs that guide specific genes of value [13]. However, their routes are often complicated control networks that are hard to grasp. Moreover, it complicates the straightforward interpretation of experimental results [27]. Many target several genes for suppression, and they seem collaboratively regulated.

Lastly, the previous theory that exosomes discharged into the body's circulation serve as a non-invasive and singular source of signaling molecules, whose abnormal expression profile mimics that of the parent cells, was supported by this review. It lends credence to the hypothesis that those produced by the placenta may be used in first-trimester screening to detect a sizable fraction of women who may later develop pre-eclampsia or gestational hypertension [21]. The only drawback of the strategy is that since the down-regulation of the same biomarkers begins early in pregnancy, the screening of C19MC microRNAs in plasma exosomes cannot distinguish between the women who will later develop hypertension and those who will have pre-eclampsia during the first trimester of pregnancy. Nevertheless, it may one day lead to the discovery of new microRNA biomarkers that may distinguish between women at risk for gestational hypertension or pre-eclampsia, allowing for the early determent of pre-eclampsia with earlier delivery of low-dose aspirin.

5. Conclusions

In conclusion, this literature review showed that circulating C19MC microRNAs may contribute to developing pre-eclampsia and prenatal hypertension in early pregnancy. In individuals with subsequent occurrences of gestational hypertension and pre-eclampsia, C19MC microRNAs were shown to be down-regulated. The circulating C19MC microRNA expression profile from the first trimester was identical to that in placental tissues collected from individuals with hypertension and pre-eclampsia. Expression analysis of maternal plasma exosomes, as opposed to entire maternal plasma samples, increased the first trimester C19MC microRNA screening's prediction accuracy for detecting hypertension and pre-eclampsia. The results require further confirmation by large-scale investigations. More first-trimester plasma samples must be gathered to achieve a sufficient number of individuals who may later suffer pregnancy-related problems, making conducting the study very difficult.

Author Contributions: Conceptualization, A.K. (Adrianna Kondracka), B.K., D.K., M.R.-K., J.S. and A.K. (Anna Kwaśniewska); methodology, A.K. (Adrianna Kondracka), B.K., I.J., K.F., A.O., A.F. and A.K. (Anna Kwaśniewska); software, B.K., I.J., K.F. and J.S.; validation, A.K. (Adrianna Kondracka), A.O., D.K., M.R.-K., A.F. and A.K. (Anna Kwaśniewska); writing—original draft preparation, A.K. (Adrianna Kondracka), B.K., I.J. and A.F.; writing—review and editing, D.K., K.F., A.O., M.R.-K., J.S. and A.K. (Anna Kwaśniewska); visualization, A.K. (Adrianna Kondracka) and B.K.; supervision, A.K. (Anna Kwaśniewska) and B.K. All authors have read and agreed to the published version of the manuscript.

Funding: The APC was funded by Medical University of Lublin.

Institutional Review Board Statement: Not applicable.

Informed Consent Statement: Not applicable.

Data Availability Statement: Not applicable.

Conflicts of Interest: The authors declare no conflict of interest.

References

1. Hromadnikova, I.; Kotlabova, K.; Ondrackova, M.; Kestlerova, A.; Novotna, V.; Hympanova, L.; Doucha, J.; Krofta, L. Circulating C19MC MicroRNAs in Preeclampsia, Gestational Hypertension, and Fetal Growth Restriction. *Mediat. Inflamm.* **2013**, *2013*, e186041. [CrossRef]
2. Špačková, K. First-Trimester Screening of Pregnancy-Related Complications Using Plasma Exosomal C19MC MicroRNAs. Ph.D. Thesis, Department of Anthropology and Human Genetics, Faculty of Science, Charles University, Prague, Czech Republic, 2019.
3. Ali, A.; Hadlich, F.; Abbas, M.W.; Iqbal, M.A.; Tesfaye, D.; Bouma, G.J.; Winger, Q.A.; Ponsuksili, S. MicroRNA–MRNA Networks in Pregnancy Complications: A Comprehensive Downstream Analysis of Potential Biomarkers. *Int. J. Mol. Sci.* **2021**, *22*, 2313. [CrossRef]
4. Cronqvist, T.; Tannetta, D.; Mörgelin, M.; Belting, M.; Sargent, I.; Familari, M.; Hansson, S.R. Syncytiotrophoblast Derived Extracellular Vesicles Transfer Functional Placental MiRNAs to Primary Human Endothelial Cells. *Sci. Rep.* **2017**, *7*, 4558. [CrossRef] [PubMed]
5. Demirer, S.; Hocaoglu, M.; Turgut, A.; Karateke, A.; Komurcu-Bayrak, E. Expression Profiles of Candidate MicroRNAs in the Peripheral Blood Leukocytes of Patients with Early- and Late-Onset Preeclampsia versus Normal Pregnancies. *Pregnancy Hypertens.* **2020**, *19*, 239–245. [CrossRef] [PubMed]
6. He, X.; Ding, D.-N. Expression and Clinical Significance of MiR-204 in Patients with Hypertensive Disorder Complicating Pregnancy. *BMC Pregnancy Childbirth* **2022**, *22*, 182. [CrossRef] [PubMed]
7. Jelena, M.; Sopić, M.; Joksić, I.; Zmrzljak, U.P.; Karadžov-Orlić, N.; Košir, R.; Egić, A.; Miković, Ž.; Ninić, A.; Spasojević-Kalimanovska, V. Placenta-Specific Plasma MiR518b Is a Potential Biomarker for Preeclampsia. *Clin. Biochem.* **2020**, *79*, 28–33. [CrossRef]
8. Jin, Y.; Jia, T.; Wu, X.; Wang, Y.; Sun, W.; Chen, Y.; Wu, G. The Predictive Value of MicroRNA in Early Hypertensive Disorder Complicating Pregnancy (HDCP). *Am. J. Transl. Res.* **2021**, *13*, 7288–7293.
9. Jing, Y.; Wang, Y.; Quan, Y.; Wang, Z.; Liu, Y.; Ding, Z. Maternal Obesity Alters C19MC MicroRNAs Expression Profile in Fetal Umbilical Cord Blood. *Nutr. Metab.* **2020**, *17*, 52. [CrossRef]
10. Légaré, C.; Desgagné, V.; Poirier, C.; Thibeault, K.; White, F.; Clément, A.-A.; Scott, M.S.; Jacques, P.-É.; Perron, P.; Guérin, R.; et al. First Trimester Plasma MicroRNAs Levels Predict Matsuda Index-Estimated Insulin Sensitivity between 24th and 29th Week of Pregnancy. *BMJ Open Diabetes Res. Care* **2022**, *10*, e002703. [CrossRef] [PubMed]
11. Li, H.; Ouyang, Y.; Sadovsky, E.; Parks, W.T.; Chu, T.; Sadovsky, Y. Unique MicroRNA Signals in Plasma Exosomes from Pregnancies Complicated by Preeclampsia. *Hypertension* **2020**, *75*, 762–771. [CrossRef]
12. Lv, Y.; Lu, C.; Ji, X.; Miao, Z.; Long, W.; Ding, H.; Lv, M. Roles of MicroRNAs in Preeclampsia. *J. Cell. Physiol.* **2019**, *234*, 1052–1061. [CrossRef]
13. Miura, K.; Higashijima, A.; Murakami, Y.; Tsukamoto, O.; Hasegawa, Y.; Abe, S.; Fuchi, N.; Miura, S.; Kaneuchi, M.; Masuzaki, H. Circulating Chromosome 19 MiRNA Cluster MicroRNAs in Pregnant Women with Severe Pre-Eclampsia. *J. Obstet. Gynaecol. Res.* **2015**, *41*, 1526–1532. [CrossRef]
14. Munjas, J.; Sopić, M.; Stefanović, A.; Košir, R.; Ninić, A.; Joksić, I.; Antonić, T.; Spasojević-Kalimanovska, V.; Prosenc Zmrzljak, U. Non-Coding RNAs in Preeclampsia—Molecular Mechanisms and Diagnostic Potential. *Int. J. Mol. Sci.* **2021**, *22*, 10652. [CrossRef]
15. Murakami, Y.; Miura, K.; Sato, S.; Higashijima, A.; Hasegawa, Y.; Miura, S.; Yoshiura, K.; Masuzaki, H. Reference Values for Circulating Pregnancy-Associated MicroRNAs in Maternal Plasma and Their Clinical Usefulness in Uncomplicated Pregnancy and Hypertensive Disorder of Pregnancy. *J. Obstet. Gynaecol. Res.* **2018**, *44*, 840–851. [CrossRef]

16. Herrera-Van Oostdam, A.S.; Toro-Ortíz, J.C.; López, J.A.; Noyola, D.E.; García-López, D.A.; Durán-Figueroa, N.V.; Martínez-Martínez, E.; Portales-Pérez, D.P.; Salgado-Bustamante, M.; López-Hernández, Y. Placental Exosomes Isolated from Urine of Patients with Gestational Diabetes Exhibit a Differential Profile Expression of MicroRNAs across Gestation. *Int. J. Mol. Med.* **2020**, *46*, 546–560. [CrossRef]
17. Qin, S.; Sun, N.; Xu, L.; Xu, Y.; Tang, Q.; Tan, L.; Chen, A.; Zhang, L.; Liu, S. The Value of Circulating MicroRNAs for Diagnosis and Prediction of Preeclampsia: A Meta-Analysis and Systematic Review. *Reprod. Sci.* **2021**, *29*, 3078–3090. [CrossRef]
18. Srinivasan, S.; Treacy, R.; Herrero, T.; Olsen, R.; Leonardo, T.R.; Zhang, X.; DeHoff, P.; To, C.; Poling, L.G.; Fernando, A.; et al. Discovery and Verification of Extracellular MiRNA Biomarkers for Non-Invasive Prediction of Pre-Eclampsia in Asymptomatic Women. *Cell Rep. Med.* **2020**, *1*, 100013. [CrossRef]
19. Ura, B.; Feriotto, G.; Monasta, L.; Bilel, S.; Zweyer, M.; Celeghini, C. Potential Role of Circulating MicroRNAs as Early Markers of Preeclampsia. *Taiwan. J. Obstet. Gynecol.* **2014**, *53*, 232–234. [CrossRef]
20. Whigham, C.-A.; MacDonald, T.M.; Walker, S.P.; Hiscock, R.; Hannan, N.J.; Pritchard, N.; Cannon, P.; Nguyen, T.V.; Miranda, M.; Tong, S.; et al. MicroRNAs 363 and 149 Are Differentially Expressed in the Maternal Circulation Preceding a Diagnosis of Preeclampsia. *Sci. Rep.* **2020**, *10*, 18077. [CrossRef]
21. Wommack, J.C.; Trzeciakowski, J.P.; Miranda, R.C.; Stowe, R.P.; Ruiz, R.J. Micro RNA Clusters in Maternal Plasma Are Associated with Preterm Birth and Infant Outcomes. *PLoS ONE* **2018**, *13*, e0199029. [CrossRef]
22. Kalluri, R.; LeBleu, V.S. Discovery of Double-Stranded Genomic DNA in Circulating Exosomes. *Cold Spring Harb. Symp. Quant. Biol.* **2016**, *81*, 275–280. [CrossRef]
23. Tkach, M.; Théry, C. Communication by Extracellular Vesicles: Where We Are and Where We Need to Go. *Cell* **2016**, *164*, 1226–1232. [CrossRef]
24. Pillay, P.; Moodley, K.; Moodley, J.; Mackraj, I. Placenta-Derived Exosomes: Potential Biomarkers of Preeclampsia. *Int. J. Nanomed.* **2017**, *12*, 8009–8023. [CrossRef]
25. Tomasetti, M.; Lee, W.; Santarelli, L.; Neuzil, J. Exosome-Derived MicroRNAs in Cancer Metabolism: Possible Implications in Cancer Diagnostics and Therapy. *Exp. Mol. Med.* **2017**, *49*, e285. [CrossRef]
26. Mavreli, D.; Papantoniou, N.; Kolialexi, A. MiRNAs in Pregnancy-Related Complications: An Update. *Expert Rev. Mol. Diagn.* **2018**, *18*, 587–589. [CrossRef]
27. Ghafourian, M.; Mahdavi, R.; Akbari Jonoush, Z.; Sadeghi, M.; Ghadiri, N.; Farzaneh, M.; Mousavi Salehi, A. The Implications of Exosomes in Pregnancy: Emerging as New Diagnostic Markers and Therapeutics Targets. *Cell Commun. Signal.* **2022**, *20*, 51. [CrossRef]
28. MacDonald, T.M.; Walker, S.P.; Hannan, N.J.; Tong, S.; Kaitu'u-Lino, T.J. Clinical Tools and Biomarkers to Predict Preeclampsia. *eBioMedicine* **2022**, *75*, 103780. [CrossRef]
29. Czernek, L.; Düchler, M. Exosomes as Messengers between Mother and Fetus in Pregnancy. *Int. J. Mol. Sci.* **2020**, *21*, 4264. [CrossRef]
30. Hornakova, A.; Kolkova, Z.; Holubekova, V.; Loderer, D.; Lasabova, Z.; Biringer, K.; Halasova, E. Diagnostic Potential of MicroRNAs as Biomarkers in the Detection of Preeclampsia. *Genet. Test. Mol. Biomark.* **2020**, *24*, 321–327. [CrossRef]

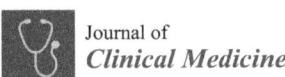

Article

The UA Doppler Index, Plasma HCY, and Cys C in Pregnancies Complicated by Congenital Heart Disease of the Fetus

Xiaona Xu [1,2,†], Baoying Ye [3,†], Min Li [1], Yuanqing Xia [1], Yi Wu [1,2,*] and Weiwei Cheng [1,2,4,*]

1. Prenatal Diagnosis Center, The International Peace Maternity and Child Health Hospital, School of Medicine, Shanghai Jiao Tong University, Shanghai 200030, China
2. Shanghai Key Laboratory of Embryo Original Diseases, Shanghai 200030, China
3. Department of Ultrasonography, The International Peace Maternity and Child Health Hospital, School of Medicine, Shanghai Jiao Tong University, Shanghai 200030, China
4. Shanghai Municipal Key Clinical Specialty, Shanghai 200030, China
* Correspondence: thomasguo1122@163.com (Y.W.); wwcheng29@shsmu.edu.cn (W.C.); Tel.: +86-021-64070434 (Y.W. & W.C.)
† These authors contributed equally to this work.

Abstract: Background: Congenital heart disease/defect (CHD) is one of the most common congenital disabilities. Early diagnosis of CHD can improve the prognosis of newborns with CHD. The aim of this study was to evaluate the relationship between the factors and the onset of fetal congenital heart disease by measuring fetal umbilical artery (UA) Doppler index, maternal HCY, and Cys C levels during pregnancy. Methods: This retrospective study analyzed 202 fetuses with CHD, including 77 cases (39.1%) of simple CHD and 120 cases (60.9%) of complex CHD. Singleton pregnant women who were examined at the same time and whose malformation screening did not suggest any structural abnormalities in the fetus were assigned to the control group ($n = 400$). The UA Doppler index, plasma HCY, and Cys C levels were compared among the pregnant women across the three groups, and logistic regression analysis was performed on statistically significant markers. The ROC of UA S/D, PI, RI, HCY, and Cys C were plotted, and the area under the ROC (AUC) was calculated. Results: The UA S/D, PI, and RI in the complex CHD group were significantly higher than those in the control group ($p < 0.05$). The levels of HCY and Cys C in the CHD group were significantly higher than those in the control group ($p < 0.05$). HCY and S/D revealed a positive correlation ($r = 0.157$), and the difference was statistically significant ($p < 0.001$). Cys C and S/D were positively correlated ($r = 0.131$), and the difference was statistically significant ($p < 0.05$). The levels of UA Doppler indices, maternal plasma HCY, and Cys C were elevated in fetuses with CHD. The AUC of the combined test of the UA index, HCY, and Cys C was higher than that of each individual test. Conclusions: Elevated levels of the UA doppler indices, HCY, and Cys C during pregnancy are positively associated with the development of congenital heart disease in offspring. The combination of HCY and Cys C was the most efficient test for the diagnosis of CHD. We are the first to report that plasma Cys C levels of women pregnant with fetuses with CHD were higher than those of women pregnant with normal fetuses.

Keywords: congenital heart disease; homocysteine; cystatin C; the UA Doppler index

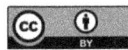

1. Introduction

Congenital heart disease/defect (CHD) is one of the most common congenital disabilities, with a prevalence rate of 1 in 100 live births. It is one of the leading causes of perinatal mortality [1]. With the rapid development of prenatal imaging technologies, the application of fetal echocardiogram to detect CHD has advanced, and the use of color Doppler noninvasive detection of fetal hemodynamic changes is also becoming gradually common. Several studies have reported [2–4] that the increase in maternal plasma homocysteine (HCY) level is closely associated with cardiac malformations in their offspring.

The maternal plasma cystatin C (Cys C) is a biomarker of early kidney injury [5] and also a novel cardiac biomarker [6] independently associated with the risk of cardiovascular anomalies and mortality. The relationship between Cys C level during pregnancy and the occurrence of fetal CHD has not been reported yet. In this study, we aimed to determine the relationship between the factors and the onset of fetal congenital heart disease by measuring fetal umbilical artery (UA) Doppler index, maternal HCY, and Cys C levels during pregnancy.

2. Materials and Methods

2.1. Patient Cohort

The present study is a retrospective study. Fetal cases diagnosed as CHD by fetal cardiography in International Peace Maternity and Child Health Hospital from January 2015 to December 2021 were enrolled in the CHD group. Fetal cases with normal anomaly scans were enrolled in the control group. Electric clinical medical charts were reviewed to obtain demographic information on maternal age and pregestational body mass index (BMI). Serological screening results of maternal plasma HCY and Cys C level at 12–14 weeks of gestation were also collected from the medical charts.

The inclusion criteria were as follows: fetuses with CHD were included in the CHD group. The control group was normal fetuses without structural malformation matched with maternal age and gestational age, and a 1:2 ratio was used. The exclusion criteria were as follows: fetuses with CHD combined with extracardiac anomalies, multiple pregnancies, and pregnancies with maternal obstetric complications.

This study was approved by the Medical Ethics Committee of the International Peace Maternity and Child Health Hospital (GKLW 2019-24). Written informed consent was obtained from the pregnant women involved in our study.

CHD was diagnosed by ultrasound and clinical diagnosis. Based on the codes of the International Classification of Diseases, Ninth Revision, Clinical Modification, complex CHD (CCHD) refers to all types of CHD except for simple CHD (SCHD). The main types of SCHD included ventricular septal defect (VSD), aortic valve stenosis, pulmonary stenosis, patent ductus arteriosus, and secundum atrial septal defects The fetal heart defects that were not included in the study were persistent left superior vena cava, simple right aortic arch, aberrant right subclavian artery, and heart tumors. The main types of CCHD include tetralogy of Fallot (TOF), tricuspid atresia and stenosis, coarctation of the aorta, hypoplastic right heart syndrome, tricuspid valve dysplasia, atrioventricular septal defect, single ventricle, interruption of aortic arch, pulmonary atresia, persistent truncus arteriosus, hypertrophic cardiomyopathy, vascular ring, hypoplastic left heart syndrome, transposition of great arteries, and double outlet right ventricle [7,8].

2.2. Fetal Echocardiogram

The gestational age range for echocardiography was 18–28 weeks. Detection of fetal echocardiography was performed based on the Guidelines of the International Society of Ultrasound in Obstetrics and Gynecology (ISUOG) [9]. Ultrasound examination was performed by radiologists with prenatal ultrasound diagnostic qualifications using GE Voluson E10 (GE Healthcare, Zipf, Austria), Philips iU Elite (Philips, Copenhagen, Denmark), or Philips iE33 (Philips, Copenhagen, Denmark). Subjects were kept a flat, lying position and exposed their lower abdomen. The number of fetuses was routinely checked, multiple pregnancies were excluded, and the fetal orientation was determined. The transverse and four-chamber heart section of the fetal abdomen was determined along with the position of the internal organs, the heart, and the cardiac axis. Based on this, the left and right ventricular outflow tract, long axis and short axis section, three-vessel section or three-vessel tracheal section, aortic arch section, ductus arteriosus arch section, and the vein-atrial connection section determined the fetal atrioventricular connection relationship. The left and right atrioventricular valves determined the fetal ventricular–artery connection relationship. The interrelationship between the great arteries, the ratio of the inner diameter of the aortic arch and the ductus arteriosus, and finally the measurement results were collected and stored.

All fetuses with CHD were diagnosed by two experienced fetal echocardiographists. Postnatal results were obtained from the newborn's examination records at the hospital or directly from the parents. For CHD cases, neonatal echocardiograpy was performed by another examiner (approximately 2–4 days after birth) prior to discharge. A clinical examination by an experienced pediatrician included auscultation of the heart murmur and oxygen saturation of the upper and lower extremities. The newborn/fetus was considered normal if no abnormalities were suspected or found.

2.3. The UA Doppler Index at 22–24 Weeks of Pregnancy

When ultrasound fetal malformation screening was performed at 22 to 24 weeks of pregnancy, after detecting the free segment of the umbilical cord, the umbilical artery blood flow spectrum was obtained. When measuring the umbilical artery spectrum, pregnant women had to hold their breath for 3–5 s to facilitate the acquisition of a stable umbilical artery spectrum. The indices of systolic/diastolic ratio (S/D), resistance index (RI), and pulsatility index (PI) were measured and recorded.

2.4. Blood Sampling and Biochemical Characteristics at 12–14 Weeks of Pregnancy

Pregnant women underwent fasting after 22:00 on the day before the first antenatal examination in the 12th to 14th weeks of pregnancy. A total of 3 mL of venous blood was drawn on an empty stomach at 08:00–10:00 on the day of examination. The serum was routinely separated, and the levels of Hcy and Cys C were measured. The automatic biochemical analyzer was used for detection, and the detection of various indicators was performed according to the instructions given in the kit.

2.5. Statistical Analysis

SPSS 25.0 statistical software was used for analysis. The measurement data following the normal distribution were expressed as a one-way analysis of variance. The data are expressed as mean ± standard deviation. The comparison of the counting data is expressed by the Wilcoxon rank sum test, and the data are expressed as frequencies. Pearson's (r) correlation was performed to analyze the correlation between maternal plasma HCY, Cys C level, and the UA doppler indices, and the logistic regression analysis of the various influencing factors of fetal congenital heart disease was performed. A p-value < 0.05 indicated that the difference was statistically significant.

3. Results

A total of 197 fetuses with CHD were assessed, which included 77 cases (39.1%) of simple CHD and 120 cases (60.9%) of complex CHD. The type of CHD is depicted in Table 1. The demographic characteristics of the patients in the CHD groups and the healthy control groups are depicted in Table 2. The mean maternal age and pregestational BMI were not significantly different between the CHD and control groups ($p > 0.05$; Table 2).

3.1. The Comparison of the UA Doppler Indices at 22–24 Weeks of Pregnancy between the CHD and Control Groups

The UA S/D, PI, and RI in the complex CHD group were significantly higher than those in the control group (3.43 ± 0.84, 1.18 ± 0.19, 0.70 ± 0.06 vs. 3.21 ± 0.57, 1.12 ± 0.16, 0.68 ± 0.05; $p < 0.05$, respectively). No statistically significant difference was noted in the UA Doppler indices between the simple CHD group and the complex CHD group. In addition, no statistically significant difference was noted in the UA Doppler indices between the simple CHD group and the control group (Table 3).

Table 1. Antenatal cardiac finding in all cases of CHD.

Groups	Type of CHD	n
Simple CHD group	VSD	74
	PS	3
Complex CHD group	TOF	29
	TGA	16
	COA	14
	HLHS	10
	DORV	9
	HRHS	6
	TVD	6
	AVSD	5
	Vascular ring	4
	SV	6
	IAA	3
	PS + VSD	3
	PA	2
	TA	2
	PTA	2
	HCM	2
	Ebstein's anomaly	1
Total		197

VSD, ventricular septal defect; COA, coarctation of the aorta; PS, pulmonary stenosis, TOF, tetralogy of Fallot; TGA, transposition of great arteries; HLHS, hypoplastic left heart syndrome; HRHS, hypoplastic right heart syndrome; DORV, double outlet of right ventricle; TVD, tricuspid valve dysplasia; AVSD, atrioventricular septal defect; SV, single ventricle; IAA, interruption of aortic arch; PA, pulmonary atresia; TA, tricuspid atresia; PTA, persistent truncus arteriosus; HCM, hypertrophic cardiomyopathy.

Table 2. Maternal characteristics of the case and control group.

Characteristics	Simple CHD Group Mean ± SD	Complex CHD Group Mean ± SD	Control Group Mean ± SD	p
Maternal age (y)	31.96 ± 5.41	31.29 ± 4.54	31.07 ± 3.70	>0.05
Pregestational BMI	21.84 ± 3.38	21.28 ± 3.01	21.31 ± 2.92	>0.05

Table 3. Comparison of the UA Doppler indices at 22–24 weeks of pregnancy.

Groups	n	UA S/D Mean ± SD	UA PI Mean ± SD	UA RI Mean ± SD
CHD group	197	3.40 ± 0.79	1.17 ± 0.21	0.69 ± 0.06
Simple CHD group	77	3.35 ± 0.70	1.16 ± 0.24	0.69 ± 0.06
Complex CHD group	120	3.43 ± 0.84	1.18 ± 0.19	0.70 ± 0.06
Control group	400	3.21 ± 0.57	1.12 ± 0.16	0.68 ± 0.05
p	Simple CHD vs. Complex CHD	0.826	0.517	0.262
	Simple CHD vs. Control group	0.288	0.055	0.254
	Complex CHD vs. Control group	0.022	0.001	0.003

3.2. The Comparison of Maternal Plasma HCY and Cys C Levels at 12–14 Weeks of Pregnancy

The levels of HCY and Cys C in the simple CHD group were significantly higher than those in the control group ($p < 0.05$). The HCY and Cys C levels in the complex CHD group were significantly higher than those in the control group, and the difference was statistically significant ($p < 0.05$). However, the difference in the HCY and Cys C levels between the simple and complex CHD groups was not statistically significant (Table 4).

Table 4. Comparison of HCY and Cys C levels at 12–14 weeks of pregnancy.

Groups		n	HCY (μmol/L) Mean ± SD	Cys C (mg/L) Mean ± SD
CHD group		197	4.56 ± 2.04	0.55 ± 0.11
Simple CHD group		77	4.35 ± 1.66	0.56 ± 0.12
Complex CHD group		120	4.69 ± 2.24	0.54 ± 0.11
Control group		400	3.78 ± 1.44	0.51 ± 0.10
	Simple CHD vs. Complex CHD		0.162	0.695
p	Simple CHD vs. Control group		0.005	0.007
	Complex CHD vs. Control group		<0.001	0.032

3.3. Correlation between the Plasma Biochemical Indicators and the UA Doppler Indices

Pearson's correlation was applied to analyze the maternal plasma HCY and Cys C levels and the UA Doppler indices. The results revealed that HCY and S/D had a positive correlation with PI (r = 0.157, 0.088; $p < 0.05$, respectively). Cys C and S/D, PI, and RI were positively correlated (r = 0.131, 0.118, 0.118; $p < 0.05$, respectively) (Tables 5–7).

Table 5. Pearson correlation of UA S/D with HCY and Cys C.

Variable	r	p
HCY	0.157	<0.001
Cys C	0.131	0.001

Table 6. Pearson correlation of UA PI and HCY with Cys C.

Variable	r	p
HCY	0.088	0.031
Cys C	0.118	0.004

Table 7. Pearson correlation of UA RI and HCY with Cys C.

Variable	r	p
HCY	0.066	0.108
Cys C	0.118	0.004

3.4. Analysis of the Influencing Factors of Fetal Congenital Heart Disease

Multifactorial logistic regression equations were constructed by including age, pregestational BMI, UA S/D, UA PI, UA RI, and maternal plasma HCY and Cys C levels with the presence or absence of CHD as the dependent variable. The results showed that the effect of UA S/D, PI, RI, and the level of maternal plasma HCY and Cys C on fetal CHD were statistically significant ($p < 0.05$). The ORs for UA RI and Cys C were especially high (69.55 and 24.75) (Table 8).

Table 8. Logistic regression analysis.

Variable	B	S.E.	Wald	p	OR	95%CI
Maternal age	0.03	0.02	1.80	0.179	1.03	0.99–1.07
Pregestational BMI	0.02	0.03	0.53	0.469	1.02	0.97–1.08
UA S/D	0.43	0.13	10.44	0.001	1.54	1.19–2.00
UA PI	1.61	0.49	10.97	0.001	5.01	1.93–12.98
UA RI	4.24	1.54	7.55	0.006	69.55	3.38–1433.25
HCY	0.31	0.06	26.40	<0.001	1.37	1.21–1.54
Cys C	3.21	0.46	27.42	<0.001	24.75	4.75–129.10

The ROC of UA S/D, PI, RI, HCY, and Cys C were plotted, and the area under the ROC (AUC) was calculated. The binary logistic regression analysis was used to obtain the cut-off value of the combined prediction probability of each index to evaluate the sensitivity and specificity of the individual and combined tests for the diagnosis of CHD. The value of the individual and combined tests for the diagnosis of CHD was analyzed. The results showed that the AUC of the combined test of HCY and Cys C was higher than that of each individual test, and its optimal cut-off value was 0.371, and the sensitivity and specificity for the diagnosis of CHD were 45.7% and 78.5%, respectively (Table 9, Figure 1).

Table 9. The area under the ROC.

Variable	Threshold	Sensitivity (%)	Specificity (%)	Area	S.E.	p	95%CI
UA S/D	3.265	51.8	59.2	0.565	0.03	0.010	0.52–0.61
UA PI	1.065	75.1	39.5	0.567	0.03	0.008	0.52–0.62
UA RI	0.685	57.9	52.2	0.564	0.03	0.011	0.52–0.61
HCY	3.850	63.5	56.0	0.626	0.02	<0.001	0.58–0.67
Cys C	0.515	60.4	54.5	0.589	0.03	<0.001	0.54–0.64
S/D + PI + RI	0.307	64.5	52.5	0.574	0.03	0.003	0.53–0.62
HCY + Cys C	0.371	45.7	78.5	0.651	0.02	<0.001	0.60–0.70

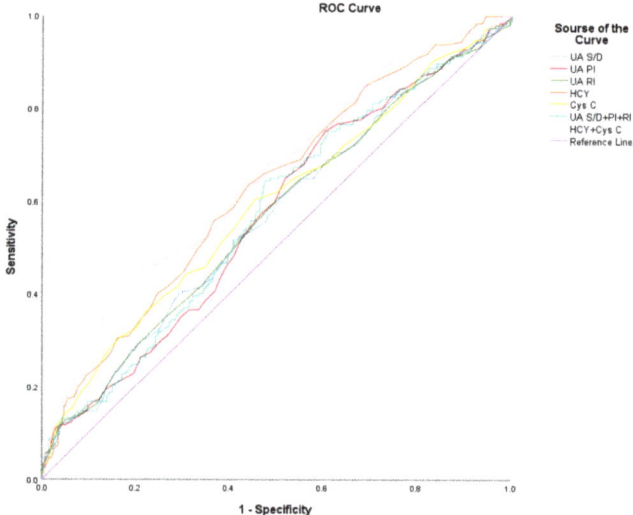

Figure 1. ROC Curve.

4. Discussion

The umbilical cord is the only channel through which any material can be transmitted between the mother and the fetus. Therefore, the umbilical artery blood contains a large amount of fetal–placental circulation information, and the UA S/D, PI, and RI reflect the placental resistance and the fetal intrauterine condition. In the first trimester of pregnancy, the resistance of umbilical artery blood flow is high. With the progression of pregnancy, to ensure the blood supply of normal fetal development, the placenta gradually matures, the villus increases and thickens, the resistance of the placental blood vessels decreases, and the blood flow increases. If the placenta function is poor, the placental vascular spasm, infarction, edema, and other conditions make the lumen narrow, which results in increased fetal–placental circulatory resistance and reduced umbilical artery blood flow. This affects the development and growth of the fetus [10]. Previous studies [11,12] have reported that in cases of isolated major fetal heart defects, maternal serum placental growth factor (PlGF) decreases at 11–13 weeks of gestation, which indicates that placental angiogenesis was impaired in the first trimester of pregnancy. Moreover, the overexpression of vascular endothelial growth factor A, soluble FMS-like tyrosine kinase-1 (sFlt-1), and soluble endocrine in fetuses with congenital heart disease were observed in their heart tissue and cord blood. Maternal blood PlGF levels were decreased, and sFlt-1 levels were increased at 18–37 weeks of gestation. This indicated that placental angiogenesis is affected when the fetus has congenital heart disease [10]. A study [13] reported that increased UA PI is associated with CHD in the fetus. Another study [14] reported that regardless of the type of congenital heart disease, the UA PI increased as the pregnancy progressed, which suggested that the degree of placental damage increased with the progression of pregnancy. We found that UA S/D, PI, and RI of the fetuses with CHD were higher than those of normal fetuses, and UA S/D, PI, and RI were particularly increased in the fetuses with complex CHD. UA hemodynamic changes are a good indicator of changes in placental functions [15], and the increase in UA Doppler indices in the second trimester in the CHD group in this study indicated possible placental function impairment in the second trimester of pregnancy, reflecting that CHD occurrence is associated with placental hypofunction, followed by placental ischemia and hypoxia and fetal ischemia and hypoxia, ultimately leading to adverse pregnancy outcomes. Based on previously reported studies, echocardiography is recommended in fetuses with increased UA Doppler indices in the second trimester to detect fetal heart defects as soon as possible and improve the prenatal diagnosis rate of fetal CHD. In case fetal echocardiography indicates a fetus with CHD, ultrasound should be performed regularly to measure the blood flow index of the UA to assess the growth and development of the fetus, monitor the intrauterine safety of the fetus, terminate the pregnancy on time, and ensure that newborns with CHD receive timely treatment.

This study also showed that the HCY of the simple CHD group was higher than that of the control group, and the difference was statistically significant ($p < 0.05$). The HCY level of the complex CHD group was significantly higher than that of the control group ($p < 0.001$). Previous studies [4,16,17] have shown that hyperhomocysteinemia in pregnant women may be associated with CHD occurrence in their offspring, and the present study also confirmed that high maternal HCY levels are associated with fetal cardiac malformation. HCY can pass through the placental barrier and exert cytotoxic effects, inducing excessive apoptosis in early embryonic cells, impairing placental functions, and causing embryonic malformations [18]. The abnormal differentiation of neural crest cells at high HCY concentrations may lead to neural tube defects and abnormal cardiac development [19]. If the maternal plasma HCY level can be determined in the first trimester of pregnancy, hyperhomocysteinemia can be detected as early as possible, and early screening for fetal congenital heart disease in pregnant women with hyperhomocysteinemia can be performed. Such women can be supplemented with an appropriate diet and nutrition.

Cys C is a non-glycosyl alkaline protein belonging to cysteine protease inhibitors. Previous studies showed [20,21] that Cys C can be reabsorbed and completely degraded at the proximal tubule after glomerular filtration; hence, Cys C is less affected by factors such as age, sex, weight, diet, lipid metabolism, and inflammation. Cys C levels may be associated with cardiovascular disease. Cys C impairs the cardiovascular system by affecting smooth muscle cell functions, coagulation, lipid peroxidation, and endothelial cell functions [22]. We found that Cys C levels of the subjects who were pregnant with fetuses with CHD were significantly higher than those of the normal control group ($p < 0.05$). Infants and children with CHD have increased Cys C levels, and Cys C can be used as a biomarker to predict postoperative complications of acute kidney injury after undergoing cardiac surgery [23,24]. The relationship between maternal plasma Cys C and fetal CHD has not been reported. To the best of our knowledge, we are the first to report that plasma Cys C levels of women pregnant with fetuses with CHD were higher than those of women pregnant with normal fetuses. Future studies are necessary for establishing a correlation between newborn plasma Cys C, placental Cys C, and maternal plasma Cys C levels in CHD for better understanding.

A strong positive correlation exists between Cys C levels and HCY. Cys C is a strong independent predictor of long-term all-cause death and major adverse cardiac events in elderly patients with acute myocardial infarction. The combined detection of Cys C and HCY further improves the predictive value [25]. Cys C can inhibit HCY decomposition, increase its concentration in blood, and interact with factors including plasma HCY and histones, thereby increasing the risk of hypertension and gestational diabetes in pregnant women and further increasing the risk of premature birth, miscarriage, and fetal intrauterine growth restriction [26]. The accumulated HCY in the body passes through the placental barrier; if the endothelial function of the blood vessels in the placenta is impaired, the vascular resistance in the placenta increases, which damages placental functions, affecting the blood flow motility of the UA and eventually increasing UA blood flow resistance. This study showed that increased UA Doppler indices and maternal plasma HCY and Cys C levels affected the fetuses suffering from CHD. A positive correlation was observed between maternal plasma HCY and Cys C levels and UA Doppler indices. From the clinical perspective, fetal echocardiography is a routine part of prenatal screening and is only added if a possible abnormality in heart development is detected during fetal systemic ultrasound or if there are high-risk factors for CHD, so some congenital heart diseases are not detected prenatally and are detected after birth due to presence of cardiac symptoms. The early detection of high HCY and Cys C levels in the first trimester of pregnancy or the high UA Doppler indices in the second trimester of pregnancy will help assist fetal echocardiography in fetal CHD diagnosis. This will improve the detection rate of fetal CHD, thereby increasing the rate of neonatal treatment and reducing neonatal mortality.

A limitation of our study was that not all heart malformations can be diagnosed by ultrasound in the fetus, which might lead to a possible statistical bias in our results. Fetal cardiac structure screening mainly relies on prenatal echocardiography. For those simple CHDs, such as isolated ventricular septal defect, the diagnostic accuracy of fetal echocardiography is not very high. This is mainly because some defects would close spontaneously during pregnancy or after birth. Echocardiography is not routinely performed on newborns after birth, but only newborns diagnosed with CHD in the fetal period require an echocardiogram after birth and a clinical examination of each newborn by an experienced pediatrician, including auscultation of heart murmurs and oxygen saturation of the upper and lower extremities. Another limitation of the present study was that the blood testing and UA Doppler were not performed in the same time, which could also cause some biases in the results. In the subsequent study design, we would consider performing the blood sampling and ultrasound in the same gestational age.

5. Conclusions

To summarize, UA S/D, PI, and RI values of the fetuses with CHD, especially complex CHD, were significantly higher than those of normal fetuses. The maternal plasma HCY and Cys C levels of women pregnant with fetuses with CHD increased significantly. Maternal plasma HCY, Cys C, and UA Doppler indices were positively correlated, which were increased in fetal CHD. The detection of increased HCY and Cys C in the first trimester of pregnancy suggests an increased risk of fetal CHD, and fetal echocardiography is required in the second trimester, indicating the screening value of increased HCY and Cys C levels in the first trimester of pregnancy. In this study, we only analyzed the relationship between maternal plasma HCY and Cys C levels in the first trimester of pregnancy, UA Doppler indices, and fetal CHD. Prospective application of these results in a validation study is still required to evaluate the clinical utility of these markers or a combination of these markers. In future large-sized studies, researchers need to investigate maternal blood indicators in the first, second, and third trimesters of pregnancy and make longitudinal comparisons to explore the correlation between various indicators and fetal CHD. A few studies on the correlation between maternal plasma Cys C and fetal CHD are available. In the future, the effect of plasma Cys C on fetal CHD can be analyzed in depth by conducting basic trials combined with prospective clinical studies, which can help to detect congenital disabilities as early as possible and reduce the incidence of adverse outcomes.

Author Contributions: Supervision, W.C.; writing—original draft, X.X.; writing—review and editing, Y.W. and B.Y.; software, Y.X.; visualization, M.L. All authors have read and agreed to the published version of the manuscript.

Funding: This research was funded by the Shanghai Committee of Science and Technology, China, grant number 18411963500.

Institutional Review Board Statement: The study was conducted in accordance with the Declaration of Helsinki and approved by the Ethics Committee of IPMCH (GKLW 2019-24).

Informed Consent Statement: Informed consent was obtained from all subjects involved in the study.

Data Availability Statement: The data presented in this study are openly available in FigShare at 10.6084/m9.figshare.21300045.

Conflicts of Interest: The authors declare no conflict of interest.

References

1. Hoffman, J.I.; Kaplan, S. The incidence of congenital heart disease. *J. Am. Coll. Cardiol.* **2002**, *39*, 1890–1900. [CrossRef]
2. Kapusta, L.; Haagmans, M.L.; Steegers, E.A.; Cuypers, M.H.; Blom, H.J.; Eskes, T.K. Congenital heart defects and maternal derangement of homocysteine metabolism. *J. Pediatr.* **1999**, *135*, 773–774. [CrossRef]
3. Verkleij-Hagoort, A.C.; Verlinde, M.; Ursem, N.T.C.; Lindemans, J.; Helbing, W.A.; Ottenkamp, J.; Siebel, F.M.H.; Gittenberger-de Groot, A.C.; De Jonge, R.; Bartelings, M.M.; et al. Maternal hyperhomocysteinaemia is a risk factor for congenital heart disease. *Bjog* **2006**, *113*, 1412–1418. [CrossRef] [PubMed]
4. Elizabeth, K.E.; Praveen, S.L.; Preethi, N.R.; Jissa, V.T.; Pillai, M.R. Folate, vitamin B12, homocysteine and polymorphisms in folate metabo-lizing genes in children with congenital heart disease and their mothers. *Eur. J. Clin. Nutr.* **2017**, *71*, 1437–1441. [CrossRef]
5. He, L.; Li, J.; Zhan, J.; Yi, F.; Fan, X.; Wei, Y.; Zhang, W. The value of serum cystatin C in early evaluation of renal insufficiency in patients undergoing chemotherapy: A systematic review and meta-analysis. *Cancer Chemother. Pharmacol.* **2019**, *83*, 561–571. [CrossRef]
6. Loew, M.; Hoffmann, M.M.; Koenig, W.; Brenner, H.; Rothenbacher, D. Genotype and plasma concentration of cystatin C in patients with coronary heart disease and risk for secondary cardiovascular events. *Arterioscler. Thromb Vasc. Biol.* **2005**, *25*, 1470–1474. [CrossRef]
7. Marelli, A.J.; Mackie, A.S.; Ionescu-Ittu, R.; Rahme, E.; Pilote, L. Congenital heart disease in the general population: Changing prevalence and age distribution. *Circulation* **2007**, *115*, 163–172. [CrossRef]
8. Matthiesen, N.B.; Henriksen, T.B.; Agergaard, P.; Gaynor, J.W.; Bach, C.C.; Hjortdal, V.E.; Østergaard, J.R. Congenital Heart Defects and Indices of Placental and Fetal Growth in a Nationwide Study of 924 422 Liveborn Infants. *Circulation* **2016**, *134*, 1546–1556. [CrossRef]
9. Carvalho, J.S.; Allan, L.D.; Chaoui, R.; Copel, J.A.; DeVore, G.R.; Hecher, K.; Lee, W.; Munoz, H.; Paladini, D.; Tutschek, B.; et al. ISUOG Practice Guidelines (updated): Sonographic screening examination of the fetal heart. *Ultrasound Obstet. Gynecol.* **2013**, *41*, 348. [CrossRef]
10. Llurba, E.; Sánchez, O.; Ferrer, Q.; Nicolaides, K.H.; Ruíz, A.; Domínguez, C.; Sánchez-de-Toledo, J.; García-García, B.; Soro, G.; Arévalo, S.; et al. Maternal and foetal angiogenic imbalance in congenital heart defects. *Eur. Heart J.* **2014**, *35*, 701–707. [CrossRef]
11. Llurba, E.; Syngelaki, A.; Sánchez, O.; Carreras, E.; Cabero, L.; Nicolaides, K.H. Maternal serum placental growth factor at 11–13 weeks' gestation and fetal cardiac defects. *Ultrasound Obstet. Gynecol.* **2013**, *42*, 169–174. [CrossRef] [PubMed]
12. Fantasia, I.; Kasapoglu, D.; Kasapoglu, T.; Syngelaki, A.; Akolekar, R.; Nicolaides, K.H. Fetal major cardiac defects and placental dysfunction at 11–13 weeks' gestation. *Ultrasound Obstet. Gynecol.* **2018**, *51*, 194–198. [CrossRef] [PubMed]
13. Yamamoto, Y.; Khoo, N.S.; Brooks, P.A.; Savard, W.; Hirose, A.; Hornberger, L.K. Severe left heart obstruction with retrograde arch flow influences fetal cer-ebral and placental blood flow. *Ultrasound Obstet. Gynecol.* **2013**, *42*, 294–299. [CrossRef] [PubMed]
14. Ruiz, A.; Cruz-Lemini, M.; Masoller, N.; Sanz-Cortés, M.; Ferrer, Q.; Ribera, I.; Martínez, J.M.; Crispi, F.; Arévalo, S.; Gómez, O.; et al. Longitudinal changes in fetal biometry and cerebroplacental hemodynamics in fetuses with congenital heart disease. *Ultrasound Obstet. Gynecol.* **2017**, *49*, 379–386. [CrossRef]
15. Dubiel, M.; Gunnarsson, G.O.; Gudmundsson, S. Blood redistribution in the fetal brain during chronic hypoxia. *Ultrasound Obstet. Gynecol.* **2002**, *20*, 117–121. [CrossRef] [PubMed]
16. Kalisch-Smith, J.I.; Ved, N.; Sparrow, D.B. Environmental Risk Factors for Congenital Heart Disease. *Cold Spring Harb. Perspect. Biol.* **2020**, *12*, a037234. [CrossRef]

17. Hobbs, C.A.; James, S.J.; Jernigan, S.; Melnyk, S.; Lu, Y.; Malik, S.; Cleves, M.A. Congenital heart defects, maternal homocysteine, smoking, and the 677 C > T polymorphism in the methylenetetrahydrofolate reductase gene: Evaluating gene-environment interactions. *Am. J. Obstet. Gynecol.* **2006**, *194*, 218–224. [CrossRef]
18. Hobbs, C.A.; Malik, S.; Zhao, W.; James, S.J.; Melnyk, S.; Cleves, M.A. Maternal homocysteine and congenital heart defects. *J. Am. Coll. Cardiol.* **2006**, *47*, 683–685. [CrossRef]
19. Huhta, J.C.; Hernandez-Robles, J.A. Homocysteine, folate, and congenital heart defects. *Fetal Pediatr. Pathol.* **2005**, *24*, 71–79. [CrossRef]
20. Vijay, P.; Lal, B.B.; Sood, V.; Khanna, R.; Alam, S. Cystatin C: Best biomarker for acute kidney injury and estimation of glomerular filtration rate in childhood cirrhosis. *Eur. J. Pediatrics* **2021**, *180*, 3287–3295. [CrossRef]
21. Levey, A.S.; Inker, L.A. Assessment of Glomerular Filtration Rate in Health and Disease: A State of the Art Review. *Clin. Pharmacol. Ther.* **2017**, *102*, 405–419. [CrossRef] [PubMed]
22. Ballew, S.; Matsushita, K. Cardiovascular Risk Prediction in CKD. *Semin. Nephrol.* **2018**, *38*, 208–216. [CrossRef] [PubMed]
23. Herbert, C.; Patel, M.; Nugent, A.; Dimas, V.V.; Guleserian, K.J.; Quigley, R.; Modem, V. Serum Cystatin C as an Early Marker of Neutrophil Gelatinase-associated Lipocalin-positive Acute Kidney Injury Resulting from Cardiopulmonary Bypass in Infants with Congenital Heart Disease. *Congenit. Heart Dis.* **2015**, *10*, E180–E188. [CrossRef] [PubMed]
24. Van den Eynde, J.; Salaets, T.; Louw, J.J.; Herman, J.; Breysem, L.; Vlasselaers, D.; Desmet, L.; Meyns, B.; Budts, W.; Gewillig, M.; et al. Persistent Markers of Kidney Injury in Children Who Developed Acute Kidney Injury After Pediatric Cardiac Surgery: A Prospective Cohort Study. *J. Am. Heart Assoc.* **2022**, *11*, e024266. [CrossRef] [PubMed]
25. Fu, Z.; Yang, X.; Shen, M.; Xue, H.; Qian, G.; Cao, F.; Guo, J.; Dong, W.; Chen, Y. Prognostic ability of cystatin C and homocysteine plasma levels for long-term outcomes in very old acute myocardial infarction patients. *Clin. Interv. Aging* **2018**, *13*, 1201–1209. [CrossRef] [PubMed]
26. Kawasaki, M.; Arata, N.; Ogawa, Y. Obesity and abnormal glucose tolerance in the offspring of mothers with diabetes. *Curr. Opin. Obstet. Gynecol.* **2018**, *30*, 361–368. [CrossRef]

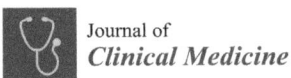

Article

A Predictive Model for Large-for-Gestational-Age Infants among Korean Women with Gestational Diabetes Mellitus Using Maternal Characteristics and Fetal Biometric Parameters

Hee-Sun Kim [1], Soo-Young Oh [2], Geum Joon Cho [3], Suk-Joo Choi [2], Soon Cheol Hong [3], Ja-Young Kwon [4] and Han Sung Kwon [5,*]

1. Division of Maternal-Fetal Medicine, Department of Obstetrics and Gynecology, Dongguk University Ilsan Hospital, Goyang 10326, Korea
2. Division of Maternal-Fetal Medicine, Department of Obstetrics and Gynecology, Samsung Medical Center, Sungkyunkwan University School of Medicine, Seoul 06351, Korea
3. Division of Maternal-Fetal Medicine, Department of Obstetrics and Gynecology, Korea University College of Medicine, Seoul 02841, Korea
4. Division of Maternal-Fetal Medicine, Department of Obstetrics and Gynecology, Yonsei University College of Medicine, Yonsei University Health System, Seoul 03722, Korea
5. Division of Maternal-Fetal Medicine, Department of Obstetrics and Gynecology, Konkuk University School of Medicine 120-1, Neungdongno, Gwangjin-gu, Seoul 05030, Korea
* Correspondence: 20050024@kuh.ac.kr; Tel.: +82-2-2030-7645; Fax: +82-2-2030-7748

Abstract: Background: With increasing incidence of gestational diabetes mellitus (GDM), newborn infants with perinatal morbidity, including large-for-gestational-age (LGA) or macrosomia, are also increasing. The purpose of this study was to develop a prediction model for LGA infants with GDM mothers. Methods: This was a retrospective case-control study of 660 women with GDM and singleton pregnancies in four tertiary care hospitals from 2006 to 2013 in Korea. Biometric parameters were obtained at diagnoses of GDM and within two weeks before delivery. These biometric data were all transformed retrospectively into Z-scores calculated using a reference. Interval changes of values between the two periods were obtained. Multivariable logistic and stepwise backwards regression analyses were performed to develop the most parsimonious predictive model. The prediction model included pre-pregnancy body mass index (BMI), head circumference (HC), Z-score at 24 + 0 to 30 + 6 weeks' gestation, and abdominal circumference (AC) Z-score at 34 + 0 to 41 + 6 weeks within 2 weeks before delivery. The developed model was then internally validated. Results: Our model's predictive performance (area under the curve (AUC): 0.925) was higher than estimated fetal weight (EFW) within two weeks before delivery (AUC: 0.744) and the interval change of EFW Z-score between the two periods (AUC: 0.874). It was internally validated (AUC: 0.916). Conclusions: A clinical model was developed and internally validated to predict fetal overgrowth in Korean women with GDM, which showed a relatively good performance.

Keywords: ultrasound; gestational diabetes mellitus; prenatal diagnosis; Z-score

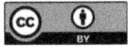

1. Introduction

Gestational diabetes mellitus (GDM) affects maternal, fetal, and neonatal well-being. The incidence of GDM has reached 14% in the United States of America [1]. It has increased from 2 to 13% worldwide [2,3]. GDM increases the risk of traumatic vaginal delivery, emergency cesarean section, postpartum hemorrhage, and large-for-gestational-age (LGA) or macrosomic infant delivery. LGA or macrosomic infants are at an increased risk of peripartum mortality due to complications such as shoulder dystocia, brachial plexus injury, bone fracture (clavicle or humerus), and birth asphyxia [4–6]. LGA newborns are also more likely to develop chronic health problems such as diabetes and metabolic diseases later in life [5–7]. Therefore, preventing fetal overgrowth through strict glycemic control and accurately predicting fetal overgrowth are crucial.

Several researchers have investigated specific equations to assess fetal growth using maternal factors and biomarkers [8,9] or to improve the predictive performance of fetal overgrowth among mothers with diabetes using biometric parameters such as abdominal circumference (AC), serial AC measurements, and estimated fetal weight (EFW) during the early third or third trimester [10–13].

Based on a comparison of weights among overweight newborns, EFW measurement at term is not as accurate as expected. Visualization of biometric parameters by ultrasonic imaging is limited due to distortion of the ultrasound beam when it penetrates deeper into the pregnant uterus of obese women [14]. Given inaccuracies caused by clinical characteristics of mothers, integration trials of clinical features to improve the prediction of LGA infant delivery are necessary.

Thus, the aim of this study was to develop a prediction model using clinical characteristics of pregnant women and fetal serial biometry based on Z-scores measured at GDM diagnosis and within two weeks before delivery to improve the detection of LGA fetus in mothers with GDM. An accurate model that could predict the risk of delivering an LGA baby would be useful for counseling women regarding risks of attempting a vaginal delivery and the timing of delivery in cases of suspected LGA infant delivery.

2. Materials and Methods

2.1. Study Design

This was a retrospective, case-control study of 660 women with GDM and singleton pregnancies at four tertiary care hospitals from 2006 to 2013 in Korea. We reviewed clinical information from medical records. Informed consent was not required due to the retrospective nature of this study. Fetal biometric parameters, such as biparietal diameter (BPD), head circumference (HC), AC, femur length (FL), and EFW measured during GDM diagnosis from 24 to 30 weeks of gestation (hereby indicated as BPD1, HC1, AC1, FL1, and EFW1), within 2 weeks before delivery at more than 34 weeks' gestation (BPD2, HC2, AC2, FL2, and EFW2), and interval changes between the two values in these values, were obtained from medical records. For example, interval changes of EFW and EFW Z-score between two periods are described as EFW/week [(EFW2 − EFW1)/(week2 − week1)] and Δ EFW Z-score.

BPD, HC, AC, and FL were converted to Z-scores and percentiles adjusted for gestational age according to reference charts and equations of Korean fetal biometry [15]. EFW was converted using INTERGROWTH-21st equation [16]. EFW as determined by ultrasonography was calculated using the Hadlock formula C [log10 EFW = 1.335 − 0.0034 (AC) (FL) + 0.0316 (BPD) + 0.0457 (AC) + 0.1623 (FL)] [17]. We then applied EFW (in grams) to the Alexander growth curve nomogram to calculate fetal weight percentage [18]. Based on the Alexander growth curve, an LGA fetus was suspected when the EFW by ultrasonography was >90%. An LGA infant at birth was defined as having a birth weight of ≥90%.

Exclusion criteria were: multiple gestations, major fetal anomalies and stillbirth, preterm birth of <34 weeks of gestation, and other medical and surgical problems except GDM. All ultrasonography examinations were routinely performed in each unit by skilled technicians or physicians. GDM was diagnosed using the Carpenter and Coustan criteria. Clinical and demographic data, including gestational age and birth weight, and specific details of neonatal outcomes were collected from medical records.

2.2. Data Analysis

Maternal demographic data were compared between LGA and appropriate-for-gestational-age (AGA) infants of mothers with GDM. Clinical variables were compared using Pearson's X^2 test, Student's t-test, and the Mann–Whitney U test. Clinically significant factors, fetal biometric parameters, and their Z-scores were analyzed to evaluate a risk an LGA infant at birth by univariate logistic regression (Table 2). For a new prediction model, a backward stepwise variable elimination procedure was used to select the best goodness-of-fit model in multivariable binary logistic regression analysis. We performed a multiple binary logistic regression analysis to identify significant risk factors and to generate the most parsimonious prediction model. The developed model was internally validated by LOOCV (leave-one-out cross-validation). Significant predictors were converted to binary variables using receiver operator characteristic (ROC) curve analysis (response variables: LGA vs. AGA). For each predictive variable, we created a binary variable defined as "low" when it was smaller than the cutoff and "high" when it was larger than the cutoff. Significance was defined at $p < 0.05$. R language version 3.3.3 (R Foundation for Statistical Computing, Vienna, Austria), T&F program version 1.6 (YooJin BioSoft, Goyang, Korea), and IBM SPSS Statistics for Windows version 23 (IBM Corp., Armonk, NY, USA) were used for all statistical analyses.

3. Results

Among 660 women with GDM and singleton pregnancies, 77 (11.6%) had an LGA infant delivery. Maternal age and height were not significant factors for predicting LGA infants (Table 1). Delivery occurred at 38.67 ± 1.22 weeks and 38.1 ± 1.19 weeks of gestation in AGA and LGA groups, respectively ($p < 0.001$). The cesarean section rate in the LGA group was 75.3%, which was higher than that (48.2%) in the AGA group. Pre-pregnancy weight and BMI were significantly higher in women who delivered an LGA fetus compared to those who delivered an AGA fetus. LGA and AGA infants had mean birth weights of 3998 g and 3214 g, respectively. The significance level of the above-mentioned variables was $p < 0.001$.

Table 1. Demographic data of pregnant women with gestational diabetes mellitus based on type of infant delivery.

Variable	AGA (n = 583)	LGA (n = 77)	p-Value
Maternal age (years) *	33.74 ± 4.08	34.53 ± 4.29	0.139
Delivery (weeks) *	38.67 ± 1.22	38.1 ± 1.19	<0.001
Delivery mode ‡			<0.001
Vaginal delivery	302 (51.8)	19 (24.7)	
Cesarean section	281 (48.2)	58 (75.3)	
Height *	160.26 ± 5.51	160.92 ± 5.93	0.512
Pre-pregnancy weight *	58.53 ± 10.53	66.73 ± 12.37	<0.001
Pre-pregnancy BMI *	22.73 ± 3.82	25.81 ± 4.45	<0.001
Birth weight (g) †	3214.32 ± 343.39	3998.77 ± 330.74	<0.001

Abbreviations: LGA, large for gestational age; AGA, appropriate for gestational age; BMI, body mass index. *,†: Values are given as mean ± standard deviation. ‡: Values are given as number (percentage). * Tested using the Mann–Whitney U test. † Tested using Student's t-test. ‡ Tested using Pearson's χ^2 test.

Results of univariate binary logistic regression using type (LGA vs. AGA) are shown in Table 2. Among statistically significant results ($p < 0.001$), parameters with the highest odd ratios (OR) were AC1 Z-score (2.015; 95% confidence interval (CI): 1.612—2.518; $p < 0.001$) in gestational diagnosis periods, AC2 Z-score (6.15; 95% CI: 4.284—8.83; $p < 0.001$) in 2 weeks before delivery periods, and the interval change of AC between two periods (AC/week) (193.31; 95% CI: 44.516—839.503; $p < 0.001$). The Δ AC Z-score had the highest OR (1.889; 95% CI: 1.509—2.366; $p < 0.001$) among Z-scores between the two periods.

Table 2. Result of univariable binary logistic regression analysis using type (LGA vs. AGA) according to gestational age.

Predictor	OR (95% CI)	p-Value
BPD1 Z-score	1.463 (1.16–1.844)	0.001
HC1 Z-score	1.449 (1.179–1.781)	<0.001 **
AC1 Z-score	2.015 (1.612–2.518)	<0.001 **
FL1 Z-score	1.086 (0.88–1.339)	0.441
EFW1 Z-score	1.935 (1.511–2.477)	<0.001 **
BPD2 Z-score	2.206 (1.643–2.962)	<0.001 **
HC2 Z-score	1.734 (1.263–2.382)	<0.001 **
AC2 Z-score	6.15 (4.284–8.83)	<0.001 **
EFW2 Z-score	8.438 (5.527–12.883)	<0.001 **
FL2 Z-score	1.91 (1.481–2.465)	<0.001 **
Pre-pregnancy BMI	1.169 (1.105–1.237)	<0.001 **
EFW2 (g)	1.002 (1.002–1.003)	<0.001 **
HC (cm)/Week	0.445 (0.07–2.847)	0.393
AC (cm)/Week	193.317 (44.516–839.503)	<0.001 **
EFW (g)/Week	1.041 (1.032–1.05)	<0.001 **
Δ HC Z-score	0.916 (0.737–1.139)	0.431
Δ AC Z-score	1.889 (1.509–2.366)	<0.001 **
Δ EFW Z-score	1.745 (1.383–2.202)	<0.001 **

**: $p < 0.001$. Abbreviations: LGA, large for gestational age; AGA, appropriate for gestational age; OR, odds ratio; 95% CI, 95% confidence interval of AUC; BMI, body mass index; BPD, biparietal diameter; HC, head circumference; AC, abdominal circumference; FL, femur length; EFW, estimated fetal weight; 1, fetal biometric parameters measured during screening of gestational diabetes mellitus; 2, fetal biometric parameters measured within 2 weeks before delivery. "Predictor/week" means predictor velocity. Predictor velocity between two scans described as predictor/week and calculated by [(predictor 2 − predictor 1)/(week2-week1)]. "Δ Predictor (Z-score)" means Z-score's interval change of predictor between gestational weeks [(predictor 2 (Z-score) − predictor 1 (Z-score)].

In Table 3, the best predictive model consisted of three predictors (HC1 Z-score, AC2 Z-score, and pre-pregnancy BMI) by multivariable binary logistic regression model to predict LGA using dichotomous predictors. As shown in Table 4, AUCs for the ability of EFW2 alone and EFW2 Z-score to predict LGA infant delivery were 0.744 (95% CI: 0.675–0.813; $p < 0.001$) and 0.874 (95% CI: 0.874–0.919; $p < 0.001$), respectively. Meanwhile, the AUC of our prediction model was 0.925, with a sensitivity of 81.1% and a specificity of 89.5% (95% CI: 0.892–0.957; $p < 0.001$). In Table 4, the prediction model was internally validated by LOOCV (AUC: 0.916), which showed a sensitivity of 81.1% and a specificity of 87.4% (95% CI: 0.880–0.953; $p < 0.001$). Additionally, several diagnostic measures of the prediction performance of the internally validated prediction model (diagnostic OR: 29.84) were shown. Figure 1 presents results of comparison of ROC with EFW2, EFW2 Z-score, and prediction model using type as binary response.

Table 3. Results of multivariable logistic regression model to predict LGA using dichotomous predictors using type (LGA vs. AGA).

Predictor	Continuous Predictors		Binary Predictors		
	OR (95% CIs)	p-Value	OR (95% CIs)	p-Value	Cut-Off
HC1 Z-score	1.358 (1.055–1.748)	0.018	2.625 (1.23–5.601)	0.013	1.439
AC2 Z-score	6.345 (3.976–10.124)	<0.001	18.083 (8.35–39.164)	<0.001	1.321
Pre-pregnancy BMI	1.153 (1.055–1.26)	0.002	4.996 (2.405–10.378)	<0.001	24.02

Abbreviations: LGA, large for gestational age; AGA, appropriate for gestational age; OR, odds ratio; CI, confidence interval; BMI, body mass index; HC, head circumference; AC, abdominal circumference; 1, fetal biometric parameters measured during screening of gestational diabetes mellitus; 2, fetal biometric parameters measured within 2 weeks before delivery. The cutoff of predictor value was used for classifying binary response of type: control response, AGA vs. case response, LGA.

Table 4. Diagnostic performance of EFW2, estimated model, and validated model using type (LGA vs. AGA).

Predictor	AUC	Lo95% CI	Up95% CI	p-Value	Acc.	Sensi	Speci	FPR	FNR	PPV	NPV	LR+	LR−	DOR	Cut-Off
EFW2	0.744	0.675	0.813	<0.001	0.798	0.623	0.822	0.178	0.377	0.316	0.943	3.495	0.458	7.623	
EFW2 Z-score	0.874	0.829	0.919	<0.001	0.809	0.805	0.811	0.189	0.208	0.357	0.967	4.199	0.256	16.394	0.108
Estimated Model	0.925	0.892	0.957	<0.001	0.884	0.811	0.894	0.106	0.189	0.5	0.973	7.642	0.211	36.20	0.165
Validated Model	0.916	0.880	0.953	<0.001	0.867	0.811	0.874	0.126	0.189	0.457	0.973	6.443	0.216	29.84	

Abbreviations: EFW2, estimated fetal weight within 2 weeks before delivery; LGA, large for gestational age; AGA, appropriate for gestational age; AUC, area under the curve; 95% CI, 95% confidence interval; Sensi, sensitivity; Speci, specificity; Acc., accuracy; FPR, false-positive rate; FNR, false-negative rate; PPV, positive predictive value; NPV, negative predictive value; LR+, positive likelihood ratio; LR−, negative likelihood ratio; DOR, diagnostic odds ratio.

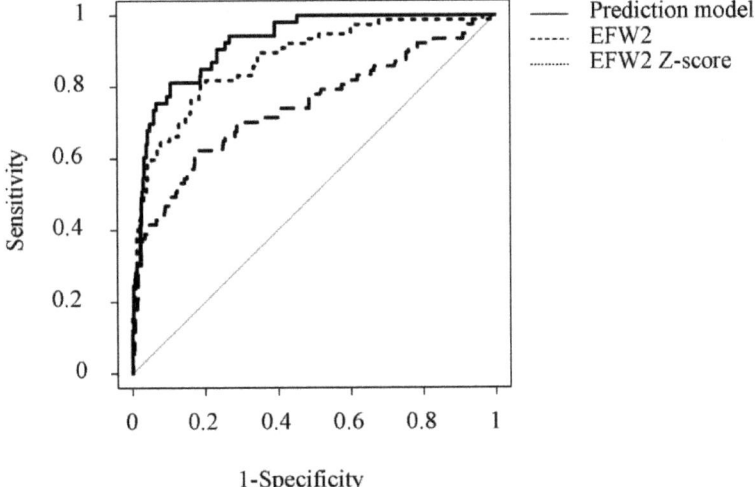

Figure 1. Comparison of ROC with EFW2 and EFW2 Z-score measured within two weeks before delivery and prediction model using type as binary response. ROC, receiver operator characteristic curve; EFW, estimated fetal weight.

Based on univariate and multivariate binary analyses, the nomogram for predicting an LGA infant using cutoff of predictors is presented in Figure 2. The probability in the nomogram was determined using the following formula:

$$P = e^{\beta X}/(1 + e^{\beta X})$$

where
$\beta X = -4.469 + C1 * HC1\ Z\text{-score} + C2 * AC2\ Z\text{-score} + C3 * \text{Pre-pregnancy BMI}$;
$C1 = \{0, 0.965\}$ when HC1 Z-score = $\{\leq 1.439, >1.439\}$;
$C2 = \{0, 2.895\}$ when AC2 Z-score = $\{\leq 1.321, >1.321\}$;
$C3 = \{0, 1.609\}$ when Pre-pregnancy BMI = $\{\leq 24, >24\}$.

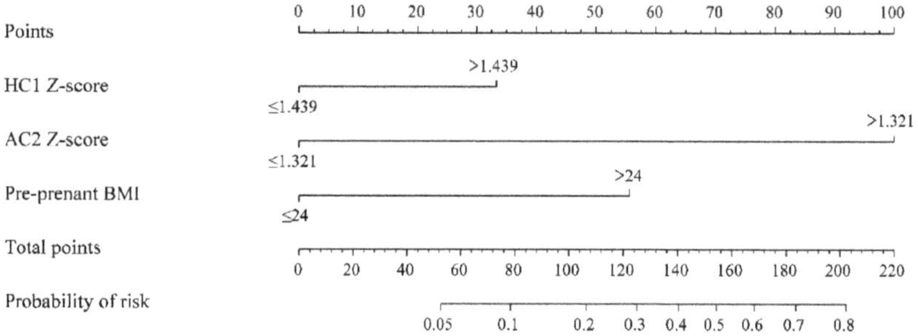

Figure 2. Nomogram for predicting an LGA infant in mothers with GDM. Directions: pre-pregnancy BMI, HC1 Z-score measured during GDM diagnosis, and AC2 Z-score measured within two weeks before delivery for an individual patient. Instructions: Each individual's risk of delivering an LGA infant was estimated by plotting on each variable axis. The nomogram was able to predict LGA babies in pregnant women with GDM at the optimal cutoff values of HC1 Z-scores > 1.439, AC2 Z-scores > 1.321, and pre-pregnancy BMIs > 24, under which AGA babies could be considered. Points from each variable value were then summed. The sum of the total points scale was located and vertically projected onto the bottom axis. A probability risk for an LGA infant was then obtained. LGA, large for gestational age; GDM, gestational diabetes mellitus; BMI, body mass index; HC, head circumference; AC, abdominal circumference.

4. Discussion

Our study has significant strengths. As mentioned above, we developed a prediction model by combining maternal pre-pregnancy BMI with biometric parameters adjusted for gestational age with Z-scores according to reference charts and equations from Korean reference data. The model with the highest diagnostic performance was selected and internally validated.

Another strength of our study was the creation of a clinically applicable nomogram. Using the nomogram, points for each category presented can be calculated and summed to assess the overall risk of LGA infant delivery in mothers with GDM. The total number of points of >0.8 and <0.05 corresponded to extremely high risk and extremely low risk, respectively. This will help improve the prediction of LGA infant delivery in women with GDM and allow clinicians to appropriately counsel women about potential risks. Moreover, compared with the predictive value of EFW or AC alone measured by ultrasonography during the third trimester, our prediction model had significantly higher predictive value for diagnosing LGA infant delivery. Although accurately estimating the fetal weight at delivery is often limited due to fetal malposition or maternal clinical status, appropriate counseling during pregnancy is possible using the created nomogram.

Previous researchers have proposed that growth acceleration of LGA infants begins in the second trimester and continues throughout the third trimester [19–21]. Considering this, we sought to create a model to predict LGA infants' delivery in mothers with GDM.

To develop a predictive model, fetal biometric parameters such as BPD, AC, FL, and EFW measured at GDM diagnosis and within two weeks before delivery and interval changes between the two periods were obtained from medical records. The addition of clinical characteristics such as pre-pregnancy BMI significantly improved the prediction. Biometric parameters and clinical risk factors were combined through multivariable logistic analysis, carefully considering each factor and their possible interrelationships.

Predictors for LGA infant delivery in our model have been determined in prior studies. In several recent studies, ultrasonography-measured EFW in the third trimester was used to predict LGA infant delivery. In one study involving 1689 pregnant women who were within 8 days of delivery after 37 weeks of gestation, the detection rate at a 5% false-positive rate (FPR) for LGA infant delivery using EFW derived from fetal AC was 54% [22]. Canavan et al. showed that an AC of >90th percentile is the best predictor of macrosomia at birth when comparing EFW, AC, and FL measured during sonographic examinations at 28–34 weeks of gestation [23]. The prediction of LGA infant delivery using only EFW in the third trimester tends to be overestimated, and the detection rate tends to be inferior. In our study, the detection rate with EFW2 was inferior to that of our new model. AUCs computed using our prediction model and EFW2 were 0.925 (95% CI: 0.892–0.957) and 0.744 (95% CI: 0.675–0.813), respectively, which were significantly different ($p < 0.001$ using DeLong's test).

Based on previous studies, attempts have been made to increase the prediction rate for LGA infant delivery by ultrasonographic findings in the third trimester as well as in the first or second trimester. Pilalis et al. reported that the detection rate for LGA infant delivery at >95th percentile is 31% at a 10% FPR using a combination of maternal weight and height, fetal crown–rump length, and delta nuchal translucency at 11–13 weeks of gestation [24]. The rate was increased to 52% after adding fetal biometry at 30–32 weeks. It was improved to 63% at 34–37 weeks in the same group [12,25]. Meanwhile, in a previous study, the ultrasonographic difference between fetal AD and BPD was used to predict macrosomia [26]. The improved accuracy of predicting LGA infant delivery could reduce the error between EFW and actual neonatal weight at delivery, thereby reducing complications that may occur during delivery and the rate of unnecessary cesarean sections.

This study had some limitations. First, GDM diagnosis in this paper is based on the Carpenter and Coustan criteria, whereas many countries are using IADPSG or WHO criteria. It should be considered that the LGA infant prediction with GDM mothers by our prediction model may perform differently used according to the IADPSG or WHO criteria. Second, the degree of glycemic control and treatment status were not included as a variable in the predictive model. This study considered HbA1C as a glycemic control variable. However, since it was conducted as a multicenter-retrospective study, the examination time of HbA1C test was different in each hospital, and many data were missing. Therefore, using it to develop a predictive model of LGA infants with HbA1C related to the degree of glycemic control had limitations. In addition, this study did not include variables between the group treated with oral hypoglycemic agents or insulin and without treatment and parameters related to adverse outcomes such as preeclampsia. Finally, the EFW Z-score calculation equation for our prediction model was applied using the INTERGROWTH 21 equation because it was not found among the Korean reference data. Considering that Asian data such as that from India, China, etc., were included compared to other studies, EFW was calculated by applying INTERGROWTH 21. We hope that as soon as the Korean reference data are developed, further study will be conducted based on them. A prospective study will be needed complementing for these limitations in the predictive model.

In conclusion, a clinical model was developed and internally validated to predict fetal overgrowth in Korean women with GDM, which showed a relatively good performance. By providing obstetricians and future mothers with an instrument in assessing fetal weight, it is expected to increase the predictive rate of LGA infants in GDM mothers. Applying clinically nomograms derived from this model will be helpful in reducing LGA births and improving a perinatal prognosis for mothers and newborns.

Author Contributions: Conceptualization, H.S.K. and H.-S.K.; formal analysis, H.-S.K.; methodology, S.-Y.O., G.J.C., S.-J.C., S.C.H., and J.-Y.K.; supervision, H.S.K.; writing—original draft preparation, H.-S.K.; writing—review, S.-Y.O., G.J.C., S.-J.C., S.C.H., J.-Y.K., and H.S.K.; editing, H.S.K. All authors have read and agreed to the published version of the manuscript.

Funding: This work was supported by Konkuk University School of Medicine, Korea University College of Medicine, Sungkyunkwan University School of Medicine, and Yonsei University College of Medicine. It was not financially supported.

Institutional Review Board Statement: This study was approved by the Ethics Committee of Konkuk University Medical Center (approval number: KUH1040055).

Informed Consent Statement: Patient consent was waived due to REASON. This study a retrospective study based on medical record analysis, we couldn't obtain consent of the participants. This has been approved by the IRB.

Data Availability Statement: Data presented in this study are available from the corresponding author upon reasonable request.

Conflicts of Interest: The authors declare no conflict of interest.

References

1. Ferrara, A.; Kahn, H.S.; Quesenberry, C.P.; Riley, C.; Hedderson, M.M. An increase in the incidence of gestational diabetes mellitus: Northern California, 1991–2000. *Obstet. Gynecol.* **2004**, *103*, 526–533. [CrossRef] [PubMed]
2. Hunt, K.J.; Schuller, K.L. The increasing prevalence of diabetes in pregnancy. *Obstet. Gynecol. Clin. N. Am.* **2007**, *34*, 173–199. [CrossRef] [PubMed]
3. Ryan, E.A. Diagnosing gestational diabetes. *Diabetologia* **2011**, *54*, 480–486. [CrossRef] [PubMed]
4. Yogev, Y.; Visser, G.H. Obesity, gestational diabetes and pregnancy outcome. *Semin. Fetal Neonatal Med.* **2009**, *14*, 77–84. [CrossRef]
5. Modanlou, H.D.; Dorchester, W.L.; Thorosian, A.N.N.A.; Freeman, R.K. Macrosomia—Maternal, fetal, and neonatal implications. *Obstet. Gynecol.* **1980**, *55*, 420–424.
6. HAPO Study Cooperative Research Group. Hyperglycemia and Adverse Pregnancy Outcome (HAPO) Study: Associations with neonatal anthropometrics. *Diabetes* **2009**, *58*, 453–459. [CrossRef]
7. Bérard, J.; Dufour, P.; Vinatier, D.; Subtil, D.; Vanderstichele, S.; Monnier, J.C.; Puech, F. Fetal macrosomia: Risk factors and outcome. A study of the outcome concerning 100 cases >4500 g. *Eur. J. Obstet. Gynecol. Reprod. Biol.* **1998**, *77*, 51–59. [CrossRef]
8. Holcomb, W.L., Jr.; Mostello, D.J.; Gray, D.L. Abdominal circumference vs. estimated weight to predict large for gestational age birth weight in diabetic pregnancy. *Clin. Imaging* **2000**, *24*, 1–7. [CrossRef]
9. Frick, A.P.; Syngelaki, A.; Zheng, M.; Poon, L.C.; Nicolaides, K.H. Prediction of large-for-gestational-age neonates: Screening by maternal factors and biomarkers in the three trimesters of pregnancy. *Ultrasound Obstet. Gynecol.* **2016**, *47*, 332–339. [CrossRef]
10. Combs, C.A.; Rosenn, B.; Miodovnik, M.; Siddiqi, T.A. Sonographic EFW and macrosomia: Is there an optimum formula to predict diabetic fetal macrosomia? *J. Matern. Fetal Med.* **2000**, *9*, 55–61.
11. Nelson, L.; Wharton, B.; Grobman, W.A. Prediction of large for gestational age birth weights in diabetic mothers based on early third-trimester sonography. *J. Ultrasound Med.* **2011**, *30*, 1625–1628. [CrossRef]
12. Pilalis, A.; Souka, A.P.; Papastefanou, I.; Michalitsi, V.; Panagopoulos, P.; Chrelias, C.; Kassanos, D. Third trimester ultrasound for the prediction of the large for gestational age fetus in low-risk population and evaluation of contingency strategies. *Prenat. Diagn.* **2012**, *32*, 846–853. [CrossRef]
13. Neff, K.J.; Walsh, C.; Kinsley, B.; Daly, S. Serial fetal abdominal circumference measurements in predicting normal birth weight in gestational diabetes mellitus. *Eur. J. Obstet. Gynecol. Reprod. Biol.* **2013**, *170*, 106–110. [CrossRef]
14. Benacerraf, B. The use of obstetrical ultrasound in the obese gravida. *Semin. Perinatol.* **2013**, *37*, 345–347. [CrossRef]
15. Jung, S.I.; Lee, Y.H.; Moon, M.H.; Song, M.J.; Min, J.Y.; Kim, J.-A.; Park, J.H.; Yang, J.H.; Kim, M.Y.; Chung, J.H.; et al. Reference charts and equations of Korean fetal biometry. *Prenat. Diagn.* **2007**, *27*, 545–551. [CrossRef]
16. Cheng, Y.K.Y.; Lu, J.; Leung, T.Y.; Chan, Y.M.; Sahota, D.S. Prospective assessment of INTERGROWTH-21st and World Health Organization estimated fetal weight reference curves. *Ultrasound Obstet. Gynecol.* **2018**, *51*, 792–798. [CrossRef]
17. Hadlock, F.P.; Deter, R.L.; Harrist, R.B.; Park, S.K. Estimating fetal age: Computer-assisted analysis of multiple fetal growth parameters. *Radiology* **1984**, *152*, 497–501. [CrossRef]
18. Alexander, G.R.; Himes, J.H.; Kaufman, R.B.; Mor, J.; Kogan, M. A United States national reference for fetal growth. *Obstet. Gynecol.* **1996**, *87*, 163–168. [CrossRef]
19. Buchanan, T.A.; Kjos, S.L.; Montoro, M.N.; Wu, P.Y.K.; Madrilejo, N.G.; Gonzalez, M.; Nunez, V.; Pantoja, P.M.; Xiang, A. Use of fetal ultrasound to select metabolic therapy for pregnancies complicated by mild gestational diabetes. *Diabetes Care* **1994**, *17*, 275–283. [CrossRef]
20. Wong, S.F.; Chan, F.Y.; Oats, J.J.; McIntyre, D.H. Fetal growth spurt and pregestational diabetic pregnancy. *Diabetes Care* **2002**, *25*, 1681–1684. [CrossRef]

21. Greco, P.; Vimercati, A.; Scioscia, M.; Rossi, A.C.; Giorgino, F.; Selvaggi, L. Timing of fetal growth acceleration in women with insulin-dependent diabetes. *Fetal Diagn. Ther.* **2003**, *18*, 437–441. [CrossRef] [PubMed]
22. Kayem, G.; Grange, G.; Breart, G.; Goffinet, F. Comparison of fundal height measurement and sonographically measured fetal abdominal circumference in the prediction of high and low birth weight at term. *Ultrasound Obstet. Gynecol.* **2009**, *34*, 566–571. [CrossRef] [PubMed]
23. Canavan, P.T.; Hill, L.M. Sonographic biometry in the early third trimester: A comparison of parameters to predict macrosomia at birth. *J. Clin. Ultrasound* **2015**, *43*, 243–248. [CrossRef] [PubMed]
24. Papastefanou, I.; Souka, A.P.; Pilalis, A.; Eleftheriades, M.; Michalitsi, V.; Kassanos, D. First trimester prediction of small- and large-for-gestation neonates by an integrated model incorporating ultrasound parameters, biochemical indices and maternal characteristics. *Acta Obstet. Gynecol. Scand.* **2012**, *91*, 104–111. [CrossRef]
25. Souka, A.P.; Papastefanou, I.; Pilalis, A.; Michalitsi, V.; Panagopoulos, P.; Kassanos, D. Performance of the ultrasound examination in the early and late third trimester for the prediction of birth weight deviations. *Prenat. Diagn.* **2013**, *33*, 915–920. [CrossRef]
26. Rajan, P.V.; Chung, J.H.; Porto, M.; Wing, D.A. Correlation of increased fetal asymmetry with shoulder dystocia in the nondiabetic woman with suspected macrosomia. *J. Reprod. Med.* **2009**, *54*, 478–482.

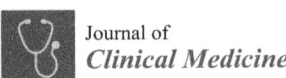

Article

Is Fetal Hydrops in Turner Syndrome a Risk Factor for the Development of Maternal Mirror Syndrome?

Ivonne Alexandra Bedei [1,*], Alexander Graf [1], Karl-Philipp Gloning [2], Matthias Meyer-Wittkopf [3], Daria Willner [4], Martin Krapp [5], Sabine Hentze [6], Alexander Scharf [7], Jan Degenhardt [8], Kai-Sven Heling [9], Peter Kozlowski [10], Kathrin Trautmann [11], Kai Jahns [12], Anne Geipel [13], Ismail Tekesin [14], Michael Elsässer [15], Lucas Wilhelm [16], Ingo Gottschalk [17], Jan-Erik Baumüller [18], Cahit Birdir [19], Felix Zöllner [1], Aline Wolter [1], Johanna Schenk [1], Tascha Gehrke [1], Corinna Keil [20], Jimmy Espinosa [21] and Roland Axt-Fliedner [1]

1. Department of Prenatal Diagnosis and Fetal Therapy, Justus-Liebig University, 35392 Giessen, Germany
2. Prenatal Medicine and Genetics München, 80639 Munich, Germany
3. Center for Prenatal Diagnosis, Mathias-Spital Rheine, 48431 Rheine, Germany
4. Center for Prenatal Medicine and Human Genetics, 20357 Hamburg, Germany
5. Center for Prenatal Medicine on Elbe, 20457 Hamburg, Germany
6. Center for Human Genetics, Cytogenetic Laboratory Heidelberg, 69120 Heidelberg, Germany
7. Center for Prenatal Medicine, 55116 Mainz, Germany
8. Praenatal Plus, Center for Prenatal Medicine and Genetics, 50672 Cologne, Germany
9. Center of Prenatal Diagnosis and Human Genetics, 10117 Berlin, Germany
10. Praenatal.de, Prenatal Medicine and Genetics Düsseldorf, 40210 Düsseldorf, Germany
11. Center for Prenatal Medicine "am Salzhaus", 60311 Frankfurt, Germany
12. Department of Internal Medicine, Johannes Gutenberg University, 55131 Mainz, Germany
13. Obstetrics and Prenatal Medicine, University Hospital Bonn, 53127 Bonn, Germany
14. Prenatal Medicine Stuttgart, 70173 Stuttgart, Germany
15. Department of Gynecology and Obstetrics, Heidelberg University Hospital, 69120 Heidelberg, Germany
16. Westend Ultrasound, Center for Prenatal Diagnosis and Fetal Echocardiography, 60325 Frankfurt, Germany
17. Division of Prenatal Medicine, Department of Obstetrics and Gynecology, University of Cologne, 50931 Cologne, Germany
18. Gynaecologikum, Frankfurt, 60389 Frankfurt, Germany
19. Department of Obstetrics and Gynecology, University Hospital Carl Gustav Carus Dresden, 01307 Dresden, Germany
20. Department of Prenatal Medicine and Fetal Therapy, Philipps University, 35041 Marburg, Germany
21. Baylor College of Medicine Department of Obstetrics and Gynecology, Division of Fetal Therapy and Surgery and Texas Children's Hospital Fetal Center, Houston, TX 77030, USA

* Correspondence: ivonne.bedei@gyn.med.uni-giessen.de; Tel.: +49-641-98559109

Abstract: Mirror syndrome is a rare and serious maternal condition associated with immune and non-immune fetal hydrops after 16 weeks of gestational age. Subjacent conditions associated with fetal hydrops may carry different risks for Mirror syndrome. Fetuses with Turner syndrome are frequently found to be hydropic on ultrasound. We designed a retrospective multicenter study to evaluate the risk for Mirror syndrome among pregnancies complicated with Turner syndrome and fetal hydrops. Data were extracted from a questionnaire sent to specialists in maternal fetal medicine in Germany. Out of 758 cases, 138 fulfilled our inclusion criteria and were included in the analysis. Of the included 138, 66 presented with persisting hydrops at or after 16 weeks. The frequency of placental hydrops/placentomegaly was rather low (8.1%). Of note, no Mirror syndrome was observed in our study cohort. We propose that the risk of this pregnancy complication varies according to the subjacent cause of fetal hydrops. In Turner syndrome, the risk for Mirror syndrome is lower than that reported in the literature. Our observations are relevant for clinical management and parental counseling.

Keywords: Mirror syndrome; fetal hydrops; Turner syndrome; monosomy X; placental hydrops; placentomegaly

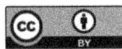

1. Introduction

Mirror syndrome was first described by John William Ballantyne in 1892 as a combination of fetal and placental hydrops as well as maternal edema and preeclampsia-like symptoms (triple edema) [1–3]. Mirror syndrome is a rare condition that is associated with immune and non-immune fetal hydrops [4,5]. The incidence is 1 in 3000 pregnancies, but it may be underestimated due to its similarity with preeclampsia [6]. Mirror syndrome has been described as early as 16 weeks of pregnancy [5,7]. Some authors proposed that placental-derived antiangiogenic factors are involved in the pathogenesis of Mirror syndrome [2,8–11]. ß-hCG may also play a role in the mechanisms of the disease since hCG seems to be markedly increased in these cases [12,13]. The frequency of maternal Mirror syndrome in cases of fetal hydrops varies between 5% and 37.8% [12,14,15]. Of note, maternal Mirror syndrome can resolve after successful in-utero treatment or delivery [4,9]. Fetal hydrops is defined as an accumulation of fluid in fetal soft tissue and body cavities. The conventional definition involves two or more abnormal fetal fluid collections (ascites, pleural effusions, pericardial effusion, and skin edema). Other frequent findings associated with fetal hydrops include polyhydramnios and placental thickening and/or edema also known as placentomegaly or placental hydrops [16]. Following the implementation of routine use of Rh(D) prophylaxis, immune fetal hydrops has dramatically decreased. Nonimmune fetal hydrops accounts now for almost 90% of cases of fetal hydrops [16,17]. Chromosomal anomalies, including Turner syndrome and Trisomy 21, are common causes of fetal hydrops [18,19].

The incidence of Turner syndrome is 1:2000 liveborn girls [20]. Prenatally, this syndrome is much more frequent, and most embryos, particularly those with the karyotype 45,X are spontaneously miscarried in the first trimester [21,22]. The rate of termination of pregnancy is high, more so in cases with fetal hydrops and other associated fetal anomalies [23]. Turner syndrome is frequently associated with early fetal hydrops [16,24]. It has been proposed that lymphatic dysplasia is the main pathophysiologic mechanism behind abnormal fluid accumulation [25]. In hydropic fetuses with Turner syndrome, hCG is increased in the second trimester; in contrast, in fetuses without hydrops, the maternal blood concentration of hCG tends to be decreased [26,27]. There is scarce literature about the placental thickness in Turner syndrome, but some reports indicate that this condition is not associated with placentomegaly [28,29]. Prenatal counseling is an important factor in parents' decision-making [30]. In the case of fetal hydrops, counseling should not only include the risk for development abnormality and fetal or neonatal death but also potential maternal risks, including the development of Mirror syndrome and/or preeclampsia with severe features, which may influence prenatal care, the timing of delivery and the nature of antenatal surveillance [31].

The conventional view is that Mirror syndrome is associated with fetal hydrops irrespective of the subjacent cause [31,32]. The aim of our study is to describe the frequency of Mirror syndrome among pregnant women with fetal hydrops associated with Turner syndrome. We hypothesize that frequency is lower than that expected in other conditions associated with fetal hydrops because the fetal fluid accumulation is largely due to lymphatic dysplasia.

2. Materials and Methods

This is an observational multicenter retrospective cohort study. We developed a questionnaire consisting of 24 items, including demographic data, information on prenatal ultrasound findings at diagnosis and during pregnancy, genetic testing, pregnancy complications, and outcomes. Question 19 asked about complications during pregnancy. An explicit distinction was made between Mirror syndrome and preeclampsia. The questionnaire forms are available to readers upon reasonable request. To ensure a homogeneous and high-quality level of fetal ultrasound, only experts with DEGUM qualification II + III (German Society for Ultrasound in Medicine) were invited to participate. Data from

21 centers in Germany were included in the analysis. Cases diagnosed between 2000 and 2022 that fulfilled the inclusion criteria were included in the analysis.

2.1. Inclusion Criteria

1. Fetal hydrops, defined as an abnormal fluid collection in two or more body compartments (ascites, pleural effusions, pericardial effusion, skin edema) at the time of diagnosis/first presentation. In the first trimester, generalized skin edema with or without cystic hygroma was also considered fetal hydrops
2. Karyotype resulting in Turner syndrome (45,X or cytogenetic variants)
3. Documented fetal cardiac activity beyond 16 weeks of gestation. This is the earliest gestational age at which Mirror syndrome has been reported [5,7].

2.2. Exclusion Criteria

1. No cytogenetic confirmation of Turner syndrome by karyotype on chorionic villous sampling or genetic amniocentesis.
2. Intrauterine demise before 16 weeks or, no documented cardiac activity at or after 16 weeks.

The maximal placental thickness measured sonographically was additionally requested and available for analysis in 37 cases. Placentomegaly was defined as a placental thickness greater than 4 cm in the second trimester or greater than 6 cm in the third trimester [16].

2.3. Outcome Measures

The frequency of maternal Mirror syndrome was determined in a prenatally diagnosed population of pregnant women, whose fetuses were affected by Turner syndrome and hydrops. The interval between the first diagnosis of/presentation with fetal hydrops and fetal death or live birth was estimated to evaluate the time that mothers were exposed to the risk for Mirror Syndrome. The median gestational age at fetal death in cases of IUFD or at delivery in cases of live birth was also calculated.

2.4. Statistical Analysis

All statistical analyses were performed using IBM SPSS Statistics for Windows®, version 26. Contingency tables were generated. Data are presented as median, minimum, and maximum.

Ethical approval was received by the ethical committee for Medicine at the Justus-Liebig University Giessen, Germany (AZ 119/19)

3. Results

We analyzed 758 cases with suspected or diagnosed Turner syndrome. Fifty-three cases were excluded because no karyotype was available, or the final karyotype was different and not Turner syndrome. Of 705 fetuses, 440 had fetal hydrops at the time of diagnosis. Of these, 302 died spontaneously or the pregnancy was terminated before 16 weeks GA or cardiac activity was not documented at or after 16 weeks. A total of 138 fetuses with hydrops and Turner Syndrome fulfilled the inclusion criteria. In 66/138 hydrops was documented at or after 16 weeks GA (Figure 1).

Table 1 shows demographic and clinical characteristics of the study population.

Twenty of the 138 (14.5%) cases were live births, 47/138 (34%) had a spontaneous abortion/intrauterine fetal demise (IUFD), and in 62/138 (44.9%) cases pregnancy was terminated (TOP) at or after 16 weeks. In 9/138 cases (6.5%) outcome information was not available.

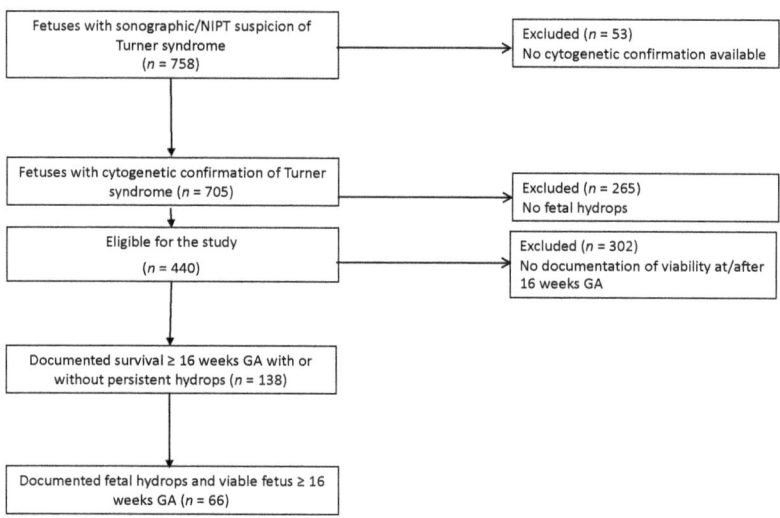

Figure 1. Selection of study cohort.

Table 1. Demographic and clinical characteristics of the study population.

Maternal Characteristics n = 138	
Age (years)	30 (17–45)
BMI (kg/m^2)	24.9 (17.8–46.3)
Mode of conception	
Spontaneous	111 (80.4%)
IVF/ICSI	8 (5.8%)
Unknown	19 (13.8%)
Fetal karyotype n = 138	
45,X	134 (97.1%)
mos 45,X/46,XX	4 (2.9%)
First diagnosis of/presentation with fetal hydrops (weeks) (n = 133)	15.4 (10.57–25.43)
GA at delivery in case of live birth (n = 20)	38 (31–42)

Data expressed as number and percentage or median, maximum and minimum. BMI (Body mass index), IVF (In-vitro-Fertilization), ICSI (Intracytoplasmic sperm injection), mos (mosaic), GA (gestational Age).

In 66/138 (47.8%) cases, cardiac activity and persistent hydrops were documented at or after 16 weeks. In 72/138 fetuses, hydrops was diagnosed in the first and early second trimester and no longer mentioned thereafter, potentially due to incomplete reporting. It is possible that hydrops also persisted in these cases; thus, we included these cases in the analysis. The highest gestational age with documented fetal hydrops in a live fetus was 25.4 weeks in the whole cohort, with a median of 18 weeks for the group with documented hydrops at or after 16 weeks GA. None of the newborn babies had hydrops at birth.

The median gestational age of delivery in the case of live birth was 38 weeks (Table 1). The median gestational age of fetal demise was 23 weeks (Table 2). One fetus died unexpectedly at 38 weeks. In this case, hydrops was diagnosed in the first trimester and resolved before 17 weeks. On fetal echocardiography, there was suspicion of hypoplastic aortic arch/CoA and small left ventricle. After an otherwise unremarkable pregnancy, the fetus died before induction of labor was scheduled.

Table 2. Clinical characteristics of cases with documented cardiac activity ≥16 weeks with hydrops.

	Median (Weeks)	Minimum and Maximum (Weeks)
GA at fetal death ($n = 29$)	23	16.14–38
Interval from diagnosis of hydrops to live birth ($n = 18$)	25.4	17.14–27.86
Interval from diagnosis of hydrops to fetal death ($n = 28$)	7.4	0.28–25.14

Data expressed as median, minimum, and maximum. Gestational Age (GA).

The median interval between diagnosis of hydrops and live birth or IUFD is shown in Table 2.

Pregnancy complications were observed in 33 (23.9%) cases, including fetal growth restriction in 27/138 (19.6%) fetuses. One case of preeclampsia and one case of HELLP syndrome were observed. Both babies were delivered after 36 weeks without signs of hydrops at birth. Of note, no cases of Mirror syndrome were observed in our study cohort (Table 3).

Table 3. Fetal/maternal complications.

	n (%)
None	105 (76.1)
IUGR	27 (19.6)
PPROM	2 (1.4)
Preexisting hypertonus	1 (0.7)
Preeclampsia/HELLP	2 (1.4)
Preterm birth <34 weeks GA	1 (0.7)
Mirror syndrome	0

IUGR (Intrauterine growth restriction), PPROM (preterm premature rupture of membranes).

Placentomegaly was observed in 8.1% (3/37) of cases whose sonographic measurements were available for analysis.

4. Discussion

No cases of Mirror syndrome were observed in our cohort of 138 hydropic fetuses with Turner syndrome, particularly in the subgroup of individuals with documented fetal cardiac activity at or after 16 weeks. Placentomegaly, a frequent and important finding in Mirror syndrome, was observed only in 8.1% of our cases with available placental thickness measurement. This is consistent with prior reports indicating that placental villous edema and placentomegaly are not frequent in cases of Turner syndrome in the second trimester [28,33]. Our results are in stark contrast to prior reports of the rates of Mirror syndrome ranging from 5% to 37.8% among fetal hydrops associated with other conditions [12,14,15]. These conditions include rhesus alloimmunization, viral infections, Ebstein's anomaly, aneurysm of the vein of Galen, sacrococcygeal teratoma (SCT), supraventricular tachycardia (SVT), twin to twin transfusion syndrome (TTTS), hemoglobin Bart's and placental chorioangioma [3,7,34–36].

The pathogenesis for the development of Mirror syndrome is still not completely understood. Placentomegaly or "placental hydrops" resulting from villous edema leads to compression of villous blood vessels and/or thicker interphase. As a result, oxygen exchange is impaired [37]. Espinoza et al. proposed that hypoxia of the villous trophoblast leads to increased release of antiangiogenic factors [2]. This seems to play an important role in the pathogenesis of Mirror syndrome [2,3,5,10].

We hypothesize that conditions with significant villous edema lead to reduced perfusion of the placental villi and reduced oxygen exchange and thereby triggering the release of antiangiogenic factors with subsequent development of Mirror syndrome. The mechanism for fetal hydrops in Turner syndrome appears to be related to lymphatic dysplasia, therefore placental hydrops is not a frequent finding in this condition [25,38,39].

The prognosis of fetuses with Turner syndrome is guarded with a high percentage of spontaneous demise and pregnancy terminations [21,23,24,30]. This is consistent with our observations. TOP was done in 44.9% and spontaneous fetal death occurred in 34%. The median gestational age of IUFD was 23 weeks. Occasionally hydropic babies with Turner syndrome survive and the hydrops resolves during pregnancy. Typical findings in these newborns are webbed neck and lymphedema of the hands and feet [40,41]. However, there is a paucity regarding prognostic factors for survival or death in these fetuses [41]. Additionally, the typical gestational age at which the hydrops resolves is not well known. In our cohort, the maximum gestational age in which hydrops was documented in a viable fetus was 25.4 weeks, with a median GA of 18 weeks.

Collectively, our results suggest that pregnant women carrying a hydropic fetus with Turner syndrome have a lower risk to develop Mirror syndrome compared to other etiologies of fetal hydrops [12,15]. This information is relevant for parental counseling and clinical management.

Strengths and Limitations

The strengths of our study include a large cohort of fetuses with Turner syndrome and hydrops. To our knowledge, this is the largest cohort published on the risk of Mirror syndrome among fetuses with hydrops and Turner syndrome. In addition, the inclusion of several academic centers increases the generalizability of our findings. The results of our study are of clinical relevance and could help to improve risk stratification and patient counseling in pregnancies with Turner syndrome.

Limitations of our study include the retrospective design as well as incomplete reporting in our questionnaire limiting the subgroup analyses. As placental thickness was only available in 8.1%, the prevalence of placentomegaly in Turner syndrome must be evaluated by a larger cohort study. In addition, placental histology to evaluate the frequency of placental villous edema was not available. Larger prospective studies are required to confirm our findings and to better characterize the natural history of fetal hydrops in fetuses with Turner syndrome.

5. Conclusions

Maternal Mirror syndrome is a severe condition complicating pregnancies with fetal hydrops of different etiologies. Our observations suggest that Mirror syndrome is rare among pregnancies complicated by fetal hydrops and Turner syndrome compared to other conditions. This information is important for patient management and parental counseling.

Author Contributions: Conceptualization, I.A.B. methodology, I.A.B.; software, J.E.; validation, I.A.B., K.-P.G. and J.E.; formal analysis, J.E.; investigation, I.A.B. and A.G. (Alexander Graf); resources, K.-P.G., M.M.-W., D.W., M.K., S.H., A.S., J.D., K.-S.H., P.K., K.T., A.G. (Anne Geipel)., K.J., I.T., M.E., L.W., I.G., J.-E.B., C.B., F.Z., A.W. and J.S.; data curation, A.G. (Alexander Graf). and T.G.; writing—original draft preparation, I.A.B.; writing—review and editing, J.E. and C.K.; supervision, R.A.-F. All authors have read and agreed to the published version of the manuscript.

Funding: This research received no external funding.

Institutional Review Board Statement: The study was conducted in accordance with the Declaration of Helsinki and approved by the Ethics Committee of Medicine at the Justus-Liebig University Giessen (AZ 119/19).

Informed Consent Statement: Patient consent was waived due to retrospective analysis of completely anonymized data.

Data Availability Statement: The data used to support the findings in this study are available from the corresponding author upon reasonable request.

Conflicts of Interest: R.A.-F. is guest editor of this special edition. This should have no influence on the content of this article.

References

1. Kaiser, I.H. Ballantyne and triple edema. *Am. J. Obstet. Gynecol.* **1971**, *110*, 115–120. [CrossRef]
2. Espinoza, J.; Romero, R.; Nien, J.K.; Kusanovic, J.P.; Richani, K.; Gomez, R.; Kim, C.J.; Mittal, P.; Gotsh, F.; Erez, O.; et al. A role of the anti-angiogenic factor sVEGFR-1 in the "mirror syndrome" (Ballantyne's syndrome). *J. Matern.-Fetal Neonatal Med.* **2006**, *19*, 607–613. [CrossRef] [PubMed]
3. Navarro-Perez, S.F.; Corona-Fernandez, K.; Rodriguez-Chavez, J.L.; Bañuelos-Franco, A.; Zavala-Cerna, M.G. Significant Clinical Manifestations in Ballantyne Syndrome, after a Case Report and Literature Review: Recognizing Preeclampsia as a Differential Diagnosis. *Case Rep. Obstet. Gynecol.* **2019**, *2019*, 2013506. [CrossRef] [PubMed]
4. Valsky, D.V.; Daum, H.; Yagel, S. Reversal of mirror syndrome after prenatal treatment of Diamond-Blackfan anemia. *Prenat. Diagn.* **2007**, *27*, 1161–1164. [CrossRef]
5. Mathias, C.R.; Rizvi, C. The diagnostic conundrum of maternal mirror syndrome progressing to pre-eclampsia—A case report. *Case Rep. Women's Health* **2019**, *23*, e00122. [CrossRef]
6. Heinonen, S.; Ryynänen, M.; Kirkinen, P. Etiology and outcome of second trimester non-immunologic fetal hydrops. *Acta Obstet. Gynecol. Scand.* **2000**, *79*, 15–18.
7. Braun, T.; Brauer, M.; Fuchs, I.; Czernik, C.; Dudenhausen, J.W.; Henrich, W.; Sarioglu, N. Mirror syndrome: A systematic review of fetal associated conditions, maternal presentation and perinatal outcome. *Fetal Diagn. Ther.* **2010**, *27*, 191–203. [CrossRef]
8. Bixel, K.; Silasi, M.; Zelop, C.M.; Lim, K.H.; Zsengeller, Z.; Stillman, I.E.; Rana, S. Placental Origins of Angiogenic Dysfunction in Mirror Syndrome. *Hypertens. Pregnancy* **2012**, *31*, 211–217. [CrossRef]
9. Llurba, E.; Crispi, F.; Verlohren, S. Update on the Pathophysiological Implications and Clinical Role of Angiogenic Factors in Pregnancy. *Fetal Diagn. Ther.* **2015**, *37*, 81–92. [CrossRef]
10. Graham, N.; Garrod, A.; Bullen, P.; Heazell, A.E.P. Placental expression of anti-angiogenic proteins in mirror syndrome: A case report. *Placenta* **2012**, *33*, 528–531. [CrossRef]
11. Katoh, Y.; Seyama, T.; Mimura, N.; Furuya, H.; Nakayama, T.; Iriyama, T.; Nagamatsu, T.; Osuga, Y.; Fujii, T. Elevation of Maternal Serum sFlt-1 in Pregnancy with Mirror Syndrome Caused by Fetal Cardiac Failure. *Oxf. Med Case Rep.* **2018**, *2018*, omx112. [CrossRef]
12. Hirata, G.; Aoki, S.; Sakamaki, K.; Takahashi, T.; Hirahara, F.; Ishikawa, H. Clinical characteristics of mirror syndrome: A comparison of 10 cases of mirror syndrome with non-mirror syndrome fetal hydrops cases. *J. Matern.-Fetal Neonatal Med.* **2016**, *29*, 2630–2634. [CrossRef] [PubMed]
13. Gherman, R.B.; Incerpi, M.H.; Wing, D.A.; Goodwin, T.M. Ballantyne syndrome: Is placental ischemia the etiology? *J. Matern.-Fetal Med.* **1998**, *7*, 227–229.
14. Gedikbasi, A.; Oztarhan, K.; Gunenc, Z.; Yildirim, G.; Arslan, O.; Yildirim, D.; Ceylan, Y. Preeclampsia Due to Fetal Non-immune Hydrops: Mirror Syndrome and Review of Literature. *Hypertens. Pregnancy* **2011**, *30*, 322–330. [CrossRef]
15. Han, Z.; Chen, X.; Wang, Q.; Zhou, J.; Guo, Y.; Hou, H.; Zhang, Y. Clinical characteristics and risk factors of mirror syndrome: A retrospective case-control study. *BMC Pregnancy Childbirth* **2021**, *21*, 660. [CrossRef]
16. Norton, M.E.; Chauhan, S.P.; Dashe, J.S. Society for Maternal-Fetal Medicine (SMFM) Clinical Guideline #7: Nonimmune hydrops fetalis. *Am. J. Obstet. Gynecol.* **2015**, *212*, 127–139.
17. Sparks, T.N.; Thao, K.; Lianoglou, B.R.; Boe, N.M.; Bruce, K.G.; Datkhaeva, I.; Field, N.T.; Fratto, V.M.; Jolley, J.; Laurent, L.C.; et al. Nonimmune hydrops fetalis: Identifying the underlying genetic etiology. *Genet. Med.* **2019**, *21*, 1339–1344. [CrossRef] [PubMed]
18. Bellini, C.; Donarini, G.; Paladini, D.; Calevo, M.G.; Bellini, T.; Ramenghi, L.A.; Hennekam, R.C. Etiology of non-immune hydrops fetalis: An update. *Am. J. Med Genet. Part A* **2015**, *167*, 1082–1088. [CrossRef] [PubMed]
19. Santo, S.; Mansour, S.; Thilaganathan, B.; Homfray, T.; Papageorghiou, A.; Calvert, S.; Bhide, A. Prenatal diagnosis of non-immune hydrops fetalis: What do we tell the parents? *Prenat. Diagn.* **2011**, *31*, 186–195. [CrossRef]
20. Gravholt, C.H. Epidemiological, endocrine and metabolic features in Turner syndrome. *Eur. J. Endocrinol.* **2004**, *151*, 657–688. [CrossRef]
21. Lin, A.E.; Prakash, S.K.; Andersen, N.H.; Viuff, M.H.; Levitsky, L.L.; Rivera-Davila, M.; Crenshaw, M.L.; Hansen, L.; Colvin, M.K.; Hayes, F.J.; et al. Recognition and management of adults with Turner syndrome: From the transition of adolescence through the senior years. *Am. J. Med. Genet. Part A* **2019**, *179*, 1987–2033. [CrossRef] [PubMed]
22. Hook, E.B.; Warburton, D. The distribution of chromosomal genotypes associated with Turner's syndrome: Livebirth prevalence rates and evidence for diminished fetal mortality and severity in genotypes associated with structural X abnormalities or mosaicism. *Hum. Genet.* **1983**, *64*, 24–27. [CrossRef] [PubMed]
23. Viuff, M.H.; Stochholm, K.; Uldbjerg, N.; Nielsen, B.B.; the Danish Fetal Medicine Study Group; Gravholt, C.H. Only a minority of sex chromosome abnormalities are detected by a national prenatal screening program for Down syndrome. *Hum. Reprod.* **2015**, *30*, 2419–2426. [CrossRef] [PubMed]
24. Surerus, E.; Huggon, I.C.; Allan, L.D. Turner's syndrome in fetal life. *Ultrasound Obstet. Gynecol.* **2003**, *22*, 264–267. [CrossRef]
25. Bellini, C.; Hennekam, R.C.; Fulcheri, E.; Rutigliani, M.; Morcaldi, G.; Boccardo, F.M.; Bonioli, E. Etiology of Nonimmune Hydrops Fetalis: A Systematic Review. *Am. J. Med. Genet. Part A* **2009**, *149*, 844–851. [CrossRef]

26. Alvarez-Nava, F.; Soto, M.; Lanes, R.; Pons, H.; Morales-Machin, A.; Bracho, A. Elevated second-trimester maternal serum β-human chorionic gonadotropin and amniotic fluid alpha-fetoprotein as indicators of adverse obstetric outcomes in fetal Turner syndrome: Biochemical screening in fetal TS. *J. Obstet. Gynaecol. Res.* **2015**, *41*, 1891–1898. [CrossRef]
27. Lambert-Messerlian, G.M.; Saller, D.N.; Tumber, M.B.; French, C.A.; Peterson, C.J.; Canick, J.A. Second-trimester maternal serum progesterone levels in Turner syndrome with and without hydrops and in trisomy 18. *Prenat. Diagn.* **1999**, *19*, 476–479. [CrossRef]
28. Benirschke, K.; Kaufmann, P. *Pathology of the Human Placenta*; Springer Science & Business Media: Berlin/Heidelberg, Germany, 2013; 891p.
29. Wegrzyn, P.; Faro, C.; Falcon, O.; Peralta, C.F.A.; Nicolaides, K.H. Placental volume measured by three-dimensional ultrasound at 11 to 13 + 6 weeks of gestation: Relation to chromosomal defects. *Ultrasound Obstet. Gynecol.* **2005**, *26*, 28–32. [CrossRef]
30. Jeon, K.C.; Chen, L.S.; Goodson, P. Decision to abort after a prenatal diagnosis of sex chromosome abnormality: A systematic review of the literature. *Genet. Med.* **2012**, *14*, 27–38. [CrossRef]
31. Burwick, R.M.; Pilliod, R.A.; Dukhovny, S.E.; Caughey, A.B. Fetal hydrops and the risk of severe preeclampsia. *J. Matern.-Fetal Neonatal Med.* **2019**, *32*, 961–965. [CrossRef]
32. Torres-Gómez, L.G.; Silva-González, M.E.; González-Hernández, R. Ballantyne syndrome or mirror syndrome. *Ginecol. Obstet. Mex.* **2010**, *78*, 621–625. [PubMed]
33. Vogel, M. *Atlas der Morphologischen Plazentadiagnostik*, 2nd ed.; Springer: Berlin/Heidelberg, Germany, 1996; 263p.
34. Chimenea, A.; García-Díaz, L.; Calderón, A.M.; Heras, M.M.D.L.; Antiñolo, G. Resolution of maternal Mirror syndrome after succesful fetal intrauterine therapy: A case series. *BMC Pregnancy Childbirth* **2018**, *18*, 85. [CrossRef] [PubMed]
35. Zhang, Z.; Xi, M.; Peng, B.; You, Y. Mirror syndrome associated with Fetal Hemoglobin Bart's disease: A case report. *Arch. Gynecol. Obstet.* **2013**, *288*, 1183–1185. [CrossRef] [PubMed]
36. Hermyt, E.; Zmarzły, N.; Jęda-Golonka, A. Mirror syndrome: A literature review. *Pediatr. Med. Rodz.* **2019**, *15*, 246–251. [CrossRef]
37. Llurba, E.; Marsal, G.; Sanchez, O.; Dominguez, C.; Alijotas-Reig, J.; Carreras, E.; Cabero, L. Angiogenic and antiangiogenic factors before and after resolution of maternal mirror syndrome. *Ultrasound Obstet. Gynecol.* **2012**, *40*, 367–369. [CrossRef]
38. Chervenak, F.A.; Isaacson, G.; Blakemore, K.J.; Breg, W.R.; Hobbins, J.C.; Berkowitz, R.L.; Tortora, M.; Mayden, K.; Mahoney, M.J. Fetal Cystic Hygroma: Cause and Natural History. *N. Engl. J. Med.* **1983**, *309*, 822–825. [CrossRef]
39. Jauniaux, E. Diagnosis and management of early non-immune hydrops fetalis. *Prenat. Diagn.* **1997**, *17*, 1261–1268. [CrossRef]
40. Atton, G.; Gordon, K.; Brice, G.; Keeley, V.; Riches, K.; Ostergaard, P.; Mortimer, P.S.; Mansour, S. The lymphatic phenotype in Turner syndrome: An evaluation of nineteen patients and literature review. *Eur. J. Hum. Genet.* **2015**, *23*, 1634–1639. [CrossRef]
41. Mostello, D.J.; Bofinger, M.K.; Siddiqi, T.A. Spontaneous resolution of fetal cystic hygroma and hydrops in Turner syndrome. *Obstet. Gynecol.* **1989**, *73 Pt 2*, 862–865.

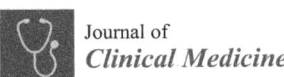

Case Report

Lethal Congenital Contracture Syndrome 11: A Case Report and Literature Review

Miriam Potrony [1,2,3], Antoni Borrell [2,4], Narcís Masoller [2,4], Alfons Nadal [3,5,6], Leonardo Rodriguez-Carunchio [5,7], Karmele Saez de Gordoa Elizalde [5], Juan Francisco Quesada-Espinosa [8,9], Jose Luis Villanueva-Cañas [10], Montse Pauta [3,4], Meritxell Jodar [1,3], Irene Madrigal [1,2,3], Celia Badenas [1,2,3], Maria Isabel Alvarez-Mora [1,2,3] and Laia Rodriguez-Revenga [1,2,3,*]

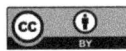

Citation: Potrony, M.; Borrell, A.; Masoller, N.; Nadal, A.; Rodriguez-Carunchio, L.; Saez de Gordoa Elizalde, K.; Quesada-Espinosa, J.F.; Villanueva-Cañas, J.L.; Pauta, M.; Jodar, M.; et al. Lethal Congenital Contracture Syndrome 11: A Case Report and Literature Review. *J. Clin. Med.* 2022, *11*, 3570. https://doi.org/10.3390/jcm11133570

Academic Editor: Roland Axt-Fliedner

Received: 17 May 2022
Accepted: 20 June 2022
Published: 21 June 2022

Publisher's Note: MDPI stays neutral with regard to jurisdictional claims in published maps and institutional affiliations.

Copyright: © 2022 by the authors. Licensee MDPI, Basel, Switzerland. This article is an open access article distributed under the terms and conditions of the Creative Commons Attribution (CC BY) license (https://creativecommons.org/licenses/by/4.0/).

1. Biochemistry and Molecular Genetics Department, Hospital Clinic of Barcelona, 08036 Barcelona, Spain; potrony@clinic.cat (M.P.); mjodar@clinic.cat (M.J.); imadbajo@clinic.cat (I.M.); cbadenas@clinic.cat (C.B.); mialvarez@clinic.cat (M.I.A.-M.)
2. CIBER of Rare Diseases (CIBERER), Instituto de Salud Carlos III, 28029 Madrid, Spain; aborrell@clinic.cat (A.B.); masoller@clinic.cat (N.M.)
3. Institut d'Investigacions Biomèdiques August Pi i Sunyer (IDIBAPS), 08036 Barcelona, Spain; anadal@clinic.cat (A.N.); mpauta@clinic.cat (M.P.)
4. BCNatal, Barcelona Center for Maternal-Fetal and Neonatal Medicine (Hospital Clínic and Hospital Sant Joan de Deu), Institut Clínic de Ginecologia, Obstetricia i Neonatologia Fetal i+D Fetal Medicine Research Center, Universitat de Barcelona, 08007 Barcelona, Spain
5. Pathology Department, Biomedical Diagnostic Center Hospital Clínic de Barcelona, 08036 Barcelona, Spain; lerodrig@clinic.cat (L.R.-C.); saezdegord@clinic.cat (K.S.d.G.E.)
6. Department of Basic Clinical Practice, Medical School, Universitat de Barcelona, 08007 Barcelona, Spain
7. Medicine Department, University of Vic-Central University of Catalonia (UVic-UCC), 08500 Barcelona, Spain
8. Genetics Department, 12 de Octubre University Hospital, 28041 Madrid, Spain; juanf.quesada@ingene.es
9. UDISGEN (Unidad de Dismorfología y Genética), 12 de Octubre University Hospital, 28041 Madrid, Spain
10. Molecular Biology CORE (CDB), Hospital Clínic de Barcelona, 08036 Barcelona, Spain; jlvillanueva@clinic.cat
* Correspondence: lbodi@clinic.cat; Tel.: +34-93-227-56-73; Fax: 34-93-451-52-72

Abstract: Lethal congenital contracture syndrome 11 (LCCS11) is caused by homozygous or compound heterozygous variants in the *GLDN* gene on chromosome 15q21. *GLDN* encodes gliomedin, a protein required for the formation of the nodes of Ranvier and development of the human peripheral nervous system. We report a fetus with ultrasound alterations detected at 28 weeks of gestation. The fetus exhibited hydrops, short long bones, fixed limb joints, absent fetal movements, and polyhydramnios. The pregnancy was terminated and postmortem studies confirmed the prenatal findings: distal arthrogryposis, fetal growth restriction, pulmonary hypoplasia, and retrognathia. The fetus had a normal chromosomal microarray analysis. Exome sequencing revealed two novel compound heterozygous variants in the *GLDN* associated with LCCS11. This manuscript reports this case and performs a literature review of all published LCCS11 cases.

Keywords: *GLDN*; arthrogryposis multiplex congenita; fetal akinesia deformation sequence

1. Introduction

Arthrogryposis is characterized by congenital joint contractures in two or more body areas resulting from reduced or absent fetal movements [1]. Once the contracture is formed, a variety of secondary deformations occur, including craniofacial changes, pulmonary hypoplasia, polyhydramnios, decreased gut mobility and shortened gut, short umbilical cord, skin changes, and multiple joints with limitation of movement. Arthrogryposis is a complex trait that exhibits phenotypic and genotypic heterogeneity with an overall incidence of 1 in 3000 to 5000 [2]. Rather than a diagnosis, arthrogryposis is a descriptive term since it encompasses more than 400 medical conditions [3]. Alternative nomenclature in the literature includes multiple congenital contractures (MCC), arthrogryposis multiplex congenita (AMC), and fetal akinesia deformation sequence (FADS) or Pena–Shokeir syndrome type I (reviewed in [4]). Prenatal ultrasound imaging is crucial in its early diagnosis by identifying fetal movement limitations and the presence of club foot or joint contractures [5]. On prenatal suspicion of arthrogryposis, genetic diagnosis is important not only for identifying the causative genetic variant(s), but also for genetic counseling in regard to the prognosis, recurrence risk, and the options of prenatal testing or reproductive choice for future pregnancies.

The use of next-generation sequencing (NGS) methods in the diagnostic workup of arthrogryposis has proved to be an efficient technology in achieving the underlying genetic causes in many cases, i.e., [6–8]. The diagnosis rates of arthrogryposis improve up to 60% when whole-exome sequencing (WES) is used [8]. In fact, this strategy has also allowed the identification of new arthrogryposis-associated genes such as *GLDN* [9].

The *GLDN* gene encodes the gliomedin protein, a secreted cell adhesion molecule involved in peripheral nervous system development. Biallelic variants in the *GLDN* gene have recently been associated with lethal congenital contracture syndrome 11 (LCCS11, OMIM # 617194), a clinically severe form of AMC [9,10]. Here, we report a prenatal diagnosis of LCCS11 detected by WES in a fetus with AMC, hydrops, and retrognathia, and a literature review of all cases reported to date. Although *GLDN* has been described as a new AMC-associated gene, we conclude that it should be better associated with FADS or Pena–Shokeir syndrome type I.

2. Case Report

A 35-year-old primigravid woman was referred at the 28th week of gestation for hydrops fetalis and arthrogryposis. Sonography examination revealed hydrothorax, subcutaneous generalized edema, short long bones, fixed limb joints, absent fetal movements, fetal growth restriction (estimated fetal weight in the 4th percentile and absent end-diastolic flow in both umbilical arteries), and polyhydramnios (amniotic fluid index 28 cm) (Figure 1). The couple was nonconsanguineous, healthy, and both showed unremarkable family history with no congenital malformations. The mother denied any exposure to alcohol, teratogenic agents, irradiation, or infectious diseases during this pregnancy. Serologic testing for TORCH (Toxoplasmosis, Rubella, Cytomegalovirus, Herpes simplex virus) infection diseases was negative. In consideration of the abnormal ultrasound findings, amniocentesis was performed and chromosomal microarray analysis (CMA) was performed using qChipPrenatal microarray (qGenomics, Spain) on uncultured amniocytes. The qChipPrenatal microarray is a genome-wide oligonucleotide array (based on an Agilent 8×60 K format) with a practical resolution of approximately 350–500 Kb throughout the entire genome and 30–100 Kb in regions associated with constitutional pathology (qChipCM, 8×60 K, qGenomics). The results revealed a normal female profile, arr(X, 1 − 22) × 2. Written informed consent was obtained from the pregnant woman.

The woman elected to terminate the pregnancy at 29 weeks of gestation. Postmortem examination was performed and findings were consistent with the prenatally observed sonographic anomalies. The autopsy revealed a slightly macerated female fetus with hydrops with subcutaneous edema and pleural effusions, distal arthrogryposis of the hands, left pes equinus, flexed elbows with preserved mobility of all major joints, fetal growth restriction, pulmonary hypoplasia with a lung to body weight ratio of 0.0058 (normal > 0.012), and retrognathia (Figure 2). Histological examination of the brain was unremarkable.

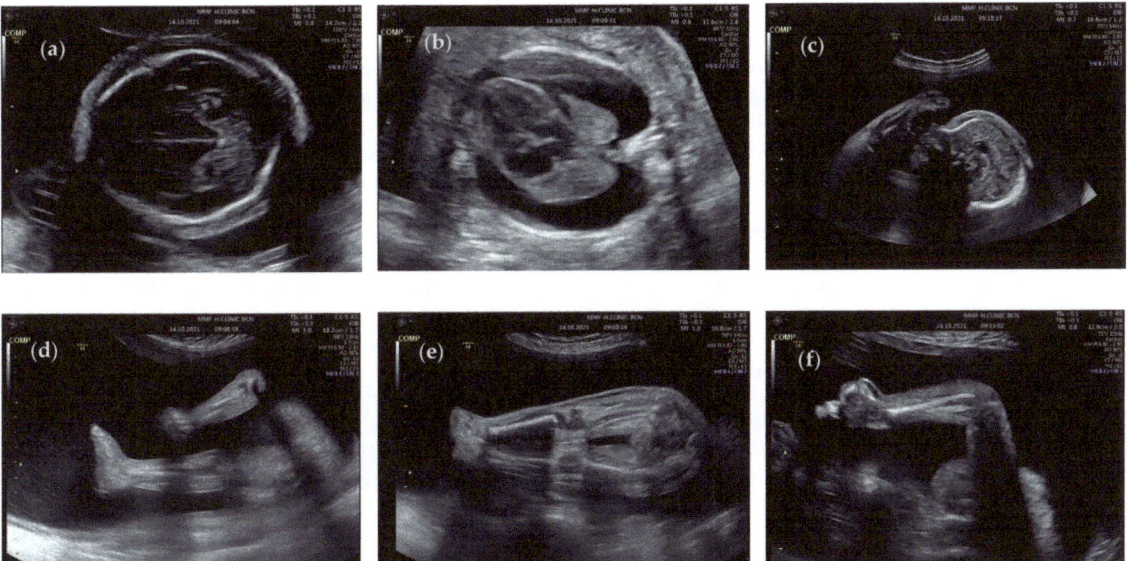

Figure 1. Transabdominal ultrasound images of the present case. Transabdominal ultrasound images of the present case showing (**a**) scalp edema, (**b**) subcutaneous edema and hydrothorax, (**c**) forehead edema, (**d**,**e**) lower extremity hyperextension, (**f**) upper extremity and hand contracture.

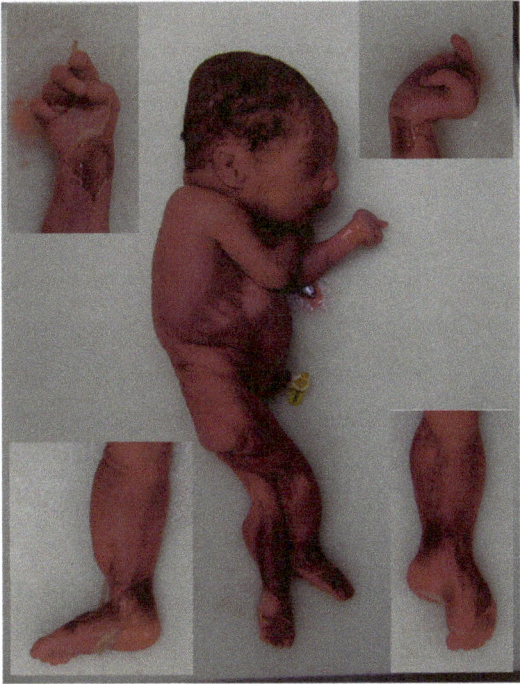

Figure 2. Lateral view of the fetus. Lateral view of the fetus shows skin slippage due to maceration. Both hands show medially overlapping fingers (**upper insets**) and left pes equinus (**lower insets**).

WES analysis was further performed. Massively parallel sequencing was performed using DNA Prep with Enrichment (Exome capture, Illumina, San Diego, CA, USA) on a NextSeq 500 sequencer (Illumina, San Diego, CA, USA), with a targeted mean coverage of 100× and a minimum of 90% of bases sequenced to at least 20×. Bioinformatic analysis consisted of alignment to the reference human genome (hg38) using BWA MEM (v0.7.17) and Bowtie2 (v2.4.1) short-read aligners, genotyping using Haplotype Caller from Genome Analysis Toolkit (v.4.2) and VarDict (v1.7.0) variant callers, and annotation using Ensembl Variant Effect Predictor (v104). Copy Number Variants (CNVs) analysis was performed using ExomeDepth R package (v1.15) for CNVs identification and AnnotSV (v2.3) for CNVs annotation. Variants that did not meet the established quality criteria were filtered out: strand bias variants or those in repetitive or high CGs content regions with low mapping quality reads. In addition, variants with frequency greater than 3% in gnomAD population database (v3.1.1) were also filtered together with those classified as benign or likely benign by multiple subscribers in the ClinVar database (March 2020 release). Variant interpretation and classification were performed according to the ACMG recommendations [11].

Results evidenced a compound heterozygous for two variants in the *GLDN* (NM_181789) gene. The maternally inherited *GLDN* variant (c.1494G>T, p.Leu498Phe) is a missense variant predicted to be damaging by the majority of in silico functional prediction programs (PolyPhen, SIFT, CADD, Mutation Taster). The leucine residue at this position has a high conservation score (phyloP and phastCons 100 vertebrates) and it is located within the conserved extracellular olfactomedin domain of gliomedin. The variant is absent in population databases (gnomAD, 1000G) and the same amino acid change has been previously reported in one LCCS11 case [12].

The paternally inherited variant is also a missense variant, c.62C>A, p.Ala21Glu, that has been detected in very low frequency in the general population (gnomAD: 4 heterozygous individuals, allele frequency 0.000058, dbSNP: rs778094534), but has not been previously detected in LCCS11-affected individuals. The affected alanine residue is partially conserved (phyloP and phastCons 100 vertebrates) and it is located within a trasmembrane domain. Although this variant did not have sufficient evidence to be classified as pathogenic in the absence of additional functional data, the phenotype of our patient is remarkably similar to that previously reported.

The publications available in the literature were reviewed, and 28 cases, belonging to 19 different families, with compound heterozygous or homozygous variants in *GLDN*, were collected in this report (Figure 3). Table 1 summarizes the sonographic, postmortem, and molecular findings.

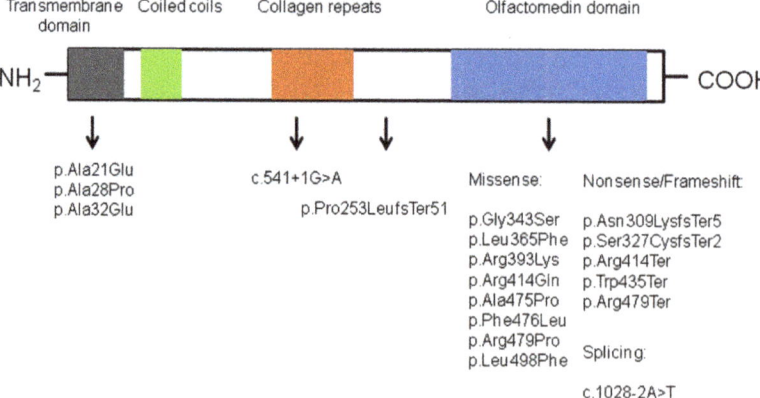

Figure 3. Location of the pathogenic/likely pathogenic variants identified in *GLDN* in AMC-affected families relative to the predicted protein domains.

Table 1. Clinical characteristics of cases with biallelic *GLDN* variants and arthrogryposis multiplex congenita (AMC).

ID	Sex	Prenatal Ultrasound Examination	Fetal Death	Postmortem Examination	Birth	Genetic Variant 1	Genetic Variant 2	Reference
Family 1 Case 1	male	32 wg: Akinesia Polyhydramnios	Exitus 33 wg	Extension of lower limbs Extension contractures of wrists Pulmonary hypoplasia	-	c.758delC p.(Pro253LeufsTer51)	c.1423G>C p.(Ala475Pro)	[9]
Family 1 Case 2	female	Akinesia Polyhydramnios	TOP 33 wg	Unremarkable histological examination of the spinal cord and skeletal muscle Reduced number of myelinated fibers	-	c.758delC p.(Pro253LeufsTer51)	c.1423G>C p.(Ala475Pro)	[9]
Family 2 Case 1	male	30 wg: Polyhydramnios Intrauterine growth retardation AMC (flexion contractures of the elbows, extension of the knees, camptodactyly, and retrognathia)	-	NI	30 wg AMC (flexion contractures of the elbows, extension of the knees, camptodactyly, and retrognathia) Exitus: day 1	c.95C>A p.(Ala32Glu)	c.95C>A p.(Ala32Glu)	[9]
Family 3 Case 1	male	28 wg: Akinesia Polyhydramnios Bilateral flexion of fingers	-	Unremarkable pathological examination of the brain and spinal cord	AMC (involving the fingers, wrists, thumbs, and knees) Pulmonary hypoplasia Exitus: day 1	c.541 + 1G>A	c.1240C>T p.(Arg414Ter)	[9]
Family 3 Case 2	male	31 wg: Polyhydramnios Bilateral flexion of fingers Reduced mobility	TOP 31 wg	AMC with microretrognathia Pulmonary hypoplasia	-	c.541 + 1G>A	c.1240C>T p.(Arg414Ter)	[9]
Family 4 Case 1	female	27 wg: Reduced mobility Polyhydramnios 29 wg: Fetal Immobility	TOP 30 wg	Unremarkable pathological examination of the brain and spinal cord	Distal arthrogryposis of the hands Bilateral club foot Pulmonary hypoplasia	c.1435C>T p.(Arg479Ter)	c.1435C>T p.(Arg479Ter)	[9]

Table 1. Cont.

ID	Sex	Prenatal Ultrasound Examination	Fetal Death	Postmortem Examination	Birth	Genetic Variant 1	Genetic Variant 2	Reference
Family 5 Case 1	male	Reduced mobility Breech		AMC Pulmonary hypoplasia and pulmonary hemorrhage Bilateral hip dislocations Fistula from the left anterior descending artery to right ventricle Bilateral small kidneys with calcifications, an ectopic right ureter without signs of obstruction, and intraventricular hemorrhage Skeletal muscle fibers were small for age and central nuclei suggested centronuclear myopathy	38 wg Respiratory failure Exitus: day 2	c.927_930del p.(Asn309LysfsTer5)	c.1436G>C p.(Arg479Pro)	[10]
Family 5 Case 2	female	Polyhydramnios Intrauterine growth restriction Bilateral club feet	-	-	37 wg Respiratory insufficiency Contractures of hips, knees fixed in extension Bilateral club feet Flexion contracture of left long finger Bilateral hip dislocation Axial and appendicular hypotonia Alive at 22 months with tracheostomy and home ventilation	c.927_930del p.(Asn309LysfsTer5)	c.1436G>C p.(Arg479Pro)	[10]
Family 5 Case 3	male	Polyhydramnios Bilateral club feet Flexed wrists Extended knees Breech Intrauterine growth restriction	-	-	39 wg Respiratory insufficiency Contractures of hips, knees Bilateral club feet Hyperextension of thumbs to radii Axial and appendicular hypotonia Undescended testes Alive at 7 months with tracheostomy and home ventilation	c.927_930del p.(Asn309LysfsTer5)	c.1436G>C p.(Arg479Pro)	[10]

Table 1. Cont.

ID	Sex	Prenatal Ultrasound Examination	Fetal Death	Postmortem Examination	Birth	Genetic Variant 1	Genetic Variant 2	Reference
Family 6 Case 1	male	Polyhydramnios	-	-	33 wg Pulmonary hypoplasia Bilateral hip dislocation Contractures of knees and wrists Bilateral club feet Progressive scoliosis, diaphragm paralysis, borderline intellectual functioning (IQ 74) Alive at age 17 years old with intermittent use of non-invasive mask ventilation	c.1305G>A p.(Trp435Ter)	c.1305G>A p.(Trp435Ter)	[10]
Family 7 Case 1	female	30 wg. Akinesia Polyhidramnios Skin edema	TOP 31 wg	NI	-	c.1305G>A p.(Trp435Ter)	c.1305G>A p.(Trp435Ter)	[10]
Family 7 Case 2	male	-	-	-	41 wg Paresis of right vocal cord and right side of the soft palate Bilateral hip flexion contractures with dislocated hips Extension contractures of kneesCalcaneovalgus deformity of feet Axial and appendicular hypotonia Atrophy of lower limbs Right-sided cryptorchidism Intubated at birth for respiratory failure Tracheostomy at 6 weeks of age Alive at 28 months without ventilatory support	c.1305G>A p.(Trp435Ter)	c.1305G>A p.(Trp435Ter)	[10]
Family 8 Case 1	male	Akinesia Flexed arms and closed hand	TOP 27 wg	Pulmonary hypoplasia Extension contractures of hip sand knees Flexion contractures of fingers	-	Unknown	Unknown	[10]

Table 1. Cont.

ID	Sex	Prenatal Ultrasound Examination	Fetal Death	Postmortem Examination	Birth	Genetic Variant 1	Genetic Variant 2	Reference
Family 8 Case 2	female	26 wg: Polyhydramnios Arthrogryposis	-	-	36 wg: Pulmonary hypoplasia Extension contractures of hips and knees Flexion contractures of elbows, wrists, and fingers Bilateral vertical talus information Diffuse muscle atrophy/hypoplasia Exitus: 12 h	c.1178G>A p.(Arg393Lys)	c.1428C>A p.(Phe476Leu)	[10]
Family 9 Case 1	male	26 wg: Multiple joint contracture Polyhydramnios	-	-	-	c.1027G>A p.(Gly343Ser)	c.1240C>T p.(Arg414Ter)	[13]
Family 9 Case 2	female	26 wg: Multiple joint contracture Polyhydramnios	-	-	-	c.1027G>A p.(Gly343Ser)	c.1240C>T p.(Arg414Ter)	[13]
Family 10 Case 1	-	NI	NI	NI	NI	c.1494G>C p.(Leu498Phe)	c.1494G>C p.(Leu498Phe)	[12]
Family 11 Case 1	female	Early fetal demise of a twin <12 wg Polyhydramnios Preterm premature rupture of membranes Breech (20 wg)	-	-	30 wg: Bilateral extension knee contractures and camptodactyly Bilateral congenital hip dysplasia and right-sided hip dislocation Hypotonia Pulmonary hypoplasia Alive at 44 months	c.1093C>T p.(Leu365Phe)	c.1178G>A p.(Arg393Lys)	[14]
Family 12 Case 1	female	Fetal akinesia	NI	NI	Joint contractures: Hips, knees, ankles, elbows, fingers Microcephaly Delayed motor development Muscular hypertonia Hip joint luxation Alive at 1 year	c.1178G>A p.(Arg393Lys)	c.1428C>A p.(Phe476Leu)	[7]
Family 13 Case 1	male	Hydrops fetalis	-	-	Subtle joint contractures Down-slanted palpebral fissures Ventilator support Care redirected towards palliation	c.980_981del p.(Ser327CysfsTer2)	c.980_981del p.(Ser327CysfsTer2)	[15]
Family 14 Case 1	male	No findings	-	-	Exitus: < 1 month	c.95C>A p.(Ala32Glu)	c.95C>A p.(Ala32Glu)	[8] *

Table 1. Cont.

ID	Sex	Prenatal Ultrasound Examination	Fetal Death	Postmortem Examination	Birth	Genetic Variant 1	Genetic Variant 2	Reference
Family 15 Case 1	female	Abnormalities	TOP	NI	-	c.1435C>T p.(Arg479Ter)	c.1435C>T p.(Arg479Ter)	[8] *
Family 16 Case 1 + Case 2	Female (2 cases)	Abnormalities	-	NI	Exitus: 2 months	c.82G>C p.(Ala28Pro)	c.1241G>A p.(Arg414Gln)	[8] *
Family 17 Case 1	-	32 wg: Polyhydramnios Missing fetal movements Facial dismorphism Lung hypoplasia Flexed knees, extended anckles, flexed elbows, fisted hands	-	-	32 wg Exitus: 1 day	c.1423G>C p.(Ala475Pro)	c.1423G>C p.(Ala475Pro)	[16]
Family 17 Case 2	-	23 wg: Polyhydramnios Missing fetal movements Microcephaly Single umbilical artery Pericardial and pleural effusion Flexed knees, flexed elbows, fisted hands	TOP 27 wg	-	-	c.1423G>C p.(Ala475Pro)	c.1423G>C p.(Ala475Pro)	[16]
Family 18 Case 1	-	NI	-	-	Flexion contracture Hydrops fetalis Pulmonary hypoplasia Pleural effusion	c.1028-2A>T	c.1028-2A>T	[17]
PRESENT CASE	female	28 wg: Hydrops fetalis Arthrogryposis	TOP 29 wg	Distal arthrogryposis of the hands Left club foot Pulmonary hypoplasia Retrognathia	-	c.62C>A p.(Ala21Glu)	c.1494G > T p.(Leu498Phe)	PRESENT STUDY

wg: weeks of gestation; TOP: termination of pregnancy, NI: no information. * Cases already reported by Maluenda et al. [9] were excluded from this table. Families and cases have been renumbered in this table based on the order of appearance in each study.

3. Discussion

Biallelic *GLDN* variants have been associated with a lethal form of AMC since most of the reported patients did not survive past neonatal ages (LCCS11) [9]. However, among the 28 herein reviewed cases, there are 6 long-term survivors (from 5 families) that, although the majority required intensive clinical support, survived beyond the neonatal period [7,10,14]. On the basis of these cases, it has been suggested that pulmonary insufficiency in patients with biallelic *GLDN* variants is not necessarily lethal [10,14]. Nevertheless, 57% (8/14) of the neonate cases died before 2 months. The remaining six cases survived beyond the neonatal period although they required intensive respiratory support.

A distinguishing clinical feature described in the majority of patients with pathogenic *GLDN* variants is pulmonary hypoplasia. To our knowledge, among the herein 28 reviewed cases, 16 reported respiratory findings, pulmonary hypoplasia being the most frequent (75%, 12/16), followed by pulmonary insufficiency or need of respiratory support. As pulmonary hypoplasia is a feature not common in AMC at large, some authors have recently suggested that AMC secondary to *GLDN* variants may be best fitted under the umbrella of FADS [14]. The FADS (ORHA:994) is characterized by multiple joint contractures, facial anomalies, and pulmonary hypoplasia. The common feature of this sequence is decreased fetal activity, which leads to a failure of normal deglutition, resulting in polyhydramnios. The lack of movement of the diaphragm and intercostal muscles leads to pulmonary hypoplasia. Finally, the lack of normal fetal movement also results in a short umbilical cord and multiple joint contractures.

Sonographic detection of AMC in a prenatal context is often missed or diagnosed during late gestation, when associated anomalies are more pronounced [18,19]. In the series herein reviewed, approximately 30–32 weeks of gestational age is the mean gestational age of prenatal diagnosis, with fetal akinesia, missing fetal movements, arthrogryposis, and polyhydramnios being the most frequently reported features. Among the 28 reviewed cases, 29% (8/28) elected to terminate pregnancy. Postmortem examination is only reported in half of them, confirming the prenatal diagnosis and expanding the associated phenotype spectrum with pulmonary hypoplasia, retrognathia, and clubfoot (Table 1).

Due to the relative rarity of this entity, few patients have been reported; this makes it difficult to establish a genotype–phenotype correlation. Among the 19 different pathogenic variants described in the *GLDN* gene (Table 1), the majority of them (68%, 13/19) correspond to missense, nonsense, or frameshift variants located within the highly conserved olfactomedin domain (aa 300–550) [20] (Figure 3). The olfactomedin domain mediates the interaction between gliomedin and NrCAM, as well as neurofascin-186 (NF186), two cell adhesion molecules expressed at the nodes of Ranvier, to induce clustering of sodium channels at heminodes of myelinating Schwann cells [20–23]. Thus, these variants might impact the formation of the NrCAM–NF186–gliomedin complex at nodes. To our knowledge, only three different missense variants (c.95C>A, c.82G>C and the c.62C>A detected in the present case) have been described outside this domain and within the transmembrane domain of gliomedin (aa 16–38) (Table 1, Figure 3) [21,22]. Although these variants might be initially classified as variants of uncertain significance (VUS), as the amino acid residues are not highly conserved, functional analyses have also revealed an abnormal localization of the resultant protein [9,14]. Western blotting experiments in transfected CHO cells with different *GLDN* variants showed similar amounts of GLDN protein [9]. Thus, it can be inferred that rather than a loss of function effect, pathogenic variants detected in the *GLDN* gene affect gliomedin's transportation to the cell surface and its binding to NF186 [9,14].

4. Conclusions

The present reported case and the literature review confirms the association of biallelic *GLDN* variants with AMC and other phenotypic spectra such as pulmonary hypoplasia, reaffirming that it should be better classified as FADS. Prenatal diagnosis of this condition is challenging since it is often missed or diagnosed in the second or third trimester. Postnatal autopsy is recommended as it confirms the prenatal diagnosis and might identify further associated congenital anomalies. Furthermore, it provides a valuable source of DNA material. Finally, and due to the high degree of genetic heterogeneity, WES should be recommended when a FADS is suspected. Once the underlying etiology is known, genetics consultation and individualized recurrence risk assessment can be offered.

Author Contributions: Conceptualization, M.P. (Miriam Potrony) and L.R.-R.; Methodology, J.F.Q.-E., J.L.V.-C., M.J., I.M. and C.B.; Formal Analysis, A.B., N.M., A.N., L.R.-C., K.S.d.G.E. and M.I.A.-M.; Data Curation, J.F.Q.-E., J.L.V.-C., A.B., N.M., A.N., L.R.-C., K.S.d.G.E., M.P. (Miriam Potrony), M.P. (Montse Pauta) and L.R.-R.; Writing—Original Draft Preparation, M.P. (Miriam Potrony) and L.R.-R.; Writing—Review and Editing, all authors. All authors have read and agreed to the published version of the manuscript.

Funding: This work was supported by grants Fundación Mutua Madrileña (Grant/Award Number: AP171442019) and AGAUR from the Autonomous Catalan Government (2017SGR1134). The CIBER de Enfermedades Raras is an initiative of the Instituto de Salud Carlos III.

Institutional Review Board Statement: Not applicable.

Informed Consent Statement: Written informed consent has been obtained from the patient(s) to perform the study.

Data Availability Statement: The analyzed data sets generated during the study are available from the corresponding author on reasonable request.

Conflicts of Interest: The authors declare no conflict of interest.

References

1. Hall, J.G.; Kimber, E.; Dieterich, K. Classification of arthrogryposis. *Am. J. Med. Genet. C Semin. Med. Genet.* **2019**, *181*, 300–303. [CrossRef] [PubMed]
2. Lowry, R.B.; Sibbald, B.; Bedard, T.; Hall, J.G. Prevalence of multiple congenital contractures including arthrogryposis multiplex congenita in Alberta, Canada, and a strategy for classification and coding. *Birth Defects Res. A Clin. Mol. Teratol.* **2010**, *88*, 1057–1061. [CrossRef] [PubMed]
3. Kiefer, J.; Hall, J.G. Gene ontology analysis of arthrogryposis (multiple congenital contractures). *Am. J. Med. Genet. C Semin. Med. Genet.* **2019**, *181*, 310–326. [CrossRef]
4. Niles, K.M.; Blaser, S.; Shannon, P.; Chitayat, D. Fetal arthrogryposis multiplex congenita/fetal akinesia deformation sequence (FADS)-Aetiology, diagnosis, and management. *Prenat. Diagn.* **2019**, *39*, 720–731. [CrossRef] [PubMed]
5. Skaria, P.; Dahl, A.; Ahmed, A. Arthrogryposis multiplex congenita in utero: Radiologic and pathologic findings. *J. Matern. Fetal Neonatal Med.* **2019**, *32*, 502–511. [CrossRef] [PubMed]
6. Ravenscroft, G.; Clayton, J.S.; Faiz, F.; Sivadorai, P.; Milnes, D.; Cincotta, R.; Moon, P.; Kamien, B.; Edwards, M.; Delatycki, M.; et al. Neurogenetic fetal akinesia and arthrogryposis: Genetics, expanding genotype-phenotypes and functional genomics. *J. Med. Genet.* **2021**, *58*, 609–618. [CrossRef] [PubMed]
7. Pergande, M.; Motameny, S.; Özdemir, Ö.; Kreutzer, M.; Wang, H.; Daimagüler, H.S.; Becker, K.; Karakaya, M.; Ehrhardt, H.; Elcioglu, N.; et al. The genomic and clinical landscape of fetal akinesia. *Genet. Med.* **2020**, *22*, 511–523. [CrossRef]
8. Laquerriere, A.; Jaber, D.; Abiusi, E.; Maluenda, J.; Mejlachowicz, D.; Vivanti, A.; Dieterich, K.; Stoeva, R.; Quevarec, L.; Nolent, F.; et al. Phenotypic spectrum and genomics of undiagnosed arthrogryposis multiplex congenita. *J. Med. Genet.* **2021**, *59*, 559–567. [CrossRef]
9. Maluenda, J.; Manso, C.; Quevarec, L.; Vivanti, A.; Marguet, F.; Gonzales, M.; Guimiot, F.; Petit, F.; Toutain, A.; Whalen, S.; et al. Mutations in GLDN, Encoding Gliomedin, a Critical Component of the Nodes of Ranvier, Are Responsible for Lethal Arthrogryposis. *Am. J. Hum. Genet.* **2016**, *99*, 928–933. [CrossRef]
10. Wambach, J.A.; Stettner, G.M.; Haack, T.B.; Writzl, K.; Škofljanec, A.; Maver, A.; Munell, F.; Ossowski, S.; Bosio, M.; Wegner, D.J.; et al. Survival among children with "Lethal" congenital contracture syndrome 11 caused by novel mutations in the gliomedin gene (GLDN). *Hum. Mutat.* **2017**, *38*, 1477–1484. [CrossRef] [PubMed]
11. Richards, S.; Aziz, N.; Bale, S.; Bick, D.; Das, S.; Gastier-Foster, J.; Grody, W.W.; Hegde, M.; Lyon, E.; Spector, E.; et al. Standards and guidelines for the interpretation of sequence variants: A joint consensus recommendation of the American College of Medical Genetics and Genomics and the Association for Molecular Pathology. *Genet. Med.* **2015**, *17*, 405–424. [CrossRef]
12. Baker, S.W.; Murrell, J.R.; Nesbitt, A.I.; Pechter, K.B.; Balciuniene, J.; Zhao, X.; Yu, Z.; Denenberg, E.H.; DeChene, E.T.; Wilkens, A.B.; et al. Automated Clinical Exome Reanalysis Reveals Novel Diagnoses. *J. Mol. Diagn.* **2019**, *21*, 38–48. [CrossRef] [PubMed]
13. Guo, W.; Lai, Y.; Yan, Z.; Wang, Y.; Nie, Y.; Guan, S.; Kuo, Y.; Zhang, W.; Zhu, X.; Peng, M.; et al. Trio-exome sequencing and preimplantation genetic diagnosis for unexplained recurrent fetal malformations. *Hum. Mutat.* **2020**, *41*, 432–448. [CrossRef] [PubMed]

14. Mis, E.K.; Al-Ali, S.; Ji, W.; Spencer-Manzon, M.; Konstantino, M.; Khokha, M.K.; Jeffries, L.; Lakhani, S.A. The latest FADS: Functional analysis of GLDN patient variants and classification of GLDN-associated AMC as a type of viable fetal akinesia deformation sequence. *Am. J. Med. Genet. A* **2020**, *182*, 2291–2296. [CrossRef] [PubMed]
15. Australian Genomics Health Alliance Acute Care Flagship; Lunke, S.; Eggers, S.; Wilson, M.; Patel, C.; Barnett, C.P.; Pinner, J.; Sandaradura, S.A.; Buckley, M.F.; Krzesinski, E.I.; et al. Feasibility of Ultra-Rapid Exome Sequencing in Critically Ill Infants and Children With Suspected Monogenic Conditions in the Australian Public Health Care System. *JAMA* **2020**, *323*, 2503–2511. [CrossRef] [PubMed]
16. Reischer, T.; Liebmann-Reindl, S.; Bettelheim, D.; Balendran-Braun, S.; Streubel, B. Genetic diagnosis and clinical evaluation of severe fetal akinesia syndrome. *Prenat. Diagn.* **2020**, *40*, 1532–1539. [CrossRef]
17. Bertoli-Avella, A.M.; Beetz, C.; Ameziane, N.; Rocha, M.E.; Guatibonza, P.; Pereira, C.; Calvo, M.; Herrera-Ordonez, N.; Segura-Castel, M.; Diego-Alvarez, D.; et al. Successful application of genome sequencing in a diagnostic setting: 1007 index cases from a clinically heterogeneous cohort. *Eur. J. Hum. Genet.* **2021**, *29*, 141–153. [CrossRef]
18. Filges, I.; Hall, J.G. Failure to identify antenatal multiple congenital contractures and fetal akinesia–proposal of guidelines to improve diagnosis. *Prenat. Diagn.* **2013**, *33*, 61–74. [CrossRef]
19. Tjon, J.K.; Tan-Sindhunata, M.B.; Bugiani, M.; Witbreuk, M.M.E.H.; van der Sluijs, J.A.; Weiss, M.M.; van Weissenbruch, M.M.; van de Pol, L.A.; Buizer, A.I.; van Doesburg, M.H.M.; et al. Care Pathway for Foetal Joint Contractures, Foetal Akinesia Deformation Sequence, and Arthrogryposis Multiplex Congenita. *Fetal Diagn. Ther.* **2021**, *48*, 829–839. [CrossRef]
20. Eshed, Y.; Feinberg, K.; Poliak, S.; Sabanay, H.; Sarig-Nadir, O.; Spiegel, I.; Bermingham, J.R., Jr.; Peles, E. Gliomedin mediates Schwann cell-axon interaction and the molecular assembly of the nodes of Ranvier. *Neuron* **2005**, *47*, 215–229. [CrossRef]
21. Eshed, Y.; Feinberg, K.; Carey, D.J.; Peles, E. Secreted gliomedin is a perinodal matrix component of peripheral nerves. *J. Cell Biol.* **2007**, *177*, 551–562. [CrossRef] [PubMed]
22. Maertens, B.; Hopkins, D.; Franzke, C.W.; Keene, D.R.; Bruckner-Tuderman, L.; Greenspan, D.S.; Koch, M. Cleavage and oligomerization of gliomedin, a transmembrane collagen required for node of ranvier formation. *J. Biol. Chem.* **2007**, *282*, 10647–10659. [CrossRef] [PubMed]
23. Labasque, M.; Devaux, J.J.; Lévêque, C.; Faivre-Sarrailh, C. Fibronectin type III-like domains of neurofascin-186 protein mediate gliomedin binding and its clustering at the developing nodes of Ranvier. *J. Biol. Chem.* **2011**, *286*, 42426–42434. [CrossRef] [PubMed]

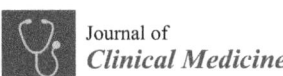

Systematic Review

Validity and Utility of Non-Invasive Prenatal Testing for Copy Number Variations and Microdeletions: A Systematic Review

Luca Zaninović [1,2], Marko Bašković [1,2,*], Davor Ježek [1,3,4] and Ana Katušić Bojanac [1,5]

1. Scientific Centre of Excellence for Reproductive and Regenerative Medicine, School of Medicine, University of Zagreb, Šalata 3, 10 000 Zagreb, Croatia; zaninovicluca@gmail.com (L.Z.); davor.jezek@mef.hr (D.J.); ana.katusic@mef.hr (A.K.B.)
2. Children's Hospital Zagreb, Ulica Vjekoslava Klaića 16, 10 000 Zagreb, Croatia
3. Department of Histology and Embryology, School of Medicine, University of Zagreb, Šalata 3, 10 000 Zagreb, Croatia
4. Department of Transfusion Medicine and Transplantation Biology, University Hospital Centre Zagreb, Kišpatićeva 12, 10 000 Zagreb, Croatia
5. Department of Medical Biology, School of Medicine, University of Zagreb, Šalata 3, 10 000 Zagreb, Croatia
* Correspondence: baskovic.marko@gmail.com; Tel.: +385-1-3636-379

Abstract: Valid data on prenatal cell-free DNA-based screening tests for copy number variations and microdeletions are still insufficient. We aimed to compare different methodological approaches concerning the achieved diagnostic accuracy measurements and positive predictive values. For this systematic review, we searched the Scopus and PubMed databases and backward citations for studies published between 2013 and 4 February 2022 and included articles reporting the analytical and clinical performance of cfDNA screening tests for CNVs and microdeletions. Of the 1810 articles identified, 32 met the criteria. The reported sensitivity of the applied tests ranged from 20% to 100%, the specificity from 81.62% to 100%, and the PPV from 3% to 100% for cases with diagnostic or clinical follow-up information. No confirmatory analysis was available in the majority of cases with negative screening results, and, therefore, the NPVs could not be determined. NIPT for CNVs and microdeletions should be used with caution and any developments regarding new technologies should undergo strict evaluation before their implementation into clinical practice. Indications for testing should be in correlation with the application guidelines issued by international organizations in the field of prenatal diagnostics.

Keywords: non-invasive prenatal testing; microdeletion; copy number variation; cell-free DNA; validity; screening; prenatal diagnosis; molecular method

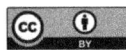

1. Introduction

In response to the growing appreciation of the incidence of and a better understanding of the importance of submicroscopic copy number variations and cytogenetic abnormalities other than common aneuploidies in recent years, laboratories have begun developing the ability to identify smaller cytogenetic changes using cell-free DNA. Fetal DNA analysis is the only method for detecting these disorders. The correlation between an elevated risk for pathological copy number variations and increased nuchal translucency, as well as altered serum levels of PAPP-A and free β-HCG, was noticed [1,2]. Other than these, the main indications for wide NIPT analysis are previous children with chromosomal alterations, the sonographic detection of fetal abnormalities, and a history of family members testing positive for chromosomal or genetic disorders [3]. Currently, there are two non-invasive approaches; one targets a handful of clinically significant microdeletions, and the other sets a size cutoff threshold for genome-wide copy number variations that are often the cause of microdeletions. Peters et al. were the first to apply this methodology in prenatal screening for fetal CNVs in 2011 [1,2,4]. In contrast to the convincing evidence for cell-free DNA-based screening for trisomies 21, 18, and 13, valid data concerning the accuracy and positive predictive values of most of these additional tests are still missing. There is a concern that a low incidence and a potentially much lower PPV for CNVs and microdeletions, resulting in a high false-positive rate, will increase the number of unnecessary invasive tests performed, especially taking into consideration that, due to the lack of official guidelines, the test is often performed on a population of pregnant women who are not preselected [2]. There are many controversies regarding this topic since clinical validation for cell-free DNA microdeletion and CNV testing has been sacrificed in a commercial race to expand indications for noninvasive testing. Many argue that the reliability and accuracy of NIPT for the detection of such conditions have not been subjected to the rigor necessary to make this a valid clinical test [5]. Any recommendations for the use of these tests should be based on clinical research evidence. There are several reviews on this topic and one systematic review that included seven cohort studies, but we intend to offer a more comprehensive and up-to-date overview of the literature available on this subject [2,6–9].

The objective of this systematic review was to evaluate the accuracy and reliability of non-invasive prenatal testing for CNVs and microdeletions and to compare different approaches, taking into account molecular methods of sample analysis and the assumed risk for the studied population of pregnant women as well as the biological characteristics of the analyzed submicroscopic anomalies.

2. Materials and Methods

2.1. Study Design and Search Strategy

The study was performed according to Preferred Reporting Items for Systematic-Reviews and Meta-Analysis (PRISMA) statement.

On 4 February 2022, we searched the Scopus and PubMed databases. The search combinations used included the Boolean operators "AND" and "OR" in combination with the following MeSH and free text terms: [(prenatal diagnoses) OR (prenatal diagnosis)] AND [(non-invas *) OR (noninvas *) OR (non invas *)] AND [(cell-free DNA) OR (cell free DNA) OR (cfDNA) OR (cffDNA)] AND [(test *) OR (valid *)] AND [(microdel *) OR (copy number varia *)]. Neither search filters nor text analysis tools were used. The study selection process is described in Figure 1.

2.2. Inclusion and Exclusion Criteria

We included a total of 32 study reports. To be included, a report had to contain information about the validity or utility of cfDNA-based non-invasive prenatal testing for fetal CNVs and microdeletions. Articles reporting solely on the application of NIPT for the detection of other chromosomal aberrations were excluded. Furthermore, reports in which the validity of the test was not confirmed by invasive testing or statistically expressed were excluded. Articles describing ethical aspects of NIPT as well as the ones addressing the usage of cfDNA-based methodology in the terms of oncology are valuable but not relevant to the topic and we, therefore, excluded them. We restricted our selection to English-language articles only and those published from 2013 onwards, as that is when this type of screening test first became clinically available.

2.3. Screening Process and Critical Appraisal

Studies were selected in a four-stage process. The first step was to assess their eligibility based on the title and abstract. Two researchers independently reviewed the titles and abstracts of half of the records each. In the second step, the same two researchers independently screened full-text articles for inclusion. In case of disagreement, the consensus was reached by discussion. Study reports were directly included in our systematic review, and a backward citation search solely for study reports was performed on the other articles (reviews, book chapters, case reports, commentaries, debate reports). As in the first step, two researchers independently reviewed titles and abstracts, then screened full-text reports. Subsequently, the data were collected by one independent researcher (see flow diagram summarizing the selection of studies for inclusion in the systematic review). The review protocol was registered with the International Prospective Register of Systematic Reviews (PROSPERO, ID334674).

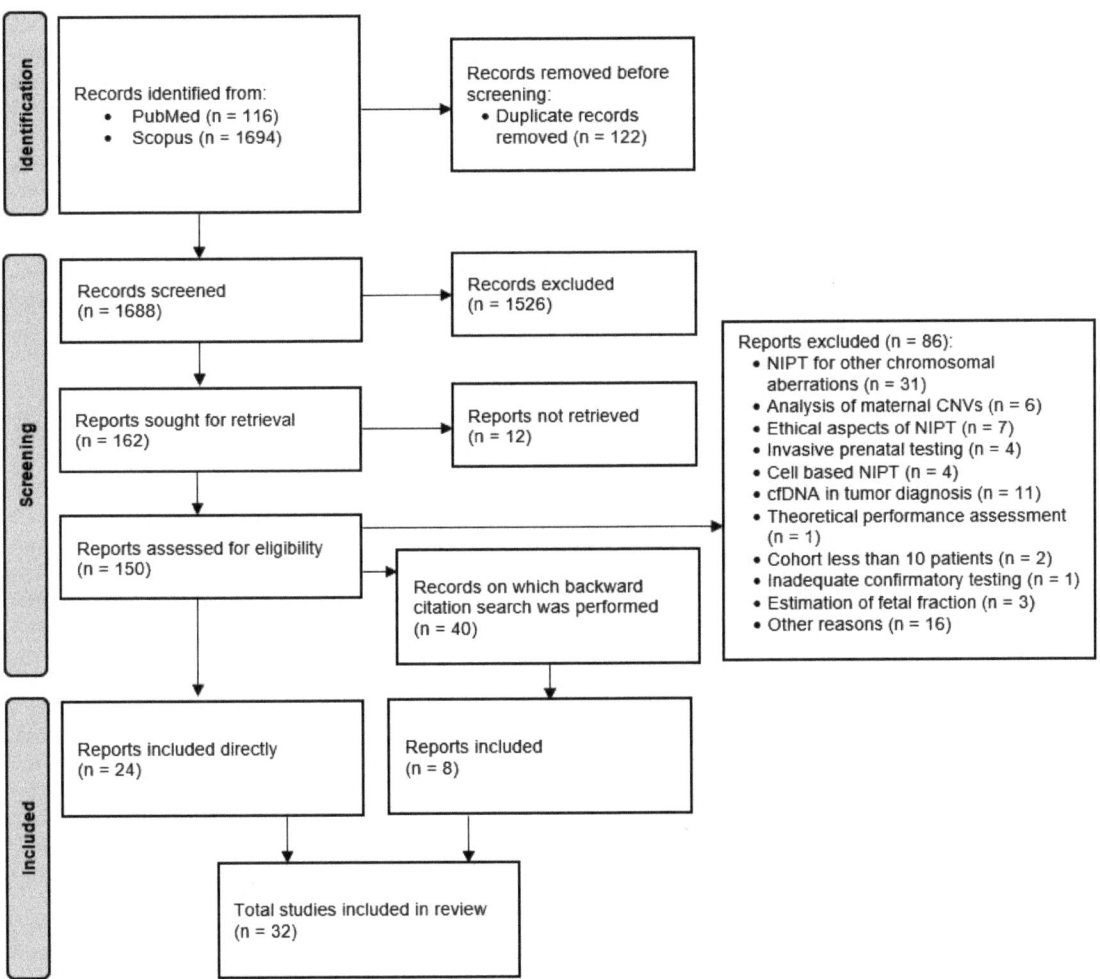

Figure 1. PRISMA flow diagram.

3. Results

3.1. Search Results

Overall, 1810 references were collected in Mendeley. After the exclusion of duplicates, 1688 articles remained. Based on the titles and abstracts, 1526 were excluded. Of the remaining 162 articles, 24 study reports were directly included, and a backward citation search was performed on the 40 selected articles, resulting in eight study reports appointed for inclusion in the review.

3.2. Chromosomal Aberrations of Interest

A total of 32 studies were included in this systematic review (Table 1). Of those, 21 studies explored screening possibilities for microdeletion syndromes using cell-free DNA. The most frequently analyzed pathologies were the DiGeorge (22q11.2 del), Cri-du-chat (5p), Prader–Willi/Angelman (15q del), 1p36 deletion, and Wolf–Hirschhorn (4p del) syndromes [10–25]. Helgeson et al. additionally screened for the 8q and 11q (Jacobsen) deletion syndromes and Koumbaris also checked for Smith–Magenis (17p del) syndrome [15,19]. Two studies focused on the Southeast Asian (SEA) deletion (20 kb size) [26,27], which is the cause of α0-thalassemia and Bart's hydrops fetalis. Three studies estimated possibilities for the genome-wide detection of microdeletions [28–30]. In addition to selected microdeletions, three studies simultaneously assessed the validity of screening tests for genome-wide copy number variations larger than 7 Mb using cfDNA, as CNVs are considered to be the cause of subchromosomal microaberrations including microdeletions [21–23]. Twelve studies solely evaluated the genome-wide detection of CNVs. Most of them screened for previously undiagnosed fetal CNVs [4,31–38], but two studies obtained samples with known CNVs and retrospectively conducted NIPT analysis [39,40].

3.3. Patient Characteristics and Acquisition of Samples

Most of the studies obtained plasma samples from the population of pregnant women who underwent NIPT without specifically defining referral indications for the screening [4,10,15,17,19–21,28,30,31,33–35,37,38]. Some included only samples of women with high-risk pregnancies (over 35 years of age), positive serum screening results, a history of aneuploidy, abnormal ultrasound findings, or simply maternal anxiety [22,32,40]. Two studies analyzed samples that showed an increased risk of chromosomal abnormalities from an NIPT which had already been performed [16,18]. Four reports took into consideration samples with already-confirmed fetal microdeletions or CNVs by invasive testing and euploid samples as controls [12,14,29,39]. Only one study explicitly analyzed twin pregnancies [13]. The most common exclusion criteria in these studies were known parental chromosomal abnormalities, multiple pregnancies, known maternal malignancy, the mother receiving an allogeneic blood transfusion, organ transplantation surgery, stem cell therapy, or immunotherapy, as well as an egg donor or surrogate pregnancies [10,13,34,36–38]. Li et al. also excluded samples whose transportation to the laboratory took more than 48 h, those with visible hemolysis, and a fetal fraction of less than 3% [40]. Due to the low prevalence of chromosomal aberrations of interest, some researchers used in vitro created plasma samples constructed by using DNA from the affected individual, with known deletion or CNV, and spiking it into the isolated plasma DNA of non-pregnant women [11,14,24,25].

3.4. Molecular Methods for cfDNA Analysis

Nowadays, there are two primary next-generation sequencing-based approaches for cfDNA testing: massively parallel shotgun sequencing (MPSS), which sequences DNA fragments from the whole genome, and targeted sequencing, which is the selective testing of targeted genomic regions. Both techniques are based on counting sequenced DNA fragments obtained from maternal blood and consider only the number of reads to identify numeric abnormalities of fetal chromosomes. Another type of targeted cfDNA testing is single-nucleotide polymorphism (SNP) sequencing, which enables a more accurate cfDNA analysis, allowing for a qualitative approach to differentiating between maternal and fetal input. SNP sequencing can rely on the allele ratio or specifically target the amplification of polymorphic loci, followed by NGS and bioinformatics analysis. In such an approach, allelic information from both parents is included in the analysis, taking into consideration different genetic inheritance patterns [41].

Table 1. Studies included in the systematic review.

Study	Country	Type of Study	Microdeletions/CNVs	Molecular Method	Number of Participants	Sample	Size	Number of Reads	TP	FP	PPV	Sensitivity	Specificity
Yang et al., 2019 [26]	China	training set-retrospective, testing set-prospective cohort	SEA deletion	targeted method (SNP-based)	878	plasma	20 kb	training set 4.84 M, testing set 5.22 M	321	16	95.25%	98.98%	96.06%
Sawakwongpra et al., 2021 [27]	Thailand	prospective cohort	SEA deletion	targeted method (droplet digital PCR)	22	plasma	20 kb					95.38%	91.01%
Gross et al., 2016 [10]	USA	retrospective cohort	DiGeorge	targeted method (SNP-based)	21,948	plasma	2.91 Mb	8.9 M	11	50	18%		
Schmid et al., 2018 [11]	UK	cross-sectional	DiGeorge	targeted method (microarray-based)	1953	plasma + artificial	1.96–3.25 Mb		97	8	92.38%	75.2%	99.6%
Ravi et al., 2018 [12]	USA	prospective cohort	DiGeorge	targeted method (SNP-based)	10 affected and 409 controls	plasma	2.55–3.16 Mb	4.7 M			19.6%	90%	99.74%
Lin et al., 2021 [13]	Taiwan	retrospective cohort	DiGeorge	MPSS	8158	plasma	3 Mb	20 M	7	6	53.85%	100%	99.92%
Wapner et al., 2015 [14]	USA	prospective cohort	microdeletions (common)	targeted method (SNP-based)	6 affected, 352 controls, 111 artificial	plasma + artificial	2.91–20 Mb	8.9 M	106	4	96.36%		
Zhao et al., 2015 [28]	USA	prospective cohort	microdeletions (genome-wide)	MPSS	178	plasma	3–40 Mb	0.2× coverage	17	1	94.4%	94.4%	99.4%
Helgeson et al., 2015 [15]	USA	prospective cohort	microdeletions (common)	MPSS	175,393	plasma					90.9%		
Yin et al., 2015 [29]	China	prospective cohort	microdeletions and microduplications (genome-wide)	MPSS	1476	plasma	0.52–84 Mb	3.5 M	56	58	49.12%	85.4%	95.7%
Petersen et al., 2017 [16]	USA	retrospective cohort	microdeletions (common)	various technologies	712	plasma	>1.5 Mb		7	45	13.4%		
Martin et al., 2018 [17]	USA	retrospective cohort	microdeletions (common)	targeted method (SNP-based)	114,616	plasma	2.91–20 Mb	>3.2 M	30	43	41.1%	96.77%	81.62%
Schwartz et al., 2018 [18]	USA	retrospective cross-sectional	microdeletions (common)	various technologies	349	plasma			25	310	7.4%		
Hu et al., 2019 [30]	China	prospective cohort	microdeletions (genome-wide)	MPSS	8141	plasma	>10, <10 Mb	4.89 M	13	23	36.11%		
Koumbaris et al., 2019 [19]	Cyprus	retrospective cohort	microdeletions (common)	targeted method (TACS)	2033	plasma			5	0	100%	100%	100%
Welker et al., 2021 [20]	USA	prospective cohort	microdeletions (common)	MPSS (FF method)	2401	plasma						97.2%	99.8%
Pescia et al., 2017 [31]	Switzerland	retrospective cross-sectional	CNVs	MPSS	6388	plasma	>10 M		7	3	70%		
Lo et al., 2016 [39]	UK	prospective cohort	CNVs	MPSS	31 affected + 534 controls	plasma	>6, <6 Mb	4–10 M			55%	83%	99.6%
Li et al., 2016 [40]	China	prospective cohort	CNVs	MPSS	117	plasma	>5, <5 Mb	3.95 M	11	4	73.33%	61.1%	95%

Table 1. Cont.

Study	Country	Type of Study	Microdeletions/CNVs	Molecular Method	Number of Participants	Sample	Size	Number of Reads	TP	FP	PPV	Sensitivity	Specificity
Lefkowitz et al., 2016 [22]	USA	retrospective cross-sectional	CNVs > 7 Mb and common microdeletions	MPSS	1166	plasma	>7 Mb + selected smaller	32 M	42	1	97.67%	97.7%	99.9%
Fiorentino et al., 2017 [32]	Italy	prospective cohort	CNVs	MPSS	12,114	plasma	>1.9 Mb	30 M	8	5	61.54%	100%	99.96%
Yu et al., 2018 [33]	China	prospective cohort	CNVs	MPSS	20,003	plasma	>10, 5–10, <5 Mb	4.2 M	29	7	80.56%	80.56%	
Liang et al., 2019 [21]	China	prospective cohort	CNVs and common microdeletions	MPSS	94,085	plasma	>10, <10 Mb	20 M	49	71	40.8%	90.74%	99.92%
Chen et al., 2019 [34]	China	prospective cohort	CNVs	MPSS	42,910	plasma	>10, 5–10, <5 Mb		20	49	28.99%		
Luo et al., 2020 [36]	China	retrospective cohort	CNVs	MPSS	40,256	plasma		>3.5 M	4	131	3%		
Pei et al., 2020 [4]	China	retrospective cohort	CNVs	MPSS	141	plasma	>20, 10–20, <10 Mb	>6 M	21	120	14.89%		
Liu et al., 2020 [37]	China	retrospective cohort	CNVs	MPSS	42,924	plasma			11	27	28.95%		
Rafalko et al., 2021 [23]	USA	prospective cohort	CNVs > 7 Mb and common microdeletions	MPSS	86,902	plasma	>7 Mb + selected smaller		181	63	74.2%		
Chen et al., 2021 [35]	China	prospective cohort	CNVs	MPSS	34,620	plasma	>5 Mb	0.1× coverage	21	20	51.22%		
Lai et al., 2021 [38]	China	prospective cohort	CNVs	MPSS	86,262	plasma	6–32.5 Mb	3 M	4	8	33.3%	20%	99.99%
Neofytou et al., 2017 [24]	Cyprus	prospective cohort	common microdeletions + Potocki Lupski	targeted method (TACS)	21 affected + 50 controls	plasma + artificial	>0.5 Mb		21	0	100%	100%	100%
Kucharik et al., 2020 [25]	Slovakia	case-control study	microdeletions (common)	MPSS	29	artificial	0.9–21 Mb	20 M	24	0	100%		

CNV—copy number variation, PPV—positive predictive value, TP—true positive, FP—false positive, SEA—Southeast Asian, SNP—single nucleotide polymorphism, PCR—polymerase chain reaction, MPSS—massively parallel shotgun sequencing, TACS—target capture sequences, FFA—fetal fraction amplification, USA—United States of America, UK—United Kingdom.

A total of 21 studies used massively parallel sequencing technology that enables the detection of microdeletions and genome-wide CNVs without prior knowledge of the event's location. After cfDNA quantification, libraries were tag-sequenced to generate 3.5 M–32 M reads per sample and aligned to the human reference genome [22,29]. Reads were then allocated to continuous non-overlapping 20 kb–100 kb bins and filtered to remove bins with abnormal GC content [13,21,33,38–40]. Next, similar statistical methods were used by five teams of researchers. They normalized the bin counts and then used the circular binary segmentation algorithm to divide each chromosome into contiguous regions of equal copy numbers. This step was followed by the identification of segments with consistently underrepresented regions indicative of a loss in the genome. Furthermore, they used decision tree analysis to differentiate whole-chromosome events from deletions [15,22,23,25,28]. Two studies also described the combination of the MPSS method with technology that leverages the reduced size of fetal-derived cfDNA fragments, in comparison to maternally derived ones, to increase the sensitivity of the test. After quantification, they performed the size selection of cfDNA libraries by removing fragments > 200 nt via gel electrophoresis. These size-selected libraries contained a higher cffDNA fraction because, after the removal of maternally derived fragments, cffDNA represented a higher share of ultimately analyzed cfDNA. Importantly, the obtained gain in a fetal fraction was molecular and not algorithmic [20,31].

Targeted or directed technologies of cfDNA testing, in contrast to massively parallel shotgun sequencing, enable the detection of microdeletions and CNVs of known pathogenicity only, instead of testing the entire genome and consequently revealing CNVs of unknown significance [41].

In six included studies, samples were analyzed using an SNP-based screening methodology. For the detection of DiGeorge-causing microdeletions, sets of pooled primers containing 672 or 1351 SNPs were designed to target the 2.91 Mb section of the 22q11.2 region that constitutes approximately 87% of all deletions detected in individuals with 22q11.2 deletion syndrome [10,12,14,17]. Wapner et al. and Martin at al. also used sets of primers designed to amplify 1152 SNPs in each of the following regions: a 10 Mb region deleted in ~60% of patients diagnosed with 1p36 deletion syndrome, a 20 Mb region deleted in ~65% of patients diagnosed with Cri-du-chat syndrome, and a 5.85 Mb region deleted in ~28% of patients diagnosed with the Prader–Willi/Angelman syndromes [14,17]. Amplified samples were sequenced to 3.2–4.7 million reads per sample [12,17]. Deletions were predicted based on the allele distribution pattern for SNPs in the regions of interest [10,12,17]. Yang et al. used the target-captured SNP sequencing of cfDNA to detect pathogenic SEA deletion—the cause of $\alpha 0$-thalassemia. Nearly 2000 SNPs were used to target the gene region of alpha-globin (HBA) and 20,000 bp upstream and downstream of the gene region [26].

The droplet digital PCR-based method for the non-invasive detection of SEA deletion was described by Sawakawongpra et al. This technique amplifies a low initial amount of target DNA molecules and itemizes different PCR products using probe-specific fluorescent signals. Two probes were designed—one to bind the genomic region inside the targeted deletion and the other one to bind just outside of the SEA locus. The first signal was expected to be detected only in cases of a wild type of the gene, whereas the other one was expected to be present both in a wild type and in cases with a SEA deletion [27].

Schmid et al. developed a targeted microarray-based cfDNA test for the detection of 22q11.2 microdeletion. Additional 500 digital analysis of selected regions (DANSR) assays, in comparison to array-based NIPT for detecting common aneuploidies, were designed against targets uniformly distributed within a 3 Mb region of interest. Each of the samples was furtherly analyzed on a single custom microarray [11]. Despite its efficiency, microarrays are not commonly used in cfDNA testing.

Koumbaris et al. and Neofytou et al. developed novel analytical approaches using target capture sequences (TACS) to enrich regions of interest associated with sought-after microdeletions. Target loci were selected based on the GC content, the distance from repetitive elements, and the absence of known surrounding complex architecture. This type of approach avoids CNVs of unknown clinical significance and has the ability to identify deletions in a fetus as small as 0.5 Mb in size [19,24].

Two studies retrospectively analyzed NIPT results obtained by various molecular methods and performed solely confirmatory testing using invasively acquired samples. In many cases, while obtaining samples, Petersen et al. were not provided with the information of the laboratory that performed the NIPT. Consequently, they used pooled data for the interpretation of the results [16]. In the other study, Schwartz et al. broadly separated results depending on the NIPT technologies used. They noticed a statistically significant difference between a PPV of 4.2%, acquired by the usage of the SNP-based approach, and one of 32.3%, acquired by MPSS technology-based tests, but noticed that this was most likely false and caused by false-positive results due to the presence of the homozygotic stretches associated with consanguinity [18].

3.5. Study Outcomes

Studies that used MPSS technology to test for common microdeletions achieved an overall sensitivity of 85.4–97.2% and a specificity of 95.7–99.8% [20,28,29].

Regarding the individuality of positive predictive values (PPVs) for certain conditions, Helgeson et al. presented individual PPVs for microdeletions ranging from 100% for the Wolf–Hirschhorn, Jacobsen and Langer–Giedion syndromes, 96.9–100% for DiGeorge syndrome and 66.7% for Cri-du-chat syndrome. While testing for DiGeorge, 20/32 detected deletions had a maternal contribution. A likely explanation for this high rate of maternal findings lies in the small size of deletions detected in the 22q11 region which represents pregnant women with mild clinical findings [15]. Others, such as Liang et al., achieved a PPV ranging from 93% for DiGeorge to 0% for 1p36 microdeletion [21].

Clearly, one of the factors that affect the detection of subchromosomal deletions and CNVs using the whole-genome sequencing approach was the size of the event of interest. The larger the CNV in the cffDNA is, the easier it is to detect it against a background of normal maternal DNA [15]. In the study by Yin et al., 93.3% of deletions/duplications larger than 5 Mb and 100% larger than 10 Mb in size were detected at 3.5 million reads per sample. In contrast, only 1.2% of deletions/duplications less than 5 Mb in size and none less than 1 Mb in size were detected at 3.5 million reads per sample. Also, 67.2% of false positives predicted a deletion/duplication less than 5 Mb in size [29]. In the study conducted by Kucharik et al. out of the 1,705,600 carried out simulations, the simulated syndrome was correctly predicted in 937,335 cases, resulting in a sensitivity of 55.0%. Importantly, the sensitivity increased to 97.1% if the read count was at least 15 M and the size of the deletion was at least 3 Mb. The mutuality between the above-mentioned deletion size and the fetal fraction percentage was found to be a key parameter in NIPT, and different combinations of them were tested from 5% to 20%. Fetal fractions lower than 5% were shown to be problematic due to an increased number of false-negative detections. This approach achieved an accuracy of 79.3% for a 10% fetal fraction with a 20 M read depth, which further increased to 98.4% if the search was only for deletions longer than 3 Mb. The results of the in silico simulated data were in accordance with an artificial laboratory sample evaluation test that correctly detected 24 out of 29 control samples [25].

A majority of the included studies investigated the genome-wide detection of CNVs. When comparing these results, there is no consistency in achieved sensitivity, specificity, and PPV rates depending on the CNV size. While Lo et al. demonstrated a significantly higher sensitivity for the detection of CNVs larger than 6 Mb (83% compared to 20% for ones smaller than 6 Mb), whereas Chen et al. achieved the highest PPV for CNVs size of 5–10 Mb [34,39]. However, this was not the case in a study conducted by Yu et al. who for CNVs 5–10 Mb achieved the highest sensitivity (100% in comparison to 92% and 68% for CNVs > 10 Mb and <5 Mb) but the lowest PPV (71% in comparison to 85% and 81% for CNVs > 10 Mb and <5 Mb) [33]. One study demonstrated a significantly lower PPV, only 3%, for CNVs greater than 10 Mb, compared with 40% for the ones less than 10 Mb [4]. In general, smaller CNVs were more likely to be confirmed than larger CNVs. Furthermore, for the cases where two or more CNVs were identified, where only one of the findings was confirmed by diagnostic testing, the smaller one was confirmed more frequently than the larger finding [23].

In another study, deeper sequencing correctly identified the fetal CNV in 9 of 11 samples where the imbalance had not been detected by the standard shallow-sequencing pipeline. The discrepancy in the count ratios decreased as the depth of sequencing increased, as demonstrated by one fetus with a 22q11.2 deletion, which was ultimately detected when the sample was sequenced to a depth of 32 million reads. In addition to identifying the CNVs, the pipeline indicated locations that were highly accurate and matched well with positions provided by microarray analysis [39]. The study by Rafalko et al. demonstrated the importance of the initial ultrasound fetal risk assessment, as cases referred to due to ultrasound findings as the sole indication for testing comprised 15% of the overall screening cohort, compared to 33% for the CNV-positive cohort. For cases in which only one of the two findings was confirmed, the detected CNV that was discordant showed sequencing data suggestive of mosaicism. This may have been caused by a segmental "rescue" event in progress, such as telomere capture, which acts to stabilize an open deletion by acquiring material from another chromosome and results in mosaicism for the "stabilizing" CNV [23].

A study which used the SNP-based approach scored detection rates of 97.8% for a 22q11.2 deletion and 100% for the Prader–Willi, Angelman, 1p36 deletion, and Cri-du-chat syndromes. The false-positive rates were 0.76% for 22q11.2 deletion syndrome and 0.24% for Ci-du-chat syndrome. No false positives occurred for the Prader–Willi, Angelman, or 1p36 deletion syndromes. An explanation for the lower DR for the 22q11.2 locus lies in the fact that the number of SNPs targeted in this region was less than for other locations. The performance of this SNP-based method for the detection of well-defined microdeletions is expected to depend primarily on the number of informative SNPs in each region of interest, which may limit its detection capabilities for small regions of interest [14]. The study by Martin et al. first achieved a positive predictive rate of 15.7% for 22q11.2 deletion syndrome, and 5.2% for the other four disorders combined. Then, the analysis of high-risk samples with a revised protocol of high-depth sequencing showed an increase in the PPV rate to 44.2% for 22q11.2 and 31.7% for the others as well as a decrease in false-positive rates [17]. In the studies analyzing only deletions characteristic of DiGeorge syndrome, a sensitivity and specificity of 90% and 99.74%, respectively, were presented [12]. Overall, the PPV was 18%. In contrast, for cases with no abnormal ultrasound findings prior to NIPT, the PPV was 4.9%. This estimate was based on a small sample size and could be subject to an ascertainment bias because information about ultrasound findings was not comprehensively gathered at the time of testing [10].

The first study to show the application of ddPCR to identify the copy number of SEA deletion in unprocessed cell-free DNA obtained from maternal plasma yielded a sensitivity of 95.38% and a specificity of 91.01% [27].

A prenatal screening test for 22q11.2 deletion using a targeted microarray-based cfDNA test achieved a sensitivity of 75.4% and a specificity of at least 99.5%. The smallest deletion size detected was 1.96 Mb. There was no interdependence between the sensitivity and deletion size. To comprehend these results, it is crucial to take into consideration the fact that this study included samples with the typical 3 Mb deletion as well as samples with smaller nested deletions, unlike the other included studies. In fact, one could argue that the sensitivity reported for comparable cfDNA tests using MPSS and SNP technologies should be adjusted if established only based on the common 3 Mb 22q11.2 deletion [11]. Both of the studies which used NIPT based on a validated targeted capture enrichment technology identified all microdeletions correctly without any false-negative events, exhibiting 100% sensitivity and 100% specificity. This type of approach avoids CNVs of unknown clinical significance and has the ability to identify deletions or duplications in a fetus as small as 0.5 Mb in size [19,24].

Studies that used retrospectively obtained data from laboratories using various NIPT platforms yielded an overall PPV of 9.2–13% [16,18]. In the study conducted by Schwartz et al., 39.3% of the cases in which microdeletion was confirmed by invasive testing had additional abnormal microarray findings. Unrelated abnormal microarray findings were detected in 11.8% of the patients in whom the screen positive microdeletion was denied and declared as false positive [18].

3.6. Limitations and Biases

The limitations of our systematic review largely reflect the shortcomings of the reports reviewed. The weaknesses of included studies arose from the their processes for gathering each cohort, choices of technology for the analysis of collected or artificially created samples, follow-up processes, as well as the biological characteristics of the subchromosomal aberrations of interest.

Firstly, diverse indications for wide NIPT performance were applied depending on the countries the studies were conducted in, and this may have influence the calculated PPVs and sensitivities. The sample size in a substantial number of the studies was too small for comprehensive analysis. In addition, the gestational age of a large number of the recruited pregnancies was in the second trimester, resulting in a higher fetal fraction than in cases of samples obtained in clinical practice [12,14,40]. As the incidence of analyzed subchromosomal aberrations is extremely low, to decrease the cost of the research, several studies included only high-risk populations and this way may have introduced bias while calculating the PPV [23]. Due to the unknown fetal prevalence of screened microdeletions and CNVs, it was difficult to estimate the PPV of the molecular methods used for the analysis [39]. In some studies, microduplication screening results were calculated in summarized PPV and sensitivity values [24,29]. The studies that evaluated prenatal screenings for CNVs where similar in this regard, since they are not only the cause of microdeletions but also other submicroscopic chromosomal rearrangements. Retrospective cohort studies often lack sufficient data such as the total number of cfDNA tests performed during a given period, meaning they lack the total denominator required for the evaluation of the test's specificity. Also, two such studies did not take into consideration differences between the testing platforms used for the analysis of samples when calculating overall statistics [16,18]. Furthermore, some of the researchers did not have the access to the clinical data to assess possible explanations for false-positive results such as the presence of a vanished twin's cfDNA in the maternal plasma, placental mosaicism, maternal chromosomal abnormalities, or maternal neoplastic conditions [16,18,22,23,36]. Studies that used artificial samples did not take into consideration real case scenario causes of inconsistent results when expressing sensitivity, specificity, and PPV [11,24,25]. Most of the included studies could correctly address the test sensitivity, as they were limited by the incomplete follow-up of the pregnancy outcome of negative cfDNA screening cases and ascertainment bias [10,11,16]. The inconsistent results may be related to the GC bias [30]. NIPT methodology in general suffers from the problem of multiple hypothesis testing, meaning that false-positive rates become additive for independently analyzed genome regions [22]. Several screen-positive cases were validated by low-pass whole-genome sequencing and fluorescence in situ hybridization rather than chromosomal microarray analysis—the gold standard diagnostic for microdeletions [10,12,33].

The extensive and systematic literature search, which included a backward citation search that yielded additional reports, is one of the strengths of this study. An assessment of the methodological quality of the included studies was not performed after taking into consideration the number of included studies and the extent of the information that would have arisen from this, which would have exceeded the scale of this systematic review. The possibility of pooling data for meta-analysis was explored but this was not pursued because of the heterogeneity of the studies with respect to the processes for gathering the cohorts, molecular methodologies used, and confirmation testing performed. Therefore, the conclusions were based on narrative synthesis. Between-study heterogeneity was not assessed quantitatively, as a meta-analysis could not be conducted.

4. Discussion

CNVs are the cause of microdeletions—structural chromosomal abnormalities whose size is less than 5 Mb—a standard resolution of karyotyping and therefore cannot be detected by this method [2]. Although individually extremely rare, with frequencies ranging from 1:4000 for DiGeorge syndrome to 1:50,000 for Cri-du-chat syndrome, the overall prevalence rate of microdeletions is considered to be around 1:2500 and is not associated with maternal age [7,42]. Hence, for the population of pregnant women younger than 35 years, fetal microdeletions are more common than Down syndrome and often show equally serious phenotypes [43]. This imposed the need for a form of preinvasive testing for these conditions. With CMA being the gold standard diagnostic method but exposing pregnant women to possible complications due to the invasive procedures involved in the obtaining of samples, NIPT technology slowly but surely became a leading method in prenatal screening for microdeletions and CNVs [40].

Cell-free DNA-based screening tests have been developed and marketed exclusively by the developers to the practitioner and patient communities without conducting independent trials and validating their performance prior to their introduction into the marketplace [43]. The process of developing a screening test from the laboratory to clinical application requires the determination of its validity and utility. In the context of NIPT, the assessment of analytical validity answers the question of whether various concentrations of placental and maternal DNA can be used to determine the presence or absence of a condition of interest. Clinical validity refers to the detection rate, sensitivity, and specificity of the evaluated test—metrics that are independent of the prevalence of the condition screened for. Clinical utility evaluates the practical usefulness of the test to the screened population, expressed through objective metrics such as the PPV and NPV. The American College of Medical Genetics and Genomics, in their position statement from 2016, claims that the previously mentioned values should be expressed for each CNV screened when reporting laboratory results [44]. Unfortunately, it is fair to say that the selection of microdeletions and CNVs included in commercial panels was often more driven by their detection feasibility than by their clinical relevance [2].

As previously mentioned in Section 3.4, there are two primary approaches for cfDNA-based screening tests. Targeted sequencing technologies that process a smaller amount of data provide better values in terms of the test's validity and utility indicators, requiring less time and expense than MPSS-based methods [7,28]. Increasing the sequencing depth is the most direct way to improve the accuracy of diagnosis. In clinical practice, this is limited by the sequencing cost. However, certain parts of the genome may not be amenable to adequate coverage because of the inherent features of DNA structure (for example GC rich regions and heterochromatin regions of repetitive DNA sequences) [29]. Kucharik et al. recommend using approximately 16 M–17 M reads per sample for analyses, due to fact that the detection rate reaches a plateau for a 10% fetal fraction and 3 Mb deletion size around this point [25].

Other than the sequencing depth, the detection capability is dependent on the variation or microdeletion size, fetal fraction, as well as the biological variability of the region of interest [7,28]. Reports claim that the detection efficiency for microdeletions and CNVs is determined mainly by their size, but in the studies by Yu et al. and Chen et al., the highest PPV and sensitivity were achieved for CNVs between 5 and 10 Mb in size in comparison to smaller and larger ones [29,33,34,39]. This may be explained by the limited number of cases identified in that subgroup and the case bias that possibly contributed to a higher sensitivity [33,34].

Although there were initially concerns that the technical aspects of the sequencing methods and bioinformatics analyses were the reason for the reduction in specificity and false-positive results, over time, it has become clear that a significant proportion of cases have an underlying biological etiology [45]. CffDNA is of placental origin, and, consequently, a confined placental mosaicism observed in around 1% of all pregnancies can be the cause of FP results. Other potential causes are maternal microdeletions and CNVs; Lo et al. described the detection of all three maternal microduplications but could not determine if the fetus had inherited them. Therefore, achieving sufficient accuracy in fetal inheritance would require knowledge of fetal fractions and the use of counting statistics [39]. Also, in the case of multiple reported abnormalities, the source of pathologically altered DNA could be apoptotic tumor cells of maternal origin [46]. Rafalko et al. reported that at least 12 of their positive cases were caused by maternal fibroids and myelodysplastic syndromes [23]. Another possible source of pathological findings is the presence of a vanished co-twin's DNA, although this extremely rare [45].

Despite the detection rates of all the cfDNA-based screening tests being high, the PPV depends on the patient's *a priori* risk for the analyzed disorder, which is primarily determined by the prevalence of an abnormality [1]. With the possible exception of 22q11.2 and 1p36 deletions, microdeletions show no phenotypic characteristics detectable by ultrasound, and screening is essentially performed on an average-risk population of pregnant women. As the adequate assessment of clinical utility is difficult while using the traditional idea of prospective randomized trials due to the rarity of the microdeletions and CNVs, study designs have used archived samples and artificial mixtures of abnormal DNA to provide at least an estimate of accuracy [11,24,25,47]. The current systematic review was unable to provide any new contributions to this topic considering that the analyzed reports included fetuses with different background risks, and, consequently, the reported PPVs may not reflect the genuine clinical utility.

None of the included studies performed systematic confirmatory analysis by CMA for negative/low-risk cases. They mostly relied on clinical follow-up. That being the case, the exact negative predictive values could not be determined. In an average-risk population, an estimated NPV of 99% is more often than not the result of the rarity of the condition rather than the test performance itself. Yaron et al. made a calculation that, given a 1.7% *a priori* risk of any clinically significant microdeletion or CNV being present in the fetus, a negative NIPT result would only modestly reduce the risk to 1.6% [47].

One of the limitations of implementing NIPT methods in clinical practice is the fact that the fetal genome is screened for specific chromosomal abnormality and not a consequently expressed clinical syndrome. For example, DiGeorge syndrome is not caused by a single chromosomal entity but rather a group of different microdeletions, all located in the 22q11.1 chromosome band. Approximately 85% of the cases are caused by a typical 3 Mb size deletion that encompasses 45 functional genes located between the low copy repeats LCR22A and LCR22D, which, respectively, correspond to the SNP coordinates 18,835,221 and 21,592,477 (based on human reference genome hg19) [10,11]. The remaining patients suffering from DiGeorge syndrome have atypical or nested microdeletions that occur between other low-copy repeats within the same region [11,48]. Even though, in the study by Schmid et al., atypical and nested deletions were covered by DANSR assays, neither of them is detectable by currently available commercial tests [11,12]. Similarly, only 65–75% of Prader–Willi cases are caused by microdeletion, whereas the remaining cases are caused by uniparental disomy or single gene disorder [8]. In addition, the variable penetrance of a considerable number of microdeletions may lead to milder phenotypic expressions of the same genetic defect [9].

The debate about the optimal way to implement wide NIPT into clinical practice to ameliorate the management of pregnancy is still ongoing. The main obstacle remains the undefined reliability of these tests. The current position of the main professional organizations, namely, the American College of Obstetricians and Gynecologists, the American Society for Human Genetics, and the European Society for Human Genetics, is that NIPT is not recommended for the detection of microdeletions. Alternatively, the American College of Medical Genetics and Genomics holds an opinion that informing women about the availability of cfDNA-based screening for selected microdeletions should be provided when specific conditions are met by both the healthcare provider and the performing laboratory [1,49]. This configures NIPT for microdeletions and CNVs as contingent tests offered in cases of pathological ultrasound findings or abnormal serum marker levels along with anamnestic indications for screening.

It is necessary to provide comprehensive genetic counseling to all pregnant women undergoing NIPT. Special attention should be paid to CNVs classified as variants of unknown significance as well as all the other limitations of the test arising from the biological characteristics of analyzed genetic abnormalities and the molecular methods used for the analysis. The main limitations to the introduction of these tests into clinical practice are the associated cost, which still exceeds those of other prenatal screening methods, and a high share of false results, leading to challenges in the management of these cases [3].

5. Conclusions

Considering the limited follow-up and validation data available at this time, NIPT for microdeletions and CNVs should be used with caution and screen-positive results confirmed by invasive testing. Any developments regarding new technologies should undergo robust evaluation in terms of validity and clinical utility. The commercial implementation of NIPT should be subordinate to the public health sector. Standards for the inclusion of cfDNA-based screening methods into national health systems should be established by major organizations in the field of prenatal diagnostics.

Author Contributions: Conceptualization, L.Z., M.B. and A.K.B.; methodology, L.Z. and M.B.; validation, D.J. and A.K.B.; formal analysis, L.Z., M.B. and A.K.B.; investigation, L.Z. and M.B.; resources, D.J. and A.K.B.; data curation, L.Z. and M.B.; writing—original draft preparation, L.Z. and M.B.; writing—review and editing, D.J. and A.K.B.; visualization, M.B. and A.K.B.; supervision, D.J. and A.K.B.; project administration, D.J. and A.K.B.; funding acquisition, D.J. All authors have read and agreed to the published version of the manuscript.

Funding: The research was supported by the Scientific Center of Excellence for Reproductive and Regenerative Medicine, Republic of Croatia, and the European Union through the European Regional Development Fund, under the contract KK.01.1.1.01.0008, project "Regenerative and Reproductive Medicine—Exploring New Platforms and Potentials".

Institutional Review Board Statement: The review protocol was registered with the International Prospective Register of Systematic Reviews (PROSPERO, ID334674).

Informed Consent Statement: Not applicable.

Data Availability Statement: The data that support the findings of this study are available upon request from the corresponding author.

Conflicts of Interest: The authors declare no conflict of interest. The funders had no role in the design of the study; in the collection, analyses, or interpretation of data; in the writing of the manuscript, or in the decision to publish the results.

References

1. Levy, B.; Wapner, R. Prenatal diagnosis by chromosomal microarray analysis. *Fertil. Steril.* **2018**, *109*, 201–212. [CrossRef] [PubMed]
2. Bedei, I.; Wolter, A.; Weber, A.; Signore, F.; Axt-Fliedner, R. Chances and Challenges of New Genetic Screening Technologies (NIPT) in Prenatal Medicine from a Clinical Perspective: A Narrative Review. *Genes* **2021**, *12*, 501. [CrossRef] [PubMed]
3. Carbone, L.; Cariati, F.; Sarno, L.; Conforti, A.; Bagnulo, F.; Strina, I.; Patore, L.; Maruotti, G.M.; Alviggi, C. Non-Invasive Prenatal Testing: Current Perspectives and Future Challenges. *Genes* **2020**, *12*, 15. [CrossRef] [PubMed]
4. Pei, Y.; Hu, L.; Liu, J.; Wen, L.; Luo, X.; Lu, J.; Wei, F. Efficiency of noninvasive prenatal testing for the detection of fetal microdeletions and microduplications in autosomal chromosomes. *Mol. Genet. Genom. Med.* **2020**, *8*, e1339. [CrossRef]
5. Yatsenko, S.A.; Peters, D.G.; Rajkovic, A. Response to Sahoo et al. *Genet. Med.* **2016**, *18*, 277. [CrossRef] [PubMed]
6. Benn, P. Expanding non-invasive prenatal testing beyond chromosomes 21, 18, 13, X and Y. *Clin. Genet.* **2016**, *90*, 477–485. [CrossRef]
7. Shi, J.; Zhang, R.; Li, J.; Zhang, R. Novel perspectives in fetal biomarker implementation for the noninvasive prenatal testing. *Crit. Rev. Clin. Lab. Sci.* **2019**, *56*, 374–392. [CrossRef]

8. Shaffer, B.L.; Norton, M.E. Cell-Free DNA Screening for Aneuploidy and Microdeletion Syndromes. *Obstet. Gynecol. Clin. N. Am.* 2018, *45*, 13–26. [CrossRef]
9. Familiari, A.; Boito, S.; Rembouskos, G.; Ischia, B.; Accurti, V.; Fabietti, I.; Volpe, P.; Persico, N. Cell-free DNA analysis of maternal blood in prenatal screening for chromosomal microdeletions and microduplications: A systematic review. *Prenat. Diagn.* 2021, *41*, 1324–1331. [CrossRef]
10. Gross, S.J.; Stosic, M.; McDonald-McGinn, D.M.; Bassett, A.S.; Norvez, A.; Dhamankar, R.; Kobara, K.; Kirkizlar, E.; Zimmermann, B.; Wayham, N.; et al. Clinical experience with single-nucleotide polymorphism-based non-invasive prenatal screening for 22q11.2 deletion syndrome. *Ultrasound Obstet. Gynecol.* 2016, *47*, 177–183. [CrossRef]
11. Schmid, M.; Wang, E.; Bogard, P.E.; Bevilacqua, E.; Hacker, C.; Wang, S.; Doshi, J.; White, K.; Kaplan, J.; Sparks, A.; et al. Prenatal Screening for 22q11.2 Deletion Using a Targeted Microarray-Based Cell-Free DNA Test. *Fetal Diagn. Ther.* 2018, *44*, 299–304. [CrossRef] [PubMed]
12. Ravi, H.; McNeill, G.; Goel, S.; Meltzer, S.D.; Hunkapiller, N.; Ryan, A.; Levy, B.; Demko, Z.P. Validation of a SNP-based non-invasive prenatal test to detect the fetal 22q11.2 deletion in maternal plasma samples. *PLoS ONE* 2018, *13*, e0193476. [CrossRef] [PubMed]
13. Lin, T.-Y.; Hsieh, T.-T.; Cheng, P.-J.; Hung, T.-H.; Chan, K.-S.; Tsai, C.; Shaw, S.W. Taiwanese Clinical Experience with Noninvasive Prenatal Testing for DiGeorge Syndrome. *Fetal Diagn. Ther.* 2021, *48*, 672–677. [CrossRef] [PubMed]
14. Wapner, R.J.; Babiarz, J.E.; Levy, B.; Stosic, M.; Zimmermann, B.; Sigurjonsson, S.; Wayham, N.; Ryan, A.; Banjevic, M.; Lacroute, P.; et al. Expanding the scope of noninvasive prenatal testing: Detection of fetal microdeletion syndromes. *Am. J. Obstet. Gynecol.* 2015, *212*, 332.e1–332.e9. [CrossRef] [PubMed]
15. Helgeson, J.; Wardrop, J.; Boomer, T.; Almasri, E.; Paxton, W.B.; Saldivar, J.S.; Dharajiya, N.; Monroe, T.J.; Farkas, D.H.; Grosu, D.S.; et al. Clinical outcome of subchromosomal events detected by whole-genome noninvasive prenatal testing. *Prenat. Diagn.* 2015, *35*, 999–1004. [CrossRef]
16. Petersen, A.K.; Cheung, S.W.; Smith, J.L.; Bi, W.; Ward, P.A.; Peacock, S.; Braxton, A.; van den Veyver, I.B.; Breman, A.M. Positive predictive value estimates for cell-free noninvasive prenatal screening from data of a large referral genetic diagnostic laboratory. *Am. J. Obstet. Gynecol.* 2017, *217*, 691.e1–691.e6. [CrossRef]
17. Martin, K.; Iyengar, S.; Kalyan, A.; Lan, C.; Simon, A.L.; Stosic, M.; Kobara, K.; Ravi, H.; Truong, T.; Ryan, A.; et al. Clinical experience with a single-nucleotide polymorphism-based non-invasive prenatal test for five clinically significant microdeletions. *Clin. Genet.* 2018, *93*, 293–300. [CrossRef]
18. Schwartz, S.; Kohan, M.; Pasion, R.; Papenhausen, P.R.; Platt, L.D. Clinical experience of laboratory follow-up with noninvasive prenatal testing using cell-free DNA and positive microdeletion results in 349 cases. *Prenat. Diagn.* 2018, *38*, 210–218. [CrossRef]
19. Koumbaris, G.; Achilleos, A.; Nicolaou, M.; Loizides, C.; Tsangaras, K.; Kypri, E.; Mina, P.; Sismani, C.; Velissariou, V.; Christopoulou, G.; et al. Targeted capture enrichment followed by NGS: Development and validation of a single comprehensive NIPT for chromosomal aneuploidies, microdeletion syndromes and monogenic diseases. *Mol. Cytogenet.* 2019, *12*, 48. [CrossRef]
20. Welker, N.C.; Lee, A.K.; Kjolby, R.A.S.; Wan, H.Y.; Theilmann, M.R.; Jeon, D.; Goldberg, J.D.; Haas, K.R.; Muzzey, D.; Chu, C.S. High-throughput fetal fraction amplification increases analytical performance of noninvasive prenatal screening. *Genet. Med.* 2021, *23*, 443–450. [CrossRef]
21. Liang, D.; Cram, D.S.; Tan, H.; Linpeng, S.; Liu, Y.; Sun, H.; Zhang, Y.; Tian, F.; Zhu, H.; Xu, M.; et al. Clinical utility of noninvasive prenatal screening for expanded chromosome disease syndromes. *Genet. Med.* 2019, *21*, 1998–2006. [CrossRef] [PubMed]
22. Lefkowitz, R.B.; Tynan, J.A.; Liu, T.; Wu, Y.; Mazloom, A.R.; Almasri, E.; Hogg, G.; Angkachatchai, V.; Zhao, C.; Grosu, D.S.; et al. Clinical validation of a noninvasive prenatal test for genome wide detection of fetal copy number variants. *Am. J. Obstet. Gynecol.* 2016, *215*, 227.e1–227.e16. [CrossRef]
23. Rafalko, J.; Soster, E.; Caldwell, S.; Almasri, E.; Westover, T.; Weinblatt, V.; Cacheris, P. Genome-wide cell-free DNA screening: A focus on copy-number variants. *Genet. Med.* 2021, *23*, 1847–1853. [CrossRef] [PubMed]
24. Neofytou, M.C.; Tsangaras, K.; Kypri, E.; Loizides, C.; Ioannides, M.; Achilleos, A.; Mina, P.; Keravnou, A.; Sismani, C.; Koumbaris, G.; et al. Targeted capture enrichment assay for non-invasive prenatal testing of large and small size sub-chromosomal deletions and duplications. *PLoS ONE* 2017, *12*, e0171319. [CrossRef]
25. Kucharik, M.; Gnip, A.; Hyblova, M.; Budis, J.; Strieskova, L.; Harsanyova, M.; Pös, O.; Kubiritova, Z.; Radvanszky, J.; Minarik, G.; et al. Non-invasive prenatal testing (NIPT) by low coverage genomic sequencing: Detection limits of screened chromosomal microdeletions. *PLoS ONE* 2020, *15*, e0238245. [CrossRef] [PubMed]
26. Yang, J.; Peng, C.F.; Qi, Y.; Rao, X.Q.; Guo, F.; Hou, Y.; He, W.; Wu, J.; Chen, Y.Y.; Zhao, X.; et al. Noninvasive prenatal detection of hemoglobin Bart hydrops fetalis via maternal plasma dispensed with prenatal haplotyping using the semiconductor sequencing platform. *Am. J. Obstet. Gynecol.* 2019, *222*, 185.e1–185.e17. [CrossRef]
27. Sawakwongpra, K.; Tangmansakulchai, K.; Ngonsawan, W.; Promwan, S.; Chanchamroen, S.; Quangkananurug, W.; Sriswasdi, S.; Jantarasaengaram, S.; Ponnikorn, S. Droplet-based digital PCR for non-invasive prenatal genetic diagnosis of α and β-thalassemia. *Biomed. Rep.* 2021, *15*, 82. [CrossRef]
28. Zhao, C.; Tynan, J.; Ehrich, M.; Hannum, G.; McCullough, R.; Saldivar, J.-S.; Oeth, P.; van den Boom, D.; Deciu, C. Detection of Fetal Subchromosomal Abnormalities by Sequencing Circulating Cell-Free DNA from Maternal Plasma. *Clin. Chem.* 2015, *61*, 608–616. [CrossRef]

29. Yin, A.H.; Peng, C.F.; Zhao, X.; Caughey, B.A.; Yang, J.X.; Liu, J.; Huang, W.W.; Liu, C.; Luo, D.H.; Liu, H.L.; et al. Noninvasive detection of fetal subchromosomal abnormalities by semiconductor sequencing of maternal plasma DNA. *Proc. Natl. Acad. Sci. USA* **2015**, *112*, 14670–14675. [CrossRef]
30. Hu, H.; Wang, L.; Wu, J.; Zhou, P.; Fu, J.; Sun, J.; Cai, W.; Liu, H.; Yang, Y. Noninvasive prenatal testing for chromosome aneuploidies and subchromosomal microdeletions/microduplications in a cohort of 8141 single pregnancies. *Hum. Genom.* **2019**, *13*, 14. [CrossRef]
31. Pescia, G.; Guex, N.; Iseli, C.; Brennan, L.; Osteras, M.; Xenarios, I.; Farinelli, L.; Conrad, B. Cell-free DNA testing of an extended range of chromosomal anomalies: Clinical experience with 6,388 consecutive cases. *Genet. Med.* **2017**, *19*, 169–175. [CrossRef] [PubMed]
32. Fiorentino, F.; Bono, S.; Pizzuti, F.; Duca, S.; Polverari, A.; Faieta, M.; Baldi, M.; Diano, L.; Spinella, F. The clinical utility of genome-wide noninvasive prenatal screening. *Prenat. Diagn.* **2017**, *37*, 593–601. [CrossRef] [PubMed]
33. Yu, D.; Zhang, K.; Han, M.; Pan, W.; Chen, Y.; Wang, Y.; Jiao, H.; Duan, L.; Zhu, Q.; Song, X.; et al. Noninvasive prenatal testing for fetal subchromosomal copy number variations and chromosomal aneuploidy by low-pass whole-genome sequencing. *Mol. Genet. Genom. Med.* **2019**, *7*, e674. [CrossRef] [PubMed]
34. Chen, Y.; Yu, Q.; Mao, X.; Lei, W.; He, M.; Lu, W. Noninvasive prenatal testing for chromosome aneuploidies and subchromosomal microdeletions/microduplications in a cohort of 42,910 single pregnancies with different clinical features. *Hum. Genom.* **2019**, *13*, 60. [CrossRef]
35. Chen, Y.; Lai, Y.; Xu, F.; Qin, H.; Tang, Y.; Huang, X.; Meng, L.; Su, J.; Sun, W.; Shen, Y.; et al. The application of expanded noninvasive prenatal screening for genome-wide chromosomal abnormalities and genetic counseling. *J. Matern.-Fetal Neonatal Med.* **2021**, *34*, 2710–2716. [CrossRef]
36. Luo, Y.; Hu, H.; Jiang, L.; Ma, Y.; Zhang, R.; Xu, J.; Pan, Y.; Long, Y.; Yao, H.; Liang, Z. A retrospective analysis the clinic data and follow-up of non-invasive prenatal test in detection of fetal chromosomal aneuploidy in more than 40,000 cases in a single prenatal diagnosis center. *Eur. J. Med. Genet.* **2020**, *63*, 104001. [CrossRef]
37. Liu, Y.; Liu, H.; He, Y.; Xu, W.; Ma, Q.; He, Y.; Lei, W.; Chen, G.; He, Z.; Huang, J.; et al. Clinical performance of non-invasive prenatal served as a first-tier screening test for trisomy 21, 18, 13 and sex chromosome aneuploidy in a pilot city in China. *Hum. Genom.* **2020**, *14*, 21. [CrossRef]
38. Lai, Y.; Zhu, X.; He, S.; Dong, Z.; Tang, Y.; Xu, F.; Chen, Y.; Meng, L.; Tao, Y.; Yi, S.; et al. Performance of Cell-Free DNA Screening for Fetal Common Aneuploidies and Sex Chromosomal Abnormalities: A Prospective Study from a Less Developed Autonomous Region in Mainland China. *Genes* **2021**, *12*, 478. [CrossRef]
39. Lo, K.K.; Karampetsou, E.; Boustred, C.; McKay, F.; Mason, S.; Hill, M.; Plagnol, V.; Chitty, L.S. Limited Clinical Utility of Non-Invasive Prenatal Testing for Subchromosomal Abnormalities. *Am. J. Hum. Genet.* **2016**, *98*, 34–44. [CrossRef]
40. Li, R.; Wan, J.; Zhang, Y.; Fu, F.; Ou, Y.; Jing, X.; Li, J.; Li, D.; Liao, C. Detection of fetal copy number variants by non-invasive prenatal testing for common aneuploidies. *Ultrasound Obstet. Gynecol.* **2016**, *47*, 53–57. [CrossRef]
41. Cogulu, O. Next Generation Sequencing as a Tool for Noninvasive Prenatal Tests. In *Clinical Applications for Next-Generation Sequencing*, 1st ed.; Demkow, U., Ploski, R., Eds.; Academic Press: Cambridge, MA, USA, 2016; pp. 171–188.
42. Wou, K.; Levy, B.; Wapner, R.J. Chromosomal Microarrays for the Prenatal Detection of Microdeletions and Microduplications. *Clin. Lab. Med.* **2016**, *36*, 261–276. [CrossRef] [PubMed]
43. Evans, M.I.; Wapner, R.J.; Berkowitz, R.L. Noninvasive prenatal screening or advanced diagnostic testing: Caveat emptor. *Am. J. Obstet. Gynecol.* **2016**, *215*, 298–305. [CrossRef] [PubMed]
44. Gregg, A.R.; Skotko, B.G.; Benkendorf, J.L.; Monaghan, K.G.; Bajaj, K.; Best, R.G.; Klugman, S.; Watson, M.S. Noninvasive prenatal screening for fetal aneuploidy, 2016 update: A position statement of the American College of Medical Genetics and Genomics. *Genet. Med.* **2016**, *18*, 1056–1065. [CrossRef]
45. Bianchi, D.W. *Cherchez la femme*: Maternal incidental findings can explain discordant prenatal cell-free DNA sequencing results. *Genet. Med.* **2018**, *20*, 910–917. [CrossRef]
46. Brady, P.; Brison, N.; Van Den Bogaert, K.; de Ravel, T.; Peeters, H.; Van Esch, H.; Devriendt, K.; Legius, E.; Vermeesch, J.R. Clinical implementation of NIPT–technical and biological challenges. *Clin. Genet.* **2016**, *89*, 523–530. [CrossRef]
47. Yaron, Y.; Jani, J.; Schmid, M.; Oepkes, D. Current Status of Testing for Microdeletion Syndromes and Rare Autosomal Trisomies Using Cell-Free DNA Technology. *Obstet. Gynecol.* **2015**, *126*, 1095–1099. [CrossRef] [PubMed]
48. Grati, F.R.; Gross, S.J. Noninvasive screening by cell-free DNA for 22q11.2 deletion: Benefits, limitations, and challenges. *Prenat. Diagn.* **2019**, *39*, 70–80. [CrossRef]
49. Advani, H.V.; Barrett, A.N.; Evans, M.I.; Choolani, M. Challenges in non-invasive prenatal screening for sub-chromosomal copy number variations using cell-free DNA. *Prenat. Diagn.* **2017**, *37*, 1067–1075. [CrossRef]

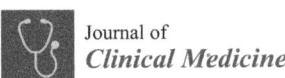

Journal of Clinical Medicine

Article

Can Thyroid Screening in the First Trimester Improve the Prediction of Gestational Diabetes Mellitus?

Zagorka Milovanović [1,2,*], Dejan Filimonović [1,2], Ivan Soldatović [2,3] and Nataša Karadžov Orlić [1,2]

1. Clinic for Gynaecology and Obstetrics Narodni Front, Kraljice Natalije 62, 11000 Belgrade, Serbia; dejan.filimonovic@gmail.com (D.F.); orlicmail@gmail.com (N.K.O.)
2. Faculty of Medicine, University of Belgrade, Dr Subotica Starijeg 8, 11000 Belgrade, Serbia; soldatovic.ivan@gmail.com
3. Institute of Medical Statistics and Informatics, Dr Subotica Starijeg 15, 11000 Belgrade, Serbia
* Correspondence: zaga_mil@yahoo.co.uk; Tel.: +381-63350015

Abstract: This study aimed to evaluate the clinical utility of the subclinical hypothyroidism (SCH) marker, elevated thyroid-stimulating hormone (TSH) and thyroid antibodies in their ability to predict subsequent gestational diabetes mellitus (GDM). In a prospective clinical trial, 230 pregnant women were screened for thyroid function during the first trimester of pregnancy. Increased TSH levels with normal free thyroxine (fT4) were considered SCH. The titers of thyroid peroxidase antibody (anti TPO Ab) at >35 IU/mL and thyroglobulin antibody (anti Tg Ab) at >115 IU/mL were considered as antibodies present. According to the OGTT results, the number of pregnant women with GDM showed the expected growth trend, which was 19%. Two groups of pregnant women were compared, one with GDM and the other without. Increased TSH levels and the presence of thyroid antibodies showed a positive correlation with the risk of GDM. TSH levels were significantly higher in pregnant women with GDM, $p = 0.027$. In this study, 25.6% of pregnant women met the diagnostic criteria for autoimmune thyroiditis. Hashimoto's thyroiditis was significantly more common in GDM patients, $p < 0.001$. Through multivariate logistic regression, it was demonstrated that patient age, TSH 4 IU/mL, and anti TPO Ab > 35 IU/mL are significant predictors of gestational diabetes mellitus that may improve first-trimester pregnancy screening performance, AUC: 0.711; 95% CI: 0.629–0.793.

Keywords: gestational diabetes mellitus; first-trimester pregnancy screening; TSH; thyroid antibodies; anti TPO Ab; anti Tg Ab

1. Introduction

First-trimester screening for chromosomal anomalies is a milestone in pregnancy monitoring. The fact that screening with a combination of fetal ultrasound, maternal serum free-beta-human chorionic gonadotropin (β-hCG) and pregnancy-associated plasma protein-A (PAPP-A) can identify 90% of fetuses with trisomy 21 and other major chromosomal abnormalities with a false-positive rate of 5% [1] has drawn doctors' and researchers' attention to the possibility of screening for other pregnancy-related conditions. Scientists worldwide have concentrated on finding the first-trimester serum markers that predict other pregnancy complications. Recent studies have shown that certain maternal conditions may be predicted in the first trimester. Screening a combination of maternal factors and measuring mean arterial pressure, uterine pulsatility index, and serum placental growth factor may predict 90% of early preeclampsia cases, before 32 weeks, and 75% of preterm preeclampsia cases, before 37 weeks, with a 10% false-positive rate [1].

Thyroid dysfunction and diabetes mellitus are the two most common endocrine disorders that occur during pregnancy [2]. Gestational diabetes mellitus (GDM) is defined as carbohydrate intolerance resulting in hyperglycemia that occurs for the first time during pregnancy [3]. International Diabetes Federation (IDF) data from 2021 indicated that the prevalence of hyperglycemia in pregnancy is 16.7%, 80.3% of which is gestational diabetes

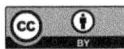

mellitus, 14% in total [4]. According to the latest recommended diagnostic criteria of the World Health Organization (WHO) and the International Association of Diabetes and Pregnancy Study Groups (IADPSG) from 2013 for hyperglycemia in pregnancy, it was expected that the GDM prevalence would rise significantly [5,6]. Pregnancy hyperglycemia is associated with numerous short- and long-term complications in the mother, fetus, and neonate [7,8]. Early diagnosis and treatment of GDM, may significantly reduce the frequency and severity of perinatal complications.

Thyroid dysfunction is the second most common endocrine disorder in women, with an incidence of about 4% in the pregnant population [9], with hypofunction being significantly more prevalent. Subclinical hypothyroidism (SCH) is defined as elevated thyroid-stimulating hormone (TSH) with normal thyroxine (T4) and triiodothyronine (T3) concentrations. According to available data from current literature, hypothyroidism prevalence in pregnant women is 2.2–5% [10–12], with subclinical hypothyroidism occurring in 3–13% [13–15]. depending on the area and population studied. In patients with sufficient iodine intake, the most common cause of hypothyroidism is autoimmune thyroiditis (Hashimoto thyroiditis) [16]. The frequency of antithyroid antibodies, thyroid peroxidase antibody-anti TPO Ab or thyroglobulin antibody-anti Tg Ab in euthyroid pregnant women, according to different authors, is about 10% (2–18%) [17–19], while the antibodies can be found in 30–60% of hypothyroid pregnant women [16]. Thyroid disorder in pregnancy is associated with an increased risk of adverse pregnancy outcomes and pregnancy complications [11,20,21]. Subclinical hypothyroidism, if not treated, may increase the risk of miscarriage, early intrauterine fetal death [10,22], pregnancy anemia, hypertension, preeclampsia [23], postpartum hemorrhage, placental abruption [11,24] and gestational diabetes mellitus [25].

The thyroid hormones directly regulate insulin secretion and glucose metabolism. Hyperthyroidism is associated with decreased insulin sensitivity and insulin resistance, which impairs glucose homeostasis and leads to hyperglycemia. There is a link between thyroid dysfunction and diabetes mellitus. Several studies have shown an increased prevalence of thyroid disorders in diabetes mellitus patients and vice versa [26]. Both disorders are part of polyglandular autoimmune syndrome (PAS). The autoimmune process causes an irreversible loss of function, while chronic autoimmune aggressions can simultaneously modify physiological processes in the affected tissue and lead to altered organ function. Early detection of specific autoantibodies and latent organ-specific dysfunction is advocated to alert physicians to take appropriate action to prevent PAS [27]. According to the available literature, studies on thyroid dysfunction and GDM incidence in different populations have shown a connection between the two entities, although the results are not consistent [26,28–32]. As thyroid and pancreatic dysfunction may be linked by the same autoimmune process, the presence of autoimmune antithyroid antibodies in the first trimester may predict impaired glucose tolerance later in pregnancy.

This study aimed to examine the association of subclinical hypothyroidism and the presence of thyroid autoantibodies in the first-trimester pregnancy with impaired glucose metabolism and to determine the potential predictive value of the elevated thyroid-stimulating hormone and the presence of antithyroid antibodies in gestational diabetes mellitus screening. Existing screening tests for gestational diabetes mellitus use maternal characteristics, family, and personal history to assess the risk of one specific condition [1]. The possibility of using screening markers of thyroid function in the early first trimester of pregnancy to assess the risk of gestational diabetes mellitus might allow one test to identify the risk for two clinically important conditions, enabling appropriate and specific treatment for pregnant women at risk.

2. Materials and Methods

2.1. Study Setting and Patients

A prospective clinical study was conducted at the University Clinic for Gynaecology and Obstetrics "Narodni Front" in Belgrade from November 2019 to November 2021, among patients on antenatal control. This research was approved by the Ethical Board of the Faculty of Medicine, Belgrade University, No. 1550/XI-39.

Included in the study were pregnant women over 18 years of age with a singleton pregnancy. Multiparity, thyroid dysfunction diagnosed before pregnancy, overt diabetes mellitus, congenital malformations of the fetus, fetal death before the planned oral glucose tolerance test, and incomplete documentation were the exclusion criteria.

The minimum number of respondents for estimating the prevalence of gestational diabetes in pregnant women, calculated based on literature data indicating a 1–14% prevalence of gestational diabetes (an assumption that in our population (in Serbia) is about 10%), with an alpha error of 0.05 and an accuracy of 5%, was 138. Considering the possibility of 10% missing data, the required minimum number of respondents for this research was 152. The study enrolled 260 patients. Twenty-five patients were excluded because of incomplete documentation, one withdrew owing to early fetal demise (miscarriage), and four patients left the study. The trial covered 230 patients.

2.2. Procedures

All the pregnant women were followed-up every 4 to 6 weeks, had at least five to six visits and underwent thyroid function screening in the first trimester and an oral glucose tolerance test (oGTT) in the late second or early third trimester of pregnancy. The first visit occurred between 5 and 11 weeks of pregnancy to determine the exact date of the pregnancy, perform the viability ultrasound scan, obtain data on the mother and her family history, perform weight and height measurements, and administer a thyroid function screening test. At the second visit, between 11 and 14 gestational weeks, first-trimester screening for chromosomal abnormality was carried out to assess the risk of chromosomal abnormality, according to the standards of the Fetal Medicine Foundation as part of the international and national guidelines, and to detect major congenital anomalies as early as possible. A detailed anatomy ultrasound scan between 20 and 24 gestational weeks was carried out on every pregnant woman as the standard of pregnancy monitoring, to check growth and exclude structural anomalies. The oGTT with 75 g, was performed between 24 and 30 gestational weeks. Growth and well-being ultrasound scans were performed between 28 and 32 gestational weeks and were repeated between 36 and 38 gestational weeks if the baby was not delivered earlier.

On her first visit to the high-risk pregnancy department, the pregnant woman's medical history was taken and stored in the hospital's electronic database ZIS (Zdravstveni Informacioni Sistem–Health information system). This information included date of birth, last menstrual period, history of chronic diseases, medication used, surgeries, previous pregnancy outcomes, births and miscarriages, and a family history of thyroid disease and diabetes mellitus (first and second-line relatives). The body height and weight of pregnant women were measured and used to calculate the body mass index (BMI) at the pregnancy's start, with the standard formula weight (kg)/height (m)^2.

Clinically confirmed pregnancy was defined as a vital after ultrasound confirmation of intrauterine pregnancy, with gestational age determined by ultrasound software in the first trimester of pregnancy. The blood was sampled, and quantitative analyses of serum TSH, fT4 and antithyroid antibodies, anti TPO Ab and anti Tg Ab, were performed with electro-chemiluminescent immunoassay, ECLIA (Roshe; Cobas blood 6000 e601 module) between 5 + 0 and 12 + 0 weeks of gestation (wg). TSH levels were measured at 8 + 6 weeks of gestation on average, the earliest at 5 + 1 weeks of gestation and the latest at 12 + 0 wg. TSH values were analyzed according to the trimester-specific reference range for gestation in the 2011 National Guideline of Good Clinical Practice for Thyroid Disorder, Republic of Serbia, and the European Thyroid Association (ETA) published in 2014 [15,33]. A TSH value of >2.5 µIU/mL in the first trimester of pregnancy with a normal fT4 value were the diagnostic criteria for subclinical hypothyroidism. According to the guidelines of the American Thyroid Association (ATA) from 2017, the diagnostic criterion for subclinical hypothyroidism is a TSH value of ≥4 µIU/mL [33]. ft4 values were analyzed according to a trimester-specific reference range. Based on available literature data (used in this study), the lower limit of the fT4 reference range in the first trimester on the 2.5th percentile as measured by immunoassay was around 10 pmol/L [16,25,34–36]. Antithyroid antibodies from pregnant women's serum were analyzed by specific ECLIA immunoassay. The values of anti TPO Ab > 35 IU/mL and anti Tg Ab > 115 IU/mL were marked as the presence of autoimmune thyroid antibodies. If women were positive for at least one antibody type, they were considered to fulfill the diagnostic criteria for chronic thyroiditis [16,37].

The oral glucose tolerance test was performed between 24 + 0 and 30 + 0 wg with an average gestation of 26 to 27 weeks. The gestational diabetes mellitus diagnosis was established using the one-step strategy according to the WHO and IADPSG recommendations for the 2 h 75 g oGTT [5,6]. Diagnostic criteria were at least one value greater than fasting glucose of 5.1 mmol/L, a 1 h glucose of 10.0 mmol/L, or a 2 h glucose of 8.6 mmol/L. Following the oGTT test, the patients were divided into two groups: one with impaired glucose homeostasis, the GDM group, and the other with regular glucose metabolism, the group without GDM.

The association of elevated TSH values and the presence of antithyroid antibodies in the first trimester of pregnancy with impaired glycemic control was investigated. The relationship between different TSH values, both cut-offs > 2.5 µIU/mL and ≥4 µIU/mL, and GDM was examined. In addition, we examined the predictive value of elevated TSH levels and antithyroid antibody levels in the first trimester for detecting gestational diabetes mellitus. Model predictive performance for early prediction of GDM was evaluated by receiver operating characteristic curves.

2.3. Statistical Analysis

The results are presented as absolute and relative numbers (%), mean ± standard deviation or median (25th–75th percentile), depending on data type and distribution. Parametric (Student's t test) and non-parametric (chi-square, Mann–Whitney U test, Fisher's exact test) tests were used to assess the significance of the difference between the groups. Univariate and multivariate logistic regression were used to assess the significance of the GDM predictor. All tests with p values of <0.05 were considered statistically significant. Data were analyzed using SPSS 20.0 (IBM Corp.2011. IBM SPSS Statistics for Windows, version 20.0. Armonk, NY, USA: IBM Corp.).

3. Results

Out of 230 pregnant women, 19.5% (45) met the oGTT-75g criteria for GDM, and 80.5% (185) of the study population had normal glycemic control. There was no difference between the two groups in the examined characteristics, body height, body weight at the beginning and end of pregnancy, weight gain, and BMI, only in the mean age of patients (33.47 (±3.86) in the GDM group and 31.82 (±4.62) in non-GDM group, $p = 0.028$). The main characteristics of the examined group are shown in Table 1.

Table 1. Maternal parameter characteristics of the study population.

Parameters	GDM Group (n = 45)	Non-GDM Group (n = 185)	p Value
age (years) *(MV ± SD)*	33.47 (±3.86)	31.82 (±4.62)	**0.028**
body height *(MV ± SD)* (cm)	168.22 (±4.61)	168.74 (±6.75)	0.540
b.w. at the pregnancy start *(MV ± SD)* (kg)	66.67 (±9.82)	64.90 (±13.19)	0.401
b.w. at delivery *(MV ± SD)* (kg)	78.98 (±11.27)	77.41 (±11.48)	0.422
weight gain *(MV ± SD)* (kg)	12.80 (±6.39)	12.92 (±4.79)	0.904
BMI *(MV ± SD)* (kg/m^2)	23.72 (±3.65)	22.79 (±4.14)	0.171

Data presented as *MV ± SD*; *MV*: mean value; *SD*: standard deviation; GDM: gestational diabetes mellitus; b.w.: body weight; BMI: body mass index.

There was no difference in the family history of hereditary conditions, diabetes mellitus and thyroid disease in the first- and second-degree relatives between groups (Table 2).

Table 2. Family history of hereditary conditions.

		Non-GDM (n = 185)	GDM (n = 45)	p Value
Family history of thyroid disorders N (N%)	no	150 (79.8%)	38 (20.2%)	0.647
	yes	35 (82.9%)	7 (17.1%)	
Family history of diabetes mellitus N (N%)	no	112 (79.4%)	29 (20.6%)	0.511
	yes	73 (83.0%)	15 (17.0%)	

Data presented as number N and percentage (%); GDM: gestational diabetes mellitus.

There was no difference in the obstetric history of previous pregnancies. The observed difference in the prevalence of miscarriages and GDM in previous pregnancies between the two groups was not of statistical significance (Table 3).

Table 3. Previous obstetric history.

		Non-GDM (n = 185)	GDM (n = 45)	p Value
Deliveries N (N%)	no	98 (79.7%)	5 (20.3%)	0.782
	yes	86 (81.1%)	20 (18.9%)	
Miscarriages N (N%)	no	135 (81.8%)	30 (18.2%)	0.369
	yes	49 (76.6%)	15 (23.4%)	
GDM in previous pregnancy	no	77 (89.54%)	16 (75.0%)	0.241
	yes	9 (10.46%)	4 (25.0%)	

Data presented as number N and percentage (%); GDM: gestational diabetes mellitus.

The mean TSH value in the GDM group was significantly higher than in the group without GDM, 2.75 µIU/mL (±2.60) compared with 1.75 µIU/mL (±1.10), $p = 0.027$. The obtained fT4 values in both groups were in the reference range for the first trimester of pregnancy, although there was a significant difference ($p = 0.021$) between the examined groups: 14.05 (±2.38) in the group with GDM and 14.98 (±2.40) in the non-GDM group (Table 4).

Table 4. Biochemical parameters in the study population.

Parameters	GDM(n = 45)	Non-GDM (n = 185)	p Value
Fasting glucose (mmol/L) (MV ± SD)	4.79 (±0.53)	4,37 (±0.37)	
Insuin fasting * (uIU/mL) M (IQ)	8.00 (5.3–11.5)	8.81 (6.6–11.8)	0.191
TSH (µIU/mL) (MV ± SD)	2.75 (±2.60)	1.75 (±1.10)	**0.027**
fT4 (pmol/L) (MV ± SD)	14.05 (±2.38)	14.98 (±2.40)	**0.021**

Data presented as MV ± SD; MV: mean value; SD: standard deviation; * Insulin levels expressed as M (IQ); M: median; IQ: interquartile range; GDM: gestational diabetes mellitus; TSH: thyroid-stimulating hormone; fT4: free thyroxine.

Using the TSH > 2.5 IU/mL criterion, we found that 25.65% of the pregnant women were diagnosed with subclinical hypothyroidism, out of which one-third (8.26%) had impaired glucose tolerance. In the group with GDM, the prevalence of TSH > 2.5 µIU/mL was 42.2%. If we applied the ATA diagnostic criterion of TSH ≥ 4.0, SCH prevalence was 7.39%, with a prevalence of 3.48% among GDM. Among patients who were diagnosed with GDM, the prevalence of SCH was 17.78% (8 out of 45). The difference for both TSH values among the examined groups was statistically significant, 0.007 for TSH ≥ 4 IU/mL and 0.005 for TSH > 2.5 IU/mL (Table 5).

Table 5. The prevalence of elevated TSH in the study population.

Parameters	GDM Group (n = 45)	Non-GDM Group (n = 185)	p Value
TSH ≥ 4.0 µIU/mL N (N%)	8 (17.8%)	9 (4.86%)	0.007
TSH > 2.5 µIU/mL N (N%)	19 (42.2%)	40 (21.6%)	0.005

Data presented as number N and percentage (%); GDM: gestational diabetes mellitus; TSH: thyroid-stimulating hormone.

In this study, 25.6% of the pregnant women had at least one type of antithyroid antibody, which met the diagnostic criteria for chronic thyroiditis, and 10% had both types of antibodies. Hashimoto's thyroiditis was diagnosed in 51.1% in the first trimester in the GDM group, compared to 19.46% in the non-GDM group, $p < 0.001$. The anti TPO Ab was detected in 19.6% of the pregnant women, and the anti Tg Ab in 15.2%. In the GDM group the anti TPO Ab was detected in 40%, while the anti Tg Ab was found in 26.67% (Table 6).

Table 6. The prevalence of antithyroid antibodies in the study population.

Parameters	GDM Group (n = 45)	Non-GDM Group (n = 185)	p Value
Hashimoto thyroiditis N (N%)	23 (51.10%)	36 (19.46%)	<0.001
Anti TPO Ab > 35 IU/mL N (N%)	18 (40.00%)	27 (14,59%)	<0.001
Anti Tg Ab > 115 IU/mL N (N%)	12 (6.67%)	23 (12.43%)	0.017

Data presented as number N and percentage (%); GDM: gestational diabetes mellitus; anti TPO Ab: anti-thyroid peroxidase antibodies; anti Tg Ab: anti-thyroglobulin antibodies.

Elevated TSH ≥ 4 and both types of antibodies (anti TPO Ab and anti Tg Ab) were present in 4.44% of the GDM group and 1.62% in the non-GDM group. In the group of pregnant women with GDM, 13.3% had an elevated value of TSH ≥ 4 µIU/mL and at least one type of antibody detected in the first trimester, compared with 2.7% in the non-GDM group.

Modeling was performed using logistic regression analysis to estimate the predictive value of the examined parameters in the study. Several steps were used to assess the most important predictors of GDM. In the first step, all significant predictors obtained from the univariable analysis and variables deemed important by expert opinion (DM in family, BMI in the pregnancy onset, age in year) were used and evaluated for multivariable analysis. Using the enter method, all predictors with a p value of <0.200 were used for multivariable modeling. In this model, age, TSH and anti TPO Ab were significant, while anti Tg Ab was not (results not presented). Then, the backward method for variable reduction in the model with $p < 0.10$ probability was employed to eliminate non-significant predictors. The model revealed age, THS ≥ 4.0 µIU/mL and anti TPO Ab > 35 IU/mL as the most important and statistically significant predictors of GDM. Using the variance inflation factor, multicollinearity was evaluated. The area under the curve was used to evaluate the discriminative power of the model. Univariable and multivariable modeling are presented in Table 7.

Table 7. Univariable and multivariable modeling.

	Univariable			Multivariable (Backward) *		
	OR (95% CI)	p Value		OR (95% CI)	p Value	
Age (yrs)	1.084 (1.008–1.167)	0.030		**1.100** (1.017–1.189)	0.017	
Age 35+	1.399 (0.709–2.759)	0.333				
BMI (kg/m²)	1.053 (0.977–1.135)	0.174				
DM in family	0.794 (0.398–1.581)	0.511				
TSH ≥ 4 µIU/mL	4.228 (1.530–11.581)	0.005		2.962 (0.992–8.846)	0.052	

Table 7. Cont.

	Univariable		Multivariable (Backward) *	
	OR (95% CI)	p Value	OR (95% CI)	p Value
TSH ≥ 2.5 µIU/mL	2.649 (1.332–5.267)	0.005		
Hashimoto Thyroiditis	4.327 (2.173–8.614)	<0.001		
Anti TPO Ab > 35IU/mL	3.901 (1.894–8.036)	<0.001	**3.627** (1.682–7.821)	**0.001**
Anti Tg Ab > 115 IU/mL	2.561 (1.160–5.655)	0.020		

* AUC of the model = 0.711 (95% CI, 0.629–0.793). BMI: body mass index; DM: Diabetes mellitus; TSH: thyroid-stimulating hormone; anti TPO Ab: anti-thyroid peroxidase antibodies; GDM: gestational diabetes mellitus; anti Tg Ab: anti-thyroid globulin antibodies.

Significant predictors of gestational diabetes mellitus were patient age, TSH ≥ 4 µIU/mL and anti TPO Ab > 35 IU/mL, as presented in Table 8.

Table 8. Significant predictors of gestational diabetes mellitus.

	OR	p Value
AGE (years)	1.100	0.017
TSH ≥ 4 µIU/mL	2.962	0.052
Anti TPO Ab > 35 IU/mL	3.627	0.001

TSH: thyroid-stimulating hormone; anti TPO Ab: anti-thyroid peroxidase antibodies; GDM: gestational diabetes mellitus.

4. Discussion

Thyroid disorders such as subclinical hypothyroidism have been associated with an increased risk of adverse pregnancy outcomes in most but not all published studies, probably because of the different criteria used to define elevated TSH levels [16,32,38,39]. TSH values in the first trimester of pregnancy normally decrease owing to the thyrotropic activity of increasing β-HCG, which has a homologous α subunit with TSH, and the free thyroxine (fT4) values increase at the same time.

In this study, the mean TSH values in the first trimester of pregnancy in GDM patients were higher than those in patients with normal glycemic control. Since 1953 in the Republic of Serbia, iodization of all salt intended for human consumption has been mandatory, so the assumption was that there were no pregnant women with iodine deficiency among the patients and that the thyroid dysfunction was not caused by that deficiency. There has been an increase in the number of patients with thyroid disorders, based on our clinical experience. To the best of our knowledge, this was the first study of its kind in the population of pregnant women in this area.

Elevated TSH levels may indicate a thyroid dysfunction that needs to be corrected to avoid maternal morbidity and to ensure normal fetal development, as well as numerous potential complications during pregnancy. Based on published studies, it has been estimated that 8–28% of pregnant women have a TSH concentration that is considered high if fixed TSH > 2.5 upper limits are used. Cut-offs set at these levels are too low and can result in overdiagnosis and overtreatment, which is unwarranted and may cause more harm than good [36,39]. New ATA guidelines from 2017 updated the recommendations by suggesting TSH values above 4.0 µIU/mL as a diagnostic criterion for subclinical hypothyroidism [16]. The percentage of patients in this study diagnosed with subclinical hypothyroidism using TSH values > 2.5 µIU/mL was 25.65%, which correlated with the findings presented in the T. Korevaar paper from 2018. That study demonstrated that with fixed TSH upper limits of 2.5 µIU/mL, 8–28% of pregnant women had a TSH concentration considered to be increased [36], in contrast to the significantly lower number of pregnant women (7.39%) diagnosed with SCH using the criterion TSH ≥ 4.0 µIU/mL. The number of patients diagnosed with GDM according to the guidelines of the WHO, IADPSG and the National Guideline for DM showed the expected growth trend, which was 19% in our study group [5,6,33].

Pregnant women with TSH > 2.5 µIU/mL in the first trimester were twice as likely to develop GDM, and pregnant women with TSH ≥ 4.0 µIU/mL were almost four times more likely to exhibit impaired glycemic control. This finding correlated with recent meta-analyses of cohort studies [40,41] and publications that suggested an association between elevated TSH and gestational diabetes mellitus [16,42]. Since thyroid hormones are involved in glucose metabolism, thyroid dysfunction during pregnancy in the form of subclinical hypothyroidism may be part of the chain of pathophysiological mechanisms in gestational diabetes mellitus onset.

The diagnosis of subclinical hypothyroidism in pregnancy is characterized by an fT4 value within the reference range for gestational age, although in this study the average value of fT4 was lower in the group of patients who developed GDM. That difference was statistically significant $p = 0.02$. This finding indicated the importance of the thyroid in glycemic control, so that lower fT4 values alone may affect the reduction in insulin sensitivity, increase insulin resistance, and result in hyperglycemia.

This research indicated a relatively high incidence of 25.6% of Hashimoto's thyroiditis in the study population. Pregnant women who were diagnosed with at least one type of thyroid antibody above the threshold at the beginning of pregnancy, regardless of the presence of other thyroid function markers, had a three times higher risk of impaired glycemia. In this population of pregnant women anti TPO Ab was more commonly diagnosed than anti Tg Ab. If anti TPO antibodies were detected in the first trimester, there was a 2.7-fold higher risk of GDM, and if anti Tg Ab was detected, there was twice the risk of GDM compared to pregnant women who had no antibodies present.

Pregnant women diagnosed with GDM were almost five times (4.9) more likely to have elevated TSH ≥ 4.0 µIU/mL and at least one type of antibody present in the titer as diagnostic criteria for autoimmune thyroiditis, compared to pregnant women with normal glycemic control.

Increased TSH levels and the presence of thyroid antibodies showed a positive correlation with the risk of GDM. The corresponding odds values for TSH and anti TPO Ab were OR 3.971, 95% CI: 1.34–11.77 and OR 4.026, CI: 1.866–8.689, respectively.

Through multivariate logistic regression, we demonstrated that significant predictors of gestational diabetes mellitus that may improve first-trimester pregnancy screening performances are patient age, TSH ≥ 4 µIU/mL and anti TPO Ab > 35 IU/mL. The receiver operating characteristic (ROC) curve for significant variables achieved an area under the curve (AUC) of 0.711; 95% confidence interval (CI) 0.629–0.793.

Increased risk of GDM in pregnant women with positive anti TPO Ab in early pregnancy and a higher rate of positive anti TPO Ab in pregnant women with GDM than in those without GDM have already been shown in publications, and that finding correlated with this study [35,43].

Insulin resistance, defined as the inability of insulin to increase glucose uptake and utilization in peripheral tissues, can be present for years before the onset of hyperglycemia, and it is known that hypothyroidism is associated with decreased insulin sensitivity since thyroid hormones directly regulate insulin secretion. The link between impaired glycemia and thyroid dysfunction may be related to an autoimmune mechanism that occurs as part of the polyglandular autoimmune syndrome, involving both the pancreas and the thyroid gland.

This study did not examine the presence of anti-insulin antibodies to prove this association, as they are an autoimmune marker of pancreatic islet cell beta cell destruction [44] and can be detected years before clinical manifestations of DM in healthy individuals or in individuals with other autoimmune disorders such as autoimmune thyroiditis. Some authors believe that the link between the two is an autoimmune inflammatory process, citing elevated serum cytokine levels in both disorders [35,45,46]. Hashimoto's disease could be considered a T helper 1 disease in which pro-inflammatory cytokines play a crucial role, and there is a connection between the level of anti TPO antibodies and pro-inflammatory cytokines that appears at higher concentrations in individuals with insulin resistance [47].

Further research is needed to better define the relationship between these two disorders in pregnant women and to better understand their pathogenetic mechanisms, allowing us to find the best possible predictor of forthcoming disorders.

Since there are many possible short and long-term complications of gestational diabetes mellitus in the mother and fetus, there is a clear need for early detection of glycemic disorders and, accordingly, adequate treatment to prevent and reduce the consequences of the disorder.

The current risk factor-based screening method estimates GDM risk by considering maternal characteristics and personal and family history. Clinical screening markers have limited diagnostic accuracy when used separately. Prediction models that include a combination of different markers may improve the sensitivity and specificity of GDM screening by risk factors. The thyroid biochemical screening markers can be used as additional markers in the first trimester since they are easily accessible and feasible. The clinical markers currently employed may be combined with thyroid markers, TSH and anti TPO Ab to improve screening performance. Numerous risk estimation models for GDM can be found in the current literature; however, most of them are based on different diagnostic criteria. Validation of predictive models in clinical practice is crucial in large cohorts and across different ethnic groups [48]. Further research is needed to confirm the benefit and effectiveness of screening strategies in the detection of GDM and prevention and reduction in perinatal complications.

There are limitations in this study that must be mentioned. The study was monocentric with a relatively small number of observation units. All patients included in our study were from the Republic of Serbia, with a certain specific genetic heritage that may differ in other populations. The research was conducted in the population of pregnant women under regular antenatal care in a tertiary institution to which patients with high-risk pregnancy gravitate, so it is possible that the actual prevalence of thyroid disease and gestational diabetes is slightly lower than in our study.

5. Conclusions

Numerous studies have evaluated new markers for first-trimester pregnancy screening to predict pregnancy complications and prevent adverse outcomes. This study suggested an association between elevated TSH values and the onset of hyperglycemia. Autoimmune thyroiditis was shown as an independent marker for GDM occurrence. According to the results of this research, elevated TSH values and anti TPO antibodies in early pregnancy might be used as additional first-trimester markers to improve screening performance for gestational diabetes mellitus.

Author Contributions: Z.M., N.K.O. and D.F., conceptualization, data curation, methodology, investigation, writing—original draft; I.S., formal analysis; N.K.O., supervision. All authors have read and agreed to the published version of the manuscript.

Funding: This research received no external funding.

Institutional Review Board Statement: The study was conducted in accordance with the Declaration of Helsinki and approved by the Ethical Board of the Faculty of Medicine, Belgrade University, No. 1550/XI-39.

Informed Consent Statement: Informed consent was obtained from all subjects involved in the study.

Data Availability Statement: Original data are available on request.

Acknowledgments: We would like to thank Aleksandra Franić for English proofreading and Aleksandar Rakić for software and technical support.

Conflicts of Interest: The authors declare no conflict of interest.

References

1. Bouariu, A.; Panaitescu, A.M.; Nicolaides, K.H. First Trimester Prediction of Adverse Pregnancy Outcomes-Identifying Pregnancies at Risk from as Early as 11–13 Weeks. *Medicina* **2022**, *58*, 332. [CrossRef] [PubMed]
2. Hage, M.; Zantout, M.S.; Azar, S.T. Thyroid Disorders and Diabetes Mellitus. *J. Thyroid. Res.* **2011**, *2011*, 1–7. [CrossRef] [PubMed]
3. Giannakou, K.; Evangelou, E.; Yiallouros, P.; Christophi, C.A.; Middleton, N.; Papatheodorou, E.; Papatheodorou, S.I. Risk factors for gestational diabetes: An umbrella review of meta-analyses of observational studies. *PLoS ONE* **2019**, *14*, e0215372. [CrossRef] [PubMed]
4. International Diabetes Federation. *IDF Diabetes Atlas*, 10th ed.; International Diabetes Federation: Brussels, Belgium.
5. Diagnostic Criteria and Classification of Hyperglycaemia First Detected in Pregnancy: A World Health Organization Guideline. *Diabetes Res. Clin. Pract.* **2014**, *103*, 341–363. [CrossRef] [PubMed]
6. International Association of Diabetes and Pregnancy Study Groups Consensus Panel; Metzger, B.E.; Gabbe, S.G.; Persson, B.; Buchanan, T.A.; Catalano, P.A.; Damm, P.; Dyer, A.R.; de Leiva, A.; Hod, M.; et al. International Association of Diabetes and Pregnancy Study Groups Recommendations on the Diagnosis and Classification of Hyperglycemia in Pregnancy. *Diabetes Care* **2010**, *33*, 676–682. [CrossRef]
7. Lende, M.; Rijhsinghani, A. Gestational Diabetes: Overview with Emphasis on Medical Management. *Int. J. Environ. Res. Public Health* **2020**, *17*, 9573. [CrossRef] [PubMed]
8. Carreiro, M.P.; Nogueira, A.I.; Ribeiro-Oliveira, A. Controversies and Advances in Gestational Diabetes-An Update in the Era of Continuous Glucose Monitoring. *J. Clin. Med.* **2018**, *7*, 11. [CrossRef]
9. Stagnaro-Green, A.; Abalovich, M.; Alexander, E.; Azizi, F.; Mestman, J.; Negro, R.; Nixon, A.; Pearce, E.N.; Soldin, O.P.; Sullivan, S.; et al. Guidelines of the American Thyroid Association for the Diagnosis and Management of Thyroid Disease During Pregnancy and Postpartum. *Thyroid.* **2011**, *21*, 1081–1125. [CrossRef]
10. Allan, W.; Haddow, J.; Palomaki, G.; Williams, J.; Mitchell, M.; Hermos, R.; Faix, J.; Klein, R. Maternal Thyroid Deficiency and Pregnancy Complications: Implications for Population Screening. *J Med. Screen* **2000**, *7*, 127–130. [CrossRef]
11. Casey, B.M.; Dashe, J.S.; Wells, C.E.; McIntire, D.D.; Byrd, W.; Leveno, K.J.; Cunningham, F.G. Subclinical Hypothyroidism and Pregnancy Outcomes. *Obstet. Gynecol.* **2005**, *105*, 239–245. [CrossRef]
12. Casey, B.M.; Dashe, J.S.; Spong, C.Y.; McIntire, D.D.; Leveno, K.J.; Cunningham, G.F. Perinatal Significance of Isolated Maternal Hypothyroxinemia Identified in the First Half of Pregnancy. *Obstet. Gynecol.* **2007**, *109*, 1129–1135. [CrossRef] [PubMed]
13. Lazarus, J.H.; Bestwick, J.P.; Channon, S.; Paradice, R.; Maina, A.; Rees, R.; Chiusano, E.; John, R.; Guaraldo, V.; George, L.M.; et al. Antenatal Thyroid Screening and Childhood Cognitive Function. *N. Engl. J. Med.* **2012**, *366*, 493–501. [CrossRef] [PubMed]
14. Potlukova, E.; Potluka, O.; Jiskra, J.; Limanova, Z.; Telicka, Z.; Bartakova, J.; Springer, D. Is Age a Risk Factor for Hypothyroidism in Pregnancy? An Analysis of 5223 Pregnant Women. *J. Clin. Endocrinol. Metab.* **2012**, *97*, 1945–1952. [CrossRef] [PubMed]
15. Lazarus, J.; Brown, R.S.; Daumerie, C.; Hubalewska-Dydejczyk, A.; Negro, R.; Vaidya, B. 2014 European Thyroid Association Guidelines for the Management of Subclinical Hypothyroidism in Pregnancy and in Children. *Eur. Thyroid. J.* **2014**, *3*, 76–94. [CrossRef] [PubMed]
16. Alexander, E.K.; Pearce, E.N.; Brent, G.A.; Brown, R.S.; Chen, H.; Dosiou, C.; Grobman, W.A.; Laurberg, P.; Lazarus, J.H.; Mandel, S.J.; et al. 2017 Guidelines of the American Thyroid Association for the Diagnosis and Management of Thyroid Disease During Pregnancy and the Postpartum. *Thyroid* **2017**, *27*, 315–389. [CrossRef]
17. Lazarus, J.H. Screening for Thyroid Dysfunction in Pregnancy: Is It Worthwhile? *J. Thyroid. Res.* **2011**, *2011*, 1–4. [CrossRef]
18. Azizi, F.; Delshad, H. Thyroid Derangements in Pregnancy. *Iran. J. Endocrinol. Metab.* **2014**, *15*, 491–508.
19. Leo, S.D.; Pearce, E.N. Autoimmune Thyroid Disease during Pregnancy. *Lancet Diabetes Endocrinol.* **2018**, *6*, 575–586. [CrossRef]
20. Gheorghiu, M.L.; Bors, R.G.; Gheorghisan-Galateanu, A.A.; Pop, A.L.; Cretoiu, D.; Varlas, V.N. Hyperthyroidism in Pregnancy: The Delicate Balance between Too Much or Too Little Antithyroid Drug. *J. Clin. Med.* **2021**, *10*, 3742. [CrossRef]
21. Harn-A-Morn, P.; Dejkhamron, P.; Tongsong, T.; Luewan, S. Pregnancy Outcomes among Women with Graves' Hyperthyroidism: A Retrospective Cohort Study. *J. Clin. Med.* **2021**, *10*, 4495. [CrossRef]
22. Abalovich, M.; Gutierrez, S.; Alcaraz, G.; Maccallini, G.; Garcia, A.; Levalle, O. Overt and Subclinical Hypothyroidism Complicating Pregnancy. *Thyroid* **2002**, *12*, 63–68. [CrossRef] [PubMed]
23. Ashoor, G.; Maiz, N.; Rotas, M.; Jawdat, F.; Nicolaides, K.H. Maternal Thyroid Function at 11 to 13 Weeks of Gestation and Subsequent Fetal Death. *Thyroid* **2010**, *20*, 989–993. [CrossRef] [PubMed]
24. Davis, L.E.; Leveno, K.J.; Cunningham, F.G. Hypothyroidism Complicating Pregnancy. *Obstet. Gynecol.* **1988**, *72*, 108–112. [PubMed]
25. Tudela, C.M.; Casey, B.M.; McIntire, D.D.; Cunningham, F.G. Relationship of Subclinical Thyroid Disease to the Incidence of Gestational Diabetes. *Obstet. Gynecol.* **2012**, *119*, 983–988. [CrossRef] [PubMed]
26. Biondi, B.; Kahaly, G.J.; Robertson, R.P. Thyroid Dysfunction and Diabetes Mellitus: Two Closely Associated Disorders. *Endocr. Rev.* **2019**, *40*, 789–824. [CrossRef] [PubMed]
27. Kahaly, G.J.; Frommer, L. Polyglandular Autoimmune Syndromes. *J Endocrinol. Investig.* **2017**, *41*, 91–98. [CrossRef]
28. Olivieri, A.; Valensise, H.; Magnani, F.; Medda, E.; Angelis, S.D.; D'Archivio, M.; Sorcini, M.; Carta, S.; Baccarini, S.; Romanini, C. High Frequency of Antithyroid Autoantibodies in Pregnant Women at Increased Risk of Gestational Diabetes Mellitus. *Eur. J. Endocrinol.* **2000**, *143*, 741–747. [CrossRef]

29. Agarwal, M.M.; Dhatt, G.S.; Punnose, J.; Bishawi, B.; Zayed, R. Thyroid Function Abnormalities and Antithyroid Antibody Prevalence in Pregnant Women at High Risk for Gestational Diabetes Mellitus. *Gynecol. Endocrinol.* **2006**, *22*, 261–266. [CrossRef]
30. Cleary-Goldman, J.; Malone, F.D.; Lambert-Messerlian, G.; Sullivan, L.; Canick, J.; Porter, T.F.; Luthy, D.; Gross, S.; Bianchi, D.W.; D'Alton, M.E.; et al. Maternal Thyroid Hypofunction and Pregnancy Outcome. *Obstet. Gynecol.* **2008**, *112*, 85–92. [CrossRef]
31. Yanachkova, V.; Kamenov, Z. The Relationship between Thyroid Dysfunction during Pregnancy and Gestational Diabetes Mellitus. *Endokrynol. Pol.* **2021**, *72*, 226–231. [CrossRef]
32. Corrales, E.P.; Andrada, P.; Aubá, M.; Zambrana, Á.R.; Grima, F.G.; Salvador, J.; Escalada, J.; Galofré, J.C. ¿Existe mayor riesgo de diabetes gestacional en pacientes con disfunción tiroidea autoinmune? *Endocrinol Nutr.* **2014**, *61*, 377–381. [CrossRef] [PubMed]
33. Републичка стручна комисија за израду и имплементацију водича добре клиничке праксе. Национални Водич Добре Клиничке Праксе За Дијагностиковање и Лечење *Diabetes Mellitus-a*, 2nd ed.; Агенција за акредитацију здравствених установа Србије: Београд, Србије, 2012; ISBN 978-86-6235-013-8.
34. Karakosta, P.; Alegakis, D.; Georgiou, V.; Roumeliotaki, T.; Fthenou, E.; Vassilaki, M.; Boumpas, D.; Castanas, E.; Kogevinas, M.; Chatzi, L. Thyroid Dysfunction and Autoantibodies in Early Pregnancy Are Associated with Increased Risk of Gestational Diabetes and Adverse Birth Outcomes. *J. Clin. Endocrinol. Metab.* **2012**, *97*, 4464–4472. [CrossRef] [PubMed]
35. Huang, K.; Xu, Y.; Yan, S.; Li, T.; Xu, Y.; Zhu, P.; Tao, F. Isolated Effect of Maternal Thyroid-Stimulating Hormone, Free Thyroxine and Antithyroid Peroxidase Antibodies in Early Pregnancy on Gestational Diabetes Mellitus: A Birth Cohort Study in China. *Endocr. J.* **2019**, *66*, 223–231. [CrossRef]
36. Korevaar, T.I.M. The Upper Limit for TSH during Pregnancy: Why We Should Stop Using Fixed Limits of 2.5 or 3.0 MU/l. *Thyroid. Res.* **2018**, *11*, 5. [CrossRef] [PubMed]
37. Pagana, K.D.; Pagana, T.J.; Pagana, T.N. *Mosby's Diagnostic and Laboratory Test Reference*, 14th ed.; Elsevier Science: Amsterdam, The Netherlands, 2019; ISBN 978-0-323-60969-2.
38. He, Y.; He, T.; Wang, Y.; Xu, Z.; Xu, Y.; Wu, Y.; Ji, J.; Mi, Y. Comparison of the effect of different diagnostic criteria of subclinical hypothyroidism and positive TPO-Ab on pregnancy outcomes. *Zhonghua Fu Chan Ke Za Zhi* **2014**, *49*, 824–828.
39. Negro, R.; Schwartz, A.; Gismondi, R.; Tinelli, A.; Mangieri, T.; Stagnaro-Green, A. Increased Pregnancy Loss Rate in Thyroid Antibody Negative Women with TSH Levels between 2.5 and 5.0 in the First Trimester of Pregnancy. *J. Clin. Endocrinol. Metab.* **2010**, *95*, E44–E48. [CrossRef]
40. Toulis, K.A.; Stagnaro-Green, A.; Negro, R. Maternal Subclinical Hypothyroidsm and Gestational Diabetes Mellitus: A Meta-Analysis. *Endocr. Pract.* **2014**, *20*, 703–714. [CrossRef]
41. Jia, M.; Wu, Y.; Lin, B.; Shi, Y.; Zhang, Q.; Lin, Y.; Wang, S.; Zhang, Y. Meta-Analysis of the Association between Maternal Subclinical Hypothyroidism and Gestational Diabetes Mellitus. *Int. J. Gynecol. Obstet.* **2018**, *144*, 239–247. [CrossRef]
42. Stohl, H.E.; Ouzounian, J.; Rick, A.-M.; Hueppchen, N.A.; Bienstock, J.L. Thyroid Disease and Gestational Diabetes Mellitus (GDM): Is There a Connection? *J. Matern.-Fetal Neonatal Med.* **2013**, *26*, 1139–1142. [CrossRef]
43. Ying, H.; Tang, Y.-P.; Bao, Y.-R.; Su, X.-J.; Cai, X.; Li, Y.-H.; Wang, D.-F. Maternal TSH Level and TPOAb Status in Early Pregnancy and Their Relationship to the Risk of Gestational Diabetes Mellitus. *Endocrine* **2016**, *54*, 742–750. [CrossRef]
44. Cai, Y.; Yan, J.; Gu, Y.; Chen, H.; Chen, Y.; Xu, X.; Zhang, M.; Yu, L.; Zheng, X.; Yang, T. Autoimmune Thyroid Disease Correlates to Islet Autoimmunity on Zinc Transporter 8 Autoantibody. *Endocr. Connect.* **2021**, *10*, 534–542. [CrossRef] [PubMed]
45. Drugarin, D.; Negru, S.; Koreck, A.; Zosin, I.; Cristea, C. The Pattern of a TH1 Cytokine in Autoimmune Thyroiditis. *Immunol. Lett.* **2000**, *71*, 73–77. [CrossRef]
46. Al-ofi, E.A. Implications of Inflammation and Insulin Resistance in Obese Pregnant Women with Gestational Diabetes: A Case Study. *SAGE Open Med. Case Rep.* **2019**, *7*. [CrossRef] [PubMed]
47. Blaslov, K.; Gajski, D.; Vucelić, V.; Gaćina, P.; Mirošević, G.; Marinković, J.; Vrkljan, M.; Rotim, K. The Association of Subclinical Insulin Resistance with Thyroid Autoimmunity in Euthyroid Individuals. *Acta Clin. Croat* **2020**, *59.*, 696–702. [CrossRef]
48. Huhn, E.A.; Rossi, S.W.; Hoesli, I.; Göbl, C.S. Controversies in Screening and Diagnostic Criteria for Gestational Diabetes in Early and Late Pregnancy. *Front. Endocrinol.* **2018**, *9*, 696. [CrossRef]

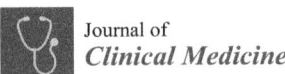

Review

Noninvasive Prenatal Testing in Immunohematology—Clinical, Technical and Ethical Considerations

Jens Kjeldsen-Kragh [1,2,*] and Åsa Hellberg [1]

1. Clinical Immunology and Transfusion Medicine, Office for Medical Services, Region Skåne, SE-221 85 Lund, Sweden; asa.hellberg@skane.se
2. Department of Laboratory Medicine, University Hospital of North Norway, N-9019 Tromsø, Norway
* Correspondence: jkk@prophylix.com; Tel.: +46-722-48-1303 or +45-4283-7300

Abstract: Hemolytic disease of the fetus and newborn (HDFN), as well as fetal and neonatal alloimmune thrombocytopenia (FNAIT), represent two important disease entities that are caused by maternal IgG antibodies directed against nonmaternally inherited antigens on the fetal blood cells. These antibodies are most frequently directed against the RhD antigen on red blood cells (RBCs) or the human platelet antigen 1a (HPA-1a) on platelets. For optimal management of pregnancies where HDFN or FNAIT is suspected, it is essential to determine the RhD or the HPA-1a type of the fetus. Noninvasive fetal RhD typing is also relevant for identifying which RhD-negative pregnant women should receive antenatal RhD prophylaxis. In this review, we will give an overview of the clinical indications and technical challenges related to the noninvasive analysis of fetal RBCs or platelet types. In addition, we will discuss the ethical implications associated with the routine administration of antenatal RhD to all pregnant RhD-negative women and likewise the ethical challenges related to making clinical decisions concerning the mother that have been based on samples collected from the (presumptive) father, which is a common practice when determining the risk of FNAIT.

Keywords: hemolytic disease of the fetus and newborn; fetal and neonatal alloimmune thrombocytopenia; noninvasive prenatal testing; polymerase chain reaction; next-generation sequencing; digital PCR; pregnancy; alloimmunization; cell-free fetal DNA; ethics

1. Introduction

A core feature of the immune system is its ability to distinguish between self from nonself. This property allows the body to mount an immune response against foreign invaders such as bacteria, fungi, viruses, etc. while being tolerant of the body's own cells and tissue. A disturbance of the immune system's balance between recognizing self and nonself can lead to a state of immunodeficiency if the nonself is not properly recognized or autoimmunity if an immune response is mounted against the body's own cells or tissue.

During normal pregnancy, the woman carries a fetus who has inherited half of its genome from the father. From an immunological point of view, is seems paradoxical that the woman's immune system does not reject the fetus since it expresses numerous antigens inherited from the father, which are foreign to the woman. The pregnant woman's immune system tolerates the fetus because numerous, primarily local, immunological mechanisms in the placenta prevent the maternal immune system from rejecting the fetus [1].

Fetal–maternal bleeding is a rather common event, particularly during the third trimester. If fetal blood cells entering the maternal circulation carry paternally inherited antigens that are foreign to the woman's immune system, her body may mount an antibody response against these paternally inherited antigens. Antibodies of the IgG class can traverse the placenta and bind to the paternally inherited antigens on the fetal cells. These sensitized fetal blood cells are then removed by the mononuclear phagocyte system in the fetus.

Three distinct clinical conditions are associated with maternal antibodies against paternally inherited antigens on red blood cells (RBCs), platelets and neutrophile granulocytes and are known as hemolytic disease of the fetus and newborn (HDFN), fetal and neonatal alloimmune thrombocytopenia (FNAIT) and neonatal alloimmune neutropenia (NAIN), respectively. If untreated, HDFN may result in severe fetal anemia that may lead to hydrops fetalis and stillbirth. Postnatally, there is severe anemia, and jaundice may lead to severe neurological damage due to deposits of bilirubin in the grey matter of the central nervous system [2]. HDFN is most commonly caused by antibodies against the RhD antigen on RBCs. FNAIT may cause severe fetal thrombocytopenia, which may lead to intrauterine death or severe neurological damage due to intracranial hemorrhage (ICH) [3]. In Whites, the most common (around 80%) and the most severe cases of FNAIT are caused by antibodies against human platelet antigen 1a (HPA-1a) [3]. NAIN can be associated with severe neutropenia, which does not have any adverse consequences in the fetus, but may leave the newborn prone to infections in the neonatal period [4]. However, NAIN usually has a benign course as infections in the neonatal period can effectively be treated with antibiotics. For this reason, we will only discuss in this review the role of noninvasive prenatal testing in relation to anti-D-associated HDFN and anti-HPA-1a-associated FNAIT.

2. Hemolytic Disease of the Fetus and Newborn
Clinical Considerations

Around five decades ago, HFDN was associated with significant mortality and morbidity. Hence, HDFN affected 150 per 100,000 births and was responsible for 10% of all perinatal deaths [2]. Within a few years after the implementation of RhD prophylaxis, there was a dramatic reduction both in the number of RhD-immunized women and in the number of HDFN cases in North America and Western Europe. Thus, RhD prophylaxis became one of the most effective immunological interventions in clinical medicine.

The RhD prophylaxis was based on the administration of a one single dose of hyperimmune anti-D IgG to all RhD-negative women within 72 h after delivery of an RhD-positive child and in relation to any event that is known to be associated with the risk of fetal–maternal bleeding. Despite this initial success, it became clear that a small proportion of RhD-negative women carrying an RhD-positive fetus still became RhD-immunized despite the administration of hyperimmune anti-D IgG after delivery. Most of these cases were due to fetal–maternal bleeding in the third trimester. This led to a modification of the RhD prophylaxis, which involved the administration of one or two doses of hyperimmune anti-D IgG in the third trimester in addition to a dose after delivery of an RhD-positive child. Although this routine was adopted by several countries such as the USA, Canada and the UK, there was one drawback: Since the fetus's RhD type is not known, it is necessary to administer hyperimmune anti-D IgG to all RhD-negative pregnant women despite the fact that around 35–40% of these women will be carrying an RhD-negative fetus, and these women can of course not be RhD-immunized in the current pregnancy or after delivery of their RhD-negative child.

With the discovery of cell-free fetal DNA (cffDNA) in the plasma of pregnant women, ref. [5] it has become possible to do noninvasive RhD typing of the fetus [6]. This technique is now used in several countries in Europe to identify which RhD-negative women are carrying an RhD-positive fetus [7–9], and these countries have changed their routine to targeted antenatal RhD prophylaxis, i.e., hyperimmune anti-D IgG is only administered to RhD-negative women carrying an RhD-positive fetus. This is reflected in several national guidelines for the care of pregnant women in many European countries [10–12].

Knowledge of the fetal RhD type is also of major importance for clinicians to manage the treatment of RhD-negative pregnant women who have become RhD-immunized in relation to a previous delivery of an RhD-positive child. If the mother's anti-D levels are high, there is a need for close clinical follow-up during pregnancy, which will involve multiple ultrasonographic assessments of the fetal blood flow as a surrogate marker for fetal anemia [13]. Further, if these examinations indicate fetal anemia, the woman will need to be referred to a specialized center that will perform an intrauterine transfusion of RhD-negative blood.

3. Technical Considerations Related to Prediction of Fetal RhD Type

The requirements of the assay performance depends on whether the assay is used for screening RhD-negative women to guide prenatal prophylaxis or whether the assay is used for determining the fetal status in an already immunized woman [14]. The main common technical challenge when using cffDNA for determination of the fetal blood group is the low concentration of fetal DNA in the maternal circulation. Hence, the absence of an RhD signal could either be interpreted as an RhD-negative fetus, or alternatively, the fetus could be RhD positive, but the very low numbers of DNA sequences from the fetal RhD gene did not allow these sequences to be amplified, resulting in a false negative result. Consequently, it is important to ensure that the preanalytical steps such as transport, storage, centrifugation and extraction are carefully monitored and validated [14]. The use of automated DNA extraction gives a standardized process. There are several robots on the market that use magnetic beads in the process of DNA extraction. The possibility to send data from the extraction robot to the analyzing instrument and the PCR result to the laboratory information system, is a key factor for a fully automated process avoiding human errors.

A fetal marker, not present in the maternal DNA, can be used for confirmation of the presence of cffDNA in the sample. Commonly used fetal markers are hypermethylated *RASSF* [15] or, for male fetuses, Y chromosome sequences [16]. Some assays instead use extraction controls by adding artificial DNA (synthetic oligonucleotide), or DNA from another species, during the extraction process to monitor the performance [17]. Hence, if the control DNA is not giving the expected result in the polymerase chain reaction (PCR), the DNA extraction should be repeated. Other assays amplify a housekeeping gene to obtain the total amount of cell-free DNA (cfDNA) of both maternal and fetal origin, applying upper and lower Ct limits, for a valid result [8]. A low Ct value indicates high levels of maternal cfDNA, which potentially can hamper the result, whereas a high Ct value indicates that too little cfDNA has been extracted. However, studies have shown that internal controls to prove the presence of fetal DNA are not necessary if the screening assay has shown sufficiently high sensitivity [18]. Nevertheless, if the assay is used to guide treatment of an immunized women, it is crucial to avoid false negative results, and the above-mentioned precautions may therefore not be considered sufficient. For immunized women, in whom the initial test showed an RhD-negative fetus, it can be recommended to repeat testing later in the pregnancy, both to reduce the risk of human error and to allow testing when the cffDNA levels have increased, which will result in increased sensitivity [14].

The RhD-negative status is most often caused by the complete deletion of the *RHD* gene; however there are numerous *RHD* variants, which can complicate prediction of the fetal RhD type. In assays for fetal *RHD* screening, the detection of two exons provides a robust assay [7,9], but tests with only one exon do also exist [8], as well as tests where more than two exons are detected [19]. Using several exons gives the possibility to distinguish between different variants including the RhD-negative pseudogene (*RHD*08N.01*).

Some laboratories offer one test for antenatal *RHD* screening and another, detecting more exons, for immunized women [20]. However, in women with *RHD* variants, the fetal *RHD* type can quite often not be determined, and RhD prophylaxis is recommended as a precautionary approach. It is important that laboratories and manufactures of assays for fetal RhD typing describe the assay limitations related to variants. Unfortunately, most studies have been performed in mainly Whites, and the implementation of *RHD* screening in nonwhite populations should be carefully validated [21]. A study performed in a mixed population of pregnant women in Argentina demonstrated that the combination of exons 5 and 10 gave conclusive results [22]. Another study from Brazil also demonstrated that the fetal RhD type can reliably be predicted in a genetically mixed population of pregnant women [23]. However, they used a more complicated set up that is not practical in large-scale screening situations [23].

Realtime PCR is the most common method used for the prediction of the fetal RhD type due to its accessibility and low cost. Yet, new techniques such as massive parallel sequencing (also called next-generation sequencing, NGS) and digital PCR (dPCR) can also be used, but are more suitable for complex cases, such as when the mother is carrying a silent *RHD* allele [24–26].

Cord blood typing has been discontinued in countries where the antenatal *RHD* screening has been implemented for routine use [27]. This means that the postnatal prophylaxis can be given without waiting for the result of the newborn's serological RhD status, i.e., anti-D IgG is often administered during delivery.

New legislation in the European Union will come into force in 2022 requiring manufacturers of in vitro diagnostic (IVD) assays to validate their assays according to these new rules [28,29]. Currently, many laboratories use their own in-house assays, which will need to be validated according to the same legislation or changed to a commercially available IVDR assay. At this time, there are four CE-marked kits according to the current European In-Vitro Diagnostic Devices Directive (IVDD 98/79/EC) available or just to be released on the market. Some characteristics of these assays are summarized in Table 1.

Table 1. Available CE/IVD kit for fetal *RHD* genotyping with real-time PCR.

	Devyser RHD	NIMoTest® Fetal RHD qPCR Kit	FetoGnost® Kit RHD	Free DNA Fetal Kit® RhD
Use for immunized women	yes	no	no	yes
Use for antenatal *RHD* screening	yes	yes	yes	yes
Detection of	Exon 4	Exons 5, 7	Exons 5, 7, 10	Exons 5, 7, 10
Extraction control	GAPDH	Synthetic DNA	FetoGnost® Kit IPC	Maize DNA
Use from gestational week	10	11	11	9
Maximal age of sample in EDTA tube	5 days	72 h	#	48 h ‡
Need to repeat negative results	no	yes ⁰	no	yes ⁰
Distinction of maternal *RHD*08N.01	no	yes	yes	yes
Suitable for automation	yes	yes	yes	yes

⁰ if performed before week 16. # not stated in kit insert. ‡ 10 days in Streck® tube.

Antenatal RhD typing and targeted RhD prophylaxis have not yet been implemented in North America. One of the reasons for this is the concern related to the ability of assays based on cffDNA to reliably predict fetal RhD in multiethnic populations. Another issue is the costs of such a program. Two studies from the US and Ontario, Canada demonstrated a significantly higher costs associated with antenatal RhD typing and targeted prophylaxis [30,31], whereas another study from Alberta, Canada reached the opposite conclusion [32]. As the prices for assays for antenatal RhD typing go down, it is possible that antenatal RhD typing and targeted RhD prophylaxis will also be implemented in North America. As discussed below, such a program also has favorable ethical implications because it will prevent anti-D to be used in women who do not need this drug.

4. Fetal and Neonatal Alloimmune Thrombocytopenia
Clinical Considerations

Although fetal thrombocytopenia is of transient nature, the clinical spectrum of FNAIT spans a continuum from no symptoms to petechiae, mucosal bleeding, hematomas, retinal bleeding and ICH that may result in stillbirth or a life-long disability. FNAIT is a rare disease because only around 2.1% are HPA-1a negative [33], which is a requirement for developing HPA-1a antibodies. Moreover, the propensity of developing anti-HPA-1a is closely linked to carriers of a particular HLA type. Women who are HLA-DRB3*01:01-positive have a 25 times higher risk of becoming HPA-1a immunized as opposed to those who do not carry this HLA type [34]. Furthermore, those few HPA-

1a and HLA-DRB3*01:01-negative women who become HPA-1a-immunized very rarely give birth to severely thrombocytopenic children, and, likewise, ICH is extremely rare in fetuses/newborns of HPA-1a and HLA-DRB3*01:01-negative women [35]. As only around 27% of Whites are HLA-DRB3*01:01-positive [36], the proportion of pregnant women who are at risk of having a fetus/newborn suffering from FNAIT is only around 0.5%. Fortunately, ICH is rare and has been estimated to occur in 1 of 10,000 unselected pregnancies [37].

FNAIT usually turns up in a term infant like a bolt from the blue without any prior suspicions during pregnancy. In a subsequent pregnancy, the woman will be offered close clinical follow-up, and most centers will start treatment with high-dose intravenous IgG (IVIg). In this context, it is prudent to mention that (1) IVIg is used off label for this indication as the efficacy in this condition has never been tested in a placebo-controlled clinical trial; (2) there is no international consensus of whom to treat, when to start treatment and dose of IVIg [38]; (3) there are significant side effects associated with IVIg treatment [39–42]; (4) this treatment is incredibly expensive and may easily exceed USD 100,000 per treated woman; (5) there is a worldwide shortage of IVIg [43]; and (6) treatment of one HPA-1a-immunized women requires tremendous donor efforts: 4.5 man-months of plasmapheresis [38].

Thus, when consulting a pregnant woman with a previous obstetric history with anti-HPA-1a-associated FNAIT, it is essential to know if the fetus is HPA-1a-positive or negative. If the fetus is HPA-1a-negative, there is of course no reason for concern in the current pregnancy. Therefore, many centers ask for a sample from the father in order to determine if he is HPA-1a-homozygous or HPA-1a/1b-heterozygous. In the first case, the fetus will be HPA-a-positive, whereas in the second case, there will be a 50% risk that the fetus will be HPA-1a-positive and hence at risk of FNAIT. With a heterozygous father, many centers determine the fetus's HPA-1 genotype by polymerase chain reaction (PCR) performed on DNA extracted from fetal cells obtained by amniocentesis.

FNAIT has not previously been considered for any prophylactic efforts similar to HDFN because it was generally believed that immunization against HPA-1a mostly occurred during the course of the first incompatible pregnancy. This view was based on data from retrospective studies, but two large prospective clinical studies conducted in England and Scotland, respectively, indicated that the majority of HPA-1a immunizations occur after a previous immunizing event, such as the delivery of an HPA-1a-positive child [44,45]. The results of a very large prospective clinical trial on FNAIT conducted in Norway between 1995 and 2004 confirmed this view [46]. In this study, it was shown that 75% of all cases of HPA-1a alloimmunization occurred in relation to the delivery rather than during pregnancy [47]. The realization that the majority of cases of alloimmunization occur after delivery of the first HPA-1a-incompatible infant paved the way for the idea of preventing HPA-1a immunization in the same manner as preventing RhD immunization by hyperimmune anti-D IgG. This idea was supported by preclinical studies in a mouse model of FNAIT in which it was documented that the administration of antibodies against paternally derived platelet antigens could suppress the development of a maternal antibody response against these antigens, reduce the number of thrombocytopenic pups and reduce the number of miscarriages and pups with ICH [48].

In past years, the EU-financed PROFNAIT consortium worked on the development a hyperimmune anti-HPA-1a IgG to be used as a prophylaxis against HPA-1a immunization, analogous to anti-D, which has been used successfully over the last 5 decades for the prevention of RhD immunization and HDFN [49]. Encouraging results from the phase 1/2 study were recently published [50]. If the results of the pivotal phase 3 study turn out successful, it will be possible to prevent HPA-1a immunization and FNAIT, and this may encourage national health authorities to add FNAIT screening to their antenatal health care programs. A screening program will most likely include maternal HPA-1a and HLA-DRB3*01:01 typing as well as fetal platelet typing. As the hyperimmune anti-HPA-1a IgG is manufactured from plasma collected from HPA-1a-immunized women, the supply of plasma for drug production is limited. Hence, it is essential to reserve the prophylactic drug for the HPA-1a-negative women with the highest risk of having a child with severe thrombocytopenia; i.e., those who are HPA-1a-negative (around 2.1%), HLA-DRB3*01:01-positive (approximately 27%) and who are carrying an HPA-1a-positive fetus (circa 85%).

Although the prediction of the fetal platelet type in principle could be performed by initial HPA-1a typing of the father followed by HPA-1a typing of the fetal DNA obtained from cells collected by amniocentesis in case the father was HPA-1a/b-heterozygous, this approach would be unpractical in a screening setting. As an alternative, several laboratories in Europe have developed noninvasive methods for fetal HPA-1 genotyping that take advantage of the presence cffDNA in the mother's plasma [51].

5. Technical Considerations Related to Prediction of Fetal HPA-1 Type

The technical challenges associated with prenatal HPA-1a typing are considerably larger than prenatal RhD typing: In contrast to fetal RhD typing, which implies detection of sequences from the *RHD* gene in the mother's plasma, there is only a single nucleotide difference between genes encoding HPA-1a and HPA-1b. Hence, the number of the fetal DNA strands in the plasma encoding HPA-1a is very low compared with the number of the maternal DNA strands encoding HPA-1b. This small amount of cffDNA in 'a large ocean' of cell-free maternal DNA represents an analytical challenge, particularly early in the pregnancy when the proportion of cffDNA is at its lowest. To address this challenge, different methods have been used to try to make fetal HPA1a typing both cost-effective and sensitive.

The first assay for fetal HPA-1 typing used a similar method with real-time PCR as for detecting the *RHD* gene. However, this was not successful without adding a pre-PCR step utilizing the restriction enzyme MspI, which recognizes and cleaves the DNA sequences encoding the maternal HPA-1b allele, hence reducing the risk of unspecific amplification [52]. The disadvantages associated with this method are the risk of incomplete enzyme digestion and the lack of internal controls for the presence of cffDNA, which could lead to a false negative result.

Another method, the coamplification at lower denaturation temperature PCR (COLD-PCR), utilizes melting temperature differences between variant and wild-type sequences, which will favor the amplification of the less abundant allele [53]. This method has been included in a workflow where first the HPA-1 status of the mother is determined by high-resolution melting (HRM) PCR, and if the mother is HPA-1-negative, COLD-PCR is applied on the same extracted DNA to determine the fetal genotype [54]. The set up shows accurate results as early as gestational week 12, but suffers from the same weakness as the previous methods since no internal control is included [54].

Novel technologies such as NGS and digital PCR are promising alternatives but involve expensive equipment not available everywhere. NGS, a technology in which millions of nucleotides are sequenced at the same time, consists of several steps: (1) DNA fragmentation, (2) adapter ligations, (3) sequencing and (4) alignment and data analysis. Currently, two main platforms using different ways of nucleotide detection are on the market. Ion Torrent™ (Themo Fischer, Waltham, MA, USA) uses a semiconductor chip where the pH change is detected when a nucleotide is incorporated, whereas the Illumina technology use fluorescence. Both whole genome sequencing and exome sequencing as well as targeted sequencing can be performed. Target enrichment of only selected parts of the genome is suitable for fetal genotyping because it increases the proportion of the targeted region [55]. Targeting can be done with an additional step using PCR (amplicon-based target enrichment) or probes (hybridization-based target enrichment) to capture target sequences.

The successful detection of fetal HPA-1a-positive sequences has been demonstrated in several studies using NGS [56,57]. The use of single-nucleotide variants (SNVs) for estimation of the fetal fraction works as an internal control, which makes NGS a reliable method [56]. To conclude, NGS is highly specific but time-consuming, and requires the analysis of several samples at the same time to be cost-effective.

Digital PCR (dPCR) is a sensitive technology based on PCR performed on partitions, i.e., the sample is separated in units, containing either zero, one or a few copies of the targeted DNA before PCR. After amplification, partitions containing target DNA are detected by fluorescence, and the positive and negative reactions are counted. To account for partitioning errors, a Poisson correction model is applied by the software. There are a number of different methods for separating the partitions such as microchambers, channels, printing-based sample dispersion and microfluidic technology, where the DNA is divided into water-in-oil droplets [58]. dPCR performs with high accuracy even when only a small volume of sample is available, which makes the method suitable for accurate noninvasive prenatal typing early in pregnancy [59]. Moreover, both *RASSF1a* and autosomal SNPs from the SNPforID panel have been used as internal controls with good results [59]. However, this method still has some disadvantages such as contamination risk, limited possibility for high-throughput, cost and lack of commercial assay kits. Table 2 summarizes some characteristics of the mentioned methods for HPA-1a typing.

Table 2. Inhouse assays for fetal HPA-1 typing.

	Realtime PCR with Digestion of Maternal Allele	Cold PCR	NGS (Targeted Massive Parallel Sequencing)	Digital PCR
Use from gestational week	18	12	13	8
Control for cffDNA	no	no	yes	yes *
Cost	low	low	high	high
Turnaround time	Medium	Medium	Long	Medium
References	[52]	[54]	[56,57]	[59]

* can be included.

Today, routine maternal HPA-1a typing is not used for identifying pregnant women at risk of having a child with FNAIT. Antenatal HPA-1a typing is only used for HPA-1a-immunized women at some centers in Europe. However, a hyperimmune anti-HPA-1a IgG is under clinical development for the prevention of HPA-1a immunization and FNAIT [50]. If the pivotal phase 3 clinical trial demonstrates that this drug can prevent HPA-1a immunization and FNAIT, there are reasons to believe that national health authorities will recommend that maternal HPA-1a typing be included in their antenatal health care program. In that case, there will also be a need for targeted HPA-1a prophylaxis. As HPA-1a immunization is primarily restricted to women who are HLA-DRB3*01:01-positive, it will only be necessary to administer the hyperimmune anti-HPA-1a IgG to those women who are HPA-1a-negative and HLA-DRB3*01:01-positive carrying an HPA-1a-positive fetus. NGS could be used to determine if a pregnant woman, who initially has been typed as HPA-1a negative, is at risk of having the pregnancy complicated with FNAIT. It is feasible to design one NGS assay that determines the maternal HPA-1 type (as a control of the initial screening), the maternal HLA-DRB3*01:01 status and fetal HPA-1 type. Since NGS is a very sensitive assay (Table 2), it could be applied late in the first trimester, and as explained below, an early answer regarding the risk of FNAIT is essential for the expecting mother. Thus, future inclusion of FNAIT screening in the antenatal health care program will hopefully go hand in hand with the development of tests that can determine the FNAIT risk status early in pregnancy.

6. Necessity of Noninvasive Prenatal Blood and Platelet Typing—Ethical Considerations

With the introduction of noninvasive prenatal testing in immunohematology, it has become possible to circumvent many ethical challenges: Many countries that have implemented antenatal RhD prophylaxis, administer hyperimmune anti-D IgG to all pregnant RhD-negative women. For 35–40% of these women, there is no risk of HDFN in the current pregnancy because they will be carrying an RhD-negative fetus. Hence, these women receive a drug for which there is no indication, which basically violates the generally accepted ethical position that a patient should not receive an unnecessary drug. Furthermore, hyperimmune anti-D IgG is a special drug as it is manufactured from plasma collected from RhD-immunized individuals. Most of these RhD-negative individuals are frequently transfused with RhD-positive RBCs in order to boost their antibody response to maximize the amount of anti-D in the plasma that is harvested from these special donors. These individuals are exposed both to the risks associated with the transfusion of RhD-positive RBCs (such as transfusion-associated infections) and the risks associated with plasmapheresis. Although both these risks are small, it is highly questionable if it can be justified to use a significant amount of the drug manufactured from plasma harvested from these special donors to patients who do not need the drug.

It also worth mentioning that while parts of the world, mainly high-income countries, are using RhD prophylaxis for women who do not need it, approximately 50% of the women around the world who require this type of immunoprophylaxis have no access to the drug. A nonprofit organization, Worldwide Initiative Rh Disease Eradication (WIRhE), has been launched to spread awareness about Rh disease and the lack of access to both blood typing and prophylaxis [60,61].

The screening programs of pregnant RhD-negative women that include noninvasive fetal RhD typing, which have been implemented in many European countries [7–9], have avoided the above-mentioned ethical challenges by identifying those RhD-negative women who should receive antenatal RhD prophylaxis to prevent RhD immunization and HDFN in subsequent pregnancies.

For an HPA-1a-immunized pregnant woman with FNAIT in her obstetric history, it is essential to know the HPA-1 type of the fetus. As a first step, it is common practice at many centers to do HPA-1a genotyping of the father, and if he is HPA-1a/b to continue with amniocentesis of the mother. Hence, the platelet type of the (presumed) father determines if the mother should undergo amniocentesis or not. This becomes an ethical challenge if the mother knows that her spouse is not the father. Furthermore, during the couple's consultation with the physician, she will be put into a very difficult situation when the physician asks for a sample from her spouse! Furthermore, the increased use of assisted reproductive technology (ART) reinforces limited use of testing the spouse [62,63].

Another ethical aspect is related to the invasive nature of amniocentesis. This procedure is associated with a risk of fetal death, which should be weighed against the risk of having a severely thrombocytopenic child. Moreover, amniocentesis may also set off fetal–maternal bleeding that could boost the mother's production of anti-HPA-1a, which in turn could worse fetal thrombocytopenia and increase the risk of severe intrauterine bleeding such as ICH.

A procedure for fetal HPA-1 determination that involves paternal HPA-1a typing, amniocentesis, expansion of fetal amniotic cells, extraction of DNA from fetal amniotic cells and finally HPA-1a typing by PCR takes a long time. This waiting time is very stressful for the expecting mother: Will the fetus be HPA-1a-positive and then at risk of FNAIT or would it be HPA-1a-negative? The latter result would be a relief for both the mother and the maternal–fetal medicine specialist, because no further follow-up during pregnancy would be necessary. Hence, it is preferable to know the fetal HPA-1 type as soon as possible after the woman has discovered she is pregnant. As explained above, some of the techniques that are used for noninvasive prenatal HPA-1 typing can be performed late in the first trimester and will minimize the waiting time for the pregnant woman. In addition, noninvasive prenatal HPA-1 typing will also avoid the other ethical challenges discussed above.

Although the results obtained from the (presumed) father should not be used for making clinical decisions for the mother, it is essential for the treating physician to know if the pregnancy is the result of ART, and if this is the case, if the conceived oocyte comes from the mother or from another woman. In the latter case, there is a risk that the fetus is homozygous for the RBC or platelet antigen to which maternal antibodies have been produced, which may increase the severity of the affected fetus. Due to the large economic and emotional costs related to these pregnancies, Curtis et al. has recommended that surrogate mothers and women who are donating oocytes for ART should be HPA-1 typed [62].

The use of noninvasive prenatal fetal RhD and HPA-1a is still limited. The reasons are both due to the technical challenges and the costs associated with these analyses. It has been argued that it is cheaper to administer anti-D to all RhD-negative women irrespective of whether or not they are carrying an RhD-positive fetus, as opposed to a program that includes noninvasive prenatal fetal RhD typing of all RhD-negative women and the administration of anti-D to only those women who need the prophylaxis.

There are reasons to believe that the use of noninvasive preclinical testing in immunohematology will increase in the near future because this will eliminate a number of ethical challenges and also because technical developments and decreasing prices will make this technology accessible to more laboratories.

7. Conclusions

In recent years, noninvasive prenatal blood and platelet typing based on cffDNA has increased considerably in immunohematology. Some of these analyses are used for rare clinical conditions and are technically challenging and are currently only performed in reference laboratories. By implementing this type of technology in immunohematology, a number of the ethical challenges associated with previous methods for fetal blood and platelet typing can be avoided. In the near future, the use of noninvasive prenatal testing will most probably increase as the costs of these assays decrease.

Funding: This research received no external funding.

Institutional Review Board Statement: Not applicable.

Informed Consent Statement: Not applicable.

Data Availability Statement: Not applicable.

Conflicts of Interest: J.K.-K. is a stockholder of Prophylix AS, a Norwegian biotech company, which has produced a hyperimmune anti-HPA-1a IgG for the prevention of HPA-1a immunization and FNAIT. J.K.-K. is currently a consultant for Rallybio (New Haven, Connecticut, US), which is developing this drug for clinical use. Å.H. does not have any competing financial interests to declare.

References

1. Kjeldsen-Kragh, J.; Skogen, B. Mechanisms and prevention of alloimmunization in pregnancy. *Obstet. Gynecol. Surv.* **2013**, *68*, 526–532. [CrossRef] [PubMed]
2. Bowman, J.M. RhD hemolytic disease of the newborn. *N. Engl. J. Med.* **1998**, *339*, 1775–1777. [CrossRef] [PubMed]
3. De Vos, T.W.; Winkelhorst, D.; de Haas, M.; Lopriore, E.; Oepkes, D. Epidemiology and management of fetal and neonatal alloimmune thrombocytopenia. *Transfus. Apher. Sci.* **2020**, *59*, 102704. [CrossRef] [PubMed]
4. Porcelijn, L.; de Haas, M. Neonatal Alloimmune Neutropenia. *Transfus. Med. Hemother.* **2018**, *45*, 311–316. [CrossRef] [PubMed]
5. Lo, Y.M.; Corbetta, N.; Chamberlain, P.F.; Rai, V.; Sargent, I.L.; Redman, C.W.; Wainscoat, J.S. Presence of fetal DNA in maternal plasma and serum. *Lancet* **1997**, *350*, 485–487. [CrossRef]
6. Lo, Y.M.; Hjelm, N.M.; Fidler, C.; Sargent, I.L.; Murphy, M.F.; Chamberlain, P.F.; Poon, P.M.; Redman, C.W.; Wainscoat, J.S. Prenatal diagnosis of fetal RhD status by molecular analysis of maternal plasma. *N. Engl J. Med.* **1998**, *339*, 1734–1738. [CrossRef]
7. Clausen, F.B.; Christiansen, M.; Steffensen, R.; Jorgensen, S.; Nielsen, C.; Jakobsen, M.A.; Madsen, R.D.; Jensen, K.; Krog, G.R.; Rieneck, K.; et al. Report of the first nationally implemented clinical routine screening for fetal RHD in D-pregnant women to ascertain the requirement for antenatal RhD prophylaxis. *Transfusion* **2012**, *52*, 752–758. [CrossRef]
8. Wikman, A.T.; Tiblad, E.; Karlsson, A.; Olsson, M.L.; Westgren, M.; Reilly, M. Noninvasive single-exon fetal RHD determination in a routine screening program in early pregnancy. *Obstet. Gynecol.* **2012**, *120*, 227–234. [CrossRef]
9. Sorensen, K.; Kjeldsen-Kragh, J.; Husby, H.; Akkok, C.A. Determination of fetal RHD type in plasma of RhD negative pregnant women. *Scand. J. Clin. Lab. Investig.* **2018**, *78*, 411–416. [CrossRef]
10. Antenatal Care. NICE Guideline. Published: 19 August 2021. Available online: http://www.nice.org.uk/guidance/ng201 (accessed on 31 March 2022).
11. Kahrs, B.H.; Tiller, H.; Haugen, G.; Bakken, K.; Akkök, Ç.A. Alloimmunisering Mot Erytrocytt-Antigener Alloimmunization against Erythroyte Antigens. Den Norske Legeforening. Available online: http://www.legeforeningen.no/foreningsledd/fagmed/norsk-gynekologisk-forening/veiledere/veileder-i-fodselshjelp/alloimmunisering-mot-erytrocytt-antigener/ (accessed on 31 March 2022).

12. Laboratoriumdiagnostiek Zwangerschap en Zwangerschapswens Laboratory Diagnostics Pregnancy and Pregnancy Wish. Nederlands Huisartsen Genootschap. Available online: http://www.nhg.org/themas/publicaties/laboratoriumdiagnostiek-zwangerschap-en-zwangerschapswens?tmp-no-mobile=1 (accessed on 31 March 2022).
13. Mari, G.; Adrignolo, A.; Abuhamad, A.Z.; Pirhonen, J.; Jones, D.C.; Ludomirsky, A.; Copel, J.A. Diagnosis of fetal anemia with Doppler ultrasound in the pregnancy complicated by maternal blood group immunization. *Ultrasound Obstet. Gynecol.* **1995**, *5*, 400–405. [CrossRef]
14. Clausen, F.B.; Hellberg, A.; Bein, G.; Bugert, P.; Schwartz, D.; Drnovsek, T.D.; Finning, K.; Guz, K.; Haimila, K.; Henny, C.; et al. Recommendation for validation and quality assurance of non-invasive prenatal testing for foetal blood groups and implications for IVD risk classification according to EU regulations. *Vox. Sang.* **2022**, *117*, 157–165. [CrossRef] [PubMed]
15. Chan, K.C.; Ding, C.; Gerovassili, A.; Yeung, S.W.; Chiu, R.W.; Leung, T.N.; Lau, T.K.; Chim, S.S.; Chung, G.T.; Nicolaides, K.H.; et al. Hypermethylated RASSF1A in maternal plasma: A universal fetal DNA marker that improves the reliability of noninvasive prenatal diagnosis. *Clin. Chem.* **2006**, *52*, 2211–2218. [CrossRef] [PubMed]
16. Zhong, X.Y.; Holzgreve, W.; Hahn, S. Risk free simultaneous prenatal identification of fetal Rhesus D status and sex by multiplex real-time PCR using cell free fetal DNA in maternal plasma. *Swiss. Med. Wkly.* **2001**, *131*, 70–74.
17. Legler, T.J.; Luhrig, S.; Korschineck, I.; Schwartz, D. Diagnostic performance of the noninvasive prenatal FetoGnost RhD assay for the prediction of the fetal RhD blood group status. *Arch. Gynecol. Obstet.* **2021**, *304*, 1191–1196. [CrossRef] [PubMed]
18. Scheffer, P.G.; de Haas, M.; van der Schoot, C.E. The controversy about controls for fetal blood group genotyping by cell-free fetal DNA in maternal plasma. *Curr. Opin. Hematol.* **2011**, *18*, 467–473. [CrossRef]
19. Papasavva, T.; Martin, P.; Legler, T.J.; Liasides, M.; Anastasiou, G.; Christofides, A.; Christodoulou, T.; Demetriou, S.; Kerimis, P.; Kontos, C.; et al. Prevalence of RhD status and clinical application of non-invasive prenatal determination of fetal RHD in maternal plasma: A 5 year experience in Cyprus. *BMC Res. Notes* **2016**, *9*, 198. [CrossRef]
20. NHS Blood and Transplant. Feral RHD Screening Test: Questions & Answers. Available online: https://nhsbtdbe.blob.core.windows.net/umbraco-assets-corp/16585/fetal-rhd-screening-test-questions-and-answers.pdf (accessed on 22 March 2022).
21. Clausen, F.B. Non-invasive foetal RhD genotyping in admixed populations. *Blood Transfus.* **2017**, *15*, 4–5. [CrossRef]
22. Blanco, S.; Giacomi, V.S.; Slobodianiuk, L.G.; Frutos, M.C.; Carrizo, L.H.; Fanin, G.E.; Culasso, J.M.; Gallego, S.V. Usefulness of Non-Invasive Fetal RHD Genotyping towards Immunoprophylaxis Optimization. *Transfus. Med. Hemother.* **2018**, *45*, 423–428. [CrossRef]
23. Boggione, C.T.; Lujan Brajovich, M.E.; Mattaloni, S.M.; Di Monaco, R.A.; Garcia Borras, S.E.; Biondi, C.S.; Cotorruelo, C.M. Genotyping approach for non-invasive foetal RHD detection in an admixed population. *Blood Transfus.* **2017**, *15*, 66–73. [CrossRef]
24. Takahashi, K.; Migita, O.; Sasaki, A.; Nasu, M.; Kawashima, A.; Sekizawa, A.; Sato, T.; Ito, Y.; Sago, H.; Okamoto, A.; et al. Amplicon Sequencing-Based Noninvasive Fetal Genotyping for RHD-Positive D Antigen-Negative Alleles. *Clin. Chem.* **2019**, *65*, 1307–1316. [CrossRef]
25. Tsui, N.B.; Hyland, C.A.; Gardener, G.J.; Danon, D.; Fisk, N.M.; Millard, G.; Flower, R.L.; Lo, Y.M. Noninvasive fetal RHD genotyping by microfluidics digital PCR using maternal plasma from two alloimmunized women with the variant RHD(IVS3 + 1G>A) allele. *Prenat. Diagn.* **2013**, *33*, 1214–1216. [CrossRef] [PubMed]
26. Eryilmaz, M.; Muller, D.; Rink, G.; Kluter, H.; Bugert, P. Introduction of Noninvasive Prenatal Testing for Blood Group and Platelet Antigens from Cell-Free Plasma DNA Using Digital PCR. *Transfus. Med. Hemother.* **2020**, *47*, 292–301. [CrossRef] [PubMed]
27. Clausen, F.B.; Steffensen, R.; Christiansen, M.; Rudby, M.; Jakobsen, M.A.; Jakobsen, T.R.; Krog, G.R.; Madsen, R.D.; Nielsen, K.R.; Rieneck, K.; et al. Routine noninvasive prenatal screening for fetal RHD in plasma of RhD-negative pregnant women-2 years of screening experience from Denmark. *Prenat. Diagn.* **2014**, *34*, 1000–1005. [CrossRef] [PubMed]
28. Bank, P.C.D.; Jacobs, L.H.J.; van den Berg, S.A.A.; van Deutekom, H.W.M.; Hamann, D.; Molenkamp, R.; Ruivenkamp, C.A.L.; Swen, J.J.; Tops, B.B.J.; Wamelink, M.M.C.; et al. The end of the laboratory developed test as we know it? Recommendations from a national multidisciplinary taskforce of laboratory specialists on the interpretation of the IVDR and its complications. *Clin. Chem. Lab. Med.* **2021**, *59*, 491–497. [CrossRef] [PubMed]
29. Publications Office of the European Union. Regulation (EU) 2017/746 of the European Parliament and of the Council of 5 April 2017 on in vitro Diagnostic Medical Devices and Repealing Directive 98/79/EC and Commission Decision 2010/227/EU (Text with EEA Relevance) Text with EEA Relevance. Available online: https://eur-lex.europa.eu/legal-content/EN/TXT/PDF/?uri=CELEX:32017R0746 (accessed on 22 March 2022).
30. Hawk, A.F.; Chang, E.Y.; Shields, S.M.; Simpson, K.N. Costs and clinical outcomes of noninvasive fetal RhD typing for targeted prophylaxis. *Obstet. Gynecol.* **2013**, *122*, 579–585. [CrossRef] [PubMed]
31. Gajic-Veljanoski, O.; Li, C.; Schaink, A.K.; Guo, J.; Shehata, N.; Charames, G.S.; de Vrijer, B.; Clarke, G.; Pechlivanoglou, P.; Okun, N.; et al. Cost-effectiveness of noninvasive fetal RhD blood group genotyping in nonalloimmunized and alloimmunized pregnancies. *Transfusion* **2022**, *62*, 1089–1102. [CrossRef] [PubMed]
32. Teitelbaum, L.; Metcalfe, A.; Clarke, G.; Parboosingh, J.S.; Wilson, R.D.; Johnson, J.M. Costs and benefits of non-invasive fetal RhD determination. *Ultrasound Obstet. Gynecol.* **2015**, *45*, 84–88. [CrossRef]
33. Kamphuis, M.M.; Paridaans, N.; Porcelijn, L.; de Haas, M.; van der Schoot, C.E.; Brand, A.; Bonsel, G.J.; Oepkes, D. Screening in pregnancy for fetal or neonatal alloimmune thrombocytopenia: Systematic review. *BJOG* **2010**, *117*, 1335–1343. [CrossRef]
34. Kjeldsen-Kragh, J.; Olsen, K.J. Risk of HPA-1a-immunization in HPA-1a-negative women after giving birth to an HPA-1a-positive child. *Transfusion* **2019**, *59*, 1344–1352. [CrossRef]

35. Kjeldsen-Kragh, J.; Fergusson, D.A.; Kjaer, M.; Lieberman, L.; Greinacher, A.; Murphy, M.F.; Bussel, J.; Bakchoul, T.; Corke, S.; Bertrand, G.; et al. Fetal/neonatal alloimmune thrombocytopenia: A systematic review of impact of HLA-DRB3*01:01 on fetal/neonatal outcome. *Blood Adv.* **2020**, *4*, 3368–3377. [CrossRef]
36. Gragert, L.; Madbouly, A.; Freeman, J.; Maiers, M. Six-locus high resolution HLA haplotype frequencies derived from mixed-resolution DNA typing for the entire US donor registry. *Hum. Immunol.* **2013**, *74*, 1313–1320. [CrossRef] [PubMed]
37. Kamphuis, M.M.; Paridaans, N.P.; Porcelijn, L.; Lopriore, E.; Oepkes, D. Incidence and consequences of neonatal alloimmune thrombocytopenia: A systematic review. *Pediatrics* **2014**, *133*, 715–721. [CrossRef] [PubMed]
38. Kjeldsen-Kragh, J.; Bengtsson, J. Fetal and Neonatal Alloimmune Thrombocytopenia-New Prospects for Fetal Risk Assessment of HPA-1a-Negative Pregnant Women. *Transfus. Med. Rev.* **2020**, *34*, 270–276. [CrossRef] [PubMed]
39. Rossi, K.Q.; Lehman, K.J.; O'Shaughnessy, R.W. Effects of antepartum therapy for fetal alloimmune thrombocytopenia on maternal lifestyle. *J. Matern.-Fetal Neonatal Med.* **2016**, *29*, 1783–1788. [CrossRef] [PubMed]
40. Wienzek-Lischka, S.; Sawazki, A.; Ehrhardt, H.; Sachs, U.J.; Axt-Fliedner, R.; Bein, G. Non-invasive risk-assessment and bleeding prophylaxis with IVIG in pregnant women with a history of fetal and neonatal alloimmune thrombocytopenia: Management to minimize adverse events. *Arch. Obstet. Gynaecol.* **2020**, *302*, 355–363. [CrossRef]
41. Rink, B.D.; Gonik, B.; Chmait, R.H.; O'Shaughnessy, R. Maternal hemolysis after intravenous immunoglobulin treatment in fetal and neonatal alloimmune thrombocytopenia. *Obstet. Gynecol.* **2013**, *121*, 471–473. [CrossRef]
42. Herrmann, A.; Samelson-Jones, B.J.; Brake, S.; Samelson, R. IVIG-Associated Maternal Pancytopenia during Treatment for Neonatal Alloimmune Thrombocytopenia. *AJP Rep.* **2017**, *7*, e197–e200. [CrossRef]
43. Nawrat, A. Why Are Patients Struggling to Access Life-Saving Immune Globulin? 2020. Available online: http://www.pharmaceutical-technology.com/features/immune-globulin-shortages/ (accessed on 2 March 2022).
44. Turner, M.L.; Bessos, H.; Fagge, T.; Harkness, M.; Rentoul, F.; Seymour, J.; Wilson, D.; Gray, I.; Ahya, R.; Cairns, J.; et al. Prospective epidemiologic study of the outcome and cost-effectiveness of antenatal screening to detect neonatal alloimmune thrombocytopenia due to anti-HPA-1a. *Transfusion* **2005**, *45*, 1945–1956. [CrossRef]
45. Williamson, L.M.; Hackett, G.; Rennie, J.; Palmer, C.R.; Maciver, C.; Hadfield, R.; Hughes, D.; Jobson, S.; Ouwehand, W.H. The natural history of fetomaternal alloimmunization to the platelet-specific antigen HPA-1a (PlA1, Zwa) as determined by antenatal screening. *Blood* **1998**, *92*, 2280–2287. [CrossRef]
46. Kjeldsen-Kragh, J.; Killie, M.K.; Tomter, G.; Golebiowska, E.; Randen, I.; Hauge, R.; Aune, B.; Oian, P.; Dahl, L.B.; Pirhonen, J.; et al. A screening and intervention program aimed to reduce mortality and serious morbidity associated with severe neonatal alloimmune thrombocytopenia. *Blood* **2007**, *110*, 833–839. [CrossRef]
47. Killie, M.K.; Husebekk, A.; Kjeldsen-Kragh, J.; Skogen, B. A prospective study of maternal anti-HPA 1a antibody level as a potential predictor of alloimmune thrombocytopenia in the newborn. *Haematologica* **2008**, *93*, 870–877. [CrossRef]
48. Tiller, H.; Killie, M.K.; Chen, P.; Eksteen, M.; Husebekk, A.; Skogen, B.; Kjeldsen-Kragh, J.; Ni, H. Toward a prophylaxis against fetal and neonatal alloimmune thrombocytopenia: Induction of antibody-mediated immune suppression and prevention of severe clinical complications in a murine model. *Transfusion* **2012**, *52*, 1446–1457. [CrossRef] [PubMed]
49. Kjeldsen-Kragh, J.; Ni, H.; Skogen, B. Towards a prophylactic treatment of HPA-related foetal and neonatal alloimmune thrombocytopenia. *Curr. Opin. Hematol.* **2012**, *19*, 469–474. [CrossRef] [PubMed]
50. Geisen, C.; Fleck, E.; Schäfer, S.M.G.; Walter, C.; Braeuninger, S.; Olsen, K.; Bhagwagar, Z.; Mortberg, A.; Wikman, A.; Kjaer, M.; et al. Rapid and complete clearance of HPA-1a mismatched platelets in a human model of fetal and neonatal alloimmune thrombocytopenia by a hyperimmune plasma derived polyclonal anti HPA-1a antibody [abstract]. *Res. Pract. Thromb. Haemost.* **2021**, *5* (Suppl. S2). Available online: https://abstracts.isth.org/abstract/rapid-and-complete-clearance-of-hpa-1a-mismatched-platelets-in-a-human-model-of-fetal-and-neonatal-alloimmune-thrombocytopenia-by-a-hyperimmune-plasma-derived-polyclonal-anti-hpa-1a-antibody/ (accessed on 31 March 2022).
51. Nogués, N. Recent advances in non-invasive fetal HPA-1a typing. *Transfus Apher Sci* **2020**, *59*, 102708. [CrossRef] [PubMed]
52. Scheffer, P.G.; Ait Soussan, A.; Verhagen, O.J.; Page-Christiaens, G.C.; Oepkes, D.; de Haas, M.; van der Schoot, C.E. Noninvasive fetal genotyping of human platelet antigen-1a. *BJOG* **2011**, *118*, 1392–1395. [CrossRef]
53. Li, J.; Wang, L.; Mamon, H.; Kulke, M.H.; Berbeco, R.; Makrigiorgos, G.M. Replacing PCR with COLD-PCR enriches variant DNA sequences and redefines the sensitivity of genetic testing. *Nat. Med.* **2008**, *14*, 579–584. [CrossRef]
54. Ferro, M.; Macher, H.C.; Fornes, G.; Martin-Sanchez, J.; Jimenez-Arriscado, P.; Molinero, P.; Perez-Simon, J.A.; Guerrero, J.M.; Rubio, A. Noninvasive prenatal diagnosis by cell-free DNA screening for fetomaternal HPA-1a platelet incompatibility. *Transfusion* **2018**, *58*, 2272–2279. [CrossRef]
55. Orzinska, A.; Kluska, A.; Balabas, A.; Piatkowska, M.; Kulecka, M.; Ostrowski, J.; Mikula, M.; Debska, M.; Uhrynowska, M.; Guz, K. Prediction of fetal blood group antigens from maternal plasma using Ion AmpliSeq HD technology. *Transfusion* **2022**, *62*, 458–468. [CrossRef]
56. Wienzek-Lischka, S.; Krautwurst, A.; Frohner, V.; Hackstein, H.; Gattenlohner, S.; Braeuninger, A.; Axt-Fliedner, R.; Degenhardt, J.; Deisting, C.; Santoso, S.; et al. Noninvasive fetal genotyping of human platelet antigen-1a using targeted massively parallel sequencing. *Transfusion* **2015**, *55*, 1538–1544. [CrossRef]
57. Orzinska, A.; Guz, K.; Uhrynowska, M.; Debska, M.; Mikula, M.; Ostrowski, J.; Ahlen, M.T.; Husebekk, A.; Brojer, E. Noninvasive prenatal HPA-1 typing in HPA-1a negative pregnancies selected in the Polish PREVFNAIT screening program. *Transfusion* **2018**, *58*, 2705–2711. [CrossRef] [PubMed]

58. Tan, L.L.; Loganathan, N.; Agarwalla, S.; Yang, C.; Yuan, W.; Zeng, J.; Wu, R.; Wang, W.; Duraiswamy, S. Current commercial dPCR platforms: Technology and market review. *Crit. Rev. Biotechnol.* **2022**, 1–32. [CrossRef] [PubMed]
59. Ouzegdouh Mammasse, Y.; Chenet, C.; Drubay, D.; Martageix, C.; Cartron, J.P.; Vainchenker, W.; Petermann, R. A new efficient tool for non-invasive diagnosis of fetomaternal platelet antigen incompatibility. *Br. J. Haematol.* **2020**, *190*, 787–798. [CrossRef] [PubMed]
60. Pegoraro, V.; Urbinati, D.; Visser, G.H.A.; Di Renzo, G.C.; Zipursky, A.; Stotler, B.A.; Spitalnik, S.L. Hemolytic disease of the fetus and newborn due to Rh(D) incompatibility: A preventable disease that still produces significant morbidity and mortality in children. *PLoS ONE* **2020**, *15*, e0235807. [CrossRef] [PubMed]
61. Visser, G.H.A.; Di Renzo, G.C.; Spitalnik, S.L. The continuing burden of Rh disease 50 years after the introduction of anti-Rh(D) immunoglobin prophylaxis: Call to action. *Am. J. Obstet. Gynecol.* **2019**, *221*, 227.e1–227.e4. [CrossRef] [PubMed]
62. Curtis, B.R.; Bussel, J.B.; Manco-Johnson, M.J.; Aster, R.H.; McFarland, J.G. Fetal and neonatal alloimmune thrombocytopenia in pregnancies involving in vitro fertilization: A report of four cases. *Am. J. Obstet. Gynecol.* **2005**, *192*, 543–547. [CrossRef]
63. Storry, J.R. Don't ask, don't tell: The ART of silence can jeopardize assisted pregnancies. *Transfusion* **2010**, *50*, 2070–2072. [CrossRef]

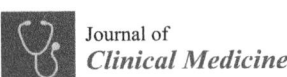

Article

First-Trimester Fetal Hepatic Artery Examination for Adverse Outcome Prediction

Bartosz Czuba [1], Piotr Tousty [2,*], Wojciech Cnota [1], Dariusz Borowski [3], Agnieszka Jagielska [1], Mariusz Dubiel [4], Anna Fuchs [5], Magda Fraszczyk-Tousty [6], Sylwia Dzidek [2], Anna Kajdy [7], Grzegorz Świercz [8,9] and Sebastian Kwiatkowski [2]

1. Department of Obstetrics and Gynecology, Medical University of Silesia, 41-703 Ruda Slaska, Poland; bartosz.czuba@sonomed.net (B.C.); woytek@eth.pl (W.C.); majonez7@wp.pl (A.J.)
2. Department of Gynecology and Obstetrics, Pomeranian Medical University, 70-111 Szczecin, Poland; sylwiadzidek@wp.pl (S.D.); kwiatkowskiseba@gmail.com (S.K.)
3. Department of Perinatology, Gynecology and Gynecologic Oncology, Collegium Medicum, Nicolaus Copernicus University, 85-821 Bydgoszcz, Poland; darekborowski@gmail.com
4. Department of Obstetrics, Gynecology and Gynecological Oncology, Jan Biziel University Hospital, Collegium Medicum, Nicolaus Copernicus University, 85-168 Bydgoszcz, Poland; profdubiel@gmail.com
5. Chair and Department of Gynecology, Obstetrics and Oncological Gynecology, Medical University of Silesia in Katowice, 40-211 Katowice, Poland; afuchs999@gmail.com
6. Department of Neonatal Diseases, Pomeranian Medical University, 70-111 Szczecin, Poland; magfraszczyk@gmail.com
7. Department of Reproductive Health, Centre of Postgraduate Medical Education, 01-004 Warsaw, Poland; anna.kajdy@cmkp.edu.pl
8. Clinic of Obstetrics and Gynecology, Provincial Combined Hospital in Kielce, 25-736 Kielce, Poland; swierczag@poczta.onet.pl
9. Collegium Medicum, Jan Kochanowski University in Kielce, 25-369 Kielce, Poland
* Correspondence: piotr.toscik@gmail.com; Tel.: +48-735-923-533

Abstract: Objective: To assess whether there are differences in first-trimester fetal hepatic artery flows depending on pregnancy outcomes. Methods: The prospective study conducted in 2012–2020 included 1841 fetuses from singleton pregnancies assessed during the routine first-trimester ultrasound examination (between 11- and 14-weeks' gestation). Also, each fetus was examined to determine their hepatic artery flows by measuring the artery's pulsatility index (HA-PI) and peak systolic velocity (HA-PSV). Results: The fetuses that were classified as belonging to the adverse pregnancy outcome group (those with karyotype abnormalities and congenital heart defects) were characterized by a significantly lower HA-PI and higher HA-PSV compared to normal outcome fetuses. Conclusion: Hepatic artery flow assessment proved to be a very useful tool in predicting adverse pregnancy outcomes, in particular karyotype abnormalities and congenital heart defects.

Keywords: adverse outcome; hepatic artery; chromosomal abnormalities; congenital heart defects

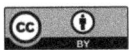

1. Introduction

Recent years have seen a continuous dynamic development in prenatal diagnosis and the discovery of increasingly improved tools for detecting congenital fetal defects, aneuploidy, or pregnant patients at risk of developing different forms of placental insufficiency [1–3]. The inversion of the pyramid of antenatal care and the focus on first-trimester screening have led to significantly improved perinatal outcomes [4]. Nowadays, no one could imagine first-semester diagnosis without the ultrasound evaluation of such parameters as nuchal translucency (NT), fetal heart rate (FHR), ductus venosus pulsatility index (DV-PI), or uterine artery pulsatility index (Ut-PI), which together with the biochemical factors, such as the β-subunit of hCG gonadotropin (beta-hCG), pregnancy-associated plasma protein A (PAPP-A), and placental growth factor (PlGF), are well-researched prognostic factors for pregnancy outcomes [1–3]. However, a continued search for new markers may contribute to improving the detection sensitivity for various abnormalities.

The liver is one of the most important organs during fetal life, where it has a hematopoietic function and regulates the entire metabolism of the fetus. Physiologically, most of the vascularity of the liver during fetal life derives from the umbilical vein and the portal vein, and only about 10% from the hepatic artery [5]. It has been proven that in the event of hypoxemia and fetal growth disorders in the second and third trimesters of pregnancy, this proportion is disturbed [6,7]. The flow through the liver coming from the veins–becoming more and more reduced under these conditions–leads to dilation of the hepatic artery related to a local increase in adenosine concentration aimed at compensating for this abnormal flow. This mechanism is known as HABR (hepatic arterial buffer response) [8].

The few reports of studies on small groups available indicate that hepatic artery flow assessment may be a predictive factor for the occurrence during pregnancy of chromosomal disorders and other adverse pregnancy outcomes [9,10].

The first aim of the study was to use ultrasound to assess the hepatic artery flow in the first trimester as a predictive factor for the occurrence of pregnancy adverse outcomes. The second aim was to identify the flow in the same artery depending on the type of karyotype abnormalities detected during pregnancy or after delivery or miscarriage.

2. Patients and Methods

The prospective study conducted in the years 2012–2020 at Sonomedico Żory and in the Clinical Department of Obstetrics and Gynecology in Ruda Śląska included 1841 fetuses from healthy singleton pregnancies during the routine first-trimester ultrasound examination (between 11- and 14-weeks' gestation) for fetal defects and the risk of aneuploidy. The patients qualified for the study had a negative history of adverse pregnancy outcomes and had no concurrent diseases. The ultrasound was performed in accordance with the Fetal Medicine Foundation (FMF) principles for first-trimester pregnancies to evaluate the anatomy of the fetus and take the following measurements: crown-rump length (CRL), nuchal translucency (NT) thickness, ductus venosus pulsatility index (DV-PI), fetal heart rate (FHR), and normal tricuspid valve flow. In addition, blood was sampled from each patient for the determination of the β-subunit of hCG gonadotropin (beta-hCG) and pregnancy-associated plasma protein A (PAPP-A). The determinations were performed using the DELFIA Xpress system (PerkinElmer Life) analyzer. Also, each fetus was examined to determine their hepatic artery flow by measuring the artery's pulsatility index (HA-PI) and peak systolic velocity (HA-PSV) according to the method described by Zvanca et al. [5]. A transabdominal transducer was used, and the blood flow parameters were measured when the fetus was not moving. In addition, the following conditions were to be met:

(1) Image magnification covering the upper torso and the lower chest of the fetus.
(2) Longitudinal plane going through the right ventricle of the fetus.
(3) Color Doppler showing the inferior vena cava, the ductus venosus and the hepatic artery.
(4) Sample volume width–1.0 mm placed in the hepatic artery.
(5) Angle of insonation < 30 degrees.
(6) Wall filter (WF) set to 120 Hz.
(7) Time-axis (sweep speed) 2–3 cm/s.
(8) Pulse repetition frequency 2.2–3.3 Hz.

Figure 1 shows an image of a normal hepatic artery flow.

Subsequently, amniocentesis (AC) was performed on patients with an elevated risk of aneuploidy (cut-off point < 1:300) detected using the FMF (Astraia software) algorithm for karyotype assessment.

Pregnancy outcome was estimated for each patient. A successful pregnancy outcome was defined as a full-term live birth, i.e., >37 gestational week, with no congenital defects of the neonate and no karyotype abnormalities diagnosed during gestation or after birth, which in the latter case were determined if dysmorphic features were observed during the newborn examination.

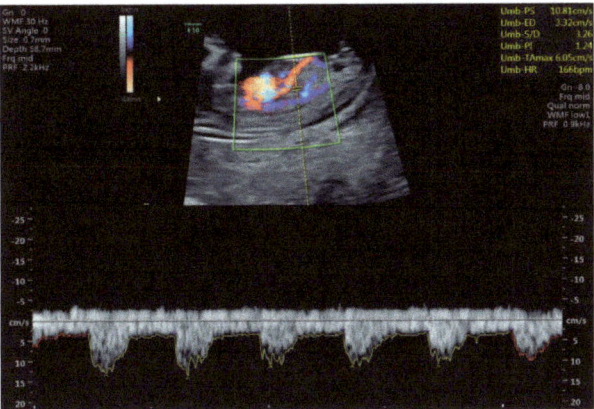

Figure 1. Longitudinal plane view of 12-week fetus showing the umbilical vein, the ductus venosus and the descending thoracic aorta on color flow. The hepatic artery is the vessel coming into close contact with the ductus venosus.

For our study, congenital defects were defined as:
(1) Congenital heart defect (CHD), being any of the following: AVSD (atrioventricular septal defect), VSD (ventricular septal defect), CoA (aortic coarctation), TAC (truncus arteriosus communis), HLHS (hypoplastic left heart syndrome), DORV (double outlet right ventricle), ToF (tetralogy of Fallot), PA (pulmonary atresia), TGA (transposition of the great vessels).
(2) Another congenital defect, being any of the following: CDH (congenital diaphragmatic hernia), omphalocele, gastroschisis, cleft lip, orofacial cleft, spina bifida, duodenal atresia.

The criteria for including a patient in the adverse pregnancy outcome group were, successively:
(1) Pregnancy ended in miscarriage, i.e., before 22 gestational week. In this case, the karyotype was additionally determined in the fetuses in which no such determination had been made during the AC.
(2) Pregnancy was terminated due to a specific chromosomal abnormality (trisomy 21, trisomy 18, trisomy 13, Turner syndrome) or congenital defects detected during first- or second-trimester ultrasound examination that provided grounds for termination.
(3) Pregnancy ended with intrauterine fetal death (IUFD).
(4) Pregnancy ended in preterm labor, i.e., before 37 gestational week.
(5) Pregnancy ended in a full-term live birth, i.e., >37 gestational week, with congenital defects or karyotype abnormalities identified.

The results were then analyzed statistically. The non-parametric Mann–Whitney U test and Kruskal–Wallis test were used to calculate the differences between the parameters tested. In addition, correlations were examined using the Spearman's rank correlation coefficient. In addition, an analysis was performed comprising multiple logistic regression and an area under curve (AUC) calculation. Statistica ver. 13 (StatSoft, Kraków, Poland) software was used for analysis. Approval from the local institutional review board was obtained for the study, and informed consent was obtained from each patient.

3. Results

In the study, 1460 (79.3%) pregnancies ended in a full-term live birth without any known chromosomal or congenital defects (the normal outcome group). Of the 381 patients qualified for the adverse pregnancy outcome group, 187 delivered prematurely (10.1%),

75 miscarried (4%), 74 had their pregnancies terminated (4%), 30 delivered full-term newborns with a diagnosed chromosomal or congenital defect (1.7%), and 15 suffered from intrauterine fetal death (0.9%).

As shown in Table 1, the fetuses with an adverse pregnancy outcome were shown to have statistically significant lower hepatic arterial pulsatility indexes and higher peak systolic velocities compared to the normal outcome fetuses. Due to the changes we observed, HA-PI values for the 5th percentile in our population (1.19) and HA-PSV values for the 95th percentile in our population (20.11) were derived for the purpose of a thorough logistic regression analysis. These cut-off points were chosen because of a lack of appropriate growth charts for the hepatic artery flow. In addition, with the help of the FMF software, we used the value for the 95th percentile for NT and DV-PI. The logistic regression revealed statistical significance for the predictive model for an adverse pregnancy outcome accounting for: NT > 95pc (OR 2.63 (1.81–3.81)), HA-PI < 5pc (OR 13.99 (4.43–44.23)), HA-PSV > 95pc (OR 11.4 (4.09–31.79)), DV-PI > 95pc (OR 22.47 (9.1–55.36)), maternal age (OR 1.033 (1.007–1.059)), and PAPP-A MoM (OR 0.73 (0.56–0.93)). The AUC for this model was 0.739. In this model, for an FPR of 5% the sensitivity was 45%, the PPV was 70.2%, and the NPV was 86.8%.

Table 1. Differences between selected first-trimester screening parameters depending on the adverse pregnancy outcome.

	Adverse Pregnancy Outcome		
	Yes (n = 381)	No (n = 1460)	p
	Median (Min–Max)	Median (Min–Max)	
FHR	161.00 (138.00–191.00)	160.00 (143.00–197.00)	0.017
NT	2.10 (1.10–13.00)	1.75 (0.80–10.50)	<0.001
HA-PI	1.43 (0.11–2.70)	1.47 (1.01–2.70)	<0.001
HA-PSV	12.27 (7.12–43.00)	11.45 (5.41–26.30)	<0.001
DVPI	1.20 (0.56–2.43)	1.10 (0.61–9.92)	<0.001
beta-HCG MoM	1.01 (0.04–7.26)	1.04 (0.17–7.68)	0.56
PAPP-A MoM	0.68 (0.05–3.54)	0.94 (0.15–4.32)	<0.001
	Mean ± SD	Mean ± SD	
Age	31.77 ± 5.97	30.5 ± 5.25	<0.001
Weight	65.05 ± 10.46	65.21 ± 7.9	0.006

Among our patients, karyotype abnormalities were found in 93 fetuses (5%), such as Down syndrome, Edwards syndrome, Patau syndrome or Turner syndrome. The fetuses affected by karyotype abnormalities had statistically significant lower hepatic artery indexes with significantly higher peak systolic velocities (Table 2). The logistic regression demonstrated statistical significance for the predictive model for karyotype abnormalities accounting for: NT > 95pc (OR 6.01 (2.95–12.23)), HA-PSV > 95pc (OR 11.36 (5.51–23.41)), DV-PI > 95pc (OR 20.11 (10.02–40.34)), and PAPP-A MoM (OR 0.26 (0.11–0.59)). The AUC for this model was 0.97. In this model, for an FPR of 5% the sensitivity was 89.2%, the PPV was 48.5%, and the NPV was 99.4%.

Our comparison of the fetuses affected by chromosomal defects with other fetuses included in the adverse pregnancy outcome group also showed statistically significant lower HA-PI and higher HA-PSV values in the former (Table 3).

Table 2. Differences between selected first-trimester screening parameters depending on the karyotype.

	Karyotype		
	Abnormal (*n* = 93)	Normal (*n* = 1741)	*p*
	Median (Min–Max)	Median (Min–Max)	
FHR	159.00 (142.00–182.00)	160.00 (138.00–197.00)	0.93
NT	4.00 (1.40–12.00)	1.80 (0.80–13.00)	<0.001
HA-PI	0.84 (0.54–2.53)	1.47 (0.11–2.70)	<0.001
HA-PSV	20.90 (7.79–43.00)	11.55 (5.41–28.70)	<0.001
DVPI	1.65 (0.78–2.43)	1.10 (0.56–9.92)	<0.001
beta-HCG MoM	1.12 (0.12–4.37)	1.03 (0.04–7.68)	0.85
PAPP-A MoM	0.44 (0.09–2.09)	0.92 (0.05–4.32)	<0.001
	Mean ± SD	Mean ± SD	
Age	32.09 ± 6.69	30.69 ± 5.35	0.14
Weight	65.15 ± 8.36	65.64 ± 10.83	0.65

Table 3. Differences between selected first-trimester screening parameters in adverse pregnancy outcome pregnancies depending on the karyotype.

	Karyotype		
	Abnormal (*n* = 93)	Normal (*n* = 288)	*p*
	Median (Min–Max)	Median (Min–Max)	
FHR	159.00 (142.00–182.00)	161.00 (138.00–191.00)	0.44
NT	4.00 (1.40–12.00)	1.90 (1.10–13.00)	<0.001
HA-PI	0.84 (0.54–2.53)	1.47 (0.11–2.70)	<0.001
HA-PSV	20.90 (7.79–43.00)	11.90 (7.12–28.70)	<0.001
DVPI	1.65 (0.78–2.43)	1.11 (0.56–2.10)	<0.001
beta-HCG MoM	1.12 (0.12–4.37)	1.01 (0.04–7.26)	0.91
PAPP-A MoM	0.44 (0.09–2.09)	0.80 (0.05–3.54)	<0.001
	Mean ± SD	Mean ± SD	
Age	32.09 ± 6.69	31.67 ± 5.72	0.96
Weight	65.15 ± 8.36	64.86 ± 10.36	0.43

A closer look at the chromosomal abnormalities and their breakdown into individual defects showed that no significant differences in the Doppler hepatic artery flow assessment existed (Table 4).

As shown in Table 5, we proved a significantly lower HA-PI in patients who were eligible for pregnancy termination compared to all the other groups. When comparing pregnancy termination patients with the other groups, HA-PSV was significantly higher in the former. In addition, HA-PSV was significantly higher in the miscarriage group compared to the preterm or full-term delivery patients.

Table 6 shows an analysis of hepatic artery flows depending on the presence of a congenital heart defect in the fetus. Fetuses with a congenital heart defect were shown to have a statistically significant lower HA-PI and higher HA-PSV compared to the fetuses without such a diagnosis. The logistic regression demonstrated statistical significance for the predictive model for CHD accounting for: HA-PI < 5pc (OR 7.73 (3.4–17.57)) and DV-PI > 95pc (OR 4.49 (1.95–10.3)). The AUC for this model was 0.75. In this model, for an FPR of 5% the sensitivity was 55.4%, the PPV was 23.1%, and the NPV was 98.5%.

Table 4. Differences between selected first-trimester screening parameters depending on the type of aneuploidy.

	Karyotype Defect				
	T13 † (n = 10)	T18 †† (n = 17)	T21 ††† (n = 57)	Turner Syndrome †††† (n = 9)	p
	Median (Min–Max)	Median (Min–Max)	Median (Min–Max)	Median (Min–Max)	
FHR	172.5 (142–182)	158 (150–169)	157 (142–182)	178 (160–180)	<0.001
NT	5.55 (2.00–8.00)	4.40 (1.70–9.60)	3.40 (1.40–9.50)	8.90 (5.80–12.00)	<0.001
HA-PI	1.04 (0.75–1.99)	0.85 (0.68–1.90)	0.82 (0.54–2.53)	0.92 (0.76–1.45)	0.098
HA-PSV	20.90 (8.57–23.10)	23.20 (19.70–43.00)	20.70 (7.79–42.20)	20.40 (10.66–33.20)	0.066
DVPI	1.56 (1.17–1.99)	1.65 (1.08–2.40)	1.65 (0.78–2.43)	1.24 (0.99–1.92)	0.3
beta-HCG MoM	0.51 (0.38–3.45)	0.45 (0.12–1.92)	1.30 (0.33–4.37)	1.50 (0.24–2.65)	<0.001
PAPP-A MoM	0.28 (0.22–1.45)	0.32 (0.09–0.73)	0.58 (0.15–2.09)	0.46 (0.22–1.52)	0.0012
	Mean ± SD	Mean ± SD	Mean ± SD	Mean ± SD	
Age	29.2 ± 6.86	29.64 ± 5.07	33.43 ± 7.08	31.44 ± 4.74	0.11
Weight	64.9 ± 8.06	67 ± 11.44	66.01 ± 11.59	61.55 ± 7.09	0.64

Post-hoc: **FHR**: † vs. ††† $p = 0.04$, †† vs. †††† $p = 0.01$, ††† vs. †††† $p = <0.001$; **NT**: ††† vs. †††† $p = <0.001$; **beta-HCG**: † vs. ††† $p = 0.01$ †† vs. ††† $p = <0.001$; **PAPP-A**: † vs. ††† $p = 0.01$ †† vs. ††† $p = 0.01$.

Table 5. Differences between selected first-trimester screening parameters depending on pregnancy outcome.

	Pregnancy Outcome					
	Labor at Term † (n = 1483)	IUFD †† (n = 15)	Miscarriage ††† (n = 75)	Terminated Pregnancy †††† (n = 74)	Preterm Labor ††††† (n = 187)	p
	Median (Min–Max)	Median (Min–Max)	Median (Min–Max)	Median (Min–Max)	Median (Min–Max)	
FHR	160 (143–197)	160 (146–177)	162 (144–190)	162 (138–191)	161 (142–189)	0.053
NT	1.80 (0.80–10.50)	1.80 (1.10–9.50)	2.00 (1.20–12.00)	4.25 (1.10–13.00)	1.90 (1.10–10.80)	<0.001
HA-PI	1.46 (0.54–2.70)	1.52 (0.72–2.66)	1.43 (0.11–2.69)	1.11 (0.68–2.58)	1.46 (0.66–2.70)	<0.001
HA-PSV	11.50 (5.41–33.20)	11.30 (7.43–41.20)	12.85 (7.54–28.70)	20.11 (7.79–42.20)	11.74 (7.12–43.00)	<0.001
DVPI	1.10 (0.61–9.92)	1.20 (0.80–1.86)	1.30 (0.70–2.43)	1.51 (0.87–2.40)	1.10 (0.56–1.95)	<0.001
beta-HCG MoM	1.04 (0.17–7.68)	0.93 (0.14–3.10)	1.09 (0.04–7.26)	1.17 (0.12–6.07)	0.99 (0.14–5.73)	0.76
PAPP-A MoM	0.94 (0.15–4.32)	0.73 (0.05–1.90)	0.59 (0.05–3.54)	0.41 (0.09–3.03)	0.84 (0.12–3.41)	<0.001
	Mean ± SD	Mean ± SD	Mean ± SD	Mean ± SD	Mean ± SD	
Age	30.59 ± 5.32	29.33 ± 6.62	33.46 ± 5.11	31.41 ± 5.88	30.84 ± 5.83	<0.001
Weight	65.21 ± 7.98	62.46 ± 10.81	64.74 ± 9.08	64.7 ± 9.88	65.51 ± 11.1	0.049

Post-hoc: **NT** † vs. ††† $p < 0.001$ † vs. †††† $p < 0.001$ † vs. ††††† $p = 0.002$; †† vs. †††† $p = 0.006$; ††† vs. †††† $p < 0.001$ ††† vs. ††††† $p = 0.02$; †††† vs. ††††† $p < 0.001$; **HA-PI** † vs. †††† < 0.001; †† vs. †††† $p = 0.02$; ††† vs. †††† $p = 0.002$; †††† vs††††† $p < 0.001$; **HA-PSV** † vs. ††† $p < 0.001$ † vs. †††† $p < 0.001$; †† vs. †††† $p = 0.02$; ††† vs. †††† $p = 0.02$ ††† vs. ††††† $p = 0.03$; †††† vs. ††††† $p < 0.001$; **DVPI** † vs. ††† $p < 0.001$ † vs. †††† $p < 0.001$; ††† vs. ††††† $p < 0.001$; †††† vs. ††††† $p < 0.001$; **PAPP-A** † vs. ††† $p < 0.001$ † vs. †††† $p < 0.001$; ††† vs. ††††† $p = 0.002$; †††† vs. ††††† $p < 0.001$; **Age** † vs. ††† $p < 0.001$; ††† vs.†††† $p = 0.002$.

Table 6. Differences between selected first-trimester screening parameters depending on present or absent fetal CHD diagnosis.

	CHD		
	Yes (*n* = 56)	No (*n* = 1785)	*p*
	Median (Min–Max)	Median (Min–Max)	
FHR	160.00 (142.00–180.00)	160.00 (138.00–197.00)	0.68
NT	2.35 (1.10–12.00)	1.80 (0.80–13.00)	<0.001
HA-PI	1.30 (0.54–2.65)	1.46 (0.11–2.70)	<0.001
HA-PSV	13.82 (7.43–43.00)	11.65 (5.41–42.20)	<0.001
DVPI	1.30 (0.78–2.11)	1.10 (0.56–9.92)	<0.001
beta-HCG MoM	0.89 (0.12–4.44)	1.04 (0.04–7.68)	0.08
PAPP-A MoM	0.63 (0.10–2.24)	0.91 (0.05–4.32)	<0.001
	Mean ± SD	Mean ± SD	
Age	32.01 ± 6.84	30.72 ± 5.37	0.18
Weight	64.66 ± 9.91	65.19 ± 8.45	0.24

Tables 7 and 8 demonstrate analyses of the correlations between hepatic flow parameters among the groups under investigation. Statistically significant negative correlations were found between nuchal translucency and the hepatic artery pulsatility index in fetuses born at term, fetuses born preterm, pregnancies ended in miscarriage, fetuses with normal karyotype, and both adverse outcome and normal outcome pregnancies. In addition, we showed positive correlation between NT and peak systolic velocity in the hepatic artery in fetuses born at term, fetuses born preterm, pregnancies ended in miscarriage, terminated pregnancies, fetuses with normal karyotype, and both adverse outcome and normal outcome pregnancies. As for the ductus venosus, statistically significant negative DV-PI correlations with the hepatic artery pulsatility index were found for fetuses born at term, pregnancies ended in intrauterine fetal death, pregnancies ended in miscarriage, terminated pregnancies, fetuses with normal karyotype, and adverse outcome pregnancies. In addition, significantly positive correlations were observed between DV-PI and peak systolic velocity in the hepatic artery for fetuses born at term, pregnancies ended in intrauterine fetal death, fetuses with normal karyotype, and both adverse outcome and normal outcome pregnancies.

Table 7. Correlations between hepatic artery flows and selected first-trimester screening parameters depending on the pregnancy outcome (ns = not significant).

		Labor at Term	IUFD	Miscarriage	Termination of Pregnancy	Preterm Labor
FHR	HA-PI	$p < 0.001$ R = 0.31	$p < 0.001$ R = 0.73	ns	ns	$p < 0.001$ R = 0.36
	HA-PSV	$p < 0.001$ R = −0.33	ns	ns	ns	$p < 0.001$ R = −0.3
NT	HA-PI	$p < 0.001$ R = −0.55	ns	$p < 0.01$ R = −0.29	ns	$p < 0.001$ R = −0.5
	HA-PSV	$p < 0.001$ R = 0.57	ns	$p < 0.001$ R = 0.61	$p < 0.001$ R = 0.38	$p < 0.001$ R = 0.56
DVPI	HA-PI	$p < 0.02$ R = −0.05	$p < 0.02$ R = −0.58	$p < 0.03$ R = −0.24	$p < 0.002$ R = −0.34	ns
	HA-PSV	$p < 0.01$ R = 0.06	$p < 0.03$ R = 0.54	ns	ns	ns
beta-HCG MoM	HA-PI	ns	ns	ns	ns	ns
	HA-PSV	ns	ns	ns	ns	ns
PAPP-A MoM	HA-PI	ns	ns	ns	ns	ns
	HA-PSV	ns	ns	ns	ns	ns

Table 8. Correlations between hepatic artery flows and selected first-trimester screening parameters depending on the karyotype and the adverse pregnancy outcome (ns = not significant).

		Abnormal Karyotype	Normal Karyotype	Adverse Outcome	Normal Outcome
FHR	HA-PI	$p < 0.01$ $R = 0.25$	$p < 0.001$ $R = 0.31$	$p < 0.001$ $R = 0.21$	$p < 0.001$ $R = 0.33$
	HA-PSV	ns	$p < 0.001$ $R = -0.3$	$p < 0.01$ $R = -0.12$	$p < 0.001$ $R = -0.34$
NT	HA-PI	ns	$p < 0.001$ $R = -0.51$	$p < 0.001$ $R = -0.47$	$p < 0.001$ $R = -0.54$
	HA-PSV	ns	$p < 0.001$ $R = 0.58$	$p < 0.001$ $R = 0.62$	$p < 0.001$ $R = 0.56$
DVPI	HA-PI	ns	$p < 0.02$ $R = -0.05$	$p < 0.001$ $R = -0.32$	ns
	HA-PSV	ns	$p < 0.001$ $R = 0.07$	$p < 0.001$ $R = 0.26$	$p < 0.03$ $R = 0.05$
beta-HCG MoM	HA-PI	ns	ns	ns	ns
	HA-PSV	ns	ns	ns	ns
PAPP-A MoM	HA-PI	ns	ns	$p < 0.001$ $R = 0.17$	ns
	HA-PSV	ns	ns	$p < 0.001$ $R = -0.17$	ns

4. Discussion

According to our knowledge, this has been the largest (1841 cases) study aiming at evaluating fetal hepatic artery flows. Our main finding was that impaired hepatic artery flows accompanied fetal adverse pregnancy outcomes, aneuploidy, and congenital heart defects.

The first reports on impaired flows in the hepatic artery were published before the year 2000, where low resistance flows in fetuses with intrauterine growth restriction were described [6]. Other authors have noted that a reduced oxygenated blood flow in the DV contributes to a compensatory increase in the hepatic artery flow aiming at maintaining constant blood flow in the organ (HABR). In their studies, however, this does not only apply to fetuses with intrauterine growth restriction, but also those affected by anemia [7,8]. This implicates that the liver is one of the organs, along with the central nervous system, the heart, and the adrenal glands, that are extremely vital for fetal survival under hypoxic conditions. This effect is probably related to the important hematopoietic function of the fetal liver. Animal studies show that a change in fetal hepatic flow increases its hematopoietic activity [11]. Interestingly, fetuses affected by Down syndrome are prenatally found to show hepatomegaly with an increased hepatic blood flow [12–14]. The authors claim that this may cause abnormal hematopoiesis and contribute to acute megakaryoblastic leukemia developing postnatally [15,16]. A similar impaired prenatal blood flow scenario may also apply to fetuses with Edwards syndrome, as postnatally they are much more frequently diagnosed with hepatoblastomas [17,18]. In connection with the above findings, the authors decided a few years ago to look into hepatic artery flows during the first-trimester ultrasound [5,9,10]. One paper shows that fetuses with an adverse pregnancy outcome had a reduced HA-PI and an increased HA-PSV compared to fetuses with normal pregnancy outcomes. However, the paper was based on a relatively small number of patients ($n = 59$) and rather focused on comparing HA flows between fetuses with a normal and an increased NT [10]. In our paper we, too, were able to show that fetuses with an adverse pregnancy outcome had a reduced HA-PI and an increased HA-PSV. In addition, it was these fetuses that we demonstrated to have multiple correlations between hepatic artery flows and the acknowledged adverse pregnancy outcome markers such as NT and DV-PI, as well as successful pregnancy outcome markers such as, say, PAPP-A. In addition, we showed that fetuses with an HA-PI of <5pc are almost 14-times more likely to experience an adverse pregnancy outcome. Fetuses with an HA-PSV >95pc are 11-times more likely to develop such complications.

It should be remembered that for all gynecologists/obstetricians, healthy pregnancy is an extremely important and satisfying part of their daily work. Nevertheless, modern practice requires doctors to reduce the risk of pregnancy complications such as, say, preterm labor or severe cases of early-onset preeclampsia, by ensuring early detection of patients carrying an elevated risk of developing these adverse states. One of the main examples is prevention making use of acetylsalicylic acid in women carrying an increased risk of preeclampsia or using progesterone in women at risk of preterm labor [19–22]. Therefore, researchers have been attempting to identify other markers causing the various forms of complications during pregnancy. The flow in the ductus venosus is an example of such a marker. An increased DV-PI, as well as the presence of a reversed a-wave in the DV, correlate significantly with pregnancy complications such as aneuploidy, miscarriage, and intrauterine fetal death [23–25].

Our results also showed that DV-PI is higher in fetuses with an adverse pregnancy outcome or those with aneuploidy. We additionally proved that a DV-PI > 95pc increases the risk of an adverse pregnancy outcome more than 22 times and the risk of aneuploidy more than 20 times.

The search for new markers for chromosomal aberrations continues, which may result in an improved detection rate of the aforementioned types of aneuploidy in the first trimester of pregnancy. So far, the evaluation proposed in 2008, which achieves a detection rate of 91% at a false-positive rate (FPR) of 5% for trisomy 21, continues to be the most effective [2]. The addition of other markers, such as the presence of the nasal bone, or tricuspid insufficiency, has been shown to improve the detection rate of aneuploidy, reducing the FPR at the same time [26–29]. Fetuses with karyotype abnormalities were reported to have a high HA-PSV and a low HA-PI. In addition, significant negative correlations were proved to exist between the hepatic artery flow and the DV flow, and positive correlations were shown to exist between it and NT [5,9,10]. In addition, two of these papers show that a higher HA-PSV and a lower HA-PI are not only found in fetuses with chromosomal abnormalities but also in fetuses in which the risk of this aneuploidy is increased, even though their karyotype is normal [5,9]. The main focus of those papers was on trisomy 21 with only a handful of other chromosomal abnormalities examined, which was an insufficient basis to assess the usefulness of hepatic artery flow measurements in such cases. As we have shown in our study, as well, HA-PI is lower and HA-PSV is higher in fetuses with confirmed chromosomal aberrations compared to fetuses with a normal karyotype. Our more detailed analysis allowed us to show that fetuses with an HA-PSV >95pc are 11 times more likely to have aneuploidy, while the AUC for our model was 0.97. When studying correlations in aneuploid fetuses, we were not able to show any significant relationships between hepatic artery flow and DV or NT. This may indicate that the flow in the hepatic artery may be an independent additional marker for these aberrations. In addition, we examined the differences in hepatic artery flows depending on the type of the chromosomal abnormality present. In this respect, we were not able to show any differences between the groups, which may mean that the presence of aneuploidy alone disturbs the normal hepatic artery flow.

Early detection of CHD is another important aspect of prenatal testing. Currently, the prenatal CHD detection rate is estimated to be approx. 60% [30,31]. So far, NT and the DV flow have been relatively well-researched as markers for the risk of developing CHD. Many authors have shown that first-trimester fetuses diagnosed with an increased NT, an elevated DV pulsatility index, or the presence of an a-wave in the DV, carry a higher risk of congenital heart defects, regardless of the risk of aneuploidy [32–34]. In the case of these fetuses, it is important that second-trimester echocardiography is performed as a follow-up.

Nevertheless, as noted above, no satisfactory CHD detection rate has been reached as yet. The flow in the hepatic artery is an additional parameter that could guide us towards obtaining a better insight into the fetus for a risk of CHD. We have been able to show that these cases of fetuses have significantly lower pulsatility index values, accompanied by significantly higher peak systolic velocities in the HA. A more thorough study of these parameters helped us note that a DV-PI > 95pc increases the risk of CHD almost 4.5 times, while an HA-PI < 5pc increases that risk more than 7 times. The AUC for this model was 0.75. However, with an assumed FPR of 5%, the sensitivity of this model was only 55.4%. Nevertheless, it should be stressed that the focus here is on the first trimester, while most CHD cases are detected much later.

In view of the above, it appears appropriate that a discussion should be started on hepatic artery flow assessments in the first trimester of pregnancy. We are aware that that beginner sonographers may find it difficult to identify the signal of the hepatic artery, especially where it indicates normal flow parameters. The fetal hepatic artery is in close proximity to the ductus venosus, which is why when imaging the ductus venosus a strong signal that corresponds to the hepatic artery is frequently observed. For persons trained in fetal ultrasound imaging, however, this assessment should not pose more difficulty than making the routine first-trimester parameter evaluations.

One of the weaknesses of our study was that no karyotype study was carried out in children born at term without dysmorphic features as this might have led to somewhat different results, but the cost of such an approach would have been unacceptable for us. In addition, due to an initial lack of reporting, we do not have accurate data about the numbers of patients excluded from the study. Certainly, if we wanted to extrapolate the detection rate of an adverse pregnancy outcome to the general population, we should also investigate patients with pre-pregnancy diseases or with a history of complications in their previous pregnancies, who according to our initial assumptions did not qualify for inclusion in the present study.

5. Conclusions

Expanding the first-trimester screening by the addition of the hepatic artery flow assessment may contribute to improving the detection rate of fetuses carrying the risk of developing adverse pregnancy outcomes. In particular cases, this could mean an ability to detect chromosomal abnormalities or congenital heart defects. However, multicenter studies would be needed to confirm our observations.

Author Contributions: Conceptualization, B.C. and M.D.; Data curation, W.C., D.B., A.J., A.F. and S.D.; Formal analysis, P.T.; Investigation, B.C., W.C., D.B., A.J. and A.F.; Methodology, B.C., W.C., D.B. and A.K.; Project administration, M.D.; Software, S.K.; Supervision, A.K. and G.Ś.; Visualization, P.T. and S.D.; Writing—original draft, P.T. and M.F.-T.; Writing—review & editing, B.C., P.T. and S.K. All authors have read and agreed to the published version of the manuscript.

Funding: This research received no external funding.

Institutional Review Board Statement: Approval from the Institutional Review Board of Medical University of Silesia was obtained for the study (number KNW/0022/KB/315/18/19).

Informed Consent Statement: Informed consent was obtained from all subjects involved in the study.

Data Availability Statement: The data presented in this study is available upon request from the author for correspondence. The data is not publicly available, as not all patients agreed to publicly disclose the data.

Conflicts of Interest: The authors declare no conflict of interest.

References

1. Karagiannis, G.; Akolekar, R.; Sarquis, R.; Wright, D.; Nicolaides, K.H. Prediction of small-for-gestation neonates from biophysical and biochemical markers at 11–13 weeks. *Fetal Diagn. Ther.* **2011**, *29*, 148–154. [CrossRef] [PubMed]
2. Kagan, K.O.; Wright, D.; Valencia, C.; Maiz, N.; Nicolaides, K.H. Screening for trisomies 21, 18 and 13 by maternal age, fetal nuchal translucency, fetal heart rate, free β-hCG and pregnancy-associated plasma protein-A. *Hum. Reprod.* **2008**, *23*, 1968–1975. [CrossRef] [PubMed]
3. Tan, M.Y.; Syngelaki, A.; Poon, L.C.; Rolnik, D.L.; O'Gorman, N.; Delgado, J.L.; Akolekar, R.; Konstantinidou, L.; Tsavdaridou, M.; Galeva, S.; et al. Screening for pre-eclampsia by maternal factors and biomarkers at 11–13 weeks' gestation. *Ultrasound Obstet. Gynecol.* **2018**, *52*, 186–195. [CrossRef]
4. Nicolaides, K.H. Turning the pyramid of prenatal care. *Fetal Diagn. Ther.* **2011**, *29*, 183–196. [CrossRef] [PubMed]
5. Zvanca, M.; Gielchinsky, Y.; Abdeljawad, F.; Bilardo, C.M.; Nicolaides, K.H. Hepatic artery Doppler in trisomy 21 and euploid fetuses at 11–13 weeks. *Prenat. Diagn.* **2011**, *31*, 22–27. [CrossRef] [PubMed]
6. Kilavuz, Ö.; Vetter, K. Is the liver of the fetus the 4th preferential organ for arterial blood supply besides brain, heart, and adrenal glands? *J. Perinat. Med.* **1999**, *27*, 103–106. [CrossRef]
7. Ebbing, C.; Rasmussen, S.; Godfrey, K.M.; Hanson, M.A.; Kiserud, T. Redistribution pattern of fetal liver circulation in intrauterine growth restriction. *Acta Obstet. Gynecol. Scand.* **2009**, *88*, 1118–1123. [CrossRef]
8. Ebbing, C.; Rasmussen, S.; Godfrey, K.M.; Hanson, M.A.; Kiserud, T. Hepatic artery hemodynamics suggest operation of a buffer response in the human fetus. *Reprod. Sci.* **2008**, *15*, 166–178. [CrossRef]
9. Togrul, C.; Ozaksit, G.M.; Seckin, K.D.; Baser, E.; Karsli, M.F.; Gungor, T. Is there a role for fetal ductus venosus and hepatic artery Doppler in screening for fetal aneuploidy in the first trimester? *J. Matern.-Fetal Neonatal Med.* **2015**, *28*, 1716–1719. [CrossRef]
10. Bilardo, C.M.; Timmerman, E.; Robles De Medina, P.G.; Clur, S.A. Low-resistance hepatic artery flow in first-trimester fetuses: An ominous sign. *Ultrasound Obstet. Gynecol.* **2011**, *37*, 438–443. [CrossRef]
11. Kunisaki, S.M.; Azpurua, H.; Fuchs, J.R.; Graves, S.C.; Zurakowski, D.; Fauza, D.O. Fetal hepatic haematopoiesis is modulated by arterial blood flow to the liver. *Br. J. Haematol.* **2006**, *134*, 330–332. [CrossRef] [PubMed]
12. Zerres, K.; Schwanitz, G.; Niesen, M.; Gembruch, U.; Hansmann, M.; Waldherr, R. Prenatal diagnosis of acute non-lymphoblastic leukaemia in Down syndrome. *Lancet* **1990**, *335*, 117. [CrossRef]
13. Hamada, H.; Yamada, N.; Watanabe, H.; Okuno, S.; Fujiki, Y.; Kubo, T. Hypoechoic hepatomegaly associated with transient abnormal myelopoiesis provides clues to trisomy 21 in the third-trimester fetus. *Ultrasound Obstet. Gynecol.* **2001**, *17*, 442–444. [CrossRef] [PubMed]
14. Hojo, S.; Tsukimori, K.; Kitade, S.; Nakanami, N.; Hikino, S.; Hara, T.; Wake, N. Prenatal sonographic findings and hematological abnormalities in fetuses with transient abnormal myelopoiesis with Down syndrome. *Prenat. Diagn.* **2007**, *27*, 507–511. [CrossRef]
15. Tunstall-Pedoe, O.; Roy, A.; Karadimitris, A.; De La Fuente, J.; Fisk, N.M.; Bennett, P.; Norton, A.; Vyas, P.; Roberts, I. Abnormalities in the myeloid progenitor compartment in Down syndrome fetal liver precede acquisition of GATA1 mutations. *Blood* **2008**, *112*, 4507–4511. [CrossRef]
16. Chou, S.T.; Opalinska, J.B.; Yao, Y.; Fernandes, M.A.; Kalota, A.; Brooks, J.S.J.; Choi, J.K.; Gewirtz, A.M.; Danet-Desnoyers, G.A.; Nemiroff, R.L.; et al. Trisomy 21 enhances human fetal erythro-megakaryocytic development. *Blood* **2008**, *112*, 4503–4506. [CrossRef]
17. Valentin, L.; Perez, L.; Masand, P. Hepatoblastoma Associated with Trisomy 18. *J. Pediatr. Genet.* **2015**, *04*, 204–206. [CrossRef]
18. Tan, Z.H.; Lai, A.; Chen, C.K.; Chang, K.T.E.; Tan, A.M. Association of trisomy 18 with hepatoblastoma and its implications. *Eur. J. Pediatr.* **2014**, *173*, 1595–1598. [CrossRef]
19. Rolnik, D.L.; Wright, D.; Poon, L.C.; O'Gorman, N.; Syngelaki, A.; de Paco Matallana, C.; Akolekar, R.; Cicero, S.; Janga, D.; Singh, M.; et al. Aspirin versus Placebo in Pregnancies at High Risk for Preterm Preeclampsia. *N. Engl. J. Med.* **2017**, *377*, 613–622. [CrossRef]
20. Romero, R.; Nicolaides, K.H.; Conde-Agudelo, A.; O'brien, J.M.; Cetingoz, E.; Da Fonseca, E.; Creasy, G.W.; Hassan, S.S.; Romero, D.R. Vaginal progesterone decreases preterm birth ≤ 34 weeks of gestation in women with a singleton pregnancy and a short cervix: An updated meta-analysis including data from the OPPTIMUM study. *Ultrasound Obstet. Gynecol.* **2016**, *48*, 308–317. [CrossRef]
21. Jarde, A.; Lutsiv, O.; Beyene, J.; McDonald, S.D. Vaginal progesterone, oral progesterone, 17-OHPC, cerclage, and pessary for preventing preterm birth in at-risk singleton pregnancies: An updated systematic review and network meta-analysis. *BJOG Int. J. Obstet. Gynaecol.* **2019**, *126*, 556–567. [CrossRef] [PubMed]
22. Likis, F.E.; Edwards, D.R.V.; Andrews, J.C.; Woodworth, A.L.; Jerome, R.N.; Fonnesbeck, C.J.; McKoy, J.N.; Hartmann, K.E. Progestogens for preterm birth prevention: A systematic review and meta-analysis. *Obstet. Gynecol.* **2012**, *120*, 897–907. [CrossRef] [PubMed]
23. Maiz, N.; Valencia, C.; Emmanuel, E.E.; Staboulidou, I.; Nicolaides, K.H. Screening for adverse pregnancy outcome by Ductus venosus Doppler at 11–13 + 6 weeks of gestation. *Obstet. Gynecol.* **2008**, *112*, 598–605. [CrossRef] [PubMed]
24. Maiz, N.; Valencia, C.; Kagan, K.O.; Wright, D.; Nicolaides, K.H. Ductus venosus Doppler in screening for trisomies 21, 18 and 13 and Turner syndrome at 11–13 weeks of gestation. *Ultrasound Obstet. Gynecol.* **2009**, *33*, 512–517. [CrossRef] [PubMed]

25. Yılmaz Baran, Ş.; Kalaycı, H.; Doğan Durdağ, G.; Yetkinel, S.; Arslan, A.; Bulgan Kılıçdağ, E. Does abnormal ductus venosus pulsatility index at the first-trimester effect on adverse pregnancy outcomes? *J. Gynecol. Obstet. Hum. Reprod.* **2020**, *49*, 101851. [CrossRef] [PubMed]
26. Kagan, K.O.; Valencia, C.; Livanos, P.; Wright, D.; Nicolaides, K.H. Tricuspid regurgitation in screening for trisomies 21, 18 and 13 and Turner syndrome at 11 + 0 to 13 + 6 weeks of gestation. *Ultrasound Obstet. Gynecol.* **2009**, *33*, 18–22. [CrossRef]
27. Kagan, K.O.; Cicero, S.; Staboulidou, I.; Wright, D.; Nicolaides, K.H. Fetal nasal bone in screening for trisomies 21, 18 and 13 and Turner syndrome at 11–13 weeks of gestation. *Ultrasound Obstet. Gynecol.* **2009**, *33*, 259–264. [CrossRef]
28. Czuba, B.; Zarotyński, D.; Dubiel, M.; Borowski, D.; Wegrzyn, P.; Cnota, W.; Reska-Nycz, M.; Maczka, M.; Wielgoś, M.; Sodowski, K.; et al. Screening for trisomy 21 based on maternal age, nuchal translucency measurement, first trimester biochemistry and quantitative and qualitative assessment of the flow in the DV—The assessment of efficacy. *Ginekol. Pol.* **2017**, *88*, 481–485. [CrossRef]
29. Czuba, B.; Nycz-Reska, M.; Cnota, W.; Jagielska, A.; Wloch, A.; Borowski, D.; Wegrzyn, P. Quantitative and qualitative Ductus Venosus blood flow evaluation in the screening for Trisomy 18 and 13—Suitability study. *Ginekol. Pol.* **2020**, *91*, 144–148. [CrossRef]
30. McBrien, A.; Sands, A.; Craig, B.; Dornan, J.; Casey, F. Major congenital heart disease: Antenatal detection, patient characteristics and outcomes. *J. Matern.-Fetal Neonatal Med.* **2009**, *22*, 101–105. [CrossRef]
31. Tegnander, E.; Williams, W.; Johansens, O.J.; Blaas, H.G.K.; Eik-Nes, S.H. Prenatal detection of heart defects in a non-selected population of 30149 fetuses—Detection rates and outcome. *Ultrasound Obstet. Gynecol.* **2006**, *27*, 252–265. [CrossRef] [PubMed]
32. Chelemen, T.; Syngelaki, A.; Maiz, N.; Allan, L.; Nicolaides, K.H. Contribution of ductus venosus doppler in first-trimester screening for major cardiac defects. *Fetal Diagn. Ther.* **2011**, *29*, 127–134. [CrossRef] [PubMed]
33. Timmerman, E.; Clur, S.A.; Pajkrt, E.; Bilardo, C.M. First-trimester measurement of the ductus venosus pulsatility index and the prediction of congenital heart defects. *Ultrasound Obstet. Gynecol.* **2010**, *36*, 668–675. [CrossRef] [PubMed]
34. Borrell, A.; Grande, M.; Bennasar, M.; Borobio, V.; Jimenez, J.M.; Stergiotou, I.; Martinez, J.M.; Cuckle, H. First-trimester detection of major cardiac defects with the use of ductus venosus blood flow. *Ultrasound Obstet. Gynecol.* **2013**, *42*, 51–57. [CrossRef]

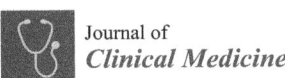

Article

Evaluation of FMR4, FMR5 and FMR6 Expression Levels as Non-Invasive Biomarkers for the Diagnosis of Fragile X-Associated Primary Ovarian Insufficiency (FXPOI)

Maria Isabel Alvarez-Mora [1,2], Ines Agusti [3], Robin Wijngaard [1], Estefania Martinez-Barrios [1], Tamara Barcos [1], Aina Borras [3], Sara Peralta [3], Marta Guimera [3], Ana Goday [3], Dolors Manau [3,†] and Laia Rodriguez-Revenga [1,2,*,†]

1. Biochemistry and Molecular Genetics Department, Hospital Clinic of Barcelona and Institut d'Investigacions Biomèdiques August Pi i Sunyer (IDIBAPS), 08036 Barcelona, Spain; mialvarez@clinic.cat (M.I.A.-M.); wijngaard@clinic.cat (R.W.); estefaniamartinezbarrios@gmail.com (E.M.-B.); tamara_barcos@hotmail.com (T.B.)
2. CIBER of Rare Diseases, Instituto de Salud Carlos III, 28029 Madrid, Spain
3. Clinical Institute of Gynecology, Obstetrics and Neonatology (ICGON), Hospital Clinic of Barcelona and Institut de Investigacions Biomèdiques August Pi iSunyer (IDIBAPS), 08036 Barcelona, Spain; iagusti@clinic.cat (I.A.); aborras1@clinic.cat (A.B.); speralta@clinic.cat (S.P.); mguimera@clinic.cat (M.G.); goday@clinic.cat (A.G.); dmanau@clinic.cat (D.M.)
* Correspondence: lbodi@clinic.cat; Tel.: +34-93-227-56-73; Fax: +34-93-451-52-72
† These authors contributed equally to this work.

Abstract: Female *FMR1* (Fragile X mental retardation 1) premutation carriers are at risk for developing fragile X-associated primary ovarian insufficiency (FXPOI), a condition characterized by amenorrhea before age 40 years. Not all women with a *FMR1* premutation suffer from primary ovarian insufficiency and nowadays there are no molecular or other biomarkers that can help predict the occurrence of FXPOI. Long non-coding RNAs (lncRNAs) comprise a group of regulatory transcripts which have versatile molecular functions, making them important regulators in all aspects of gene expression. In recent medical studies, lncRNAs have been described as potential diagnostic biomarkers in many diseases. The present study was designed to determine the expression profile of three lncRNAs derived from the *FMR1* locus, FMR4, FMR5 and FMR6, in female *FMR1* premutation carriers in order: (i) to determine a possible role in the pathogenesis of FXPOI and (ii) to investigate whether they could serve as a biomarker for the diagnosis of FXPOI. FMR4, FMR5 and FMR6 transcripts levels were evaluated in total RNA extracted from peripheral blood by digital droplet PCR and compared between *FMR1* premutation carriers with FXPOI and without FXPOI. The diagnostic value of lncRNAs was evaluated by receiver operating characteristic (ROC) analysis. Results revealed a significant association between FXPOI and high expression levels of FMR4. No association was obtained for FMR5 or FMR6. ROC curve analysis revealed that FMR4 can distinguish *FMR1* premutation carrier with FXPOI with a diagnostic power of 0.67. These findings suggest a potential role of FMR4 as a possible biomarker for FXPOI.

Keywords: FMR4; FMR5; FMR6; *FMR1* gen; CGG repeat; *FMR1* premutation and FXPOI

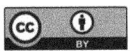

1. Introduction

The *FMR1* (Fragile X mental retardation 1) gene (OMIM*309550) contains a CGG trinucleotide repeat in the 5′ untranslated region [1–3]. Among individuals in the general population, the number of CGG repeats is polymorphic and varies between 6 and 44. In this situation the *FMR1* gene is active and there is synthesis of the Fragile Mental Retardation Protein (FMRP). Repeats in this size interval are stable when transmitted from generation to generation. In contrast, when the number of CGGs exceeds 200 repeats (full mutation) the *FMR1* gene is silenced resulting in the absence of FMRP and the clinical manifestations of fragile X syndrome (FXS, OMIM#300624; ORPHA:908): intellectual disability and characteristic dysmorphic features [4]. Finally, individuals with alleles between 55 and 200 CGG repeats are the so-called *FMR1* premutation carriers. In this situation, there is increased transcription of the *FMR1* mRNA transcript, and slightly reduced synthesis of FMRP [5]. These repeat alleles are unstable and tend to increase in each cell division, conferring an increased risk of having FXS affected offspring.

FMR1 premutation occurs in the general population with an estimated frequency that range from 1 in 800 to 1200 males and from 1 in 250 to 400 females [6]. These individuals are at risk for fragile X-associated premature ovarian insufficiency (FXPOI) in females [7], and fragile X-associated tremor/ataxia syndrome (FXTAS) in both, males and females [8].

FXPOI symptoms include the cessation of ovarian function before the age of 40 years, ovarian dysfunction, and decreased fertility as evidenced by abnormal ovarian reserve biomarkers and reduced ovarian response to controlled ovarian hyperstimulation [9–11]. FXPOI occurs in ~20% of women with the *FMR1* premutation, compared to only 1% of the general population [12]. Women with the *FMR1* premutation not only struggle with the possibility of developing FXPOI but also with the risk of passing on the full mutation to their offspring.

Long non-coding RNAs (lncRNAs), defined as untranslated RNA molecules greater than 200 nucleotides in length, can be derived from sense or antisense strands within protein-coding genes, intergenic regions, or pseudogenes [13–15]. A lot of evidence has been accumulated showing that lncRNAs have versatile molecular functions, making them important regulators in all aspects of gene expression (reviewed in [16]). The biological mechanisms of lncRNAs are multiple. They can interact with DNA, RNA and protein as well as with other biological molecules, regulating the gene expression trough controlling processes such as protein synthesis, RNA maturation and transport, or the chromatin structure [17]. Moreover, lncRNAs participate in diverse biological processes, such as development, differentiation, energy metabolism, apoptosis and angiogenesis; controlling every level of gene expression pathway [18]. These particularities make them good candidate biomarkers for several diseases.

Several lncRNAs are derived from the *FMR1* gene locus: FMR4, FMR6 and the ASFMR1 in the antisense direction and FMR5 in the sense direction (reviewed in [19]). Previous studies have described different expression levels of these lncRNAs among *FMR1* permutation carriers, suggesting a functional association with fragile X-associated disorders [20–24]. Although the *FMR1* premutation is the major risk factor for developing FXPOI, there are still some unknown genetic, epigenetic or environmental factors that might be affecting gene penetrance. On the basis of this observation, we aim to determine the expression profile of FMR4, FMR5 and FMR6 in female *FMR1* premutation carriers in order to determine a possible role in the pathogenesis of FXPOI.

2. Material and Methods

2.1. Subjects

For this study, 36 female *FMR1* premutation carriers registered in the FXS database from the Department of Biochemistry and Molecular Genetics, Hospital Clinic of Barcelona were selected. The cases met the following criteria: 20 women diagnosed with FXPOI (development of amenorrhea due to disruption of ovarian function before the age of 40 years) carrying the *FMR1* premutation (CGG repeats between 55–200) and 16 non-FXPOI *FMR1* premutation carriers with a reported normal ovarian function (regular cycles between 24–35 days) over the age of 40 years. This study was approved by the Institutional Ethical Review Board of Hospital Clinic, Barcelona. All patients that were included in this study signed a written informed consent.

2.2. RNA Extraction and cDNA Synthesis

Total RNA isolation was performed from blood using the PAXgene® Blood RNA Kit (Qiagen, Hilden, Germany) according to the manufacturer's protocols. A Qubit RNA IQ assay (ThermoFisher Scientific, Waltham, MA, USA) was used to determine the RNA concentration. Its integrity was verified with the Bioanalyzer 2100 (Agilent, Santa Clara, CA, USA). The cDNA was synthesized from 350 ng RNA using the High-Capacity cDNA reverse transcription Kit (Applied Biosystems, Waltham, MA, USA), following the manufacturer's instructions.

2.3. Digital Droplet Polymerase Chain Reaction (ddPCR)

LncRNA expression analysis was performed by ddPCR technology, which is an improvement of conventional PCR. Using a droplet generator, the sample is diluted and divided into multiple aliquots and subjected to endpoint PCR. Amplification occurs in each individual partition, which contains an individual nucleic acid molecule. A fluorescence signal is produced in each droplet with the target molecule. Quantification of cDNA molecules relies on the ability of the ddPCR system to determine the number of target molecules by the Poisson statistical analysis of "positive" (containing amplified target) and "negative" (no amplified target detected) droplets [25]. The assay was performed using the QX200™ ddPCR™ EvaGreen Supermix (Bio-Rad, Hercules, CA, USA), 100 nM specific primers targeted to FMR4 (f:5'-ACCAAACCAAACCAAACCAA-3' and r:5'-GTGGGAAATCAAATGCATCC-3'), FMR5 (f:5'-AATGCTGGCAGTCGTTTCTT-3' and r:5'-TTGACGGAGCATCTATCGTG-3'), FMR6 (f:5'-AGCACTTCAGGGCAGATTTT-3' and r:5'-TGGTGAATGATCACCCAATG-3') and the housekeeping gene GAPDH (f:5'-TCTCCTCTGACTTCAACAGCGAC-3' and r:5'- CCCTGTTGCTGTAGCCAAATTC-3') and 9 µL of the diluted cDNA sample. Droplet emulsion formation was performed by mixing 20 µL of reaction with 70 µL of droplet generation oil using a microfluidic droplet generation cartridge and QX200 Droplet Generator (Bio-Rad). End-point PCR amplification was performed using a C1000 Thermal Cycler (Bio-Rad). Primers for FMR5 and GAPDH were designed with Primer-3 (http://bioinfo.ut.ee/primer3-0.4.0/) (accessed on 10 May 2019). Primer sequences for FMR4 and FMR6 were extracted from Elizur and co-workers [24]. In order to normalize lncRNAs copies relative to nuclear DNA, the *GAPDH* gene was used as reference gene.

Results were analyzed with QuantasoftTM Software (Bio-Rad). Target RNA concentrations were calculated using the Poisson statistics and the expression of the lncRNA was reported as [copies/cell] corrected for the expression of the reference gene *GAPDH*. Expression levels are shown as transcripts per ten thousand cells.

2.4. FMR1 Molecular Parameters

CGG repeat analysis and X-chromosome inactivation (XCI) pattern were determined using the AmplideX® PCR/CE *FMR1* and AmplideX® mPCR *FMR1* kits, following manufacturer's recommendations (Asuragen, Austin, TX, USA). Skewed XCI status was considered with a threshold value greater than 90% [26]. *FMR1* mRNA quantification was performed as previously described [27].

2.5. Statistical Analysis

Statistical analysis was carried out using the IBM® SPSS® Statistics software version 25 (SPSS, Chicago, IL, USA) and the open-source computing environment R version 4.0.2 (R Foundation for Statistical Computing, Vienna, Austria). The pROC, ggplot2, MASS and caret R packages were used for assessment of the expression data. Results were expressed as mean ± standard deviation (SD). Statistical significance of differences between means or medians was examined using the parametric *t*-test or the non-parametric Mann–Whitney U test. The discriminatory ability of the lncRNAs to separate FXPOI from non-FXPOI women was assessed using receiver operating characteristic (ROC) curves and by calculating the area under the curve (AUC). Cut-off values were decided based on the optimal combined sensitivity and specificity threshold (Youden Index). The Odds Ratio (OR) was calculated to assess the association between the increased biomarker and FXPOI. Additionally, a multivariate logistic regression model was generated including FMR4 expression levels corrected by CGG repeats. Significance was accepted for *p*-value < 0.05.

3. Results

3.1. Expression Levels of FM4, FMR5 and FMR6 in FMR1 Premutation Carriers

Thirty-six *FMR1* premutation female carriers were recruited; 20 with FXPOI and 16 without FXPOI. There were no differences between the two groups regarding patients' CGG repeat expansion or *FMR1* mRNA expression levels (Table 1). As for the patients' age at time of analysis, statistically significant differences were obtained ($p = 0.03$). This difference can be attributed to a bias in the recruitment of women without FXPOI. Older women were included in this cohort in order to make sure that they did not have ovarian dysfunction. X-chromosome inactivation (XCI) pattern was also examined and compared between the FXPOI and non-FXPOI groups. Results evidenced that both groups showed a similar random XCI pattern (data not shown).

Table 1. Clinical and molecular characteristics of individuals recruited in the study.

	FMR1 Premutation with FXPOI (n = 20)	*FMR1* Premutation without FXPOI (n = 16)	*p*-Value
Age (mean ± SD, years)	41 ± 6.9	47 ± 8.3	0.03 *
CGG repeat (mean ± SD)	100 ± 35	88 ± 26	0.3
FMR1 mRNA (mean ± SD)	1.5 ± 0.8	1.8 ± 1.3	0.3

Significance: * $p < 0.05$. The exact *p*-values were calculated with the U-Mann Whitney test.

FMR4, FMR5 and FMR6 transcripts levels were evaluated in total RNA extracted from peripheral blood by ddPCR and compared between *FMR1* premutation carriers with FXPOI and without FXPOI. Results showed no significant differences between groups for none of the lncRNAs analyzed ($p = 0.09$ for FMR4; $p = 0.46$ for FMR5 and $p = 0.56$ for FMR6) (Figure 1 and Table S1). Subsequently, and since the expression of the three lncRNAs varies over a wide range, we compared *FMR1* premutation carriers with and without FXPOI among stratified subgroups based on expression levels. These subgroups consisted of low, medium and high expression levels for FMR4, FMR5 and FMR6. When comparing the distribution of lncRNAs expression levels (low, medium and high) between *FMR1* premutation carrier groups (with and without FXPOI), significant results were obtained for FMR4 ($p = 0.039$). As shown in Table 2, while 30% (6/20) of FXPOI women showed high levels of FMR4 expression, only 10% (2/16) of women without FXPOI were found to have similar levels. Therefore, evidence was obtained for an association between FMR4 transcript levels and the development of FXPOI. A similar association was also found for FMR5, although not statistically significant. Contrary, for FMR6, no significant evidence of an association was obtained (Table 2).

In addition, the correlation between the expression levels of FMR4, FMR5, FMR6 and the *FMR1* gene was appraised among the total number of female *FMR1* premutation carriers as well as in the distinct groups with and without FXPOI (Figure 2). A high correlation was found between FMR5 and FMR6 expression levels while the correlation of these two lncRNAs with FMR4 was lower. All lncRNAs correlated negatively with respect to *FMR1* expression. The correlation pattern did not change when FXPOI and non-FXPOI females were considered separately, suggesting that their relative expression behavior is not substantially affected by the presence of FXPOI.

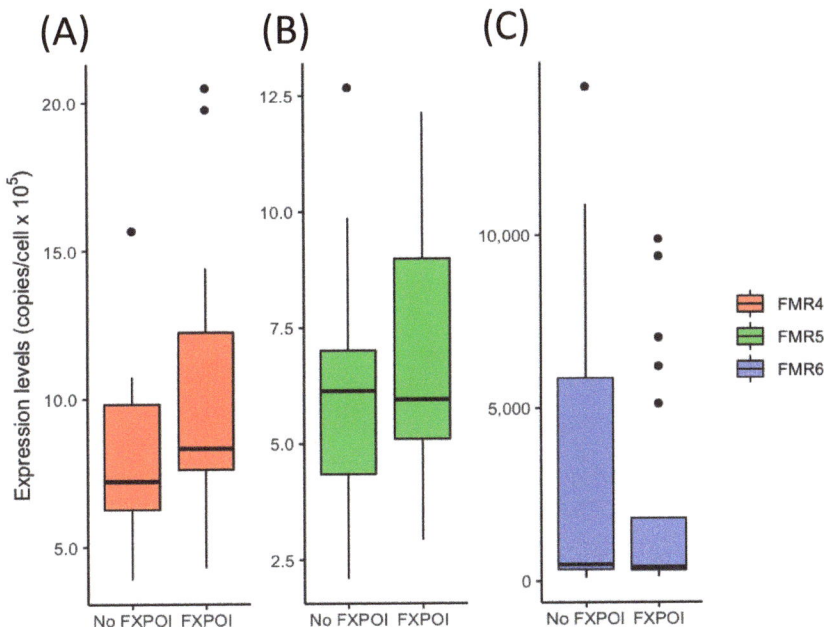

Figure 1. Expression levels of FMR4, FMR5 and FMR6 were compared between *FMR1* premutation carriers with FXPOI and without FXPOI. (**A**) The expression level of FMR4, (**B**) The expression level of FMR5 and (**C**) The expression level of FMR6. None of the comparisons were statistically significant ($p > 0.05$).

Table 2. Distribution of *FMR1* premutation carriers with and without FXPOI based on FMR4, FMR5 and FMR6 expression levels.

	FMR4 expression level			*p*-Value
	1–7	7–12	>12	
FXPOI (n = 20)	2 (10%)	12 (60%)	6 (30%)	0.039 *
No FXPOI (n = 16)	7 (44%)	8 (50%)	1 (6%)	
	FMR5 expression level			
	1–5	5–10	>10	
FXPOI (n = 20)	5 (25%)	10 (50%)	5 (25%)	0.14
No FXPOI (n = 16)	7 (44%)	8 (50%)	1 (6%)	
	FMR6 expression level			
	<400	400–1000	>1000	
FXPOI (n = 20)	10 (50%)	5 (25%)	5 (25%)	0.556
No FXPOI (n = 16)	6 (38%)	5 (31%)	5 (31%)	

Significance: * $p < 0.05$. The exact *p*-values were calculated with the Fisher exact test.

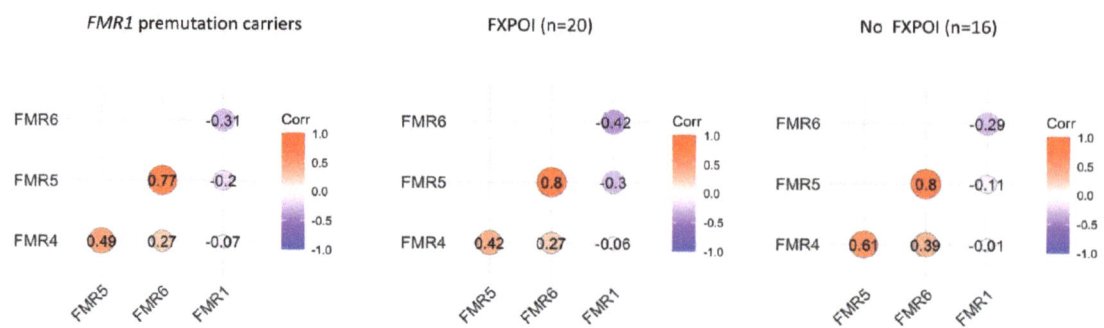

Figure 2. Correlation between expression levels of FMR4, FMR5 and FMR6 was evaluated among total *FMR1* premutation carriers as well as groups of women with FXPOI and without FXPOI.

3.2. Diagnostic Value of FMR4 for FXPOI

Since significant differences were obtained in the distribution of FMR4 expression levels between women with FXPOI and without FXPOI, the diagnostic value of FMR4 was assessed by establishing a ROC curve. As can be observed in Figure 3, the curve had an AUC value of 0.67 (95% CI 0.45–0.86). A sensitivity of 0.80 and specificity of 0.63 were achieved at the optimal threshold. These data indicate that FMR4 expression levels had a certain diagnostic value for FXPOI. FMR4 levels above the established threshold conferred a significantly increased risk of developing FXPOI (OR: 6.67 95% CI: 1.5–29.63, $p = 0.016$).

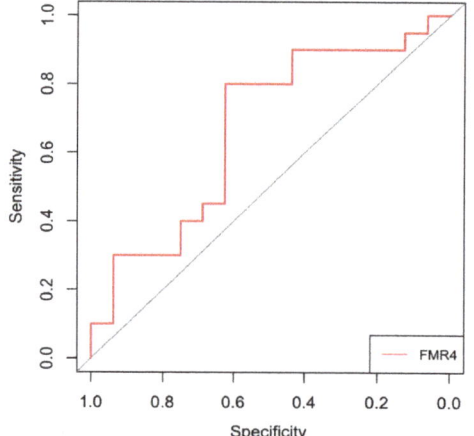

AUC: 0.6688 (95% CI: 0.4818 – 0.8557)

Best threshold: 7.542085

Odds Ratio: 6.67 (1.50 – 29.63); $p = 0.016$

Figure 3. ROC curve for assessment of diagnostic power of FMR4 among total *FMR1* premutation female carriers. The area under the curve (AUC) was 0.67.

3.3. Association of lncRNAs Expression Levels with FMR1 CGG Repeat Size

We evaluated the correlation between the expression levels of the lncRNAs and the CGG repeat size (Figure 4). Expression of FMR4 and FMR5 showed a non-linear distribution, although the association was only statistically significant for FMR4 ($p = 0.037$). The highest levels of FMR4 were detected in women with 80–99 CGG repeats (Figure 4A). For FMR6, as the expression levels showed a wide distribution range, no evidence of an association was inferred ($p = 0.9$) (Figure 4C).

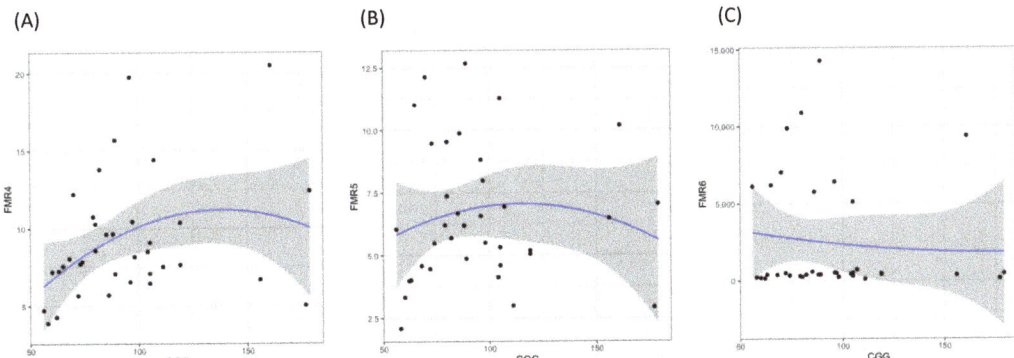

Figure 4. lncRNAs expression level in peripheral blood of *FMR1* premutation carriers according to the number of CGG repeats. (**A**) FMR4 expression levels, (**B**) FMR5 expression levels, and (**C**) FMR6 expression levels.

A multivariate logistic regression analysis was performed to explore whether the correction of FMR4 expression levels for the number of CGG repeats (as a curvilinear confounder) could improve the prediction of FXPOI. Although, the inclusion of both parameters also showed a similar 0.67 AUC, FMR4 expression did not show a significant adjusted odds ratio in the model ($p = 0.15$).

4. Discussion

Little is known about the disease pathology underlying FXPOI. Although the *FMR1* premutation is the major risk factor, there are still some unknown genetic, epigenetic or environmental factors that might be affecting gene penetrance. Current research aims to identify molecular or other biomarkers that can predict the occurrence of FXPOI and help women with the *FMR1* premutation to make decisions regarding their reproductive and family planning. LncRNAs have attracted a lot of attention in recent medical studies since emerging evidence suggests that they could be used as diagnostic biomarkers in many diseases such as cancer [28], cardiovascular or neurodegenerative disorders [29,30]. FMR4, FMR5 and FMR6 comprise a group of *FMR1*-derived lncRNAs which might partake to aspects of the clinical presentation of the Fragile X-associated disorders [21–24]. In fact, it has been described that the expression of these lncRNAs is different in both FXS patients and *FMR1* premutation carriers. In brain tissue from FXS patients both, FMR4 and FMR6 expression have been found to be down-regulated [21,22]. On the other hand, in *FMR1* premutation carriers whereas the FMR4 expression has been described up-regulated [22], the FMR6 expression has been found down-regulated [21].

On the basis of these observations, this study investigated FMR4, FMR5 and FMR6 expression levels in peripheral blood of female *FMR1* premutation carriers with and without FXPOI in order to explore their feasibility as potential biomarkers of FXPOI. For this purpose, the ddPCR technique was used, as it is a highly sensitive and specific method for absolute quantification of transcript gene expression per cell.

The results showed a wide range of expression levels for all three lncRNAs analyzed, leading to a non-significant difference when comparing mean expression levels between female *FMR1* premutation carriers with FXPOI and without FXPOI. We further assessed pairwise correlation between the expression of FMR4, FMR5, FMR6 and *FMR1* mRNA transcripts. Again, no differences were observed when comparing women with FXPOI and without FXPOI; suggesting that pairwise correlations between expressions of these lncRNAs and the *FMR1* gene might not be affected by the presence of FXPOI (Figure 2). However, a statistically significant difference was obtained for FMR4 ($p = 0.039$) when comparing both groups stratified by expression levels (low, medium or high), indicating a disequilibrium in the distribution. Among all the *FMR1* premutation carriers presenting higher FMR4 expression levels, 86% (6/7) developed FXPOI whereas only 29% (1/6) did not. ROC curve analysis revealed that FMR4 can modestly distinguish female *FMR1* premutation carriers with and without FXPOI with an AUC of 0.67. Although caution must be taken due to the limited sample size, our results showed an association between high FMR4 expression levels and FXPOI (OR 6.67, 95% CI = 1.5–29.63, p = 0.016), suggesting that this lncRNA could be a possible marker for FXPOI among female *FMR1* premutation carriers.

To date, only CGG repeat size has been associated with the risk of developing FXPOI in a non-linear way [31–33]; leading to the highest risk for FXPOI in the mid-range of the repeat expansion (~80–99 CGG). Interestingly, our findings, although not statistically significant, also showed a non-linear correlation between the FMR4 and FMR5 expression levels and the *FMR1* repeat size; yielding higher levels of both, FMR4 and FMR5 expression, in the mid-range. This correlation was not detected for FMR6 (Figure 4C). Nevertheless, since FMR6 showed the highest range of expression levels, it cannot be completely discarded. To our knowledge, only Elizur and co-workers [24] have previously analyzed the transcript levels of FMR4 and FMR6 in granulosa cells of *FMR1* premutation carriers in order to determine a putative role in the pathogenesis of FXPOI. Contrary to our results, the authors did not observe any association neither between granulosa cells FMR4 expression levels nor between the number of CGG repeats in the *FMR1* gene. On the other hand, whereas the FMR6 expression levels were not significantly different between *FMR1* permutation carriers and controls, they reported a significant non-linear association between the number of CGG repeats and FMR6 levels in the granulosa cells [24]. Although these results are not in line with ours, it has to be taken into consideration that the methodology and tissue used to measure the lncRNAs levels were different. Whereas Elizur et al. [24] used qRT-PCR and granulosa cells, we used peripheral blood and ddPCR. Moreover, although the sample size was similar in both studies, they compared *FMR1* premutation carriers against controls and we compared *FMR1* premutation carriers with FXPOI against those without FXPOI. Finally, another important difference is that their cohort lack of *FMR1* premutation carriers with *FMR1* repeat size above 150 CGGs, which could somehow bias the results.

Our study, although exploratory, has two main limitations. First, the sample size, which is not large enough to provide reliable evidence for an association between FMR4, FMR5 and FMR6 expression levels and FXPOI. However, our study provides statistically significant results, highlighting a potential role of FMR4 in predicting FXPOI. Second, the age differences between groups and the fact that *FMR1* premutation women with FXPOI had already developed ovarian dysfunction. Thus, it would be necessary to replicate our findings in other female *FMR1* premutation cohorts and, ideally, in a longitudinal study, in order to make sure that age is not affecting lncRNAs expression levels. If validated in other populations, these results might provide evidence of a potential role of FMR4 as a possible biomarker for FXPOI.

Supplementary Materials: The following supporting information can be downloaded at: https://www.mdpi.com/article/10.3390/jcm11082186/s1, Table S1: Expression levels of FMR4, FMR5 and FMR6 measured in peripheral blood of *FMR1* premutation carriers with and without FXPOI.

Author Contributions: M.I.A.-M.: substantial contributions to conception and design, acquisition of data, analysis and interpretation of data. Final approval of the version to be published. I.A.: substantial contributions to conception and design, acquisition of data, or analysis and interpretation of data. Final approval of the version to be published. R.W.: substantial contributions to conception and design, acquisition of data, or analysis and interpretation of data. Final approval of the version to be published. E.M.-B. and T.B.: acquisition, analysis and interpretation of data. Drafting the article and final approval of the version to be published. A.B., S.P., A.G. and M.G.: acquisition, analysis and interpretation of data. Final approval of the version to be published. D.M.: revising the work critically for important intellectual content and final approval of the version to be published. L.R.-R.: drafting the work or revising it critically for important intellectual content and final approval of the version to be published. All authors have read and agreed to the published version of the manuscript.

Funding: This study was supported by Fundación Merck Salud (19-FE-011) and the Instituto de Salud Carlos III (ISCIII) (through the project (PI21/01085), co-funded by the European Union, and AGAUR from the Autonomous Catalan Government (2017SGR1134).

Institutional Review Board Statement: The study was conducted in accordance with the Declaration of Helsinki, and approved by the Institutional Review Board (or Ethics Committee) of the Hospital Clinic Barcelona (protocol code HCB/2021/1030 at 21 January 2022).

Informed Consent Statement: Informed consent was obtained from all subjects involved in the study.

Data Availability Statement: The analyzed data sets generated during the study are available from the corresponding author on reasonable request.

Acknowledgments: We want to thank the Fragile X families, the "Associació Catalana Síndrome X fràgil", and the Federación Española del Síndrome X Frágil for their cooperation. This study was supported by Fundación Merck Salud (19-FE-011), the Instituto de Salud Carlos III (ISCIII) (through the project (PI21/01085), co-funded by the European Union, and AGAUR from the Autonomous Catalan Government (2017SGR1134). The CIBER de Enfermedades Raras is an initiative of the Instituto de Salud Carlos III.

Conflicts of Interest: The authors have no conflict of interest.

References

1. Verkerk, A.J.; Pieretti, M.; Sutcliffe, J.S.; Fu, Y.H.; Kuhl, D.P.; Pizzuti, A.; Reiner, O.; Richards, S.; Victoria, M.F.; Zhang, F.P.; et al. Identification of a gene (FMR-1) containing a CGG repeat coincident with a breakpoint cluster region exhibiting length variation in fragile X syndrome. *Cell* **1991**, *65*, 905–914. [CrossRef]
2. Oberle, I.; Rousseau, F.; Heitz, D.; Kretz, C.; Devys, D.; Hanauer, A.; Boue, J.; Bertheas, M.F.; Mandel, J.L. Instability of a 550-base pair DNA segment and abnormal methylation in fragile X syndrome. *Science* **1991**, *252*, 1097–1102. [CrossRef] [PubMed]
3. Yu, S.; Pritchard, M.; Kremer, E.; Lynch, M.; Nancarrow, J.; Baker, E.; Holman, K.; Mulley, J.C.; Warren, S.T.; Schlessinger, D.; et al. Fragile X genotype characterized by an unstable region of DNA. *Science* **1991**, *252*, 1179–1181. [CrossRef] [PubMed]
4. Sutcliffe, J.S.; Nelson, D.L.; Zhang, F.; Pieretti, M.; Caskey, C.T.; Saxe, D.; Warren, S.T. DNA methylation represses FMR-1 transcription in fragile X syndrome. *Hum. Mol. Genet.* **1992**, *1*, 397–400. [CrossRef] [PubMed]
5. Kenneson, A.; Zhang, F.; Hagedorn, C.H.; Warren, S.T. Reduced FMRP and increased FMR1 transcription is proportionally associated with CGG repeat number in intermediate-length and premutation carriers. *Hum. Mol. Genet.* **2001**, *10*, 1449–1454. [CrossRef] [PubMed]
6. Tassone, F.; Iong, K.P.; Tong, T.H.; Lo, J.; Gane, L.W.; Berry-Kravis, E.; Nguyen, D.; Mu, L.Y.; Laffin, J.; Bailey, D.B.; et al. FMR1 CGG allele size and prevalence ascertained through newborn screening in the United States. *Genome Med.* **2012**, *4*, 100. [CrossRef]
7. Sherman, S.L. Premature ovarian failure in the fragile X syndrome. *Am. J. Med. Genet.* **2000**, *97*, 189–194. [CrossRef]
8. Hagerman, P.J.; Hagerman, R.J. The fragile-X premutation: A maturing perspective. *Am. J. Hum. Genet.* **2004**, *74*, 805–816. [CrossRef]
9. Wheeler, A.C.; Raspa, M.; Green, A.; Bishop, E.; Bann, C.; Edwards, A.; Bailey, D.B., Jr. Health and reproductive experiences of women with an FMR1 premutation with and without fragile X premature ovarian insufficiency. *Front. Genet.* **2014**, *5*, 300. [CrossRef]
10. Rohr, J.; Allen, E.G.; Charen, K.; Giles, J.; He, W.; Dominguez, C.; Sherman, S.L. Anti-Mullerian hormone indicates early ovarian decline in fragile X mental retardation (FMR1) premutation carriers: A preliminary study. *Hum. Reprod.* **2008**, *23*, 1220–1225. [CrossRef]
11. Bibi, G.; Malcov, M.; Yuval, Y.; Reches, A.; Ben-Yosef, D.; Almog, B.; Amit, A.; Azem, F. The effect of CGG repeat number on ovarian response among fragile X premutation carriers undergoing preimplantation genetic diagnosis. *Fertil. Steril.* **2010**, *94*, 869–874. [CrossRef] [PubMed]
12. Allingham-Hawkins, D.J.; Babul-Hirji, R.; Chitayat, D.; Holden, J.J.; Yang, K.T.; Lee, C.; Hudson, R.; Gorwill, R.; Nolin, S.L.; Glicksman, A.; et al. Fragile X premutation is a significant risk factor for premature ovarian failure: The International Collaborative POF in Fragile X study—Preliminary data. *Am. J. Med. Genet.* **1999**, *83*, 322–325. [CrossRef]
13. Mercer, T.R.; Dinger, M.E.; Mattick, J.S. Long non-coding RNAs: Insights into functions. *Nat. Rev. Genet.* **2009**, *10*, 155–159. [CrossRef] [PubMed]
14. Wilusz, J.E.; Sunwoo, H.; Spector, D.L. Long noncoding RNAs: Functional surprises from the RNA world. *Genes. Dev.* **2009**, *23*, 1494–1504. [CrossRef] [PubMed]
15. Derrien, T.; Johnson, R.; Bussotti, G.; Tanzer, A.; Djebali, S.; Tilgner, H.; Guernec, G.; Martin, D.; Merkel, A.; Knowles, D.G.; et al. The GENCODE v7 catalog of human long noncoding RNAs: Analysis of their gene structure, evolution, and expression. *Genome Res.* **2012**, *22*, 1775–1789. [CrossRef]
16. Yao, R.W.; Wang, Y.; Chen, L.L. Cellular functions of long noncoding RNAs. *Nat. Cell Biol.* **2019**, *21*, 542–551. [CrossRef]
17. Wang, K.C.; Chang, H.Y. Molecular mechanisms of long noncoding RNAs. *Mol. Cell* **2011**, *43*, 904–914. [CrossRef]

18. Wapinski, O.; Chang, H.Y. Long noncoding RNAs and human disease. *Trends Cell Biol.* **2011**, *21*, 354–361. [CrossRef]
19. Huang, G.; Zhu, H.; Wu, S.; Cui, M.; Xu, T. Long Noncoding RNA Can Be a Probable Mechanism and a Novel Target for Diagnosis and Therapy in Fragile X Syndrome. *Front. Genet.* **2019**, *10*, 446. [CrossRef]
20. Ladd, P.D.; Smith, L.E.; Rabaia, N.A.; Moore, J.M.; Georges, S.A.; Hansen, R.S.; Hagerman, R.J.; Tassone, F.; Tapscott, S.J.; Filippova, G.N. An antisense transcript spanning the CGG repeat region of FMR1 is upregulated in premutation carriers but silenced in full mutation individuals. *Hum. Mol. Genet.* **2007**, *16*, 3174–3187. [CrossRef]
21. Khalil, A.M.; Faghihi, M.A.; Modarresi, F.; Brothers, S.P.; Wahlestedt, C. A novel RNA transcript with antiapoptotic function is silenced in fragile X syndrome. *PLoS ONE* **2008**, *3*, e1486. [CrossRef] [PubMed]
22. Pastori, C.; Peschansky, V.J.; Barbouth, D.; Mehta, A.; Silva, J.P.; Wahlestedt, C. Comprehensive analysis of the transcriptional landscape of the human FMR1 gene reveals two new long noncoding RNAs differentially expressed in Fragile X syndrome and Fragile X-associated tremor/ataxia syndrome. *Hum. Genet.* **2014**, *133*, 59–67. [CrossRef] [PubMed]
23. Peschansky, V.J.; Pastori, C.; Zeier, Z.; Motti, D.; Wentzel, K.; Velmeshev, D.; Magistri, M.; Bixby, J.L.; Lemmon, V.P.; Silva, J.P.; et al. Changes in expression of the long non-coding RNA FMR4 associate with altered gene expression during differentiation of human neural precursor cells. *Front. Genet.* **2015**, *6*, 263. [CrossRef] [PubMed]
24. Elizur, S.E.; Dratviman-Storobinsky, O.; Derech-Haim, S.; Lebovitz, O.; Dor, J.; Orvieto, R.; Cohen, Y. FMR6 may play a role in the pathogenesis of fragile X-associated premature ovarian insufficiency. *Gynecol. Endocrinol.* **2016**, *32*, 334–337. [CrossRef] [PubMed]
25. Zmienko, A.; Samelak-Czajka, A.; Goralski, M.; Sobieszczuk-Nowicka, E.; Kozlowski, P.; Figlerowicz, M. Selection of Reference Genes for qPCR- And ddPCR-Based Analyses of Gene Expression in Senescing Barley Leaves. *PLoS ONE* **2015**, *10*, e0118226. [CrossRef] [PubMed]
26. Amos-Landgraf, J.M.; Cottle, A.; Plenge, R.M.; Friez, M.; Schwartz, C.E.; Longshore, J.; Willard, H.F. X chromosome-inactivation patterns of 1005 phenotypically unaffected females. *Am. J. Hum. Genet.* **2006**, *79*, 493–499. [CrossRef] [PubMed]
27. Tassone, F.; Hagerman, R.J.; Taylor, A.K.; Gane, L.W.; Godfrey, T.E.; Hagerman, P.J. Elevated levels of FMR1 mRNA in carrier males: A new mechanism of involvement in the fragile-X syndrome. *Am. J. Hum. Genet.* **2000**, *66*, 6–15. [CrossRef]
28. Yan, X.; Hu, Z.; Feng, Y.; Hu, X.; Yuan, J.; Zhao, S.D.; Zhang, Y.; Yang, L.; Shan, W.; He, Q.; et al. Comprehensive Genomic Characterization of Long Non-coding RNAs across Human Cancers. *Cancer Cell* **2015**, *28*, 529–540. [CrossRef]
29. Haemmig, S.; Feinberg, M.W. Targeting LncRNAs in Cardiovascular Disease: Options and Expeditions. *Circ. Res.* **2017**, *120*, 620–623. [CrossRef]
30. Zhang, M.; He, P.; Bian, Z. Long Noncoding RNAs in Neurodegenerative Diseases: Pathogenesis and Potential Implications as Clinical Biomarkers. *Front. Mol. Neurosci.* **2021**, *14*, 685143. [CrossRef]
31. Sullivan, A.K.; Marcus, M.; Epstein, M.P.; Allen, E.G.; Anido, A.E.; Paquin, J.J.; Yadav-Shah, M.; Sherman, S.L. Association of FMR1 repeat size with ovarian dysfunction. *Hum. Reprod.* **2005**, *20*, 402–412. [CrossRef] [PubMed]
32. Ennis, S.; Ward, D.; Murray, A. Nonlinear association between CGG repeat number and age of menopause in FMR1 premutation carriers. *Eur. J. Hum. Genet.* **2006**, *14*, 253–255. [CrossRef] [PubMed]
33. Allen, E.G.; Sullivan, A.K.; Marcus, M.; Small, C.; Dominguez, C.; Epstein, M.P.; Charen, K.; He, W.; Taylor, K.C.; Sherman, S.L. Examination of reproductive aging milestones among women who carry the FMR1 premutation. *Hum. Reprod.* **2007**, *22*, 2142–2152. [CrossRef] [PubMed]

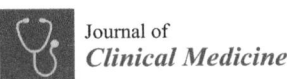

Article

Analysis of Preventable Risk Factors for *Toxoplasma gondii* Infection in Pregnant Women: Case-Control Study

Carlo Bieńkowski [1,2,3,*], Małgorzata Aniszewska [2,3], Monika Kowalczyk [4], Jolanta Popielska [2,3], Konrad Zawadka [2,3], Agnieszka Ołdakowska [2,3] and Maria Pokorska-Śpiewak [2,3]

1. Doctoral School, Medical University of Warsaw, Żwirki i Wigury 61, 02-091 Warsaw, Poland
2. Department of Children's Infectious Diseases, Medical University of Warsaw, Wolska 37, 02-091 Warsaw, Poland; malgorzata.aniszewska@wum.edu.pl (M.A.); jolanta.popielska@wum.edu.pl (J.P.); konrad.zawadka@wum.edu.pl (K.Z.); agnieszka.oldakowska@wum.edu.pl (A.O.); mpspiewak@gmail.com (M.P.-Ś.)
3. Hospital of Infectious Diseases, 01-201 Warsaw, Poland
4. Department of Epidemiology of Infectious Diseases and Surveillance, National Institute of Public Health NIH—National Research Institute, 00-791 Warsaw, Poland; mkkowalczyk1@gmail.com
* Correspondence: carlo.bienkowski@gmail.com

Abstract: Background: *Toxoplasma gondii* (TG) is a parasitic protozoon that may cause miscarriages or birth defects if the infection occurs during pregnancy. The study's aim was to evaluate the risk factors associated with TG infection in pregnant women. Materials: Medical charts for all 273 pregnant women with suspected TG infection consecutively admitted to the Hospital of Warsaw between 2019 and 2020 were retrospectively analyzed. The presumptive TG diagnosis was verified by a serologic assessment of IgM and IgG titers, and IgG affinity tests. Results: The median age was 32 years (range: 19–42 years). The diagnosis of primary TG infection was confirmed in 74/273 (27.1%) women. In 114/273 (41.8%) there was evidence of past infection. In 71/273 (26%) women, an infection was excluded. In 172/273 (62%) women the recommended testing for other infectious diseases putting fetus development at risk was performed correctly. Logistic regression model analysis revealed that living in rural areas and eating raw meat were independent factors associated with increased risk of TG infection during pregnancy (OR 2.89, 95% CI: 1.42–5.9, $p = 0.004$; and OR 2.07, 95% CI: 1.03–4.18, $p = 0.04$, respectively). Conclusions: The independent risk factors for TG infection during pregnancy include living in rural areas and eating raw meat. The physician's educational role here is crucial for the efficient prevention of congenital toxoplasmosis.

Keywords: toxoplasmosis; pregnancy; congenital infection; zoonosis

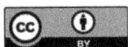

1. Introduction

Toxoplasma gondii (TG) is a parasitic protozoon. Its life cycle includes sexual reproduction in the final hosts (felids), where epithelial cells of the small intestine are infected; following the infestation, oocysts are then excreted with the feces [1]. Under appropriate environmental conditions, oocysts transform into sporocysts and can maintain their invasive potential even for several years. Vegetative reproduction takes place in intermediate hosts (humans, other mammals, and birds) where TG is spread by lymphatic and blood vessels (in monocytes and granulocytes) to distant organs and tissues. Tachyzoites form in large numbers and destroy the host cells, and then, in people with properly functioning immune systems, they are converted into resting forms—tissue cysts [2,3].

The two major routes of infection in humans include oral (via contaminated meat, hands, soil, cat feces) and transplacental transmission, resulting in acquired or congenital infection, respectively. Rare instances of transmission include organ transplant recipients who get infected by receiving organs from *Toxoplasma*-positive donors. The incidence of congenital toxoplasmosis is estimated at 1–4/1000 newborns [4].

The course of the infection in adults is usually asymptomatic or mild. However, it may pose a risk for the fetus's development of abnormalities if a pregnant woman becomes infected. The risk of transplacental infection increases with the duration of pregnancy. However, the consequences for the fetus are most severe when an infestation occurs during the first months of pregnancy. In the first trimester, the probability of TG transmission is lowest and estimated at 17–25%, however, if the parasite is transmitted, this often leads to miscarriage [4]. In the second and third trimesters of pregnancy, the likelihood of tachyzoites infesting the fetus increases (25–50% and 60–90%, respectively), and as a consequence, severe abnormalities, such as hydrocephalus, intracerebral calcification or sight damage may occur [4].

The aim of this study was to evaluate the potential risk factors associated with TG infection in pregnant women.

2. Material and Methods

The authors retrospectively analyzed the medical charts of all pregnant women, referred by their gynecologists to the Regional Hospital of Infectious Diseases in Warsaw due to suspected TG infection (based on a positive serologic assessment of anti-TG antibody titers) between 1 September 2019 and 14 March 2020. All patients in the above category referred to the hospital within these dates, in the order they were referred, were included in the study. The final study group consisted of women with a confirmed primary *Toxoplasma gondii* infection, while the control group consisted of women for whom the infection had been excluded. Women with evidence of past infection and women with inconclusive results were excluded from the final analysis.

The analysis included anamnesis data on potential risk factors for TG infection, such as age, socioeconomic status, history of miscarriage, caring for domestic and/or wild cats currently or in the past, long-distance travels, gardening without gloves, eating unwashed vegetables, or eating raw meat currently or in the past. In addition, implementation of screening testing towards other infections, including human immunodeficiency virus (HIV), hepatitis B virus (HBV), hepatitis C virus (HCV), cytomegalovirus (CMV), syphilis, and rubella were also included in the analysis. The presumptive diagnosis of TG infection was verified by a serologic assessment of immunoglobulin M (IgM) and immunoglobulin G (IgG) titers, and IgG affinity tests using Enzyme-Linked Fluorescent Assay (ELFA) by VIDAS® (bioMérieux, Lyon, France). The diagnostic algorithm for TG infection evaluation is presented in Figure 1.

An infection was excluded when both IgM and IgG antibody titers were negative. When IgM was positive and IgG negative, a primary infection was possible and another assessment was needed after 1–3 weeks. When both IgM and IgG were positive, an infection was suspected and an IgG affinity assessment was required. When IgM was negative and IgG positive, an infection had possibly occurred in the past, and an IgG affinity assessment was necessary. Low affinity indicated a primary infection, high affinity revealed an infection that had occurred in the past, while other results needed had to be reassessed. All women diagnosed with toxoplasmosis were referred for amniocentesis, but as no further observation was performed, there were no data confirming the congenital toxoplasmosis. The testing scheme for vertical infections was considered correctly implemented if the first testing towards toxoplasmosis, rubella, HIV, HCV, and syphilis were performed before the tenth week of gestation. If the first tests for TG were negative, reassessment was recommended between the twenty-first and twenty-sixth week of gestation. Moreover, testing for HBV and HIV was recommended between the thirty-third and thirty-seventh week of gestation (Table 1).

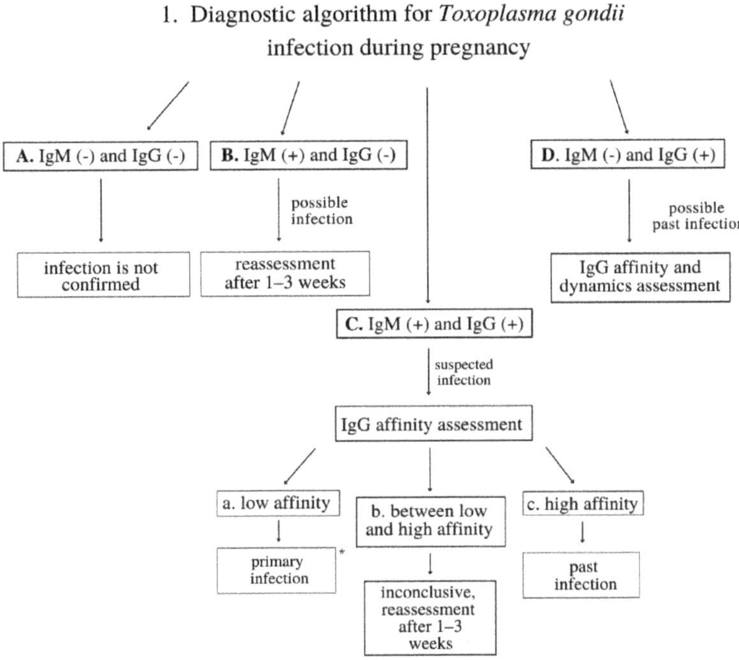

1. Diagnostic algorithm for *Toxoplasma gondii* infection during pregnancy

```
        ┌──────────────────┬─────────────────────┬──────────────────────┐
        │                  │                     │                      │
A. IgM (-) and IgG (-)   B. IgM (+) and IgG (-)              D. IgM (-) and IgG (+)
        │                  │                                            │
        │            possible infection                            possible past infection
        │                  │                                            │
infection is not      reassessment                               IgG affinity and
  confirmed          after 1–3 weeks                            dynamics assessment

                    C. IgM (+) and IgG (+)
                            │
                      suspected infection
                            │
                    IgG affinity assessment
            ┌───────────────┼────────────────┐
      a. low affinity   b. between low    c. high affinity
            │           and high affinity       │
        primary            │                 past
       infection      inconclusive,        infection
                      reassessment
                      after 1–3 weeks
```

Figure 1. The diagnostic algorithm for *Toxoplasma gondii* infection during pregnancy. * All women diagnosed with toxoplasmosis were referred for amniocentesis, but no further observation was carried out.

Table 1. Recommendations concerning diagnostic testing for infectious diseases during pregnancy according to the Polish Journal of Laws.

Examination Date	Diagnostic Tests
Up to the 10th week of gestation or at the time of first reporting	1. VDRL test. * 2. Human immunodeficiency virus (HIV) and Hepatitis C virus (HCV) testing. 3. Testing for toxoplasmosis (IgG **, IgM ***) unless the pregnant woman shows a result confirming the presence of IgG antibodies from before pregnancy. 4. Rubella test (IgG, IgM), if the pregnant woman has not been ill or has not been vaccinated or in the absence of information.
Week 21–26th of gestation	1. In women with negative results in the first trimester—testing for toxoplasmosis (IgM).
Week 33–37th of gestation	1. Testing the HBs **** antigen presence. 2. HIV testing. 3. Vaginal and rectal culture for B-hemolytic streptococci (weeks 35–37 of gestation). 4. VDRL and HCV studies in a group of women with an increased risk of infection.

* VDRL—venereal disease research laboratory (testing for syphilis); ** IgG—immunoglobulin G; *** IgM—immunoglobulin M; **** HBs—hepatitis B virus antigen.

3. Statistical Analysis

The normality of continuous variables was tested using the Shapiro–Wilk's test. The Mann–Whitney U test was used to compare continuous variables and the Chi^2 test was used to evaluate categorical variables. A p-value of <0.05 was considered significant. Multivariate analysis was performed using a logistic regression model, where candidate predictors were entered into the model irrespective of the results of the univariate analysis. After entering all variables into the model, the variables that showed the least significant associations were subsequently excluded until all variables remained significant ($p < 0.05$). Statistical analysis was performed with Medcalc ver. 20.009, Ostend, Belgium.

Ethical Statement

The design of the work conforms to standards currently applied in the Medical University of Warsaw's Bioethics Committee. Approval number: AKBE/132/2021.

4. Results

The medical records of 273 pregnant women with suspected TG infections were analyzed. The median age was 32 years (range: 19–42 years). In 119/273 (43.6%) of the participants, the place of residence was in a rural area, 44/273 (16.1%) had a history of miscarriage, and 21/273 (7.7%) had a history of long-distance travel. Chronic diseases were reported in 69/273 (25.3%) of pregnant women and 53/273 (19.4%) had autoimmune diseases.

Women with confirmed toxoplasmosis were younger than the women in the control group (28 years (IQR: 24–32 years) vs. 32 years (IQR 29–35 years), $p < 0.001$). Moreover, women with a TG infection were more likely to live in rural areas (55.4% vs. 28.2%, $p < 0.001$), more often ate raw meat before their pregnancy (58.1% vs. 38.0%, $p = 0.016$), and more often gave care to cats during pregnancy (35.1% vs. 16.9%, $p = 0.01$) (Table 2). Multivariate logistic regression revealed that living in a rural area (OR 2.89, 95% CI 1.42–5.9, $p = 0.004$), and eating raw meat (OR 2.07, 95% CI: 1.03–4.18, $p = 0.04$) were independent risk factors for TG infection during pregnancy (Table 3).

Table 2. Baseline characteristics and clinical data on women with a confirmed diagnosis of primary toxoplasmosis compared to the control group of women where the infection was excluded.

Characteristic	Total $n = 273$	TG+ * $n = 74$	TG− ** $n = 71$	*p*-Value
Age in years, median (IQR) ****	30 (26–33)	28 (24–32)	32 (29–35)	<0.001
Living in rural areas, *n* (%)	119 (43.6)	41 (55.4)	20 (28.2)	<0.001
History of miscarriage, *n* (%)	44 (16.1)	12 (16.2)	15 (21.1)	0.45
Good socioeconomic status, *n* (%)	267 (97.8)	72 (97.3)	71 (100)	0.58
Long-distance travels, *n* (%)	21 (7.7)	4 (5.4)	5 (7)	0.68
Chronic diseases, *n* (%)	69 (25.3)	20 (27)	22 (31)	0.6
Autoimmune diseases, *n* (%)	53 (19.4)	15 (20.3)	18 (25.4)	0.5
Gardening without gloves, *n* (%)	29 (10.6)	7 (9.5)	2 (2.8)	0.1
Eating habits				
• unwashed vegetables, *n* (%)	34 (12.5)	7 (9.5)	4 (5.6)	0.38
• raw meat before pregnancy, *n* (%)	150 (55)	43 (58.1)	27 (38)	0.016
• raw meat during pregnancy, *n* (%)	55 (20.1)	17 (23)	9 (12.7)	0.1
Caring for cats				
• during pregnancy, *n* (%)	91 (33.3)	26 (35.1)	12 (16.9)	0.01
• in the past, *n* (%)	106 (38.8)	30 (40.5)	19 (26.8)	0.08
• domestic cats, *n* (%)	96 (35.2)	25 (33.8)	13 (18.3)	0.03
• wild cats, *n* (%)	80 (29.3)	23 (31.1)	12 (16.9)	0.046
Correctly implemented testing for other infectious diseases ***, *n* (%)	172 (63)	45 (60.8)	51 (71.8)	0.16
Clinical evaluation				
Correct ultrasound result, *n* (%)	251 (91.9)	68 (91.9)	66 (93)	0.8
Lymphadenopathy, *n* (%)	14 (5.1)	6 (8.1)	2 (2.8)	0.16
Influenza-like symptoms, *n* (%)	35 (12.8)	12 (16.2)	8 (11.3)	0.4
Both lymphadenopathy and influenza-like symptoms, *n* (%)	41 (15)	4 (5.4)	1 (1.4)	0.19

* TG+—primary toxoplasmosis; ** TG−—excluded toxoplasmosis.; *** Women who had been correctly tested according to Polish recommendations (presented in Table 1). **** IQR—interquartile range.

Table 3. Univariate and Multivariate logistic regression analyses of factors associated with primary *Toxoplasma gondii* infection.

Factor	Odds Ratio	Univariate 95% Confidence Interval	p-Value	Odds Ratio	Multivariate 95% Confidence Interval	p-Value
Living in rural areas	3.17	1.59–6.32	0.001	2.89	1.42–5.90	0.004
Eating raw meat	2.25	1.59–4.38	0.017	2.07	1.03–4.18	0.04
Caring for wild cats	2.22	1.00–4.90	0.049	1.72	0.72–4.10	0.22
Caring for domestic cats	2.27	1.05–4.92	0.03	1.83	0.79–4.27	0.16

Data are presented as odds ratio (95% CI), *p*-value. Candidate predictors were entered into the model irrespective of the results of the univariate analysis. After entering all variables into the model, the variables that showed least significant associations were subsequently excluded until all variables remained significant ($p < 0.05$).

The diagnosis of primary TG infection was confirmed in 74/273 (27.1%) women, who were then treated with spiramycin. In 114/273 (41.8%) women, there was evidence of past infection. In 71/273 (26%) women, infection was excluded. The remaining women (14/273, 5.1%) had inconclusive results, and reassessment was recommended.

The clinical evaluation of the pregnant women did not reveal any significant differences between women with confirmed TG infection when compared to the control group regarding fetal ultrasound results (91.9% vs. 93%, $p = 0.8$), and the presence of lymphadenopathy (8.1% vs. 2.8%, $p = 0.16$), the presence of influenza-like symptoms (16.2% vs. 11.3%, $p = 0.4$), or both symptoms combined together (5.4% vs. 1.4%, $p = 0.19$).

In 172/273 (62%) women, the recommended testing procedures for other infectious diseases dangerous for the fetus's development were carried out correctly.

5. Discussion

The risk of transplacental TG infection increases with the duration of pregnancy. However, the consequences for the fetus are most severe when an infestation occurs in the first months of pregnancy. Therefore, knowledge about TG risk factors seems to have an influence on the prevention of TG infection during pregnancy [3]. However, Serdarian et al., who analyzed 653 pregnant women with IgG detected in their serum and the B1 gene of *T. gondii* found in their placental tissue using a nested-PCR assay, concluded that the detection of the B1 gene in placental tissues of the healthy newborn infants reiterates that the presence of *T. gondii* in the placenta does not always result in congenital toxoplasmosis [5].

Ferguson et al. investigated a cohort of mothers who vertically infected their children, and they revealed that 73% of the women lacked knowledge concerning the risk factors for TG infection or its potential threat to the fetus [6]. Therefore, the analysis of preventable risk factors for TG infection during pregnancy seems to be important in this matter. As in our cohort, dwelling place and eating habits increased the risk of infection during pregnancy by 2.89 times and 2.07 times, respectively.

Awareness of local seroprevalence trends, particularly in the women of childbearing age, may allow proper public health policies to be applied, targeting, in particular, seronegative women of childbearing age in high seroprevalence areas [7]. Rostami et al., in their meta-analysis, investigated geo-climatic factors and the prevalence of chronic toxoplasmosis in pregnant women. They concluded that different regions of the world may benefit from different types of interventions, and thus, novel preventive measures for a region should be developed according to local climate, agricultural activities, and the peoples' cultural attitudes [8]. However, no studies to date have included living in rural areas as a potential risk factor for TG infection.

In our analysis, older women were more likely to have a TG infection excluded (they were seronegative), which is contrary to results obtained by Fanigiulio et al., where seropositivity was more common in older women [9]. Further analyses in this matter are needed.

Tarekegn et al., in a systematic review and meta-analysis of the potential risk factors associated with seropositivity for TG among pregnant women and HIV-infected individuals, analyzed 24 reports, which included 6003 individuals (4356 pregnant women and 1647 HIV-infected individuals). They concluded that a significant overall effect of anti-*Toxoplasma gondii* seropositivity among pregnant women ($p < 0.05$) was associated with age, abortion history, contact with cats, cat ownership, having knowledge about toxoplasmosis, being a housewife, and having unsafe water sources [10].

In our analysis, the factors that independently increase TG infection risk among the population of pregnant women in our region include living in rural areas and eating raw meat. Living in the countryside may be influenced by a lot of factors and may be difficult to change. However, avoiding raw meat in the daily diet can be implemented by women planning a pregnancy or while pregnant.

Cerro et al. investigated the seroprevalence of TG among cats in Peru and revealed that it is associated with a cat's eating habits. Those fed with raw meat were more exposed compared to those fed with commercial cat food ($chi^2 = 9.50, p = 0.004$) or with homemade food ($chi^2 = 4.1, p = 0.027$) [11]. In our study, caring for cats was significantly associated with TG infection during pregnancy, but there was no difference between domestic cats and wild cats. Hence, we cannot be certain of these cats' eating habits. Moreover, Cerro et al. showed that 88% of cats were diagnosed with the chronic phase of TG infection; [11] therefore, every unknown cat, whether living at home or outdoors, poses a potential threat to previously uninfected women from TG infection.

Wei et al., in their systematic review and meta-analysis of the efficacy of anti-TG medicines in humans, concluded that the risk of vertical transmission of TG was approximately 9.9% when the infected mother received the necessary treatment with spiramycin alone or combined with pyrimethamine-sulfadiazine, against *T. gondii* [12]. However, Thiebaut et al., in their meta-analysis of the effectiveness of prenatal treatment for congenital toxoplasmosis, found only weak evidence of an association between early treatment and a reduced risk of congenital toxoplasmosis [13]. In addition, we revealed that 74/273 (27.1%) participants in our cohort had their diagnoses confirmed, and they were treated accordingly (with spiramycin). However, we lost the patients to follow-up (our hospital was transformed into a COVID-19-only hospital), therefore, we could not perform further analysis on the treatment's efficacy.

Wallon et al. proved that introducing monthly prenatal screening and improving antenatal diagnosis was associated with a significant reduction in the rate of congenital infection [14]. In our study, only 62% of women had the recommended testing scheme carried out correctly, which included performing tests for TG according to the Polish recommendations presented in Table 1.

The limitations of our study include a non-detailed differentiation of potential risk factors for TG infection, and there are no time frames for the occurrence of some of the risk factors. The data were collected from medical records retrospectively, and the medical records were prepared by more than one physician. However, for finding a cause and effect relationship between TG infection during pregnancy and its risk factors, a case-control study is methodologically justified.

To conclude, the independent risk factors for TG infection in pregnancy in our region include living in rural areas and eating raw meat. Twenty-six percent of women who were suspected of having toxoplasmosis by their gynecologists were not infected. Only 62% of women had the recommended testing scheme carried out correctly. The educational role of a physician in these matters is crucial for the effective prevention of congenital toxoplasmosis. Further studies are recommended to deepen the analysis of important risk factors for TG during pregnancy in order to support the development of more cost-effective preventive strategies.

Author Contributions: Conceptualization, C.B., M.A. and M.P.-Ś., Methodology, C.B., M.P.-Ś., Software, C.B. and M.P.-Ś., Validation, C.B., M.A. and M.P.-Ś., Formal analysis, C.B. and M.P.-Ś., Investigation, C.B., M.A., M.K., J.P., K.Z., A.O. and M.P.-Ś., Resources, C.B., M.A., M.K., J.P., K.Z., A.O. and M.P.-Ś., Data curation C.B., M.A. and M.P.-Ś., Writing—original draft preparation, C.B. and M.P.-Ś., Writing—review and editing, C.B. and M.P.-Ś., Visualization, C.B., M.K. and M.P.-Ś., Supervision, M.P.-Ś., Project administration, C.B. and M.P.-Ś. All authors have read and agreed to the published version of the manuscript.

Funding: This research received no external funding.

Institutional Review Board Statement: Approval number: AKBE/132/2021.

Informed Consent Statement: Not applicable.

Data Availability Statement: Available on reasonable request to the Corresponding Author.

Conflicts of Interest: The authors declare no conflict of interest.

References

1. Saadatnia, G.; Golkar, M. A review on human toxoplasmosis. *Scand. J. Infect. Dis.* **2012**, *44*, 805–814. [CrossRef] [PubMed]
2. Centers for Disease Control and Prevention, Toxoplasma Gondii Life Cycle. Available online: https://www.cdc.gov/parasites/toxoplasmosis/biology.html (accessed on 25 October 2021).
3. Chaudhry, S.A.; Gad, N.; Koren, G. Toxoplasmosis and pregnancy. *Can. Fam. Physician* **2014**, *60*, 334–336. [PubMed]
4. Drapała, D. Diagnosis of toxoplasmosis in a pregnant woman, fetus and infant—Current study and new possibilities. *Forum Med. Rodz.* **2013**, *7*, 176–184.
5. Sardarian, K.; Maghsood, A.H.; Farimani, M.; Hajiloii, M.; Saidijam, M.; Farahpour, M.; Mahaki, H.; Zamani, A. Detection of Toxoplasma gondii B1 gene in placenta does not prove congenital toxoplasmosis. *Hum. Antibodies* **2019**, *27*, 31–35. [CrossRef] [PubMed]
6. Ferguson, W.; Mayne, P.D.; Cafferkey, M.; Butler, K. Lack of awareness of risk factors for primary toxoplasmosis in pregnancy. *Ir. J. Med. Sci.* **2011**, *180*, 807–811. [CrossRef] [PubMed]
7. Pappas, G.; Roussos, N.; Falagas, M.E. Toxoplasmosis snapshots: Global status of Toxoplasma gondii seroprevalence and implications for pregnancy and congenital toxoplasmosis. *Int. J. Parasitol.* **2009**, *39*, 1385–1394. [CrossRef] [PubMed]
8. Rostami, A.; Riahi, S.M.; Gamble, H.R.; Fakhri, Y.; Shiadeh, M.N.; Danesh, M.; Behniafar, H.; Paktinat, S.; Foroutan, M.; Mokdad, A.H.; et al. Global prevalence of latent toxoplasmosis in pregnant women: A systematic review and meta-analysis. *Clin. Microbiol. Infect.* **2020**, *26*, 673–683. [CrossRef] [PubMed]
9. Fanigliulo, D.; Marchi, S.; Montomoli, E.; Trombetta, C.M. Toxoplasma gondii in women of childbearing age and during pregnancy: Seroprevalence study in Central and Southern Italy from 2013 to 2017. *Parasite* **2020**, *27*, 2. [CrossRef] [PubMed]
10. Tarekegn, Z.S.; Dejene, H.; Addisu, A.; Dagnachew, S. Potential risk factors associated with seropositivity for Toxoplasma gondii among pregnant women and HIV infected individuals in Ethiopia: A systematic review and meta-analysis. *PLoS Neglected Trop. Dis.* **2020**, *14*, e0008944. [CrossRef] [PubMed]
11. Cerro, L.; Rubio, A.; Pinedo, R.; Mendes-De-Almeida, F.; Brener, B.; Labarthe, N. Seroprevalence of Toxoplasma gondii in cats (Felis catus, Linnaeus 1758) living in Lima, Peru. *Rev. Bras. Parasitol. Vet.* **2014**, *23*, 90–93. [CrossRef] [PubMed]
12. Wei, H.-X.; Wei, S.-S.; Lindsay, D.S.; Peng, H.-J. A Systematic Review and Meta-Analysis of the Efficacy of Anti-Toxoplasma gondii Medicines in Humans. *PLoS ONE* **2015**, *10*, e0138204. [CrossRef] [PubMed]
13. Thiebaut, R.; Leproust, S.; Chene, G.; Gilbert, R. Effectiveness of prenatal treatment for congenital toxoplasmosis: A meta-analysis of individual patients' data. *Lancet* **2007**, *369*, 115–122. [CrossRef] [PubMed]
14. Wallon, M.; Peyron, F.; Cornu, C.; Vinault, S.; Abrahamowicz, M.; Kopp, C.B.; Binquet, C. CongenitalToxoplasmaInfection: Monthly Prenatal Screening Decreases Transmission Rate and Improves Clinical Outcome at Age 3 Years. *Clin. Infect. Dis.* **2013**, *56*, 1223–1231. [CrossRef] [PubMed]

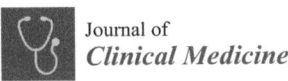 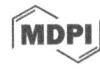

Review

Ultrasound Markers for Complex Gastroschisis: A Systematic Review and Meta-Analysis

Rui Gilberto Ferreira [1,2,*], Carolina Rodrigues Mendonça [1], Carolina Leão de Moraes [1], Fernanda Sardinha de Abreu Tacon [1], Lelia Luanne Gonçalves Ramos [3], Natalia Cruz e Melo [4], Lourenço Sbragia [5], Waldemar Naves do Amaral [1] and Rodrigo Ruano [6,*]

1. Postgraduate Program in Health Sciences, Universidade Federal de Goiás, Goiânia 74650-050, GO, Brazil; carol_mendonca85@hotmail.com (C.R.M.); carolina.leao.moraes@gmail.com (C.L.d.M.); fernandabreu2010@yahoo.com.br (F.S.d.A.T.); dr@waldemar.med.br (W.N.d.A.)
2. Department of Obstetrics and Gynaecology, Hospital das Clínicas, Universidade Federal de Goiás, Goiânia 74605-020, GO, Brazil
3. Hospital das Clínicas, Universidade Federal de Goiás, Goiânia 74605-020, GO, Brazil; leliabiomed@gmail.com
4. Departamento de Ginecologia, Universidade de São Paulo, São Paulo 04024-002, SP, Brazil; cruz.melo20@gmail.com
5. Division of Pediatric Surgery, Department of Surgery and Anatomy, Ribeirão Preto Medical School, University of Sao Paulo (USP), Ribeirão Preto 14049-900, SP, Brazil; sbragia@fmrp.usp.br
6. Division of Maternal-Fetal Medicine, Department of Obstetrics, Gynecology and Reproductive Sciences, University of Texas Health Science Center Houston (UTHealth), Houston 77030, TX, USA
* Correspondence: dr.ruigilberto@gmail.com (R.G.F.); rodrigoruano@hotmail.com (R.R.)

Abstract: Although gastroschisis is often diagnosed by prenatal ultrasound, there is still a gap in the literature about which prenatal ultrasound markers can predict complex gastroschisis. This systematic review and meta-analysis aimed to investigate the ultrasound markers that characterize complex gastroschisis. A systematic review of the literature was conducted according to the guidelines of PRISMA. The protocol was registered (PROSPERO ID CRD42020211685). Meta-analysis was displayed graphically on Forest plots, which estimate prevalence rates and risk ratios, with 95% confidence intervals, using STATA version 15.0. The combined prevalence of intestinal complications in fetuses with complex gastroschisis was 27.0%, with a higher prevalence of atresia (about 48%), followed by necrosis (about 25%). The prevalence of deaths in newborns with complex gastroschisis was 15.0%. The predictive ultrasound markers for complex gastroschisis were intraabdominal bowel dilatation (IABD) (RR 3.01, 95% CI 2.22 to 4.07; I^2 = 15.7%), extra-abdominal bowel dilatation (EABD) (RR 1.55, 95% CI 1.01 to 2.39; I^2 = 77.1%), and polyhydramnios (RR 3.81, 95% CI 2.09 to 6.95; I^2 = 0.0%). This review identified that IABD, EABD, and polyhydramnios were considered predictive ultrasound markers for complex gastroschisis. However, evidence regarding gestational age at the time of diagnosis is needed.

Keywords: gastroschisis; prenatal diagnosis; ultrasound; congenital anomalies; fetal surgery; fetal intervention

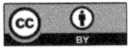

1. Introduction

Gastroschisis (GS) is an abdominal wall defect diagnosed in prenatal care in more than 90% of cases [1,2]. The diagnosis is usually made by ultrasound in the second trimester of pregnancy to detect floating intestinal loops in the uterine cavity [2]. Gastroschisis can be simple GS or complex GS and the intestinal condition at birth is an important prognostic factor for neonatal comorbidities [3,4]. The two types are differentiated due to the presence of complications in the gastrointestinal area that occurs in complex GS [3].

Complex GS is defined by the presence of congenital intestinal atresia, necrosis, stenosis, perforation, or volvulus [5,6]. Often, more than one complication coexists [5]. Newborns with complex GS stay longer in the hospital, are more likely to be discharged from the hospital with enteral tube feeding and parenteral nutrition, have more morbidities, and mortality is almost 7.6 times higher than in those with simple GS [7].

Although GS is often diagnosed from prenatal ultrasound (US) [8], attempts have been made to correlate US findings with neonatal outcomes in pregnancies with fetal GS [4,9]. However, there is still a gap in the literature about which markers of prenatal US can differentiate complex GS and predict adverse results [10]. Therefore, the objective of this systematic review and meta-analysis is to investigate the ultrasound markers that characterize complex GS and can assist in screening, prenatal counseling, and medical treatment in order to minimize postnatal complications of complex GS.

2. Materials and Methods

This systematic review was carried out according to the guidelines of the Preferred Reporting Items for Systematic Reviews and Meta-Analyzes—PRISMA [11] and was registered with the International Prospective Register of Systematic Reviews (PROSPERO) (protocol number: CRD42020211685). No ethical approval or patient consent was required.

2.1. Data Sources and Research

The electronic search was carried out in December 2020 in the CINAHL, Embase, and MEDLINE/PubMed databases. Reference lists of eligible studies were also searched, and authors were contacted to obtain unpublished data. The search terms were: (Gastroschisis OR Complex Gastroschisis OR Vanishing gastroschisis) AND (Ultrasound Markers OR Markers ultrasonography OR Sonographic Markers).

All stages of screening the articles were carried out using the Rayyan software [12], which allows a quick exploration and filtering of the eligible studies. The analysis of titles and abstracts was carried out by two researchers independently and the disagreements were resolved by a third researcher. The full reading was performed by two researchers independently. The research was limited to studies carried out in humans.

The criteria to include the patients and studies in the present systematic review were: (1) pregnant women in any gestational week; (2) fetuses with an ultrasound diagnosis of complex GS; (3) studies that reported on ultrasound markers to detect structural anomalies; (4) observational and intervention studies; (5) articles in English; (6) no restriction regarding the year of publication. The presence of intestinal atresia, stenosis, volvulus, necrosis, or intestinal perforation at birth was defined as complex GS [6]. The exclusion criteria were as follows: the use of markers other than ultrasound, studies that did not differentiate simple GS from complex GS in the results of ultrasound markers, case reports or reviews on the diagnosis of complex GS, conference abstracts, experimental research, or in vitro studies.

After reading the studies (manuscripts) in full, the following data were collected: authors and year of publication, study design, country where the study was conducted, sample size, age, gestational age at the time of delivery, ultrasound markers, and outcomes. The variables investigated for ultrasound markers were intraabdominal bowel dilatation (IABD), extra-abdominal bowel dilatation (EABD), intrauterine growth restriction, polyhydramnios, intestinal wall thickness, bowel dilatation, liver and bladder herniation, delta dilatation and final bowel dilatation, abdominal circumference, herniation, dilation of the stomach, size, and position of stomach, size of the abdominal wall defect, description of mesenteric circulation, collapsed extra-abdominal bowel, description of peristalsis and volvulus.

2.2. Bias Risk and Quality Assessment

The risk of bias assessment was analyzed using the tool "A Cochrane Risk of Bias Assessment Tool for Non-Randomized Studies" [13] using the ROBINS-I software [14]. Eight methodological domains were evaluated: (1) bias due to confounding, (2) bias in selection of participants into the study, (3) bias in measurement of interventions, (4) bias due to departures from intended interventions, (5) bias due to missing data, (6) bias in measurement of outcomes, (7) bias in selection of the reported result, and (8) overall bias.

Each domain was assigned a "low risk of bias", "moderate risk of bias", "serious risk of bias", and "critical risk of bias" judgment.

The quality of the studies was assessed using the Grading of Recommendations, Assessment, Development, and Evaluations (GRADE) [15]. The quality of the study's evidence was classified into four categories: high, moderate, low, or very low [15,16].

2.3. Statistical Analysis

Meta-analysis was conducted using the random-effects model on coded data stratified by complex GS characteristics, mortality rate, complex GS ultrasound markers, and comparison of ultrasound markers in SCG and complex GS. The data were displayed graphically in Forest plots, which estimate prevalence rates and risk ratios, with 95% confidence intervals (CI). The statistical values I^2 were calculated to quantify the degree of heterogeneity between studies, where values of 25–50% represented moderate heterogeneity and values of >50% great heterogeneity between studies [17]. Publication bias was assessed using the Egger test. All analyzes were conducted using STATA version 15.0 (StataCorp, College Station, TX, USA).

3. Results

3.1. Search Results

The initial search identified 238 articles. After excluding duplicate articles ($n = 35$), the titles and abstracts of 204 articles were read. Of these, 18 were selected for full reading. A total of 13 articles met the inclusion criteria [1,3,6,8,9,18–25]. The study selection flowchart is shown in Figure 1.

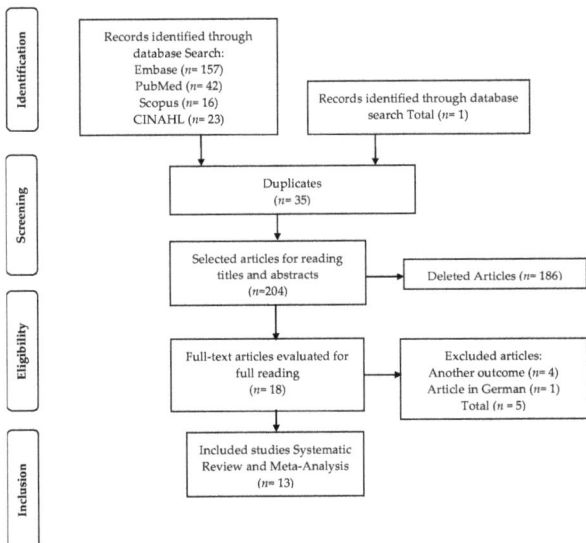

Figure 1. Flowchart of study selection.

3.2. General Characteristics

The 13 studies that met the inclusion criteria involved a total of 1440 fetuses with GS, with 274 fetuses (19.02%) with complex GS. The average weight of fetuses with complex GS was 2341 g. The average maternal age was 23.8 years, and the average gestational age at delivery was 35.5 weeks. Details on the characteristics of the studies are presented in Table 1 and Table S1.

Table 1. Characteristics of studies included in the systematic review.

Author, Year	Country	Study Design	Sample Size	Fetuses Complex Gs (n) Birth Weight, G	Gestational Age At Delivery, Weeks	Complex Gastroschisis	Diagnostic	Mean Age Of Mother (Years)	Mortality Rate	Risk Of Bias (GRADE)
Andrade et al., 2019 [18]	UK	Retrospective cohort study January 2005 and December 2018	n = 174	n = 39 (22.4%) complex GS. 2240 (2041–2678) g	35.7 (34.8–37.0)	NR	Ultrasound	20 (19.0–24.0)	17.9% (7/39)	⊕⊕⊕◯ Moderate
Andrade et al., 2018 [19]	Brazil	Retrospective cohort study January 2005 and December 2015	n = 186	n = 30 (16.1%) complex GS. 2357 ± 461 g	36.1 ± 1.5	Atresia 18/30 (60%) Necrosis 13/30 (43.3%) Perforation 8/30 (26.6%) Volvulus 3/30 (10%) Stenosis 1/30 (3.3%)	Ultrasound	20.98 ± 4.2	13.4% (25/186)	⊕⊕⊕◯ Moderate
Dewberry et al., 2020 [20]	USA	Retrospective cohort study 2007 to 2017	n = 55	n = 16 complex GS. 2300 g	36 (35–37)	Atresia 6/16 (37.5%) Necrosis 5/16 (31.25%) Perforation 1/16 (6.25%) Cases of vanishing gastroschisis 3/16 (18.75%)	Ultrasound	21 (19–24)	4% (2/55)	⊕⊕⊕◯ Moderate
Fisher et al., 2020 [8]	Indiana	Retrospective cohort study 2010 to 2018	n = 134	n = 24 complex GS. 2369.1 ± 685.2 g	NR	Atresia and perforation 3/24 (12.5%) Atresia only 16/24 (66.6%) Perforation only 3/24 (12.5%) Other indications of complex gastroschisis (matted bowel, primary bowel dysfunction) 2/24 (8.33%)	Ultrasound	NR	NR	⊕⊕◯◯ Low
Geslin et al. 2017 [21]	France	Retrospective cohort multicentre study January 2000 to October 2013	n = 200	n = 52 complex GS. NR	35.3 ± 1.5	Bowel atresia 10/52 (19.23%) Stenosis 8/52 (15.38%) Volvulus 4/52 (7.69%) Ischemia 2/52 (3.84%) Fibrous bands responsible for bowel wall compromise 24/52 (46.15%)	Ultrasound	24.3 ± 5.0	7.7% (4/52)	⊕⊕⊕◯ Moderate
Marinović et al., 2018 [25]	Sérvia	Retrospective cohort study NR	n = 65	n = 15 (23.7%) Complex GS. 2351.33 ± 633.8 g	36.16 ± 1.4	Bowel Atresia = 5/15 (7.69%) Stenosis, Perforation e Necrosis = 9/15 (60%) Gastrosquise de fechamento = 1/15 (6.66%)	Ultrasound	NR	20% (3/15)	⊕⊕⊕◯ Moderate
Martillotti et al., 2016 [23]	Canada	Retrospective cohort study over 11 years January 2000 and January 2011	n = 117	n = 16 complex GS. 2633 (2272–2782) g	35.6 (32.8–37.3)	Volvulus 6/16 (37.5%) Bowel Atresia 5/16 (31.2%) Bowel necrosis 6/16 (37.5%) Bowel perforation 1/16 (6.2%)	Ultrasound	22.8 (19.7–27.5)	56.3% (9/16)	⊕⊕⊕◯ Moderate
Hijkoop et al., 2019 [1]	The Netherlands	Prospective cohort study June 2010 and April 2015	n = 79 fetuses	n = 9 complex GS. 2220 (1840–2800) g	35.4 (33.5–37.0)	Intestinal atresia 6/9 (66.66%) Intestinal atresia + perforation 1/9 (11.11%) Intestinal atresia + necrosis 1/9 (11.11%) Intestinal atresia + necrosis + volvulus 1/9 (11.11%)	3D ultrasound	24 (22–29)	11% (1/9)	⊕⊕◯◯ Low
Hijkoop et al., 2018 [22]	The Netherlands	Retrospective cohort analysis 2000 to 2012	n = 61	n = 10 complex GS. 2385 (2228–2525) g	36.8 (36.4–37.4)	Bowel atresia 3/10 (30%) Intestinal atresia + necrosis 2/10 (20%) Intestinal atresia + perforation 1/10 (10%) Necrosis 1/10 (10%) Necrosis + volvulus 1/10 (10%) Perforation 2/10 (20%)	Ultrasound	30.1 (29.7–31.1)	NR	⊕⊕◯◯ Low

Table 1. Cont.

Author, Year	Country	Study Design	Sample Size	Fetuses Complex Gs (n) Birth Weight, G	Gestational Age At Delivery, Weeks	Complex Gastroschisis	Diagnostic	Mean Age Of Mother (Years)	Mortality Rate	Risk Of Bias (GRADE)
Kuleva et al., 2012 [6]	France	Retrospective case-control study 1999 to 2010	n = 103	n = 14 complex GS. 2325 (2005–2700) g	35.7 ± 1.5 weeks	Bowel atresia 7/14 (6.5%) Bowel perforation 3/14 (2.9%) Colonic diverticulum 1/14 (1.0%) Bowel necrosis 2/14 (2.9%) Duodenal volvulus 1/14 (0.97%)	Ultrasound	25.7 ± 4.7	14.28% (2/14)	⊕⊕⊕○ Moderate
Robertson et al., 2017 [24]	Australia	Retrospective cohort analysis January 2000 and June 2013	n = 101	n = 19 complex GS. NR	35.8 (median = 36.6 range = 24.1–41.1)	NR	Ultrasound	23.9	31.57% (6/19)	⊕⊕⊕○ Low
Lap et al., 2020 [9]	The Netherlands	Prospective cohort 2010 and 2015	n = 131	n = 19 complex GS. 2372 ± 403 g	36.0 (32.3–37.6)	Atresia 18/19 (94.7%) Antenatal volvulus 1/19 (5.3%) Necrosis 3/19 (15.8%) Perforation 3/19 (15.8%)	Ultrasound using a GE Voluson 730 or E8 (GE Healthcare, Zipf, Austria) ultrasound machine, with a 4–8 MHz transabdominal transducer.	26.9 ± 4.9	10.5% (2/19)	⊕⊕⊕○ Moderate
Nitzsche et al., 2020 [3]	Germany	Retrospective cohort analysis 2007 and 2017	n = 34	n = 11 complex GS. 2190 (1370–2985) g	33 + 6 (33 + 0–34 + 5)	NR	Ultrasound	23 (between 17 and 37)	NR	⊕⊕○○ Low

GS: gastroschisis; NR: not reported.

3.3. Assessment of Quality and Risk of Bias

A total of 12 cohort studies and a case-control study were assessed using the GRADE quality assessment tool (Table 1) and risk of bias by the Cochrane tool for non-randomized studies (Figure 2). The GRADE score indicated that five studies showed low quality of evidence [1,3,8,22,24] and eight studies with moderate quality of evidence [6,9,18–21,23,25].

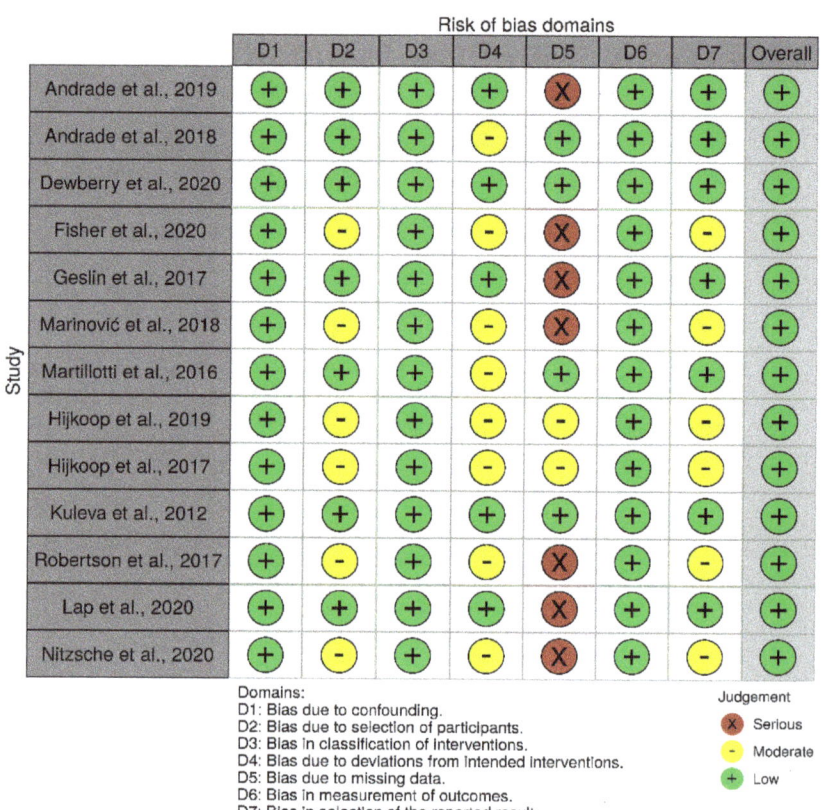

Figure 2. Assessment of the risk of bias.

The results of the risk of bias assessment of the included studies are shown in Figure 2. Although the risk of bias in general was considered moderate to low, in some studies we identified a serious risk of bias, as the studies did not meet the bias criterion due to missing data. The assessment of quality and risk of bias was influenced by the lack of information and the small sample size.

3.4. Ultrasound Markers for Complex Gastroschisis

Data on the definition of complex GS, scan, and ultrasound markers are shown in Table S1. Eight studies reported that IABD measurement is useful in predicting complex GS [6,9,18–21,23,25]. Four studies reported that the presence of EABD proved to be statistically significant in predicting complex GS [3,9,19,24]. Two studies indicated that the presence of polyhydramnios was shown to be statistically significant in predicting complex GS [8,19]. Two studies reported that US markers could not reliably distinguish between simple GS and complex GS [1,22].

3.5. Meta-Analysis

Figure 3 shows the combined prevalence of intestinal complications including atresia, necrosis, perforation, volvulus, and stenosis that are predictors for complex gastroschisis. The combined prevalence was 27.0% (95% confidence interval (CI), 0.18–0.36). Statistical heterogeneity was high (I^2 = 91.76%, p < 0.000). Thus, we performed a meta-regression analysis (tau^2 = 21.49, I^2 = 91.38%, Adj R-squared = 11.44%). The analysis showed that heterogeneity had an influence on the analysis result. Using Egger's regression test, we found evidence of publication bias in the meta-analysis of the combined prevalence of atresia, necrosis, perforation, volvulus, and stenosis (p = 0.044).

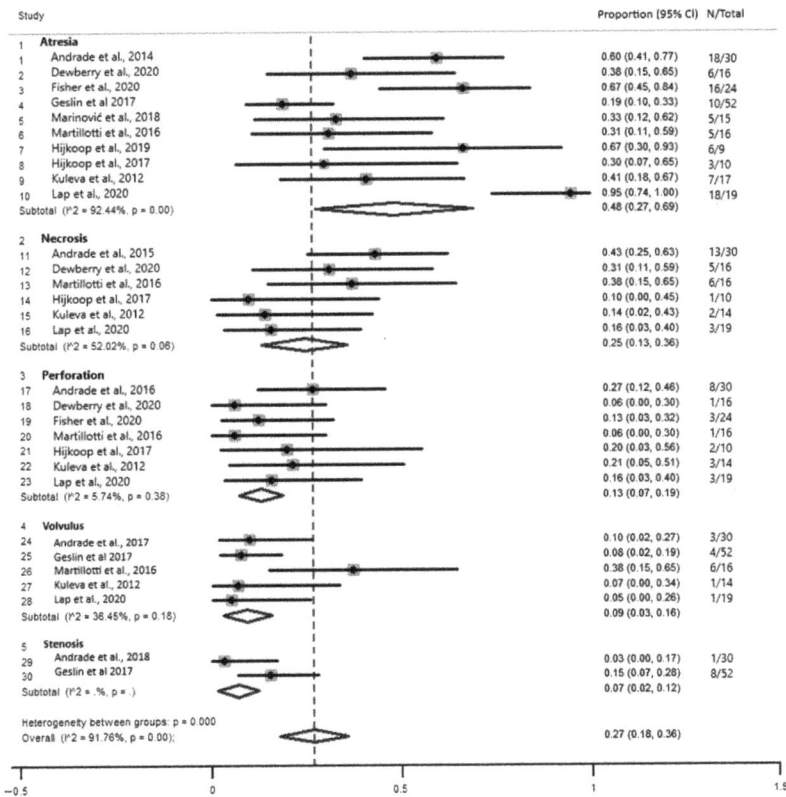

Figure 3. Forest plot of the combined prevalence of atresia, necrosis, perforation, volvulus, and stenosis in fetal complex gastroschisis.

Figure 4 indicates a prevalence of 15.0% (95% confidence interval (CI), 0.08–0.21) of deaths in newborns with complex GS. Statistical heterogeneity was high (I^2 = 69.34%, p = 0.00). Therefore, we performed a meta-regression analysis (tau^2 = 0, I^2 = 0.00%). The analysis showed that heterogeneity had no influence on the result of the analysis. Using Egger's regression test, we found no evidence of publication bias in the meta-analysis of the prevalence of mortality from complex GS (p = 0.520).

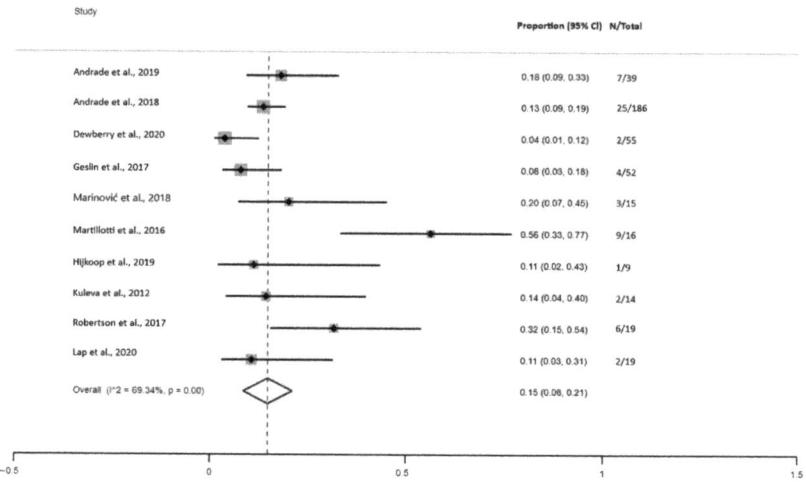

Figure 4. Forest plot of the prevalence of mortality in complex gastroschisis.

3.6. Fetal Ultrasound Evaluation

Figure 5 indicates the combined prevalence of prediction of complex GS with intraabdominal bowel dilatation (IABD), extra-abdominal bowel dilatation (EABD), and polyhydramnios. The meta-analysis indicated that the combined prevalence of ultrasound predictors for complex GS was 50.0% (95% confidence interval (CI), 0.38–0.61). There was a higher prevalence of the EABD ultrasound marker with a prevalence of 58.0% (95% confidence interval (CI), 0.37–0.79), followed by a 49.0% IABD (95% confidence interval (CI), 0.35–0.62) and polyhydramnios was 25.0% (95% confidence interval (CI), 0.07–0.43). The statistical heterogeneity was substantial ($I^2 = 82.45\%$, $p = 0.00$). The meta-regression showed that heterogeneity had an influence on the results of the analysis ($tau^2 = 13.42$, $I^2 = 85.26\%$, Adj R-squared = 57.61%).

Figures 6–8 show the results of comparisons between complex GS and simple GS for the ultrasound markers IABD, EABD, and polyhydramnios, respectively.

3.6.1. IABD

Seven studies were included in the meta-analysis comparing the use of the IABD ultrasound marker in fetuses with complex GS and simple GS. In total, 52/111 (46.84%) fetuses with complex GS had IABD while 86/562 (15.30%) fetuses with simple GS had IABD. The meta-analysis indicated that the risk of predicting IABD is higher in fetuses with complex GS (RR 3.01, 95% CI 2.22 to 4.08; $I^2 = 16\%$, $p = 0.310$). The non-significance of the heterogeneity test suggests that the differences between the studies are explained by random variation. Using Egger's regression test, we found no evidence of publication bias in the meta-analysis ($p = 0.168$) (Figure 6).

3.6.2. EABD

Seven studies were included in the meta-analysis evaluating the presence of EABD in prenatal ultrasound examinations in fetuses with complex GS and simple GS. In total, 56/109 (51.37%) fetuses with complex GS had EABD while 190/448 (42.41%) fetuses with simple GS had EABD. The meta-analysis indicated that the risk of predicting EABD is greater in fetuses with complex GS (RR 1.55, 95% CI 1.01 to 2.39; $I^2 = 77\%$, $p = 0.000$). The results revealed significant heterogeneity between studies ($I^2 = 77\%$), so we performed a meta-regression analysis to examine possible sources of heterogeneity. The analysis showed that no heterogeneity and no inconsistency had any influence on the results of the analysis (tau^2 = 0, I^2 = 0.00%). Using Egger's regression test, we found no evidence of publication bias in the meta-analysis (p = 0.945) (Figure 7).

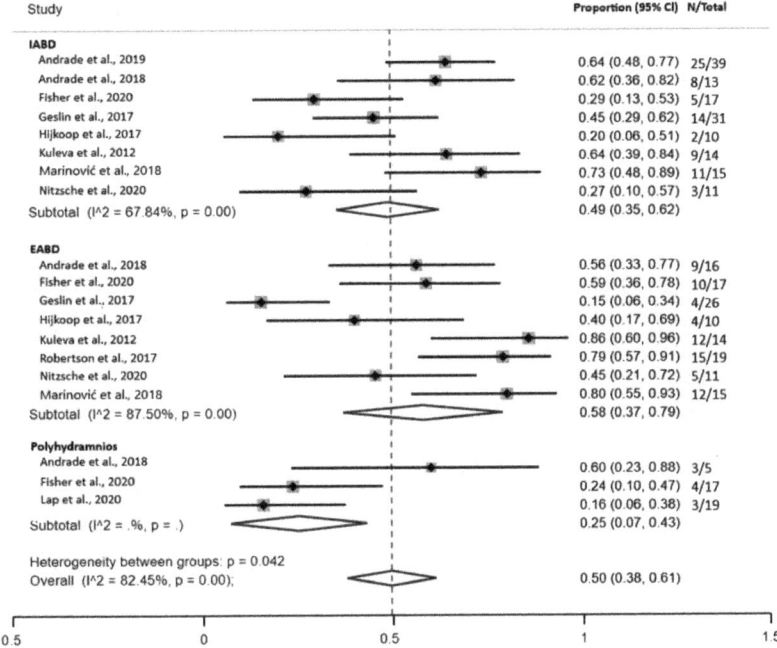

Figure 5. Forest plot of the prediction of complex gastroschisis with intraabdominal bowel dilatation (IABD), extra-abdominal bowel dilatation (EABD), and polyhydramnios.

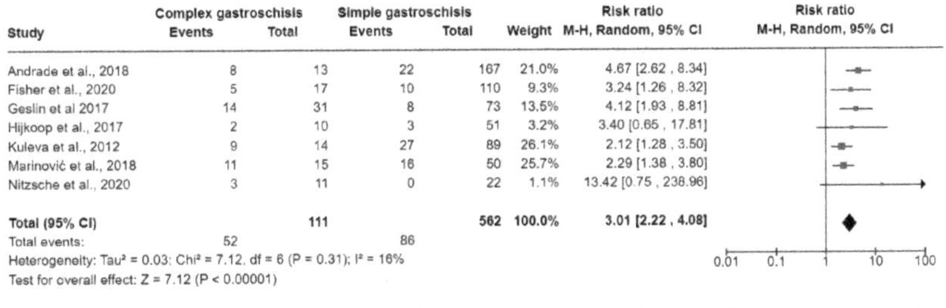

Figure 6. Forest plot between simple and complex gastroschisis for IABD ultrasound markers.

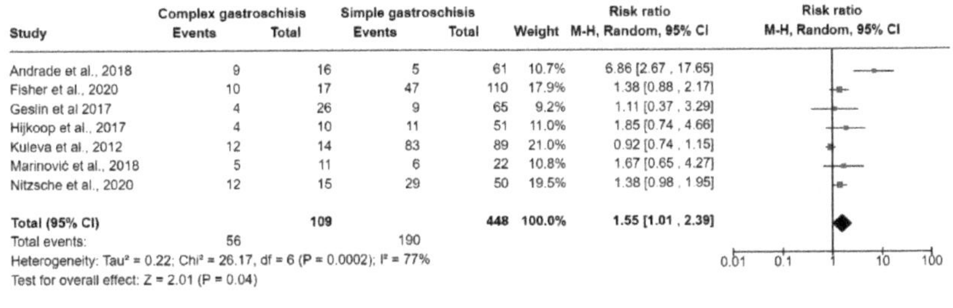

Figure 7. Forest plot between simple and complex gastroschisis for EABD ultrasound markers.

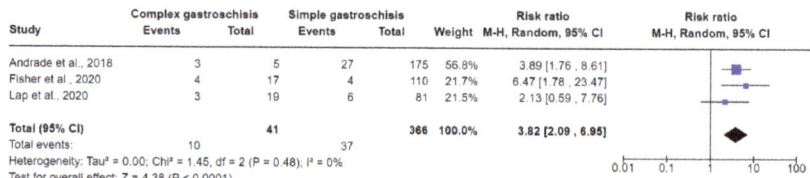

Figure 8. Forest plot between simple and complex gastroschisis for polyhydramnios ultrasound markers.

3.6.3. Polyhydramnios

Three studies were included in the meta-analysis evaluating the presence of polyhydramnios on ultrasound examination in fetuses with complex GS and simple GS. In total, 10/41 (24.39%) fetuses with complex GS had polyhydramnios while 37/366 (10.10%) fetuses with simple GS had polyhydramnios. The meta-analysis indicated that the risk of predicting polyhydramnios is greater in fetuses with complex GS (RR 3.82, 95% CI 2.09 to 6.95; I^2 = 0.0%, tau^2 = 0). Values of I^2 and Tau^2 are consistent with no heterogeneity and no inconsistency (Figure 8).

4. Discussion

Here, through systematic review and meta-analysis, we reviewed the evidence available on ultrasound markers that characterize complex gastroschisis. Thirteen cohort and case-control studies carried out in different countries and with moderate to low risk of bias, were included. The ultrasound markers that showed to be statistically significant in predicting complex GS were IABD [6,9,18–21,23,25], EABD [3,9,19,24], and polyhydramnios [8,19].

Complex GS is known to be associated with greater morbidity and mortality than simple GS. Thus, prenatal prediction of intestinal complications in infants with complex gastroschisis is important to identify cases that may benefit from early obstetric intervention [9]. Bergholz et al. and D'Antonio [7,10] initially explored gastroschisis in systematic review and meta-analysis studies. Bergholz et al. described that infants with complex GS start enteral nutrition later and take longer to complete nutrition and consequently a longer duration of parenteral nutrition. The risk of sepsis, short bowel syndrome, and necrotizing enterocolitis is also greater, as is a longer hospital stay [7]. Furthermore, D'Antonio et al. investigated prenatal risk factors and gastroschisis outcomes. These authors found significant positive associations between IABD and intestinal atresia, polyhydramnios, intestinal atresia, and gastric dilatation, and neonatal death [10].

Other prognostic factors related to mortality in neonates with gastroschisis, from prenatal care to corrective surgery, include inadequate prenatal care, low birth weight, gestational age, severity of intestinal injury, infection, and sepsis [26]. Screening of the severity of the intestinal injury is performed by fetal US in prenatal care and allows early determination of parental counseling and optimal perinatal management [27]. US scans can diagnose gastroschisis as early as 12 weeks of gestation [28]. Fetal magnetic resonance imaging can be a complement to US, providing global and detailed anatomical information, assessing the extent of defects, and also contributing to confirming the diagnosis in doubtful cases [27]. Postnatal surgical management is aimed at reducing herniated viscera and closing the abdominal wall. However, the prognosis depends on the condition of the bowel at birth. Infants with significant intestinal damage at birth are "at risk" of premature death or adverse long-term outcomes [28].

It is important to highlight that although there was an attempt to investigate different markers that could predict complex gastroschisis, US markers that showed to be statistically significant in predicting complex GS were IABD, EABD, and polyhydramnios. Furthermore, in the present study, about 46.84% of fetuses with complex GS and 15.30% of fetuses with simple GS had IABD on ultrasound. Regarding EABD, about 51.37% of fetuses with complex GS and 42.41% of fetuses with simple GS had this US finding. Polyhydramnios was detected via ultrasound in 24.39% of fetuses with complex GS and in 10.10% of fetuses with simple GS.

The meta-analysis also indicates that the combined prevalence of intestinal complications in fetuses with complex GS was 27.0%, particularly with a higher prevalence of atresia (about 48%), followed by necrosis (about 25%) and perforation (about 13%). In addition to the presence of these complications, the prevalence of deaths in newborns with complex GS was 15.0%. We did not identify other meta-analyses that reported the combined prevalence of complications in fetuses with complex GS. However, a meta-analysis reported similar results regarding the mortality rate in newborns with complex GS (16.67%) [7]. Although, it is important to note that there was an important variation in the mean gestational age (GA) at the time of ultrasound reported by these studies, but it generally occurred in pregnancies over 26 weeks. It was not possible to predict the influence of the gestational age at the time of diagnosis in predicting complex GS.

4.1. Implications for Practice

US is a great tool in the diagnosis of GS. The presence of complications in fetuses with complex GS includes atresia, necrosis, perforation, volvulus, and stenosis and the predictive ultrasound markers are IABD, EABD, and polyhydramnios.

4.2. Implications for Research

Future studies evaluating different US markers (IABD, EABD, intrauterine growth restriction, polyhydramnios, intestinal wall thickness, bowel dilatation, liver, and bladder herniation, delta dilatation and final bowel dilatation, abdominal circumference, herniation, dilation of the stomach, size, and position of stomach, size of the abdominal wall defect, description of mesenteric circulation, collapsed extra-abdominal bowel, description of peristalsis and volvulus) in fetuses with complex GS should report the mean gestational age at the time of US diagnosis to evaluate the impact of the time of the presence of those ultrasound markers in predicting complex GS. Larger, well-designed prospective studies that recruit a representative sample of participants are also still necessary. The role of US as diagnostic and predictor strategies should be evaluated, as well as the incorporation of US markers for the diagnosis of complex GS.

4.3. Strengths and Limitations

The strengths of this review include a current, comprehensive, and detailed search according to literature and standardized data extraction and the performance of meta-analysis which can to helpful fundament clinical decisions and prevent severe complications of complex GS. The main limitations of the review were the exclusion of studies in languages other than English [29]. Another limitation concerns the sample size of fetuses with complex GS in each study. However, from evidence from previous studies, we recommend that future studies include a more robust sample of fetuses with complex GS.

5. Conclusions

Intraabdominal bowel dilatation, extra-abdominal bowel dilatation, and polyhydramnios were considered predictive US markers of complex gastroschisis. However, in view of the fact that we were unable to identify the gestational age at the time of the diagnosis of these findings, we recommend future studies that assess diagnostic accuracy and include sensitivity and specificity tests.

Supplementary Materials: The following are available online at https://www.mdpi.com/article/10.3390/jcm10225215/s1, Table S1: Definition, scan, and ultrasound markers of complex gastroschisis.

Author Contributions: Conceptualization, R.G.F., C.R.M., F.S.d.A.T., L.L.G.R., W.N.d.A. and R.R.; methodology, R.G.F., C.R.M., C.L.d.M., F.S.d.A.T., L.L.G.R., N.C.e.M., L.S., W.N.d.A. and R.R.; formal analysis, R.G.F., C.R.M., C.L.d.M., F.S.d.A.T., L.L.G.R., N.C.e.M., L.S., W.N.d.A. and R.R.; investigation, R.G.F., C.R.M., C.L.d.M., F.S.d.A.T., L.L.G.R., N.C.e.M., L.S., W.N.d.A. and R.R.; data curation,

R.G.F. writing—original draft preparation, R.G.F., C.R.M., C.L.d.M., F.S.d.A.T., L.L.G.R., N.C.e.M., L.S., W.N.d.A. and R.R.; writing—review and editing, R.G.F., C.R.M., C.L.d.M., F.S.d.A.T., L.L.G.R., N.C.e.M., L.S., W.N.d.A. and R.R.; visualization, R.G.F., C.R.M., C.L.d.M., F.S.d.A.T., L.L.G.R., N.C.e.M., L.S., W.N.d.A. and R.R.; supervision, W.N.d.A. and R.R.; project administration, R.G.F., W.N.d.A. and R.R.; funding acquisition, W.N.d.A. All authors have read and agreed to the published version of the manuscript.

Funding: This research received no external funding.

Data Availability Statement: The data presented in this study are available on request from the corresponding author.

Conflicts of Interest: The authors declare no conflict of interest.

References

1. Hijkoop, A.; Lap, C.C.M.M.; Aliasi, M.; Mulder, E.J.H.; Kramer, W.L.M.; Brouwers, H.A.A.; van Baren, R.; Pajkrt, E.; van Kaam, A.H.; Bilardo, C.M.; et al. Using three-dimensional ultrasound in predicting complex gastroschisis: A longitudinal, prospective, multicenter cohort study. *Prenat. Diagn* **2019**, *39*, 1204–1212. [CrossRef]
2. Rentea, R.M.; Gupta, V. Gastroschisis. Available online: https://www.ncbi.nlm.nih.gov/books/NBK557894/ (accessed on 5 April 2021).
3. Nitzsche, K.; Fitze, G.; Rüdiger, M.; Birdir, C. Prenatal Prediction of Outcome by Fetal Gastroschisis in a Tertiary Referral Center. *Diagnostics* **2020**, *10*, 540. [CrossRef]
4. Page, R.; Ferraro, Z.M.; Moretti, F.; Fung Kee Fung, K. Gastroschisis: Antenatal Sonographic Predictors of Adverse Neonatal Outcome. *J. Pregnancy* **2014**, *2014*, 239406. [CrossRef]
5. Emil, S. Surgical strategies in complex gastroschisis. *Semin. Pediatr. Surg.* **2018**, *27*, 309–315. [CrossRef] [PubMed]
6. Kuleva, M.; Khen-Dunlop, N.; Dumez, Y.; Ville, Y.; Salomon, L.J. Is complex gastroschisis predictable by prenatal ultrasound? *BJOG Exch.* **2012**, *119*, 102–109. [CrossRef] [PubMed]
7. Bergholz, R.; Boettcher, M.; Reinshagen, K.; Wenke, K. Complex gastroschisis is a different entity to simple gastroschisis affecting morbidity and mortality: A systematic review and meta-analysis. *J. Pediatr. Surg.* **2014**, *49*, 1527–1532. [CrossRef] [PubMed]
8. Fisher, S.G.; Anderson, C.M.; Steinhardt, N.P.; Howser, L.A.; Bhamidipalli, S.S.; Brown, B.P.; Gray, B.W. It Is Complex: Predicting Gastroschisis Outcomes Using Prenatal Imaging. *J. Surg. Res* **2021**, *258*, 381–388. [CrossRef]
9. Lap, C.C.M.M.; Pistorius, L.R.; Mulder, E.J.H.; Aliasi, M.; Kramer, W.L.M.; Bilardo, C.M.; Cohen-Overbeek, T.E.; Pajkrt, E.; Tibboel, D.; Wijnen, R.M.H.; et al. Ultrasound markers for prediction of complex gastroschisis and adverse outcome: Longitudinal prospective nationwide cohort study. *Ultrasound Obs. Gynecol* **2020**, *55*, 776–785. [CrossRef] [PubMed]
10. D'Antonio, F.; Virgone, C.; Rizzo, G.; Khalil, A.; Baud, D.; Cohen-Overbeek, T.E.; Kuleva, M.; Salomon, L.J.; Flacco, M.E.; Manzoli, L.; et al. Prenatal Risk Factors and Outcomes in Gastroschisis: A Meta-Analysis. *Pediatrics* **2015**, *136*, e159. [CrossRef]
11. Moher, D.; Liberati, A.; Tetzlaff, J.; Altman, D.G. Preferred reporting items for systematic reviews and meta-analyses: The PRISMA statement. *Int. J. Surg.* **2010**, *8*, 336–341. [CrossRef]
12. Ouzzani, M.; Hammady, H.; Fedorowicz, Z.; Elmagarmid, A. Rayyan—A web and mobile app for systematic reviews. *Syst. Rev.* **2016**, *5*, 210. [CrossRef] [PubMed]
13. Sterne, J.; Higgins, J. Reeves BC on Behalf of the Development Group for ACROBAT-NRSI. A Cochrane Risk of Bias Assessment Tool: For Non-Randomized Studies of Interventions (*ACROBAT-NRSI*). 2014. Available online: https://www.bristol.ac.uk/media-library/sites/social-community-medicine/images/centres/cresyda/ACROBAT-NRSI%20Version%201_0_0.pdf (accessed on 1 November 2021).
14. Sterne, J.A.C.; Hernán, M.A.; Reeves, B.C.; Savović, J.; Berkman, N.D.; Viswanathan, M.; Henry, D.; Altman, D.G.; Ansari, M.T.; Boutron, I.; et al. ROBINS-I: A tool for assessing risk of bias in non-randomised studies of interventions. *BMJ* **2016**, *355*, i4919. [CrossRef] [PubMed]
15. Guyatt, G.; Oxman, A.D.; Akl, E.A.; Kunz, R.; Vist, G.; Brozek, J.; Norris, S.; Falck-Ytter, Y.; Glasziou, P.; deBeer, H.; et al. GRADE guidelines: 1. Introduction; GRADE evidence profiles and summary of findings tables. *J. Clin. Epidemiol.* **2011**, *64*, 383–394. [PubMed]
16. Balshem, H.; Helfand, M.; Schünemann, H.J.; Oxman, A.D.; Kunz, R.; Brozek, J.; Vist, G.E.; Falck-Ytter, Y.; Meerpohl, J.; Norris, S.; et al. GRADE guidelines: 3. Rating the quality of evidence. *J. Clin. Epidemiol.* **2011**, *64*, 401–406. [CrossRef] [PubMed]
17. Higgins, J.P.T.; Thompson, S.G.; Deeks, J.J.; Altman, D.G. Measuring inconsistency in meta-analyses. *BMJ* **2003**, *327*, 557. [CrossRef]
18. Andrade, W.S.; Brizot, M.L.; Francisco, R.P.V.; Tannuri, A.C.; Syngelaki, A.; Akolekar, R.; Nicolaides, K.H. Fetal intra-abdominal bowel dilation in prediction of complex gastroschisis. *Ultrasound Obstet. Gynecol.* **2019**, *54*, 376–380. [CrossRef] [PubMed]
19. Andrade, W.S.; Brizot, M.L.; Rodrigues, A.S.; Tannuri, A.C.; Krebs, V.L.; Nishie, E.N.; Francisco, R.P.V.; Zugaib, M. Sonographic Markers in the Prediction of Fetal Complex Gastroschisis. *Fetal Diagn. Ther.* **2018**, *43*, 45–52. [CrossRef]

20. Dewberry, L.C.; Hilton, S.A.; Zaretsky, M.V.; Behrendt, N.; Galan, H.L.; Marwan, A.I.; Liechty, K.W. Examination of Prenatal Sonographic Findings: Intra-Abdominal Bowel Dilation Predicts Poor Gastroschisis Outcomes. *Fetal Diagn. Ther.* **2020**, *47*, 245–250. [CrossRef]
21. Geslin, D.; Clermidi, P.; Gatibelza, M.-E.; Boussion, F.; Saliou, A.-H.; Le Manac'h Dove, G.; Margaryan, M.; De Vries, P.; Sentilhes, L.; Levard, G.; et al. What prenatal ultrasound features are predictable of complex or vanishing gastroschisis? A retrospective study. *Prenat. Diagn.* **2017**, *37*, 168–175. [CrossRef]
22. Hijkoop, A.; Ijsselstijn, H.; Wijnen, R.M.H.; Tibboel, D.; van Rosmalen, J.; Cohen-Overbeek, T.E. Prenatal markers and longitudinal follow-up in simple and complex gastroschisis. *Arch. Dis. Child Fetal Neonatal. Ed.* **2018**, *103*, F126. [CrossRef]
23. Martillotti, G.; Boucoiran, I.; Damphousse, A.; Grignon, A.; Dubé, E.; Moussa, A.; Bouchard, S.; Morin, L. Predicting Perinatal Outcome from Prenatal Ultrasound Characteristics in Pregnancies Complicated by Gastroschisis. *Fetal Diagn. Ther.* **2016**, *39*, 279–286. [CrossRef]
24. Robertson, J.A.; Kimble, R.M.; Stockton, K.; Sekar, R. Antenatal ultrasound features in fetuses with gastroschisis and its prediction in neonatal outcome. *Aust. N. Z. J. Obstet. Gynaecol.* **2017**, *57*, 52–56. [CrossRef] [PubMed]
25. Marinović, V.M.; Grujić, B.; Stojanović, A.; Sabbagh, D.; Rašić, P. Gastroschisis: Prenatal Diagnosis and Outcome. *Embryo Neonate* **2018**, *231*. [CrossRef]
26. Badillo, A.T.; Hedrick, H.L.; Wilson, R.D.; Danzer, E.; Bebbington, M.W.; Johnson, M.P.; Liechty, K.W.; Flake, A.W.; Adzick, N.S. Prenatal ultrasonographic gastrointestinal abnormalities in fetuses with gastroschisis do not correlate with postnatal outcomes. *J. Pediatr. Surg.* **2008**, *43*, 647–653. [CrossRef]
27. Torres, U.S.; Portela-Oliveira, E.; Braga Fdel, C.; Werner, H., Jr.; Daltro, P.A.; Souza, A.S. When Closure Fails: What the Radiologist Needs to Know About the Embryology, Anatomy, and Prenatal Imaging of Ventral Body Wall Defects. *Semin. Ultrasound CT MR* **2015**, *36*, 522–536. [CrossRef] [PubMed]
28. Bhat, V.; Moront, M.; Bhandari, V. Gastroschisis: A State-of-the-Art Review. *Children* **2020**, *7*, 302. [CrossRef]
29. Kargl, S.; Wertaschnigg, D.; Scharnreitner, I.; Pumberger, W.; Arzt, W. Closing gastroschisis: A distinct entity with high morbidity and mortality. *Ultraschall Med.* **2012**, *33*, E46–E50.